PLURAL+PLUS

COMPANION WEBSITE

Purchase of *Neuroanatomy and Neurophysiology for Speech and Hearing Sciences* comes with access to supplementary student and instructor materials on a PluralPlus companion website.

The companion website is located at:

http://www.pluralpublishing.com/publication/nnshs

STUDENTS:

To access the **student** materials, you must register on the companion website and log in using the access code below.*

Access Code: NNSHS-C6HNJTF

INSTRUCTORS:

To access the **instructor** materials, you must contact Plural Publishing, Inc. to be verified as an instructor and receive your access code.

Email: information@pluralpublishing.com
Tel: 866-758-7251 (toll free) or 858-492-1555

Note for students: If you have purchased this textbook used or have rented it, your access code will not work if it was already redeemed by the original buyer of the book. Plural Publishing does not offer replacement access codes for used or rented textbooks.

NEUROANATOMY AND NEUROPHYSIOLOGY

for Speech and Hearing Sciences

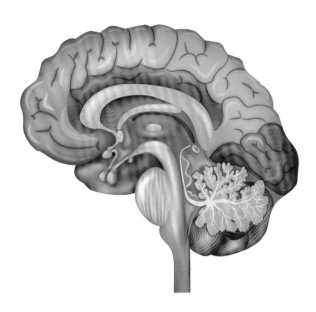

NEUROANATOMY AND NEUROPHYSIOLOGY
for Speech and Hearing Sciences

J. ANTHONY SEIKEL, PhD • KOSTAS KONSTANTOPOULOS, PhD • DAVID G. DRUMRIGHT, BS

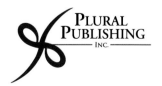

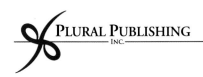

5521 Ruffin Road
San Diego, CA 92123

e-mail: information@pluralpublishing.com
website: http://www.pluralpublishing.com

Typeset in 10/12 Minion Pro by Flanagan's Publishing Services, Inc.
Printed in China by Spectrum Printing, LLC

Library of Congress Cataloging-in-Publication Data

Names: Seikel, John A., author. | Konstantopoulos, Kostas, author. |
  Drumright, David G., author.
Title: Neuroanatomy and neurophysiology for speech and hearing sciences / J.
  Anthony Seikel, Kostas Konstantopoulos, David G. Drumright.
Description: San Diego, CA : Plural, [2020] | Includes bibliographical
  references and index.
Identifiers: LCCN 2018021961| ISBN 9781635500714 (alk. paper) | ISBN
  1635500710 (alk. paper)
Subjects: | MESH: Speech—physiology | Hearing—physiology | Nervous
  System—anatomy & histology
Classification: LCC QP306 | NLM WV 501 | DDC 612.7/8—dc23
LC record available at https://lccn.loc.gov/2018021961

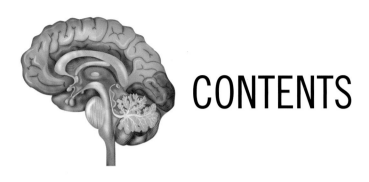

CONTENTS

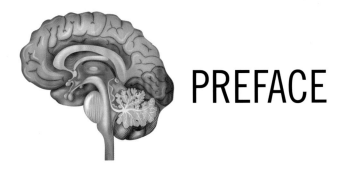

PREFACE

The study of the brain and its functions is at the heart of communication sciences and its disorders. While there are many neurological conditions that immediately come to mind when we think of maladies affecting the brain, the nervous system is intrinsically involved in most of the activities of our field, from the cognitive and motoric aspects of phonology or the impact of myelination on normal language development to (central) auditory processing disorder. All human actions arise from processes of the nervous system, and we can trace many of the deficits treated in our professions to some type of failure affecting this nervous system.

It is with this understanding that we sought to create this textbook and study materials. Neuroscience is the study of what is arguably the most complex phenomenon in the known universe, the nervous system. We, as humans, have brains that are uniquely complex in structure and, most importantly, in function. The human brain has evolved to work in complex networks that entrain multiple areas of the brain, giving it a capacity for problem solving that outstrips our nearest evolutionary neighbors.

As audiologists, speech-language pathologists, and speech and hearing scientists we are in a position to see the inner workings of the brain firsthand through the many neuropathologies with which we are presented. The basal ganglia circuits are uniquely revealed in the tremor, hyperkinesia, and hypokinesia of conditions such as Parkinson's disease, Huntington's disease, or hepatolenticular degeneration. The impact of disease conditions such as multiple sclerosis on hearing function, cognition, and speech production can provide evidence for site of lesion activity if we are able to recognize the signs and symptoms related to the brain region affected. We are challenged on a daily basis to provide meaningful therapy to individuals who have suffered cerebrovascular accident or trauma, and we must work to provide treatment to help overcome the life-changing effects of those lesions. To do this requires a deep knowledge of this extraordinarily complex nervous system but also requires that the clinician develop the intention to continually learn about the nervous system and new treatments that emerge. As an example, behavioral treatments are emerging that have been shown to differentially increase the brain volume and function in areas shown to be active during attention activities, expression of compassion, and awareness of others (theory of mind). Therapies directed toward these dysfunctions could directly affect the lives of those with right hemisphere dysfunction, and the wise clinician will keep a close eye on developments such as these. To do this requires knowledge, desire, and intention. It is our deep hope that these materials can provide at least some of the motivation for a lifetime of study in neuroscience. A central component of this text is the Neuroquest software. We owe a deep debt of gratitude to Dr. Sadanand Singh, who, many years ago as our first publisher of another book, insisted that study software was a critically important component of any text. Now, 20 years later, we are pleased and humbled to continue with his charge to make the current textbook as powerful a learning tool as we can.

The purpose of this textbook is to help the undergraduate and graduate student of speech-language pathology learn about the structure and function of the brain. This knowledge will aid not only in accurate clinical diagnosis but also in the correct use of evidence-based practice methods for speech therapy. There are many neurological diseases in which the primary signs and symptoms are within the domains of speech, language, or hearing disorders, so there is fertile ground for application of the knowledge acquired through study of neuroscience. We have included a number of clinical cases at the end of each chapter to prime the student's problem-solving clinical skills in his or her future profession. Most of the cases include neurological assessments that were performed over the course of treatment (sometimes even 10 years after initial neurological diagnosis), which we have included to help the reader recognize the timing of the speech/language disorder as related to the timing of the other neurological symptomatology.

This textbook is divided into 11 chapters. Chapter 1 briefly overviews the nervous system, starting from embryonic development to aging and including disorders of speech and language that the students in audiology and speech-language pathology need to be aware of. Chapters 2 and 3 discuss the structure and function of cellular components of the central nervous system, including how the signals are propagated (Chapter 2) and the function of basic reflexes (Chapter 3). Chapter 4 discusses the cerebral cortex, including landmarks and components and their relation to our disciplines. Chapters 5 and 6 discuss areas and structures beneath the cortex (subcortex), including the basal ganglia, hippocampus, thalamus (Chapter 5), brainstem (Chapter 6), as well as their associated connections to the cortex. Chapter 7 is dedicated to presentation of the cranial nerves, many of which are critical to hearing and speech. Chapters 8 and 9 discuss the cerebellum, the spinal cord, and their fiber connections. Chapter 10 focuses on the cerebrovascular supply to the brain, elaborating on the vascular supply critical for speech, language, and hearing. Chapter 11 aims to provide to the student the knowledge about the function for the neural control of speech and swallowing, including theoretical models of speech production.

J. Tony Seikel is co-author of two textbooks in anatomy and physiology of speech, hearing, and language and has taught neuroscience and neurogenic coursework for 30 years. Kostas Konstantopoulos is an assistant professor in the European University Cyprus and teaches all neurogenic courses and neuroanatomy. He currently serves as the coordinator for the Bachelor's degree of Speech and Language Therapy and is the coordinator for the Master's degree in Speech Language Pathology. He has extensive clinical and research experience in neurogenic communication disorders spanning 15 years. For the past 6 years he has provided clinical assessment and treatment of speech and dysphagia at the Cyprus Institute of Neurology and Genetics (CING). The majority of the case histories utilized in the chapters have been drawn from his files and referred from all four neurology clinics in the Cyprus Institute of Neurology and Genetics. David Drumright is co-author of two textbooks in anatomy and papers on pedagogy, and has developed software for study of anatomy (*Anima* and *Anatesse* for anatomy and physiology, *Audin* for auditory physiology, and now *Neuroquest* for study of neuroscience).

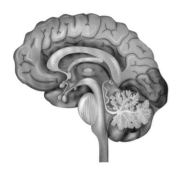

ACKNOWLEDGMENTS

We owe a tremendous debt of gratitude to many people who have contributed to the creation of this textbook. First, we wish to acknowledge our friends at Plural Publishing who have made this textbook possible. There is a deep satisfaction in "returning to our roots" by becoming Plural authors, as its predecessor publisher, Dr. Sadanand Singh, gave us our first inspiration and opportunity to publish in the field. We are deeply indebted to Angie Singh, Kalie Koscielak, and Valerie Johns for their tireless work and cheerful encouragement in this process, as well as to those unnamed individuals working in the background to make this endeavor a reality. The case studies found in this text have come directly from the clinical practice of Dr. Konstantopoulos, as well as from the neurosurgical practice of Dr. Paraskeva, resident in neurosurgery at Nicosia General Hospital in Cyprus and from the cases of Dr. Tanteles, consultant in Clinical Genetics and Head of Clinical Genetics at the Cyprus Institute of Neurology and Genetics. We owe a tremendous debt of gratitude to Drs. Paraskeva and Tanteles for their willingness to share their experiences and expertise with our students. The artwork was created by Mr. Bekoulis, a student at the Athens School of Fine Arts, Greece, and the photographs were the creation of Eric Gordon and the Idaho State University Photographic Services. Finally, we owe a deep debt of gratitude to our students in the United States, Greece, and Cyprus who continue to inspire us with their intelligence, drive, and most of all, compassion.

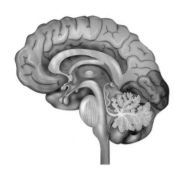

CONTRIBUTORS

Kyriakos Paraskeva, MD
Resident of Neurosurgery
Nicosia General Hospital
Cyprus
Case Studies

George A. Tanteles, MD, DM
Consultant in Clinical Genetics CCT(UK)
Head of Clinical Genetics
The Cyprus Institute of Neurology & Genetics
Cyprus
Case Studies

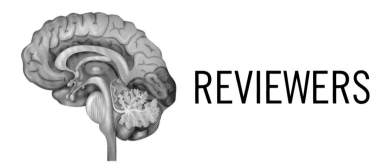

REVIEWERS

Plural Publishing, Inc. and the authors would like to thank the following reviewers for taking the time to provide their valuable feedback during the development process:

Robert Ackerman, PhD, CCC-SLP
Professor
Communication Sciences and Disorders
East Stroudsburg University
East Stroudsburg, Pennsylvania

June Graham Bethea, PhD, CCC-SLP
Adjunct Lecturer
Communication Disorders
North Carolina Agricultural and Technical State University
Greensboro, North Carolina

Ann Cralidis, PhD, CCC-SLP
Assistant Professor
Department of Social Work and Communication Sciences
   and Disorders
Longwood University
Farmville, Virginia

Tamara B. Cranfill, PhD, CCC-SLP
Associate Professor
Communication Disorders
Eastern Kentucky University
Richmond, Kentucky

Melissa Johnson, PhD, CCC-SLP
Assistant Professor
Communication Sciences and Disorders
Nazareth College
Rochester, New York

Joni Mehrhoff, MS, CCC-SLP
Assistant Professor/Clinical Supervisor
Speech, Language, Hearing Sciences
Minnesota State University Moorhead
Moorhead, Minnesota

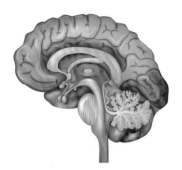

ABOUT THE AUTHORS

J. Anthony (Tony) Seikel, PhD, is emeritus faculty at Idaho State University, where he taught graduate and undergraduate coursework in neuroanatomy and neuropathology over the course of his career in Communication Sciences and Disorders. He is co-author of numerous chapters, books and research publications in the fields of speech-language pathology and audiology. His current research is examining the relationship between orofacial myofunctional disorders and oropharyngeal dysphagia.

Kostas Konstantopoulos, PhD, is assistant professor in the speech language pathology program at the European University Cyprus and serves as a program coordinator for the master's degree in speech language pathology. From 1996 to 2018 he has worked as a clinician in various neurology departments in Greece and Cyprus including the Navy Hospital of Athens and the Cyprus Institute for Neurology and Genetics. Dr. Konstantopoulos's research involves motor speech disorders and the relationship between speech and cognition.

David G. Drumright, BS, grew up in Oklahoma and Kansas, taught electronics at DeVry for several years, then spent 20 years as a technician in acoustics and speech research. He developed many programs and devices for analysis and instruction in acoustics and speech/hearing. He has been semi-retired since 2002, working on graphics and programming for courseware.

The authors wish to dedicate this book to the students in speech-language pathology and audiology who have chosen to spend their lives helping others with communication difficulties. The programmer (D.G.D.) dedicates this software to Professor Merle Phillips, who taught him something about audiology and a lot about life. K.K. would like to dedicate his work to the memory of his mother, whose philosophy was that there is no such thing as "I can't do it." For her "I can't do it" meant "I don't want to do it." J.A.S. wishes to dedicate his efforts to the memory of David Sorensen of Idaho State University, a great friend and colleague.

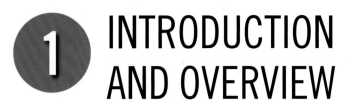

1 INTRODUCTION AND OVERVIEW

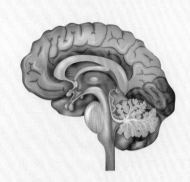

Welcome to the world of neuroscience! The nervous system is the most complex structure in nature, and perhaps in the known universe. We, your authors, remain awed and humbled by this structure and its functions, and hope that we can convey a tiny bit of that to you as you begin your studies into the world of the brain.

Neuroscience is a lot like a metropolitan area: there are marvelous sites to see, but you have to choose which road to take to get to them. You may be coming from out of town, or you may live there. In either case, you find the roads that lead you where you want to go and then you take them. In many ways, this concept reflects our motivation for writing this text. We have chosen a path to your learning that will take you from an understanding of structure at the smallest levels to a knowledge of the larger structure and, ultimately, the regional functionality of that structure. We have focused on the structures of audiology and speech-language pathology in this text, much as you might choose the Museum of Modern Art over the Guggenheim if you lived in New York.

Our part of neuroscience, as members of the communication sciences and disorders community, contains some of the most important structures and functions of the brain. We don't make this claim lightly or from an arrogant point of view. Audiologists and speech-language pathologists work with people with diseases that affect the very heart of what we consider to be our most human traits. Cognitive deficits arising from dementias, such as those caused by Alzheimer's disease, rob a person of his or her memory, personality, and communication ability. Auditory function, which is so critical to development of speech and language, can be severely compromised through small lesions to the temporal lobe, thalamus, or auditory pathway. Left hemisphere stroke can eliminate the ability to communicate, while right hemisphere stroke can strike at a person's ability to develop connectedness with others and even compassion. Damage to subcortical structures such as the basal ganglia can result in movement disorders that significantly alter quality of life, while damage to the right parietal lobe can result in significant deficits in the ability to attend to a stimulus or even recognize one's own body parts. All of these areas fall within our domains as audiologists and speech-language pathologists. We, your authors, have felt both awed and honored to be in professions that bring us so close to the epicenter of what it is to be human. The other half of this is that we feel a deep responsibility to our students and their future clients. We must never forget the awesome responsibility we have toward improvement of the lives of our clients. Welcome to the nervous system!

We begin our discussion in this chapter with an overview of the anatomy of the brain and basic functioning, followed by examination of the systems of the brain and brain development. We'll discuss some important details about terminology before starting our journey through the nervous system itself.

- Discuss the role of the extrapyramidal system in fine motor control and muscle tone maintenance.

- State the role of body sensors and the cerebellum in support of skilled movement.

- Explain the role of executive functions in completing actions.

- Recognize the difference between deep and superficial sensation.

- Identify the differences among somatic, kinesthetic, and special sensations.

- Define the difference between anatomy and physiology.

- Define the differences between autonomic and somatic nervous systems.

- Identify the differences between sympathetic and parasympathetic systems.

- Recognize the relevance of

flexures to the developing nervous system.

- Explain the differences between the pharyngeal arches in terms of their ultimate derivatives.

- Define the terminology of anatomy and physiology as they relate to the study of the nervous system.

- Define specific terminology in the fields of speech-language pathology and audiology as they relate to neuropathology.

OVERVIEW OF THE NERVOUS SYSTEM

The nervous system and its proper function are essential to all of the work of our professions, whether we work with auditory function, speech, swallowing, cognition, or language. Our field is communication science, and the nervous system is all about communication.

At the most basic level, the nervous system is composed of billions of component parts termed neurons. **Neurons** (also known as nerve cells) are cells that are specialized for communication. The sheer numbers of neurons and complexity of their interactions are the means by which cognition, language, speech, and auditory processing developed in humans (Amaral & Strick, 2013).

Neurons receive information and convey it to the next neuron (Figure 1–1). Generally, neurons have a **dendrite** (the receptive component), a **soma** or body (the portion responsible for metabolic functions), and an **axon** (the portion responsible for exciting the next neuron). When information of sufficient strength is received at the dendrite, a **miniature excitatory postsynaptic potential** is generated that passes to a point of the axon where an action potential is generated. This action potential releases **neurotransmitter substance** into the synapse or gap between the axon and the dendrite of the next neuron in the chain, and this causes ions to pass into the dendrite, stimulating it to excitation. Thus, information can pass through the neural chain from one neuron to another, with the purpose of activating muscle, conveying sensory information, or solving some complex computational problem. While we'll discuss generation of the action potential and communication between neurons in depth in the next chapter, please

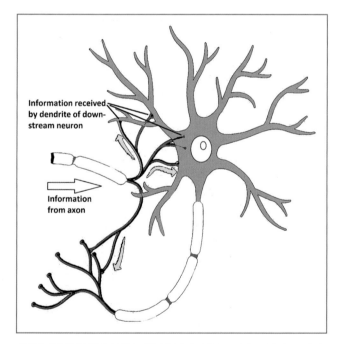

Information received by dendrite of down-stream neuron

Information from axon

FIGURE 1–1. Information from a neuron is conveyed from the axon of that neuron to the dendrite or the body of the down-stream neuron. *Source:* Adapted from Seikel, Drumright, and King (2016). *Anatomy & physiology for speech, language and hearing* (5th ed.). Clifton Park, NY: Cengage Learning.

realize that this is the basic *functional* element of the brain. With this basic process, all neurons communicate to accomplish the many tasks we demand of the nervous system.

In anatomy we refer to **organs** as groups of cells with functional unity. This holds for the anatomy of the nervous system as well. There are many types of neurons with varied functions that combine to form nuclei within the nervous system and that perform specific functions. The sensory systems provide the best examples of this: the cochlear nucleus of the auditory nervous system is the first site of feature extraction for the auditory signal transduced within the cochlea. In this case, the cochlear nucleus is something of an analytical filter. The next nucleus in the chain (superior olive) is responsible for localizing sound in space. In both cases, these two **nuclei** are made up of neurons with special functions. The nervous system has many similar nuclei with wide varieties of functions, and by studying those nuclei we can start to see how the nervous system accomplishes its tasks (e.g., Baehr & Frotscher, 2012; Pickles, 2012).

As we'll discuss in the next section, the nervous system can be broadly broken down into the **central nervous system** (CNS) and the **peripheral nervous system** (PNS) (Tables 1–1 and 1–2). The CNS consists of the cerebral cortex and other subcortical structures, brainstem, cerebellum, and spinal cord. The PNS consists of the cranial and spinal nerves.

The **cerebral cortex** stands alone in the nervous system as the site of both voluntary action and cognition (Brodal, 2004). It is where information is processed consciously and decisions are made about action. The **cerebrum** is the home to language processing and planning, as well as execution of speech, and is the site of all complex conscious activities. In a sense, you can think of it as the awakened brain. Let's review both motor execution and sensory processing as a means of discussing the nervous system components.

Motor activity is initiated in the frontal lobe of the cerebral cortex, at an area known as the **motor strip**. As an example, your cognitive processes might provide you with the motivation to bend your finger. That intention is conveyed as a motor plan to the neurons of the brain on the motor strip that are associated with activating the muscles of the finger. The impulse to flex your finger passes out of the cerebrum on efferent projection fibers whose axons pass through the brainstem and into the spinal cord. **Efferent** neurons are those whose role is to "cause an effect," as in to activate muscle. These particular fibers will terminate in the thoracic region, where they will synapse with neurons of the peripheral nervous system, and those neurons will activate muscles to cause the flexing that was planned by the cortex. While this simplification ignores some very large details, the concept holds firm: the cerebral cortex is responsible for the concept that activates the voluntary action of moving your muscles, and the peripheral nervous system (in the form of spinal or cranial nerves) is responsible for direct execution.

Conscious processing follows a reverse path. If a mosquito walks on that same finger of your hand, the pressure associated with the mosquito's movement may be sufficient to activate a sensory neuron, and the impulse from that activation enters the spinal cord in an afferent neuron. **Affer-**

TABLE 1–1.	Major Structures of the Central Nervous System and Peripheral Nervous System
Central nervous system	Subcomponents
Cerebrum	Frontal lobe
	Parietal lobe
	Occipital lobe
	Temporal lobe
	Insular cortex
	Limbic system
	Hippocampus
Brainstem	Medulla oblongata
	Pons
	Midbrain
	Cerebral peduncles
	Brainstem pathways and nuclei
Subcortex	Thalamus
	Subthalamus
	Epithalamus
	Hypothalamus
	Basal ganglia
Cerebellum	Cerebellar cortex
	Cerebellar nuclei
	Superior, middle, inferior cerebellar peduncles
Spinal cord	Spinal cord afferent and efferent pathways
Peripheral nervous system	
Cranial nerves	Cranial nerve nuclei
Spinal nerves	Spinal nerve nuclei

ent neurons have the role of taking information from the periphery and conveying it to the central nervous system. In this case, the information about the mosquito will be conveyed up through the spinal cord and to nuclei within the brainstem. Those nuclei convey the sensation to the thalamus (the sensory clearing house at the base of the brain), which conveys the information to the somatosensory strip of the parietal lobe. In this way, sensory information at your fingertip becomes a conscious sensation in the cerebral cortex, and you can choose to move your finger to scare away the insect.

Not all actions are conscious and not all sensations reach consciousness, and that begins our discussion of everything

TABLE 1–2.	Structures of the Nervous System, Based on Complexity
Structure	**Function**
Glial cells	Nutrients to neurons, support, phagocytosis, myelin, long-term memory
Neuron	Communicating tissue
Single segment reflexes	Subconscious response to environment
Multi-segment reflexes	Subconscious response to environment
Maturational reflexes (e.g., righting reflex)	Subconscious response to environment
Central pattern generators	Complex pattern generation utilizing sensory and motor nuclei to accomplish sequential activities; driven by sensation and utilizing combinations of more basic reflexive responses
Ganglia and nuclei	Aggregates of cell bodies with functional unity
Tracts	Aggregates of axons that transmit functionally united information; spinal cord
Structures of the brainstem	Aggregates of ganglia, nuclei, and tracts that mediate high-level reflexes and mediate the execution of cortical commands
Diencephalon	Aggregates of nuclei and tracts that mediate sensory information arriving at the cerebrum and provide basic autonomic responses for body maintenance
Cerebellum	Aggregates of nuclei, specialized neurons, and tracts that integrate somatic and special sensory information with motor planning and command for coordinated movement
Cerebrum	All conscious sensory awareness and conscious motor function, including perception, awareness, motor planning and preparation, cognitive function, attention, decision making, voluntary motor inhibition, language function, speech function

Source: Based on data of Seikel, Drumright, & King (2016).

below the level of the cerebrum. **Reflexes** are hard-wired responses of the nervous system that are responsible for automated, involuntary responses to environmental or other stimuli. As an example, you likely have had experience with a physician tapping your knee to activate the patellar tendon reflex. When your knee is tapped, your leg kicks as a result of a reflexive response that we'll talk about in Chapter 4. For now, realize that your body is endowed with innumerable reflexes that provide involuntary response to stimuli. Reflexes that are present in the early postnatal period are inhibited as the cortex matures so they don't interfere with voluntary actions, but the circuits are always there and are always available if needed. Some hard-wired responses, such as those associated with the complex processes of swallowing, remain active throughout life, while other reflexes, such as

the sucking reflex of early postnatal life, are inhibited as we gain voluntary control of the processes of eating.

Reflexes are the domain of the spinal cord and brainstem (Saper, Anderw, Lumsden, & Richerson, 2013). The spinal cord is home to the basic **spinal reflex arc**, as well as more complex spinal reflexes. The brainstem is involved in complex reflexive and motor patterns associated with life, such as respiration, deglutition, mastication, vomiting, and others. This hierarchy reflects the organization of the brain, with the most basic and simple responses at the lower-level spinal level, the more organized responses to the environment higher in the nervous system at the brainstem level, and the highest level of response being the conscious level of the cerebral cortex.

As infants, well before we have any voluntary function, we will manifest a *walking reflex*. It is elicited by holding the infant upright and dragging the infant's toes on a tabletop, causing stepping action to occur in the early postnatal stage. We lose that reflexive response as our nervous systems develop, but the motor pattern is retained, and our cerebral cortex uses that pattern to help us walk. To demonstrate this to yourself, actually have your cerebrum do the micromanaging. Walk slowly, intently, and focused on your feet and their movement. You will immediately notice that you lose your focus on your feet and go to another thought or sensation, and it takes a lot of effort to keep focused on the act of walking. The casual stroll of the adult doesn't require a lot of thought on your part: one foot puts itself in front of the other without your cortex having to micromanage the process. The cerebrum is very busy and is more than happy to allow these motor pattern subsystems to help you go about your daily life. This is automaticity.

Automaticity is supported by the ongoing and automatic control of background musculature. Similar to reflexes, background neural activity includes maintaining muscle tone that precisely counterbalances the desired activity. As an example, if you are reaching for a hidden birthday present that you need to wrap, and it is at the top of the closet just out of your range, you will stand on your tiptoes, extend forward a little while you reach, and will counteract your movement by extending your other arm and leg back to keep from losing your balance. Much of this is embedded within vestibular reflexes that you developed in the first six to eight months of your life and which are also within the automatic domain. In this case, these background activities support the foreground movement. You may recall from your anatomy course the discussion about **agonists** and **antagonists**. This is that same discussion, but from a neurophysiological perspective.

Part of this background response is to maintain **muscle tone**. Balanced muscle tone provides us with the right amount of counterforce to control the agonistic movement and allows our musculature to be ready for contraction at any desired instant. In the sleep state, your muscles become flaccid, or low-tone, which is normal and natural, but when you are awake and alert, you maintain a level of muscle tone that balances the needs of your voluntary system. This tone is regulated by the indirect motor system, also known as the extrapyramidal system, a primary job of the basal ganglia and the red nucleus and their pathways. The **basal ganglia** are sets of nuclei found above the level of the brainstem that are responsible for some stereotyped movements but are also importantly involved in regulation of background movements and of muscle tone.

The **motor speech system** capitalizes on automaticity in the same way: we don't overthink these processes or we get into trouble. If we were to really focus on each movement of our articulators, we would take a very long time to say anything. Be aware of this, however: when you are learning a task, such as walking, reaching, or speaking, you will put a great deal of focus on learning the motor act, paying very

close attention to what your body is telling you about the action (as we'll discuss in Chapter 11). The tactile, muscle, and joint **sensors** we discuss in Chapter 3 give you information about where your tongue and mandible are in space, how fast they are moving, and where they make contact. You pay attention to this *feedback* from the sensors and use that information to correct the movement so you make a more accurate attempt the next time. You learn, and then eventually you can automatize.

Motor learning is a significant feat of attending to the feedback from your body, and you get a great deal of help in the learning process from the **cerebellum**, the most densely packed structure of the central nervous system. The cerebellum is responsible for coordinating all motor activity as well as for integrating the diverse inputs from the body's sensors into a cohesive map of what is happening in your body at any moment for the purpose of motor control. Again, as you reach to the top shelf of that closet, you stretch and lean forward and counterbalance your actions through opposite limb extension. This is a highly coordinated activity that requires smooth interaction of a large number of agonists and antagonists, as well as input from the muscles, joints, tactile sensors, and vestibular mechanism. All of this information gets integrated as a dynamic whole in the cerebellum, providing your motor system with the data it needs to successfully reach that hidden birthday present on the shelf. If the vestibular system information isn't integrated, you'll lose your balance. If your tactile information is incorrect, you may squeeze too hard on the package, breaking its contents. If your righting reflexes aren't controlled, you may extend your counterbalancing leg too far back and become unstable. The fact is that none of these problems befalls you, typically because your nervous system is continually monitoring the condition of your body relative to your motor activity, and it is continually updating and correcting those body responses to keep everything in balance with the desires of your cerebrum. You can probably guess, however, that if any one of these components fails for some reason (such as cerebrovascular accident), the resulting imbalance in the system will require the careful efforts of a skilled clinician to reprogram these circuits. That is why you are in this field.

Information about your body's condition at any moment travels to your cerebrum by means of pathways. Nervous system pathways (**efferent** and **afferent**) provide the superhighways for information that will be used by your CNS to control movements, have thoughts, and make sense of the world. Efferent pathways provide the means for moving muscles, once the decision has been made to do so. In Chapter 4, we will introduce you to two major motor pathways (the corticospinal and corticobulbar tracts) and then provide in-depth discussion of many others in Chapter 9.

We haven't talked about the complex processes of **cognition**, which are the specific and sole domain of the cerebral cortex. These root processes include memory, attention, perception, visuospatial processes, and linguistic processes. This amazing cerebrum takes these "basic" cognitive processes and uses them to get its goals accomplished, through executive functions. **Executive functions** are called metacognitive processes, in that they are the processes that control the way we use our cognitive functions in problem-solving situations. For instance, if I have the sense of hunger, I must develop a plan for satisfying this need. Unless there is a box of *bon-bons* in easy reach, I may have to actually *plan* how to feed myself, perhaps including calling to see if the pizza joint is open, grabbing my money, and driving to town. All of this takes a great deal of cognitive engineering, and it depends very strongly on executive function. We will talk much more about this later when we discuss cortical function.

All of the information coming to the cerebral cortex arises from sensors. The body's sensors are how we know our world. The cerebral cortex is responsible for creating a "worldview" based on its sensory input. For our purposes in the fields of audiology and speech-language pathology, the special senses associated with hearing and balance are critical elements in this whole-body image, as they both provide rich information about the movement and the environment (Goldberg, Walker, & Hudspeth, 2013; Hudspeth, 2013). There are general body senses and specific senses, as we'll discuss in Chapters 3 and 7.

General somatic sensations include both superficial and deep sensation. **Superficial sensations** are those sensed at the periphery of your body, such as pain, pressure, and temperature. **Deep sensation** includes the senses associated with muscles and their tension, tendons, muscle pain, deep vibration, and others. We are able to combine sensations below the level of the cerebral cortex in order to form a richer perception. One of these combinations is termed stereognosis, which is the ability to recognize ("gnosis") the shape or form of an object ("stereo") through tactile sensation alone.

There are different types of sensation, including somatic sense, kinesthetic sense, and the special senses. **Somatic sense** (body sense) includes the sensations associated with pressure (deep and light) and thermal stimulation (cold and hot). Somatic sense also includes joint position sense, muscle tension, and tendon tension. **Kinesthetic sense** is one of those combined senses, resulting in the perception of your body moving in space. **Special sense** includes the sense of hearing, vision, smell, and taste (gustation). All of these will be discussed in detail later.

Intrinsic to all sensors is the specificity of stimulus. Pressure sensors of the skin won't respond to thermal stimulation, and retinal cells won't respond to auditory stimuli. Interestingly, nociceptors (pain sensors) are the same as thermal sensors, but individual sensors still differentiate between the two types of sensation. All sensors signal the nervous system in a similar way by means of a generator potential.

All somatic senses are routed through the **thalamus** on their way to the cerebral cortex. As we'll discuss when we examine consciousness, it is the presence of these sensory inputs that allows us to know that we exist. We "create" a perception of ourselves as a unified entity based on coordinating these inputs to form an integrated whole. The absence of sensation in a modality changes our perceptions of ourselves in space. Sensation is critically important to our well-being, and understanding of sensation and the effects of deficits is critical to the therapeutic process (Moller, 2003).

In summary,

- Neurons are cells that are specialized for communication. Neurons receive information and convey it to the next neuron. Neurons have a dendrite, soma, and axon.
- An action potential releases neurotransmitter substance into the synapse between the axon and the dendrite of the next neuron, causing ions to pass into the dendrite and stimulating it to excitation.
- Nuclei are made up of neurons with special functions.
- The central nervous system (CNS) consists of the cerebral cortex, brainstem, cerebellum, spinal cord, and other subcortical structures. The peripheral nervous system (PNS) consists of the cranial and spinal nerves.
- The cerebral cortex is where information is processed consciously and decisions are made about action. Functions include language processing, execution of speech, and all complex conscious activities. Motor activity is initiated in the frontal lobe at the motor strip. Efferent neurons are responsible for motor activity. Sensations from the periphery of the body arise in the cortex by means of afferent nerves.
- Reflexes are hard-wired responses of the nervous system that are responsible for automated, involuntary responses to environmental or other stimuli. Automaticity is supported by the ongoing and automatic control of background musculature. Background neural activity includes maintaining muscle tone that precisely counterbalances the desired activity. The tactile, muscle, and joint sensors provide somatic information about position and state of the body in space. The cerebellum is responsible for coordinating all motor activity as well as for integrating the inputs from the body's sensors.
- Efferent pathways provide the means for moving muscles once the decision has been made to do so, while afferent pathways provide information from the body's sensors to the cortex.
- Cognition involves memory, attention, visuospatial processes, perception, and linguistic processes, which are the domain of the cerebrum.
- Somatic sense includes the sensations associated with pressure (deep and light) and thermal stimulation (cold and hot), while kinesthetic sense is the perception of the body moving in space. Special senses include the sense of hearing, vision, smell, and taste.

DIVISIONS OF THE NERVOUS SYSTEM

The nervous system consists of a large number of structures that work together to accomplish survival and higher function of the organism. We are predominantly symmetrical on gross examination, with left and right arms, legs, and eyes. The symmetry that you see in the mirror is reflected at the gross levels of the nervous system as well. We have two cerebral hemispheres, two cerebellar hemispheres, two thalami, and even paired pathways descending through the spinal column. We have pairs of cranial nerves serving each side of the head, and left and right spinal nerves as well. Perhaps nature "recognized" the need for redundancy, giving us symmetrical structures as backup for the times when damage occurs.

This is a good time to remind ourselves of the difference between anatomy and physiology. **Anatomy** is the study of the structure of the organism, while **physiology** is the study of the function. **Clinical anatomy** is the study of the pathological entity, and that often includes discussion of altered or pathological physiology. The nervous system can be viewed either as a set of structures or as a set of functions. When viewed as structures (anatomy), we divide the nervous system into central and peripheral components. The **central nervous system** (CNS) consists of the cerebral cortex (or cerebrum), the brainstem, the basal ganglia, cerebellum, spinal cord, thalamus and subthalamus, nuclei and tracts within these structures, and so on. The **peripheral nervous system** (PNS) consists of the 31 spinal nerves and the 12 cranial nerves that emerge from the CNS.

The nervous system can also be organized based on function. We divide the nervous system into autonomic and somatic systems.

Autonomic Nervous System

The **autonomic nervous system** (ANS) is responsible for involuntary functions of the body, including contraction of smooth muscle, glandular secretion, and digestive and cardiac function. The autonomic nervous system includes a separate subdivision, the enteric nervous system (ENS). The ENS is responsible for digestive processes themselves.

The ANS has two responsive systems: sympathetic and parasympathetic. The **sympathetic system** (also known as the **thoracolumbar system** because of its relationship to the body's trunk) responds to stimulation by expending energy. If you have a close call while driving, you'll very quickly notice an increase in heart rate, alertness, and sweating. You'll experience increased blood pressure due to vasoconstriction, dilation of the pupils, and goose bumps. These responses are your body's way of preparing to meet some unexpected and frightening challenge, and the sympathetic system is responsible for this "flight, freeze, or fight" reaction. We now know

that these physically stressful crisis moments release norepinephrine into your system in response to danger, but we also are aware that this is more than just energy expenditure. Stress takes a tremendous toll on structures of the nervous system, literally shortening the life of the person who lives in this state constantly. The **parasympathetic system** counteracts these stress responses by slowing the heart rate, constricting the pupils, and lowering blood pressure.

The ANS is designed to maintain homeostasis of the body. You can think of it as a very complex environmental control system, much like thermostats that keep room temperature within an operationally defined limit. The values of your body's system must change to meet a crisis, and when the crisis is over they should return to a default mode. When food enters the digestive system, a set of actions need to take place, some resulting in muscular contraction and others resulting in secretion of enzymes. Some actions, such as esophageal peristalsis, are caused by stimulation of mechanoreceptors, while others are responses initiated by chemoreceptors that are sensing the need to regulate the environment by increasing or decreasing acids. The key word to keep in mind concerning the autonomic nervous system is regulation: it has responsibility for keeping the systems of the body in harmony with the external environment's demands. When those demands change, the autonomic nervous system changes in response. It's an elegant "operating system" for the body, and it's entirely involuntary.

The ANS arises from the prefrontal region of the cerebral cortex, as well as subcortical structures including the thalamus, hypothalamus, hippocampus, brainstem, spinal cord, and cerebellum. These represent control centers for the ANS, and are connected by means of afferent (sensory) and efferent (motor) tracts.

There are peripheral components to the ANS as well. These include a pair of sympathetic trunk ganglia running external to the vertebral column, as well as ganglia (groups of cell bodies with common function) and plexuses (networks of nerves that combine for common purpose or goal).

Somatic Nervous System

The somatic nervous system is critically important to audiologists and speech-language pathologists, as it governs voluntary, conscious activity. All skeletal muscles (also known as somatic muscles) contract through action of the somatic nervous system, and the decision to contract these muscles arises from conscious activity of this system. The impulse to contract the superior longitudinal muscle of the tongue (to elevate the tip) comes from the motor region of the frontal lobe, in response to the need to move the tongue. The impulse is carried on neural pathways from cerebrum to brainstem and is ultimately conveyed to a cranial nerve responsible for the action. Sensory feedback from sensors within the muscle and the tissue around it helps regulate the force and rate of contraction, much like the homeostasis of the autonomic nervous system. In this case, however, the conscious and creative cerebral cortex has generated its own stimulus to which it responds: it thinks of a word to say, and a set of complex processes are set into action to reach stasis between conception (the idea to say the word) and execution. In the case of "speech homeostasis," we are aligning the target state (accurately spoken speech sound) with our perception of that spoken utterance. If our perception of the executed speech sound differs from our internal stimulus, we will attempt to correct the production to match the model. We'll discuss this further when we talk about motor control for speech. This notion of "creating our own stimulus" underscores the critical difference between the autonomic and somatic nervous systems. The somatic system is considered the voluntary and conscious system of control, and we are therefore capable of modifying the activities in which it engages. It is largely the somatic nervous system with which you work in therapy, whether you are fitting a hearing aid or correcting a misarticulation. It also emphasizes the element that is so splendidly human, which is our cognitive capacity to self-reflect and self-correct.

The actions of the somatic nervous system are the results of motor responses governed by two mechanisms: the pyramidal and extrapyramidal systems. The **pyramidal system** is involved in direct activation of skeletal muscle and arises from the pyramidal cells of the precentral and premotor gyri of the frontal lobe. The **extrapyramidal system** (also known as the **indirect system**) governs background movements and muscle tone and supports the actions of the primary muscles for a given action. In the above speech example, the superior longitudinal muscle is the **prime mover** or **agonist**, since it is being contracted to accomplish the goal. There are muscles that support this activity by helping to maintain the tongue body posture, elevating the mandible slightly, or counteracting the force of the tip on the roof of the mouth. These "background" muscles consist of both **antagonists** (muscles that oppose the movement) and **synergists** (muscles that support the movement) which are responsible for providing the muscular environment that allows the goal to be completed. The extrapyramidal system arises from the premotor region of the frontal lobe of the cerebrum and projects to the basal ganglia and reticular formation of the brainstem.

In summary, the nervous system can be viewed either as a set of structures or as a set of functions.

- In a structural view, we divide the nervous system into the central nervous system (CNS) and the peripheral nervous system (PNS). The CNS includes the cerebral cortex, brainstem, basal ganglia, cerebellum, spinal cord, thalamus and subthalamus, and nuclei and tracts within these structures. The PNS consists of the 31 spinal nerves and the 12 cranial nerves that emerge from the CNS. Functional division of the nervous system includes the autonomic and somatic systems.
- The autonomic nervous system is responsible for involuntary function of the body, including contraction of smooth muscle, glandular secretion, and digestive and cardiac function, and includes the enteric nervous system (ENS). The ENS is responsible for digestive processes themselves.
- The ANS has two responsive systems: sympathetic and parasympathetic. The sympathetic system is responsible for metabolic activities that prepare for a response to a stimulus in the environment. The parasympathetic system counteracts these responses. The ANS is designed to maintain homeostasis of the body.
- The ANS arises from the prefrontal region of the cerebral cortex and thalamus, hypothalamus, hippocampus, brainstem, spinal cord, and cerebellum.
- All skeletal muscles contract through action of the somatic nervous system, and conscious activity is the domain of the somatic nervous system. The pyramidal system is involved in direct activation of skeletal muscle, and the extrapyramidal system governs background movements and muscle tone.

DEVELOPMENTAL ORGANIZATION

The anatomy of the nervous system arises from the complex processes of prenatal development. As the brain develops, it passes through several stages that reflect its long evolution. **Phylogeny** refers to the evolution of a species, while **ontogeny** refers to the development of the organism. In prenatal development, we will see that the evolutionarily newer structures will develop later. We are concerned about the timing of development of the CNS because of the potential effects of injury from toxins or from physical insult (Table 1–3). One of the very sobering aspects of prenatal development is that the nervous system is considered vulnerable throughout development, and thus there are no safe times for insult or injury. Let's briefly examine development of the CNS.

Development

Neural development is an unfolding, moving from simple to complex. Weeks 1 through 8 following fertilization of the egg are termed the **embryonic** period, while weeks 9 through 37 are the **fetal** period. The fetal period is the time of very rapid growth, cell proliferation, and differentiation, and this is reflected in the changes seen in the nervous system (Alberstone, 2009). You may want to refer to Figures 1–2 and 1–3, as well as Table 1–4 as we discuss this development.

The entire nervous system is derived from the embryological neural plate. Folding of the neural plate is induced by the notochord, and by the end of the first month after conception (gestational age [GA]) the neural tube is formed.

TABLE 1–3. **Agents of Congenital Malformation**

Established teratogens	Potential Effects
1. Antineoplastic agents (Busulfan)	Severe skeletal growth anom: corneal opacity, cleft palate, organ hypoplasia
1a. Folic acid antagonists (aminopterin, methotrexate)	Multiple severe anomalies
2. Antimetabolites, amethopterin, fluorouracil, 6-azauridine	Multiple anomalies
3. Estrogens	Vaginal adenocarcinoma in daughters, later years
3a. Progestogens and estrogen taken before know pt. is pregnant	VACTERL syndrome: vertebral, anal, cardiac, tracheo, esophageal, renal, limb malformations
4. Androgens, progestogens (sex hormones), ethisterone, norethisterone, testosterone	Masculinization, advanced bone age
5. Thalidomide	Fetal death, deafness, multiple anomalies: rudimentary limbs, absence or ext./inner ear, heart, urinary defect
6. Organic mercury	Cerebral palsy, MR, blindness, cerebral atrophy, seizures
7. Polychlorinated biphenyls (PCBs)	Developmental defects (PCB contaminants in cooking oil, sports fish, rice)
8. Alcohol	Fetal alcohol syndrome (FAS) (mental retardation [MR], microcephaly, ocular, palpebral, joint anomalies, maxillary hypoplasia; FAS is the most common cause of MR)
9. Aminopterin	Skeletal defects, CNS meroanencephaly (portion of brain absent)
10. Phenytoin (dilantin)	Fetal hydantoin syndrome: intrauterine growth restriction, MR, inner epicanthal folds, ptosis, broad nasal bridge
11. Lithium carbonate (antipsychotic)	Heart and other vascular deficits
11a. Diazepam	Cleft lip or lip/palate
12. Methotrexate	Multiple malformations: skeletal of face, limbs, vertebral column
13. Vitamin A (low dose)	2nd to 5th weeks: facial abnormalities, including cleft palate, neural tube defect (e.g., spina bifida cystica)
14. Tetracyclines	Dental discoloration, enamel hypoplasia, and birth abnormalities, deafness
15. Trimethadione	Developmental delay, Vshaped eyebrows, lowset ears, cleft lip and/or palate

Infectious agents as teratogens	Potential Effects
1. Cytomegalovirus	Microcephaly, hydrocephaly microphthalmia, microgyria, MR, cerebral calcifications, fetal death
2. Herpes simplex virus	Microcephaly, microphthalmia, retinal dysplasia
3. Rubella virus (German measles)	Cataracts, glaucoma, chorioretinitis, deafness, microphthalmia, congenital heart defects
4. Varicella (chicken pox)	Intrautarine growth restriction low birth rate, prematurity
4a. Herpes zoster (shingles)	Skin scarring, muscle atrophy, MR
5. Venezuelan equine encephalitis	Cataracts, brain destruction
6. Toxoplasma gondii (intracellular parasite): eating raw meat (pork, mutton), close contact with cat feces, dogs, rabbits, etc.	Microcephaly, MR, hydrocephaly microphthalmia, chorioretinitis, cerebral calcifications

continues

TABLE 1–3.	*continued*
7. Treponema pallidum	Hydrocephalus, deafness, MR, abnormal teeth and bones
8. Ionizing radiation	Severe malformation in cases of maternal radiation therapy for cervical cancer. Microcephaly, MR, skeletal malformations, fetal death. From Nagasaki and Hiroshima: to 16 weeks after fertilization is most sensitive. Single diagnostic irradiation probably does not cause damage.
9. Syphilis	Serious malformations after week 20: MR, hydrocephalus, deafness, bone anomalies: palate, nasal, and dental destruction, saddlenose, poorly developed maxilla
Suspected teratogens	
1. LSD	Fractured chromosome abnormalities (limb, CNS)
2. Insulin (high dose)	Abnormalities
3. Vitamin D	Cardiopathies
4. Corticosteroids	Cleft palate, cardiac arrest in mice
5. Phencyclidine (PCP, "angel dust")	Severe malformations
6. Iodides: potassium iodide (cough medicine), radioactive iodine, iodine deficiency	Cretinism: MR, arrested development
Fetotoxins	
1. Analgesics, narcotics (heroin, morphine, excessive salicylates [aspirin])	Neonatal death, convulsions, bleeding, tremors
2. Cardiovascular drugs: ammonium chloride, hexamethonium, reserpine	Acidosis, neonatal ileus, nasal congestion
3. Anticoagulants	Fetal death or hemorrhage
4. Poliomyelitis immunization	Death/neurologic damage
5. Sedatives, hypnotics Tranquilizers: meprobamate Phenobarbital, phenothiazines	Retarded development, neonatal bleeding, hyperbilirubinemia
6. Smallpox vaccination	Death or fetal vaccinia
7. Thiazides	Thrombocytopenia
8. Tobacco smoking	Undersized babies
9. Excessive vitamin K	Hyperbilirubimenia

Source: Based on data of Krupp & Chatton (1982) and Moore (2015).

This tube will ultimately make up the structures of the nervous system, while the cells peripheral to the tube (neural crest cells) will migrate to form the cranial nerves and structures of the face and head related to those nerves. Around the fourth week GA, the neural tube becomes pinched in two places, forming three distinct pouches. These pouches or bulges are termed the prosencephalon, mesencephalon, and rhombencephalon. The **prosencephalon** begins differentiation into the **telencephalon** and **diencephalon**, while the **rhombencephalon** begins differentiation into the **metencephalon** (hindbrain) and **myelencephalon** (sometimes called the afterbrain). Around five weeks GA the process of segmentation begins, in which the primordial components start differentiating to form what will ultimately be the cor-

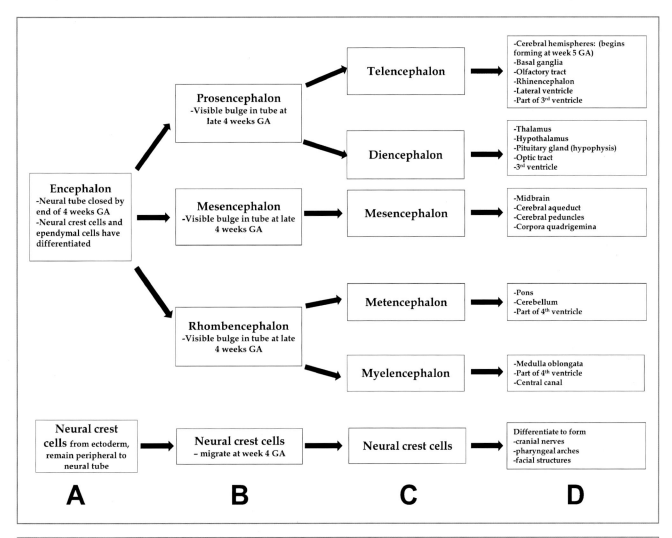

FIGURE 1–2.   Differentiation of the nervous system during development. **A.** The neural tube develops from folding of the neural plate by the end of the fourth week of gestational age (GA). Neural crest and ependymal cells remain peripheral to the neural tube. **B.** Toward the end of the fourth week GA, the encephalon has differentiated into visible representations of the prosencephalon, mesencephalon, and rhombencephalon. Neural crest cells begin migration. **C.** Around the fifth week GA, the prosencephalon differentiates into the telencephalon and diencephalon. The rhombencephalon differentiates into the metencephalon and myelencephalon. **D.** The telencephalon differentiates to become the cerebral hemispheres, the basal ganglia, olfactory tract, rhinencephalon, the lateral ventricle, and part of the third ventricle. The diencephalon differentiates to become the thalamus, hypothalamus, pituitary gland, optic tract, and remainder of the third ventricle. The mesencephalon differentiates to become the midbrain, cerebral aqueduct, cerebral peduncles, and corpora quadrigemina. The metencephalon differentiates to become the pons, cerebellum, and a portion of the fourth ventricle. The myelencephalon ultimately becomes the medulla oblongata, the remainder of the fourth ventricle, and the central canal of the brainstem and spinal cord. The neural crest cells differentiate to become five components of cranial nerves and facial primordia.

tical and subcortical structures. The telencephalon begins differentiation into the cerebral hemispheres, basal ganglia, olfactory tract, rhinencephalon, and the lateral ventricle and a portion of the third ventricle. The diencephalon differentiates to form the thalamus and hypothalamus, the hypophysis (pituitary gland), optic tract, and third ventricle. The mesencepha-

lon begins forming the midbrain, cerebral peduncles, cerebral aqueduct, and corpora quadrigemina. The metencephalon begins differentiating into the pons, cerebellum, and portion of the fourth ventricle, while the myelencephalon becomes the medulla oblongata, the remainder of the fourth ventricle, and the central canal of the brainstem and spinal cord.

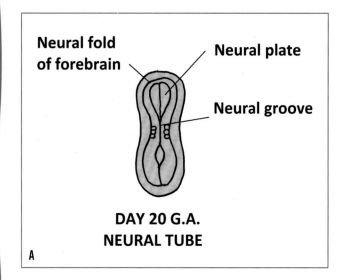

Neural fold of forebrain

Neural plate

Neural groove

DAY 20 G.A. NEURAL TUBE

A

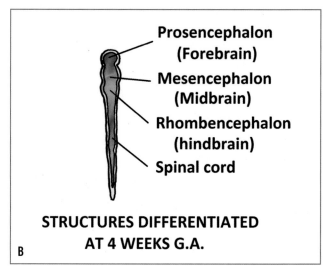

Prosencephalon (Forebrain)

Mesencephalon (Midbrain)

Rhombencephalon (hindbrain)

Spinal cord

STRUCTURES DIFFERENTIATED AT 4 WEEKS G.A.

B

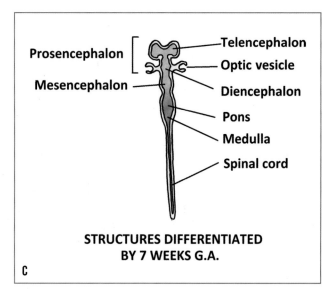

Prosencephalon

Mesencephalon

Telencephalon

Optic vesicle

Diencephalon

Pons

Medulla

Spinal cord

STRUCTURES DIFFERENTIATED BY 7 WEEKS G.A.

C

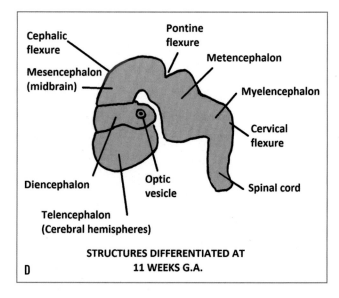

Cephalic flexure

Mesencephalon (midbrain)

Pontine flexure

Metencephalon

Myelencephalon

Cervical flexure

Diencephalon

Optic vesicle

Spinal cord

Telencephalon (Cerebral hemispheres)

STRUCTURES DIFFERENTIATED AT 11 WEEKS G.A.

D

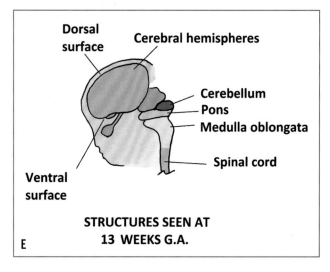

Dorsal surface

Cerebral hemispheres

Cerebellum

Pons

Medulla oblongata

Spinal cord

Ventral surface

STRUCTURES SEEN AT 13 WEEKS G.A.

E

FIGURE 1–3. Various stages of embryonic development. **A.** At 20 day gestational age (GA), the neural tube is forming from the neural plate. **B.** At 4 weeks GA, the neural tube has developed enlargements for the prosencephalon (forebrain), mesencephalon (midbrain), and rhombencephalon (hindbrain). The spinal cord is apparent. **C.** By 7 weeks GA, the prosencephalon has differentiated, revealing the two cerebral hemispheres. The diencephalon, pons, and medulla are apparent. **D.** At 11 weeks GA, the cervical, pontine, and cephalic flexures have further differentiated the nervous system. **E.** At 13 weeks GA, the cerebral cortex has flexed so that the dorsal surface is now at the rostral extreme.

TABLE 1–4.	**Components of the Encephalon**
Telencephalon	Cerebral hemispheres
	Basal ganglia
	Olfactory tract
	Rhinencephalon
	Lateral ventricle, portion of third ventricle
Diencephalon	Thalamus
	Hypothalamus
	Pituitary gland (hypophysis)
	Optic tract
	Third ventricle
Mesencephalon	Midbrain
	Cerebral aqueduct
	Cerebral peduncles
	Corpora quadrigemina
Metencephalon	Pons
	Cerebellum
	Portion of fourth ventricle
Myelencephalon	Medulla oblongata
	Portion of fourth ventricle

Source: Based on data of Seikel, Drumright, & King (2016).

During the fifth week GA, two flexures develop in the neural tube. The **cervical flexure** is a bend at the juncture of the brain and spinal cord, and the **cephalic** (or midbrain) **flexure** is a bend that develops between the midbrain (mesencephalon) and hindbrain (rhombencephalon).

The **neural crest cells** begin migrating at the same time (fourth week GA). These cells differentiate to form the pharyngeal arch system (Table 1–5). This migration is critically important for the development of structures of the face, and you will inevitably cross the neural crest cells in your study of craniofacial anomalies. The mandibular arch (Arch 1) gives rise to the V trigeminal nerve, as well as the musculature it will innervate. Notably, it also gives rise to the cartilage that will ultimately differentiate into the incus and malleus. The hyoid arch (Arch 2) gives rise to the VII facial nerve, as well as muscles of the face and other muscle that it will innervate and the primordial cartilage that will become the stapes and portions of the hyoid. From the Third Arch arises the IX glossopharyngeal nerve and the muscle it innervates, as well as the cartilage that will form the rest of the hyoid. The Fourth Arch will give rise to the pharyngeal and superior laryngeal nerves of the X vagus, as well as the extrinsic laryngeal muscles and others, while the Sixth Arch will differentiate into the recurrent laryngeal nerve of the X vagus, intrinsic laryn-

geal muscles, and the arytenoid cartilages. Humans have no derivatives from the Fifth Arch.

Waardenburg Syndrome

Waardenburg syndrome is an autosomal dominant condition arising from alterations in the migration of neural crest cells (Poswillo, 1973; Variant, 1994). First arch syndromes such as Waardenburg occur when neural crest cells fail to migrate successfully to the mandibular arch (also known as the first pharyngeal arch) in embryonic development. The tensor veli palatini muscle and muscles of mastication, as well as the V trigeminal nerve, develop from this arch. The neural crest cells of the first arch also give rise to pigment cells, and therein lies the basis for the physical signs of Waardenburg syndrome (Read & Newton, 1997). Individuals with this condition may have a prominent white streak in their hair and **heterochromia irides** (one eye has normal pigment while the other is pale blue). This rare condition occurs in 1 in 212,000 live births.

One important result of the pigment failure is deafness, since cochlear hair cells have their embryonic origin in pigment cells. Because autosomal dominant conditions can be passed from generation to generation, it is important for audiologists to be aware of this syndrome so they can refer clients for genetic counseling.

Individuals with Waardenburg syndrome may have other conditions related to the failed migration. Since the first arch is the primordial source for the mandibular tissue, there can be deficiencies related to the tensor veli palatini, muscles of mastication, and vestibular mechanism. Cleft lip and/or cleft palate may occur, as well as mandibular hypoplasia.

Interestingly, first arch syndromes such as Waardenburg are seen also in non-humans. If you see a white horse or cat with very pale blue eyes, there is a good chance that the animal will be deaf (e.g., Omenn, McKusick, & Gorlin, 1979).

The cervical flexure mentioned above can lead to some confusion in terminology related to the structures of the head and, most importantly, the cerebrum. The cervical flexure at the seventh embryonic week results in a tipping of the cerebrum, so that the dorsal (back) surface of the tube flexes to become the superior surface. In this same way, the superior surface of the tongue becomes the dorsal surface, with the inferior surface being the ventral (**belly**) surface. Likewise, the inferior surface of the cerebrum becomes the ventral surface. The brainstem immediately below the cerebrum was not involved in the flexure, so the anterior surface of the brainstem remains the ventral surface, and the posterior surface is the dorsal surface.

TABLE 1–5.	Pharyngeal Arches Derived from Neural Crest Cells		
Pharyngeal arch number and name	**Muscle**	**Nerve**	**Cartilage**
1 Mandibular	- Tensor tympani - Muscles of mastication - Mylohyoid - Anterior digastricus - Tensor veli palatini	V trigeminal nerve, mandibular branch	- Incus - Malleus - Anterior ligament of malleus - Spine of sphenoid - Sphenomandibular ligament - Genial tubercle of mandible
2 Hyoid	- Stapedius - Stylohyoid - Facial muscles - Posterior digastricus	VII facial nerve	- Stapes - Styloid process of temporal bone - Stylohyoid ligament - Lesser horn and upper part of corpus hyoid
3 Third	- Stylopharyngeus	IX glossopharyngeal nerve	- Greater horn and lower portion of hyoid
4 Fourth	- Pharyngeal extrinsic laryngeal muscles - Levator veli palatini	X vagus nerve, superior pharyngeal nerve, pharyngeal branch	- Thyroid cartilage - Corniculate cartilage - Cuneiform cartilage
6 Sixth	- Intrinsic laryngeal muscles	X vagus nerve, recurrent laryngeal branch	- Arytenoid cartilages

Genetic Terminology

Genetics refers to the study of genes and how traits are transmitted from generation to generation. Genes are sequences of deoxyribonucleic acid (DNA) that code for heritable traits. Genes make up the 23 pairs of chromosomes of the human DNA sequence, and recombination of genes during the embryonic phase of development allows traits to be transferred between generations. The newly formed embryo will contain genetic material from both parents. There are 22 pairs of somatic chromosomes, and 1 pair of sex chromosomes, so in classical Mendelian genetics, traits can be inherited as either somatic or sex linked.

A dominant gene is one that will be manifest in the individual's phenotype (observable characteristics) if it has been transmitted by either parent (Figure 1–4). If an embryo carries an autosomal dominant gene, it will be seen in the phenotype if only one copy of the gene is present. Thus, if one parent has a dominant gene, the probability is that half of the offspring will also have that gene. For example, the gene coding for facial dimples is a dominant gene. If one of your parents had dimples, 50% of the children would have dimples. Some genetic diseases have autosomal dominant inheritance. As an example, Huntington's disease is an autosomal dominant trait, so 50% of the children of a parent with the disease will also inherit the disease.

An autosomal recessive gene is one that will only be manifest in the phenotype if a person receives two copies of the gene (one from each parent). For instance, right-handedness is a dominant trait, but left-handedness is a recessive trait (see Figure 1–4B). So, for a child to be left handed, he or she must receive the autosomal recessive gene for left-handedness from both parents. The pattern of inheritance depends on the genotype (genetic makeup) of each parent. In the handedness example, if each parent carries one recessive (left-handed) and one dominant (right-handed) gene for handedness, then the chances are that one

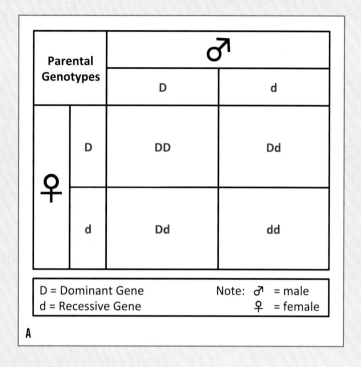

Parental Genotypes		♂	
		D	d
♀	D	DD	Dd
	d	Dd	dd

D = Dominant Gene   Note: ♂ = male
d = Recessive Gene   ♀ = female

A

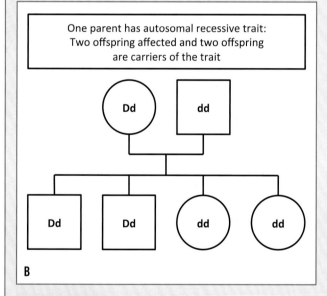

One parent has autosomal recessive trait:
Two offspring affected and two offspring
are carriers of the trait

B

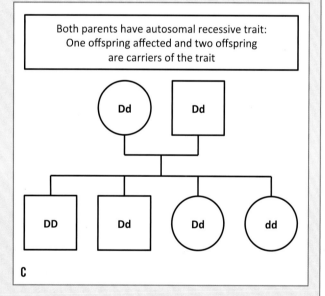

Both parents have autosomal recessive trait:
One offspring affected and two offspring
are carriers of the trait

C

FIGURE 1—4. Basic considerations for genetic inheritance. **A.** Each parent has two genes for a given trait. The gene for a trait can dominant (represented by capital "D") or recessive (represented by lower-case "d"). For instance, right-handedness is a dominant trait, while left-handedness is a recessive trait. In the case of this table, both parents have both the dominant and recessive gene for this trait. Both parents are right-handed, and three out of four children will display the dominant right-handed trait. One child (receiving the two recessive genes) will display the recessive left-handed trait. **B.** In this case, one parent has both dominant and recessive genes, while the other has two copies of the recessive gene. Two out of four children will have the dominant trait, and two will have the recessive trait. **C.** In this case, both parents have a copy of the dominant and recessive genes, so the probability is that three out of four will have the dominant trait, and one will have the recessive trait.

in four children will receive a "double dose" of the recessive gene, thereby being left-handed. The chances are that two out of four offspring will carry the recessive gene but that it won't be manifest in the phenotype. In this case, those two children are carriers for the trait. As an example, autosomal recessive cerebellar ataxia is a recessive trait. In a family in which one family member carries the trait but does not have the condition, while the other doesn't have the trait, none of the offspring will have the phenotype, but two of them will be carriers. Should a carrier marry another carrier, the chances are that 25% of the children will have the disease.

Sex-linked inheritance refers to transfer of traits that are carried on either the X or Y chromosomes. Males have an X and Y chromosome, while females have two X chromosomes. X-linked recessive traits are recessive genes that are carried on the X chromosome. The trait will be manifest if both parents carry the trait on the X chromosome, and it can affect either male or female offspring. If a parent has an X-linked dominant trait, 50% of offspring may get the trait. If a trait is present on the Y chromosome, it will be manifest in only male offspring, and female offspring will be neither affected nor carriers.

In summary, the anatomy of the nervous system arises from the complex processes of prenatal development.

- Phylogeny refers to the evolution of a species, while ontogeny refers to the development of the organism. Neural development is an unfolding, moving from simple to complex. Weeks 1 through 8 following fertilization of the egg are termed the embryonic period, while weeks 9 through 37 are the fetal period.
- The nervous system is derived from the neural plate. The neural tube has formed by four weeks gestational age (GA). Three pouches in the neural tube form the prosencephalon, mesencephalon, and rhombencephalon. The prosencephalon begins differentiation into the telencephalon and diencephalon, while the rhombencephalon begins differentiation into the metencephalon and myelencephalon. Around five weeks GA the primordial components start forming the cortical and subcortical structures.
- The telencephalon forms the cerebral hemispheres, basal ganglia, olfactory tract, and rhinencephalon, the lateral ventricle, and a portion of the third ventricle. The diencephalon forms the thalamus and hypothalamus, the hypophysis, optic tract, and third ventricle. The mesencephalon forms the midbrain, cerebral peduncles, cerebral aqueduct, and corpora quadrigemina. The metencephalon forms the pons, cerebellum, and portion of the fourth ventricle. The myelencephalon becomes the medulla oblongata, the remainder of the fourth ventricle, and the central canal of the brainstem and spinal cord.
- The cervical flexure forms at the fifth week GA at the juncture of the brain and spinal cord, and the cephalic flexure develops between the midbrain and hindbrain.
- The neural crest cells begin migrating at the fourth week GA and will form the pharyngeal arch system. The mandibular arch (Arch 1) gives rise to the V trigeminal nerve and the musculature it innervates. The hyoid arch (Arch 2) gives rise to the VII facial nerve and its muscles. The Third Arch gives rise to the IX glossopharyngeal nerve and its muscle, while the Fourth Arch gives rise to the pharyngeal and superior laryngeal nerves of the X vagus and their

muscles. The Sixth Arch becomes the recurrent laryngeal nerve of the X vagus, intrinsic laryngeal muscles, and the arytenoid cartilages.
- The cervical flexure results in the cerebrum being tipped so that the dorsal surface of the cerebrum is the superior surface.

TERMINOLOGY RELATED TO NEUROANATOMY AND NEUROPHYSIOLOGY

We will be introducing terminology in context throughout the text, but there are some terms that you already know from your study of anatomy. This is a good time to review them and to introduce a few terms that will permeate our discussion of neuroanatomy and neurophysiology.

The anatomical position is very specific, and examining it will help you understand the peculiarity we mentioned concerning the dorsal surface of the cerebrum. If you look at Figure 1–5, you can see the anatomical position, which is an erect posture with palms facing forward. There are axes related to the body and brain. Axes are imaginary midlines that run through a body or structure. In the human, we talk about the skeletal axis, which is an axis running through the vertebral column and including the head and trunk. The neuraxis is a special case for humans. Because of the embryonic flexure we discussed earlier, the neuraxis is in something of a "T" formation. The spinal cord and brainstem have dorsal surfaces that correspond to the back of the body, but because of the flexure during embryonic development the telencephalon folds forward so that the ventral surface is now the inferior aspect of the cerebrum. This is illustrated in Figure 1–6.

Three very important terms are sagittal, coronal, and transverse. A **sagittal** section or view refers to a dissection from front to back of a structure. So, a sagittal section of the body would divide the body into right and left portions. A midsagittal section would divide the body into left and right halves. A **coronal** or **frontal** section is more or less in

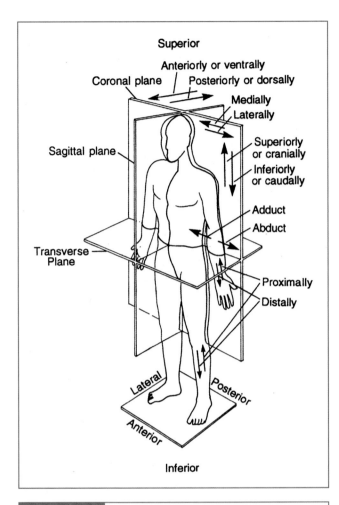

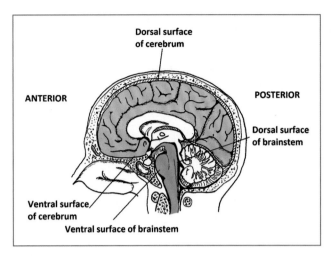

FIGURE 1–6. Orientation of the cerebrum as a result of cervical flexure during embryonic development. Note that the dorsum of the cerebrum is at the rostral end of the body, while the dorsum of the brainstem is aligned with the dorsum of the body.

parallel to the coronal suture of the head, dividing the body into front and back portions. A **transverse** section divides the body into upper and lower portions. These specific terms will come in very handy while describing sections of the brain.

There are a few more anatomical terms that we will use a lot in our discussion. **Anterior** refers to the front surface of a body and **posterior** refers to the back of the body. This is in contrast to the **dorsal** and **ventral** surfaces, which are referred to as the dorso-ventral axis rather than presenting surface. The dorsum of the human body is the back or posterior surface, but the dorsum of the cerebrum is the upper (superior) surface. The ventral surface of the body includes the abdomen, anterior thorax, etc. The ventral surface of the cerebrum is the inferior surface. **Superior** refers to the upper surface and **inferior** refers to the lower surface. **Rostral** refers

to "toward the beak," as in toward the nose, while **cranial** means "toward the skull."

Medial (or mesial) refers to being situated toward the middle, while **lateral** refers to being situated away from the midline. For an appendage (such as an arm), you will refer to **proximal** (toward the root) and **distal** (away from the root). **Superficial** means "toward the surface," while **deep** means "away from the surface" or closer to the middle of the body. The term **prone** refers to a position of lying on the belly, while **supine** refers to lying on the back.

Hands and feet have some special terms. The "belly" or ventral surface of the hand (the palm) is termed the **palmar** surface. The top of the foot is the dorsal surface. The sole of the foot is termed the **plantar** surface (you can think of "planting your feet" firmly on the ground).

Terms of Movement

There are specific terms of movement that are clinically useful. **Extension** refers to the process of increasing the angle between two structures. **Flexion**, then, is moving a structure so that the angle between them is decreased. Bending your elbow is an act of flexion, while reaching out to shake someone's hand is an extension. **Hyperextension** is extension beyond the normal limits. **Abduction** is the processing of moving a structure away from midline, as in the process of abducting the vocal folds. **Adduction** brings a structure toward midline. When speaking of the feet, one refers to the plantar surface as the sole of the foot, which is also the flexor surface. When you flex your feet, you basically curl your toes and increase the arch magnitude. Flexion would be, for instance, rising on your toes or extending your foot. A **plantar grasp reflex** is that which curls the toes to "grasp." Palmar refers to the "belly" or ventral surface of the hand, and a **palmar grasp reflex** would be an act of flexion that curled the fingers to grasp.

Pronation of the hand is rotation of the hand so that the palm of the hand is turned downward, while **supination** of the hand turns the palm superiorly (as in holding your hand out to receive something). Pronation of the foot is rotation of the foot so that it turns out, while supination rotates it to turn in.

It is useful to examine word components so that unique combinations can be parsed out as you confront them. The combining form **ipsi** means same, so **ipsilateral** refers to same side, or staying on the same side. **Contra** refers to other or opposite, so **contralateral** refers to opposite side. We'll run across the term "decussation" frequently in the nervous system. **Decussation** refers to crossing, and in neuroanatomy we see pathways that cross from the left to the right side of the body and vice versa.

Terms of Neuropathology in Speech-Language Pathology

Neurology refers specifically to the study of the diseases of the nervous system, and there are special terms for the pathologies that arise from neurological conditions. Let's review a few of these. We will talk about these disorders and their anatomical underpinnings in detail in later chapters.

Aphasia refers to a deficit of language expression or comprehension, typically arising from neurological insult. We will often refer to **nonfluent aphasia** as Broca's aphasia, a nod to Paul Broca, who is credited for first identifying the site of lesion responsible for it. Similarly, we talk about **Wernicke's aphasia**, which is a **fluent aphasia** that disturbs language comprehension. Carl Wernicke found the prominent site of lesion for this disorder (Wernicke's area). We now know that these areas are only part of the language deficit picture, but these two great scientists led the way to our understanding of the site and extent of lesion required to produce these two disorders. **Conduction aphasia** is a deficit in the ability to repeat information heard auditorily, and **global aphasia** refers to a significant loss of language reception and expression. **Transcortical sensory aphasia** will result in poor auditory comprehension with intact repetition, while **transcortical motor aphasia** produces an aphasia similar to nonfluent aphasia, but with retained repetition ability. **Anomic aphasia** is a deficit in the ability to retrieve words despite the individual feeling that he or she knows the word, while **anomia** (word-finding difficulty) is a feature of all of the forms of aphasia.

We can think of speech as the oral manifestation of language. The process of speech involves the effectors we discussed above, so the entire motor mechanism of the brain related to speech can be involved in one way or another. **Apraxia** is a deficit in planning and programming for execution of a motor act in the absence of paralysis or paresis. Any complex motor act requires planning. We can have dressing apraxia, which refers to a deficit in the ability to plan the act of dressing. **Apraxia of speech** (or verbal apraxia) is a deficit in the planning and programming of the articulators of speech, resulting in a constellation of problems that includes inconsistent articulatory errors, articulatory breakdown, halting speech, and articulatory groping, coupled with less difficulty with automatized speech, such as counting or reciting the days of the week. **Oral apraxia** is a deficit in the planning and programming of the articulators for nonspeech activities.

Dysarthria refers to difficulty speaking as a result of loss of muscle strength, alteration in muscle tone, or reduced coordination. The result may be loss of articulatory precision, altered rate of production, and changes in vocal intensity. **Paralysis** (loss of the ability to move a muscle) or **paresis** (muscular weakness) is often a contributor to dysarthria. **Flaccid dysarthria** refers to the low-tone condition of the affected articulators or speech system. **Spastic dysarthria** refers to a condition that includes high muscle tone. **Hyperkinetic dysarthria** always includes extraneous movement, while **hypokinetic dysarthria** results in a paucity of movement in the context of high muscle tone. **Ataxic dysarthria** results in loss of coordination of articulators and often low muscle tone.

The term **gnosis** refers to "knowing," so **agnosia** (a = absent or from) means not knowing something. We speak of **verbal agnosia** as losing the knowledge of words. The sensory system is intact (I can hear) but I cannot comprehend speech. In **tactile agnosia,** I have lost the ability to know the nature of an object through the sense of touch: if I am presented with a set of keys with my eyes closed I will not be able to recognize them. **Visual agnosia** is a deficit in which an object presented visually is not recognized. Gnosis goes beyond sensory reception: in the case of auditory agnosia, hearing may be demonstrably intact, but the person cannot comprehend speech.

Dementia is a condition arising typically from brain deterioration and resulting in confusion, loss of memory, personality change, and reduced reasoning capacity. There are several etiologies (causes) of dementia, but **dementia of Alzheimer's type** (DAT) is the most common. **Confabulation** is a condition in which the individual fabricates information (such as recalled memories of events) without the intention to deceive.

This list of terms within the profession is really quite limited but does provide us with a common framework from which to work in our discussion of the nervous system. Let's move on and begin that process!

In summary, the anatomical position is an erect posture with palms facing forward.

- Axes are imaginary midlines that run through a body or structure. The skeletal axis runs through the vertebral column and includes the head and trunk. The neuraxis in humans has two perpendicular elements. The spinal cord and brainstem are parallel to the skeletal axis, with dorsal surfaces that correspond to the back of the body. The cerebrum has an anterior-posterior axis, such that the ventral surface is now the inferior aspect of the cerebrum.
- A sagittal section or view divides the body into right and left portions, and a coronal or frontal section divides the body into front and back portions. A transverse section divides the body into upper and lower portions.
- Anterior refers to the front surface of a body and posterior refers to the back of the body. The dorsum of the human body is the back or posterior surface, but the dorsum of the cerebrum is the superior surface. The ventral surface of the body includes the abdomen, anterior thorax, and so on. The ventral surface of the cerebrum is the inferior surface.
- Superior refers to the upper surface and inferior refers to the lower surface. Rostral refers to "toward the nose," while cranial means "toward the skull."
- Medial or mesial refers to being situated toward the middle, and lateral refers to being situated away from the midline. When talking about appendages such as arms, we refer to proximal (toward the root of a free extremity) and distal (away from the root).
- Superficial means "toward the surface" and deep means "away from the surface" or closer to the axis of the body. The term "prone" refers to a position of lying on the belly, while "supine" refers to lying on the back.
- The ventral surface of the hand (the palm) is termed the palmar surface and the back is the dorsal surface. The top of the foot is the dorsal surface and the "belly" of the foot is termed the plantar surface.
- Extension refers to the process of increasing the angle between two structures, and flexion decreases the angle. Hyperextension is extension beyond the normal limits. Abduction is moving a structure away from midline, and adduction brings a structure toward midline. The plantar surface of the foot is also the flexor surface. A plantar grasp reflex curls the toes to grasp, while a palmar grasp reflex curls the fingers to grasp.
- Pronation of the hand is rotation of the hand so that the palm of the hand is turned downward, while supination of the hand turns the palm superiorly. Pronation of the foot is rotation of the foot so that it turns out, while supination rotates it to turn in.
- The combining form ipsi means "same," so ipsilateral refers to staying on the same side. Contra refers to other or opposite, so contralateral refers to the opposite side. Decussation refers to crossing.
- Neurology refers specifically to study of the diseases of the nervous system. Aphasia is a deficit of language expression or comprehension. Nonfluent or Broca's aphasia results in halting speech with significantly reduced syntactic depth, but with relatively retained comprehension. Fluent or Wernicke's aphasia disturbs language comprehension, with speech consisting of mostly meaningless jargon. Conduction aphasia is a deficit in the ability to repeat information heard auditorily, and global aphasia refers to a significant loss of language reception and expression. Transcortical sensory aphasia will result in poor auditory comprehension with intact repetition, while transcortical motor aphasia is similar to nonfluent aphasia with retained repetition ability. Anomic aphasia is a deficit in the ability to retrieve words, and anomia or word-finding difficulty is a feature of all of the forms of aphasia.
- Apraxia is a deficit in planning and programming for execution of a motor act in the absence of paralysis or paresis. Apraxia of speech or verbal apraxia is a deficit in the planning and programming of the articulators of speech, while oral apraxia is a deficit in the planning and programming of the articulators for nonspeech activities.
- Dysarthria refers to difficulty speaking as a result of loss of muscle strength, alteration in muscle tone, or reduced coordination. Paralysis is loss of the ability to move a muscle, and paresis is muscular weakness.
- Flaccid dysarthria arises from lower motor neuron damage and refers to the low-tone condition of the affected structures or speech system. Spastic dysarthria arises from upper motor neuron damage and results in high muscle tone. Hyperkinetic dysarthria arises from lesion to the basal ganglia and always includes extraneous movement, while hypokinetic dysarthria results in a paucity of movement. Ataxic dysarthria arises from damage to the cerebellum, its nuclei, or its pathways, and results in loss of coordination of articulators and often low muscle tone.
- Verbal agnosia is loss of knowledge of words without sensory involvement. In tactile agnosia, a person loses the ability to recognize an object through touch. In visual agnosia, an object presented visually is not recognized.
- Dementia is a condition that typically arises from brain deterioration and results in confusion, loss of memory, personality change, and reduced reasoning capacity. There are several etiologies (causes) of dementia, but Dementia of Alzheimer's Disease (DAT) is the most common.
- Confabulation is a condition in which the individual fabricates information (such as recalled memories of events) without the intention to deceive.

CHAPTER SUMMARY

Neurons are cells that are specialized for communication, receiving information and conveying it to the next neuron. Neurons have a dendrite, a soma, and an axon. An action potential releases neurotransmitter substance into the synapse causing ions to pass into the dendrite of the downstream neuron and, in turn, stimulating it to excitation. Nuclei are made up of neurons with special functions. The central nervous system (CNS) consists of the cerebral cortex, brainstem, cerebellum, spinal cord, and other subcortical structures. The peripheral nervous system (PNS) consists of the cranial and spinal nerves. The cerebral cortex is the seat of consciousness, as well as language processing, execution of speech, and all complex conscious activities. Motor activity is initiated in the frontal lobe at the motor strip. Efferent neurons are responsible for motor activity, and sensations from the periphery are conveyed to the cortex by afferent nerves. Reflexes are hard-wired responses that provide automated and involuntary responses to stimuli. Background neural activity includes maintaining muscle tone to counterbalance the desired activity. Tactile, muscle, and joint sensors provide somatic information about position and state of the body in space. The cerebellum coordinates all motor activity and integrates inputs from the body's sensors. Cognition involves memory, attention, visuospatial processes, and linguistic processes, which are the domain of the cerebrum. Somatic sense includes the sensations associated with pressure and thermal stimulation. Kinesthetic sense is the perception of the body moving in space. Special senses include hearing, vision, smell, and taste.

The central nervous system consists of the cerebral cortex, brainstem, basal ganglia, cerebellum, spinal cord, thalamus and subthalamus, nuclei, and tracts within these structures. The peripheral nervous system consists of the 31 spinal nerves and the 12 cranial nerves that emerge from the CNS. The autonomic nervous system is responsible for involuntary function of the body, including contraction of smooth muscle, glandular secretion, and digestive and cardiac function. A subsystem of the autonomic nervous system is the enteric nervous system, which is responsible for digestion. The sympathetic nervous system is responsible for metabolic activities that prepare for a response to a stimulus in the environment, while the parasympathetic system counteracts these responses. The autonomic nervous system arises from the prefrontal region of the cerebral cortex and thalamus, hypothalamus, hippocampus, brainstem, spinal cord, and cerebellum. All skeletal muscle activity and conscious activity is the domain of the somatic nervous system. The pyramidal system is involved in direct activation of skeletal muscle, and the extrapyramidal system governs background movements and muscle tone.

Neural development is an unfolding process, moving from simple to complex. Weeks 1 through 8 following fertilization of the egg are termed the embryonic period, while weeks 9 through 37 are the fetal period. The nervous system is derived from the neural plate. The neural tube has formed by four weeks gestational age (GA). Three pouches in the neural tube form the prosencephalon, mesencephalon, and rhombencephalon. The prosencephalon begins differentiation into the telencephalon and diencephalon, while the rhombencephalon begins differentiation into the metencephalon and myelencephalon. Around five weeks GA, the primordial components start forming the cortical and subcortical structures. The telencephalon forms the cerebral hemispheres, basal ganglia, olfactory tract, and rhinencephalon, the lateral ventricle and a portion of the third ventricle. The diencephalon forms the thalamus and hypothalamus, the hypophysis, optic tract, and third ventricle. The mesencephalon forms the midbrain, cerebral peduncles, cerebral aqueduct, and corpora quadrigemina. The metencephalon forms the pons, cerebellum, and a portion of the fourth ventricle. The myelencephalon becomes the medulla oblongata, the remainder of the fourth ventricle, and the central canal of the brainstem and spinal cord. The cervical flexure forms at the fifth week GA at the juncture of the brain and spinal cord, and the cephalic flexure develops between the midbrain and hindbrain. The neural crest cells begin migrating at the fourth week GA and will form the pharyngeal arch system. The mandibular arch (Arch 1) gives rise to the V trigeminal nerve and the musculature it innervates. The hyoid arch (Arch 2) gives rise to the VII facial nerve and its muscles. The Third Arch gives rise to the IX glossopharyngeal nerve and its muscle, while the Fourth Arch gives rise to the pharyngeal and superior laryngeal nerves of the X vagus and their muscles. The Sixth Arch becomes the recurrent laryngeal nerve of the X vagus, intrinsic laryngeal muscles, and the arytenoid cartilages. The cervical flexure results in the cerebrum being tipped so that the dorsal surface of the cerebrum is the superior surface.

The anatomical position is an erect posture with palms facing forward. Axes are imaginary midlines that run through a body or structure. The skeletal axis runs through the vertebral column and includes the head and trunk. The neuraxis in humans has two perpendicular elements. The spinal cord and brainstem are parallel to the skeletal axis, with dorsal surfaces that correspond to the back of the body. The cerebrum has an anterior-posterior axis, such that the ventral surface is now the inferior aspect of the cerebrum. A sagittal section or view divides the body into right and left portions, and a coronal or frontal section divides the body into front and back portions. A transverse section divides the body into upper and lower portions. Anterior refers to the front surface of a body, and posterior refers to the back of the body. The dorsum of the human body is the back or posterior surface, but the dorsum of the cerebrum is the superior surface. The ventral surface of the body includes the abdomen, anterior thorax, etc. The ventral surface of the cerebrum is the inferior surface. Superior refers to the upper surface and inferior refers to the lower surface. Rostral refers to "toward the nose," while cranial means "toward the skull."

Medial or mesial refers to being situated toward the middle, and lateral refers to being situated away from the midline. When talking about appendages such as arms we refer to proximal (toward the root of a free extremity) and distal (away from the root). Superficial means "toward the surface" and deep means "away from the surface" or closer to the axis of the body. The term "prone" refers to a position of lying on the belly, while supine refers to lying on the back. The ventral surface of the hand (the palm) is termed the palmar surface and the back is the dorsal surface. The top of the foot is the dorsal surface and the sole of the foot is termed the plantar surface. Extension refers to the process of increasing the angle between two structures, and flexion decreases the angle. Hyperextension is extension beyond the normal limits. Abduction is moving a structure away from midline, and adduction brings a structure toward midline. The plantar surface of the foot is also the flexor surface. A plantar grasp reflex curls the toes to grasp, while a palmar grasp reflex curls the fingers to grasp. Pronation of the hand is rotation of the hand so that the palm of the hand is turned downward, while supination of the hand turns the palm superiorly. Pronation of the foot is rotation of the foot so that it turns out, while supination rotates it to turn in. The combining form ipsi means "same," so ipsilateral refers to staying on the same side. Contra refers to other or opposite, so contralateral refers to opposite side. Decussation refers to crossing. Neurology refers specifically to the study of the diseases of the nervous system. Aphasia is a deficit of language expression or comprehension. Nonfluent, or Broca's, aphasia results in halting speech with significantly reduced syntactic depth, but with relatively retained comprehension, while fluent, or Wernicke's, aphasia disturbs language comprehension, with mostly meaningless jargon. Conduction aphasia is a deficit in the ability to repeat information heard auditorily, and global aphasia refers to a significant loss of language reception and expression. Transcortical sensory aphasia will result in poor auditory comprehension with intact repetition, while transcortical motor aphasia is similar to nonfluent aphasia with retained repetition ability. Anomic aphasia is a deficit in the ability to retrieve words, and anomia or word-finding difficulty is a feature of all of the forms of aphasia. Apraxia is a deficit in planning and programming for execution of a motor act in the absence of paralysis or paresis. Apraxia of speech or verbal apraxia is a deficit in the planning and programming of the articulators of speech, while oral apraxia is a deficit in the planning and programming of the articulators for nonspeech activities. Dysarthria refers to difficulty speaking as a result of loss of muscle strength, alteration in muscle tone, or reduced coordination. Paralysis is loss of the ability to move a muscle, and paresis is muscular weakness. Flaccid dysarthria arises from lower motor neuron damage and refers to the low-tone condition of the affected structures or speech system. Spastic dysarthria arises from upper motor neuron damage and results in high muscle tone. Hyperkinetic dysarthria arises from a lesion to the basal ganglia and always includes extraneous movement, while hypokinetic dysarthria results in a paucity of movement. Ataxic dysarthria arises from damage to the cerebellum, its nuclei, or its pathways, and results in loss of coordination of articulators and often low muscle tone. Verbal agnosia is loss of word knowledge without sensory involvement. In tactile agnosia, a person loses the ability to recognize an object through touch. In visual agnosia, an object presented visually is not recognized. Dementia is a condition that typically arises from brain deterioration and results in confusion, loss of memory, personality change, and reduced reasoning capacity. There are several etiologies of dementia, but dementia of Alzheimer's disease is the most common. Confabulation is a condition in which the individual fabricates information such as recalled memories of events without the intention to deceive.

CASE STUDY 1–1

Physician's Notes on Initial Physical Examination and History

The patient is a 26-year-old right-handed male (see Table 1–6 for terminology. Note that we are presenting the data of this case in chronological order to show the emerging speech and language signs and symptoms as the condition progresses). The patient reported gait unsteadiness over the last several years that progressively worsened, as well as upper and lower limb weakness, especially distally. He also admitted to having difficulties in opening his fist, suggestive of myotonia, but he denied any swallowing problems. According to his mother, the patient was born prematurely and exhibited learning difficulties as a child. His past medical history involves surgery for an abdominal cyst seven years ago. The patient was single and was working as a barber. He **denied** smoking and said that he drinks on social occasions. The family history involves a father in his middle 50s diagnosed with depression, and his mother is a female in her late 40s who, during the examination, had the same clinical presentation as her son. The patient has one older sister who is healthy and one older brother who shows the same signs as he does. On examination, the patient appeared alert and **oriented X3** with normal short-term and long-term memory. The examination of the cranial nerves did not disclose significant findings except for the sternocleidomastoid and temporalis muscles bilaterally. Muscle strength was decreased distally and proximally on the upper limbs, with arm abduction and flexion 4/5 and wrist flexion and extension 3/5 **MRC**

| TABLE 1–6. | Terminology for Case Study 1–1 |

"b-c" score	Scoring on the *Frenchay Dysarthria Assessment* (FDA). See Table 1–8 for details of the Frenchay scoring.
4/5	This is part of a muscle strength rating scale, standardized by the Medical Research Council. See Table 1–7 for specification of the terminology.
Aspiration	Pathological admission of food or liquid into the airway below the level of the vocal folds.
Bolus	Ball, typically referring to the ball of food or liquid being swallowed.
Breathy voice	Voice characterized by excessive air wastage, sometimes caused by vocal fold paralysis.
Cardiac echo	Echocardiography using ultrasound to visualize heart chambers, valves, etc.
CTG repeats	Refers to genetic disorder with repeated trinucleotide repetitions.
DAB	Classification system for dysarthria, referring to the pioneering work of Darley, Aronson, and Brown at Mayo Clinic. For further information, see Darley, Aronson, & Brown, (1969).
Deep tendon reflexes	Reflexes mediated by muscle spindle receptors, including patellar and Achilles tendon reflexes.
Denies	When used in the medical context, this simply means that the patient stated that whatever was being asked was not the case. Note that in this context, the term "denies" does not carry the accusatory tone of non-medical usage.
Dysarthria	Motor speech disorder involving muscular weakness, dyscoordination, and alteration of muscle tone.
Dysphagia	Difficulty with one of the stages of swallowing.
FBC	In laboratory testing, refers to full blood count.
Flaccid dysarthria	Dysarthria characterized by low tone, paralysis, or muscle weakness, and arising from lower motor neuron lesion.
Flexor plantar response	The plantar reflex in infants is stimulated by rubbing a blunt object on the sole of the foot with moderate force. Normal plantar response includes extension (dorsiflexion) of the big toe and abduction or fanning of the other toes. This reflex is inhibited by cortical control around 6 months of age, and is only seen in pathological conditions in adults.
Gait	Gait refers to the manner of walking of an individual.
HbAc1	Glycated hemoglobin, wherein red blood cells join with glucose.
Mastication	Chewing.
MRC	Medical Research Council system of measuring muscle strength. For more information, you may see Ciesla et al., 2011 and Table 1–7.
Myotonia	Tonic muscle spasm.
Myotonic dystrophy type 1 [DM1]	Myotonic dystrophy arising from genetic mutations of the DMPK gene.
Myotonic dystrophy	Myotonic dystrophy is an autosomal dominant genetic disorder resulting in myotonic muscle response, in which a muscle group contracts and fails to relax, producing a tonic muscle spasm. Individuals with myotonic dystrophy have a constellation of physical signs, including balding, cataracts, cognitive difficulties associated with executive function, and cardiac problems. Muscular weakness generally progresses from the hands, neck or face to include all muscles of the body, including the heart.

continues

TABLE 1–6.	*continued*
Oral phase of swallowing	The stage of swallowing in which food is prepared (chewed) and then propelled to the pharyngeal space for swallowing.
Oriented X3	This is shorthand for the results of cognitive screening, indicating that the person is "oriented to person, place, and time."
Oropharyngeal dysphagia	Dysphagia involving oral or pharyngeal structures and functions.
Percussion	Sharp and even tapping on the surface of the body.
Pharyngeal phase of swallowing	Stage of swallowing that involves moving the bolus of food or liquid through the pharynx to the esophagus, and involving protection of the airway.
Phonatory incompetence	Deficit in voicing along one of many parameters, including vocal intensity, fundamental frequency range and control, etc.
Pinprick sense	Sensation of pin prick on the skin, mediated by the spinothalamic pathway.
Polyneuropathy	Peripheral nerve damage involving more than one peripheral nerve.
Ptosis	Drooping of eyelids.
Residue	In dysphagia, food remaining in the pharynx, pyriform sinuses of valleculae after swallowing.
Rhythm Holter	Wearable cardiac monitor used to record cardiac activity.
Stocking distribution	Pattern found during neurological testing that reveals a sharp margin for areas sensing pain, temperature, touch, position and vibrations sense. This is accompanied by weakness, atrophy, and loss of deep tendon reflexes, and is indicative of distal pathology affecting specific nerves.
Tandem	Walking pattern in which toes of one foot touch heel of the other.
Thenal	Referring to the palm of hand or the base of the thumb.

TABLE 1–7.	**Examining Muscle Strength**

When examining a patient, identifying specific areas of muscular weakness helps to localize the site of lesion. Strength testing is completed for each muscle group, making sure that you test one side and then the next for each group, so you can compare strength for the two sides. Here is a muscle strength rating scale.

0/5	No contraction of muscle
1/5	Indication of muscle flicker, but no movement noted
2/5	Movement occurs, but not against gravity when tested in the horizontal plane
3/5	Movement occurs against, but not when there is resistance provided by the the examiner
4/5	Movement occurs against some resistance provided by the examiner
5/5	Normal strength

(see Table 1–7 for definitions of muscle testing). There was myotonia evoked by **percussion** on the **thenal** bilaterally. On the lower limbs, there was decreased muscle strength at the foot **dorsiflexion** bilaterally. The **deep tendon reflexes** were obtainable but decreased in all four extremities with **flexor plantar response** bilaterally. On sensory examination, there was reduced **vibration** and pinprick sense in **stocking distribution**. There was gait unsteadiness especially on **tandem**, wherein the patient was unable to walk with his toes touching his heels. The genetic analysis showed abnormally expanded **CTG repeats** (>50 repeats) in the sample of this individual, thus confirming the diagnosis of **myotonic dystrophy type 1 [DM1]**.

Medical Diagnosis

Myotonic dystrophy type 1 [DMI]

Impression

The patient presented muscle weakness of the upper and lower limbs and myotonia, consisting of muscular cramping. He also presented sensory disturbances with gait unsteadiness. The patient was to be evaluated with electromyography (EMG) and nerve conduction study (NCS) to rule out **polyneuropathy** and was scheduled to have blood examination for biochemistry, **FBC**, thyroid hormones, and **HbAc1**. A **cardiac echo and rhythm Holter** were prescribed and he was referred to a cardiologist and an ophthalmologist.

Swallowing Examination

The patient is a 28-year-old man referred for swallow function evaluation. His main complaint is that he occasionally chokes with solid food. This phenomenon has become worse in the last year. The oral motor examination showed bilateral facial weakness with eyelid **ptosis**, facial asymmetry noted at rest and right lip weakness. There were also found mildly decreased lingual strength and speed. The **oral phase of swallowing** showed slow, somewhat ineffective chewing effort, **mastication** mostly on the left side, and no rotary movement on the lower jaw, resulting in impaired **bolus** formation and **transfer** posteriorly. Solids were processed in rather large pieces. The **pharyngeal phase of swallowing** was within functional limits, the swallow response was timely, and there were no found overt symptoms/signs of **aspiration** of any consistency. However, there was found possible pharyngeal **residue** of solids as patient complains of food sticking high in his throat. The clinical impression is of mild oropharyngeal dysphagia mostly for solid food consistencies mainly due to ineffective oral preparation of bolus resulting in possible pharyngeal residue. Recommendations for thin liquids and soft solids, mashed with fork in the plate, moist diet, and processing in small bites.

The *Frenchay **Dysarthria** Assessment* was given to the patient. The results showed a mild to moderate difficulty, **"b-c" score**, with signs of **flaccid dysarthria**. The **DAB** classification shows a cluster of speech characteristics (**phonatory incompetence**). This cluster involves **breathy voice**, audible inspiration, and short phrases as well as slow rate (see Table 1–8 for details of Frenchay scoring).

Summary and Conclusion

The patient under examination showed signs consistent with the diagnosis of myotonic dystrophy type 1, includ-

TABLE 1–8.	Frenchay Scoring Details

The *Frenchay Dysarthria Assessment* (FDA) utilizes a rating scale for all testing.

a score	Normal for age
b score	Mild abnormality noticeable to skilled observer
c score	Obvious abnormality but the patient can perform task/movements with reasonable approximation
d score	Some production of task but poor in quality, unable to sustain, inaccurate, or extremely labored
e score	Unable to undertake task/movement/sound

ing myotonic responses of hands, arms, and legs. His speech was characterized by mild flaccid dysarthria that focused on dysphonia. The characteristics of the dysphonia included breathiness, audible inspiration, reduced phrase length and slowed rate. Swallowing was compromised, as the patient has difficulty masticating food. The patient also showed residue in the pharyngeal cavity following the swallow.

Speech-Language Diagnosis

Mild flaccid dysarthria and oropharyngeal dysphagia

Questions Concerning This Case

1. Why was a Holter monitor ordered for this patient? How does that relate to the diagnosis?
2. There was reduced sensation revealed in the examination. Why is this an important piece of information for the speech-language pathologist?

Case provided by Dr. Kostas Konstantopoulos, European University Cyprus.

CASE STUDY 1–2

Physician's Notes on Initial Physical Examination and History

This male child was the third child born to healthy non-consanguineous parents of Cypriot descent. There were no antenatal concerns, no history of a maternal **intercurrent infection** or known exposure to

teratogens (see Table 1–9 for terminology. Note that we are presenting the data of this case in chronological order to show the emerging speech and language signs and symptoms as the condition progresses). At birth, the child was in good condition apart from being slightly underweight compared with his siblings. A heart murmur was noted at the routine neonatal checkup and he was referred for

TABLE 1–9.	Terminology for Case Study 1–2
22q11.2 microdeletion	Genetic syndrome arising from a deletion from chromosome 22, near the middle, in the location designated as q11.2. Many of the problems arising from 22q11.2 deletion syndrome involve speech, language, and hearing.
Dysmorphic features	Unexpected variation in body features.
Echocardiogram (heart sonogram)	Use of sonography to image the heart.
Fluorescence in situ hybridization (FISH)	Genetic testing to identify specific genes on the chromosome. FISH is used to diagnose genetic mutations and chromosomal anomalies.
Intercurrent infection	Disease that interferes in the course of another disease condition.
Karyotype	Number and appearance of chromosomes.
Nasopharyngeal insufficiency (a.k.a., velopharyngeal insufficiency)	Inadequate closure of the velum, allowing communication between nasal and oral cavities during speech and swallowing.
Teratogen	Agent that causes malformation in embryonic development.
Ventricular septal defect (VSD)	Congenital hole in septum of heart.

a pediatric cardiology evaluation. An **echocardiogram** revealed a small **ventricular septal defect (VSD)**, and re-evaluation was organized. By the age of 2½ years, the murmur had disappeared and a repeat echo showed that the VSD had closed. The child was late with his developmental milestones and in particular his speech. He had some single words but his speech was described as nasal. He started speech and language therapy and his general pediatrician requested an evaluation by a clinical geneticist. The combination of slow development, particularly speech delay along with a cardiac defect, **nasopharyngeal insufficiency**, and mild **dysmorphic features** led the geneticist to request a **karyotype** analysis and a fluorescence in situ hybridization (**FISH**) test looking for a **22q11.2 microdeletion**. Karyotype analysis was normal but the FISH test revealed a 22q11.2 microdeletion in the child, a finding that completely explained his clinical presentation.

Medical Diagnosis

22q11.2 deletion syndrome

Speech-Language Implications

22q11.2 deletion syndrome arises from a deletion from chromosome 22, near the middle, in the location designated as q11.2. A variety of signs and symptoms is associated with 22q11.2 deletion syndrome, making diagnosis without genetic workup difficult. Many of the problems arising from 22q11.2 deletion syndrome involve speech, language, and hearing.

Commonly, people with this syndrome have heart abnormalities present from birth, cleft palate, and facial dysmorphias. These individuals will frequently have immune disorders, including rheumatoid arthritis and Graves' disease. In addition, there may be organ problems, including kidney, blood disorders, low blood calcium resulting in seizures, significant pediatric feeding difficulties, and hearing loss. There may also be skeletal anomalies, such as malformation of vertebrae. It is common for a child with 22q11.2 deletion syndrome to have developmental delays, which can include speech and language development and learning disabilities. The child may demonstrate attention deficit hyperactivity disorder (ADHD) and autism spectrum disorder. Later-life problems may include mental illnesses (such as schizophrenia, depression, anxiety, and bipolar disorder).

The disorder has been given a variety of names, arising from the multiple and diffuse problems associated with the deletion. Some of these include DiGeorge syndrome, velocardiofacial syndrome (Shprintzen syndrome), and conotruncal anomaly face syndrome. The preferred name is 22q11.2 deletion syndrome.

Questions Concerning This Case

1. We break hearing into conductive and sensorineural components. Could you see where there could be both types of losses with this syndrome? How would that occur?
2. We think of speech/language pathology as involving speech, language, and swallowing. Can you identify at least one correlate within this list of signs for each of these areas?

From the case book of Dr. George A. Tanteles, MD, MRCPCH DM, Consultant in Clinical Genetics CCT (UK), Head of Clinical Genetics, The Cyprus Institute of Neurology & Genetics.

CHAPTER 1
STUDY QUESTIONS

1. The cells responsible for communication in the nervous system are called _____.

2. The input to a neuron is by means of the _____ (structural component of the neuron).

3. The output of a neuron is by means of the _____ (structural component of a neuron).

4. Another term for neuron body is _____.

5. An action potential releases _____ substance into the synapse.

6. _____ refers to a group of cells with functional unity.

7. Organized groups of neurons with special function in the peripheral nervous system are called _____.

8. Organized groups of neurons with special function in the central nervous system are called _____.

9. The _____ _____ system consists of the cerebral cortex, brainstem, cerebellum, spinal cord, and other subcortical structures.

10. The _____ _____ system consists of the cranial and spinal nerves.

11. The _____ _____ (structure of the nervous system) is the home to language processing and planning, as well as execution of speech, and it is the site of all complex conscious activities.

12. _____ neurons are those that cause some action.

13. _____ neurons are those that carry sensation to the central nervous system.

14. _____ are hard-wired responses of the nervous system.

15. A general term for muscles that are prime movers is _____. These are opposed by antagonist muscles.

16. A general term for muscles that oppose agonists is _____.

17. _____ sensations are those sensed at the periphery of your body, such as pain, pressure, and temperature.

18. _____ sensation includes senses associated with muscles and their tension, tendons, muscle pain, and deep vibration.

19. _____ sense refers to "body sense," and includes sensations associated with pressure, thermal stimulation, joint position sense, muscle tension, and tendon tension.

20. _____ sense is a combined sensation including perception of the body moving in space.

21. _____ sense includes the sense of hearing, vision, smell, and taste (gustation).

22. The term _____ refers to the study of the structure of the organism.

23. The term _____ refers to the the study of the function of an organism.

24. The _____ nervous system consists of the 31 spinal nerves and the 12 cranial nerves that emerge from the CNS.

25. The _____ nervous system is responsible for involuntary functions of the body, including contraction of smooth muscle, glandular secretion, and digestive and cardiac function.

26. In the autonomic nervous system, the _____ system responds to stimulation by expending energy.

27. In the autonomic nervous system, the _____ system counteracts the action of the sympathetic nervous system.

28. Weeks 1 through 8 of prenatal development are termed the _____ period.

29. Weeks 9 through 37 of the prenatal period are termed the _____ period.

30. The prosencephalon differentiates into the _____ and the _____.

31. The rhombencephalon differentiates into the _____ and _____.

32. The _____ differentiates to form the thalamus and hypothalamus, the hypophysis (pituitary gland), optic tract, and third ventricle.

33. _____ _____ cells begin migrating at the fourth week gestational age and will differentiate to form the pharyngeal arch system that involves development of many cranial nerves and speech and hearing structures.

34. The _____ axis runs through the vertebral column and includes the head and trunk.

35. A _____ section or view divides the body into right and left portions.

36. A _____ section divides the body into front and back portions.

37. A _____ section divides the body into upper and lower portions.

38. _____ refers to the front surface of a body, and _____ refers to the back of the body.

39. The dorsum of the cerebrum is the superior/inferior (circle one) surface.

40. The ventral surface of the cerebrum is the superior/inferior (circle one) surface.

41. _____ refers to "toward the surface."

42. Pronation/supination (circle one) of the hand is rotation of the hand so that the palm of the hand is turned downward.

43. What does the combining form ipsi mean? _____

44. The term _____ means crossing over.

45. In speech-language pathology, the term _____ refers to an acquired neurogenic deficit of language expression or comprehension.

46. In speech-language pathology, the term _____ _____ _____ refers to an acquired neurogenic deficit in planning and programming of the articulators of speech.

REFERENCES

Alberstone, C. D. (2009). *Anatomic basis of neurologic diagnosis*. New York, NY: Thieme.

Amaral, D. G., & Strick, P. L. (2013). The neural bases of cognition. In E. R. Kandel, J. H. Schwartz, T. M. Jessell, S. A. Siegelbaum, & A. J. Hudspeth (Eds.), *Principles of neural science* (5th ed., pp. 337–355). New York, NY: McGraw-Hill, Health Professions Division.

Baehr, M., & Frotscher, M. (2012). *Duus' topical diagnosis in neurology: Anatomy, physiology, signs, symptoms* (5th ed.). New York, NY: Thieme.

Brodal, P. (2004). *The central nervous system: Structure and function*. New York, NY: Oxford University Press.

Ciesla, N., Dinglas, V., Fan, E., Kho, M., Kuramoto, J., & Needham, D. (2011). Manual muscle testing: A method of measuring extremity muscle strength applied to critically ill patients. *Journal of visualized experiments: JoVE*, (50).

Darley, F. L., Aronson, A. E., & Brown, J. R. (1969). Differential diagnostic patterns of dysarthria. *Journal of Speech, Language, and Hearing Research*, 12(2), 246–269.

Goldberg, M. E., Walker, M. F., & Hudspeth, A. J. (2013). The vestibular system. In E. R. Kandel, J. H. Schwartz, T. M. Jessell, S. A. Siegelbaum, & A. J. Hudspeth (Eds.), *Principles of neural science*

(5th ed., pp. 917–934). New York, NY: McGraw-Hill, Health Professions Division.

Hudspeth, A. J. (2013). The inner ear. In E. R. Kandel, J. H. Schwartz, T. M. Jessell, S. A. Siegelbaum, & A. J. Hudspeth (Eds.), *Principles of neural science* (5th ed., pp. 654–681). New York, NY: McGraw-Hill, Health Professions Division.

Krupp, M. A., & Chatton, M. J. (Eds.). (1982). *Current medical diagnosis and treatment*. Los Altos, CA: Lange Medical.

Møller, A. R. (2003). *Sensory systems: Anatomy and physiology*. Boston, MA: Academic Press.

Moore, K. L. (2015). *The developing human* (10th ed.). Philadelphia, PA: Saunders.

Omenn, G. S., McKusick, V. A., & Gorlin, R. J. (1979). The association of Waardenburg syndrome and Hirschsprung megacolon. *American Journal of Medical Genetics Part A*, 3(3), 217–223.

Pickles, J. O. (2012). *An introduction to the physiology of hearing* (4th ed.). London, UK: Academic Press.

Poswillo, D. (1973). The pathogenesis of the first and second branchial arch syndrome. *Oral Surgery, Oral Medicine, Oral Pathology*, 35(3), 302–328.

Read, A. P., & Newton, V. E. (1997). Waardenburg syndrome. *Journal of Medical Genetics*, 34(8), 656–665.

Saper, C. B., Andrew, G. S., Lumsden, G. S., & Richerson, G. B. (2013). The sensory, motor, and reflex functions of the brain stem. In E. R. Kandel, J. H. Schwartz, T. M. Jessell, S. A. Siegelbaum, & A. J. Hudspeth (Eds.), *Principles of neural science* (5th ed., pp. 1019–1037). New York, NY: McGraw-Hill, Health Professions Division.

Seikel, J. A., Drumright, D. G., & King, D. W. (2016). *Anatomy & physiology for speech, language and hearing* (5th ed.). Clifton Park, NY: Cengage Learning.

Variant, W. S. (1994). A gene for Waardenburg syndrome type 2 maps close to the human homologue of the microphthalmia gene at chromosome 3p12–p14.1. *Nature Genetics, 7*(7), 509–512.

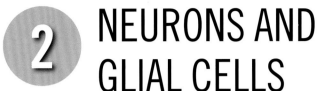

NEURONS AND GLIAL CELLS

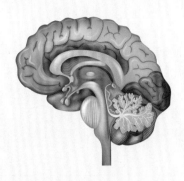

INTRODUCTION

The nervous system is a beautifully organized set of very complex tissues that consists of neurons and glial cells. These same components are found in even the most complex parts of the brain. Realize that these building blocks are exceedingly small: the adult cerebral cortex contains between 20 and 25 billion neurons, depending on age, and is housed within a volume of 489 cubic centimeters (think of a cube of about 5″ × 5″ × 5″ to get an idea of this small size). The cells of the brain are packed to extraordinary density: one cubic centimeter (1 cm × 1 cm × 1 cm) contains on the order of 40,000 neurons (Pakkenberg & Gunderson, 1997). The greatest cerebral cortex cannot have thoughts, dreams, and aspirations if the building blocks are not functioning, and it is the immeasurable interaction of these building blocks that produces these complex processes. That having been said, we continue to learn the nature of these components. As scientists and students, our understanding of these components is absolutely critical to discussing how the most complex components function. Let us talk about neurons, glial cells, and their roles in the basic function of the nervous system.

NEURONS

The smallest functional unit of the nervous system (NS) is the neuron, also known as the nerve cell. Each neuron consists of a **soma** (cell body) and **cell processes** (Figure 2–1A and Table 2–1). The soma includes all the organelles (Figure 2–1B) that are found in a typical animal cell, specifically the nucleus, nucleolus, cytoplasm, endoplasmic reticulum (ER), ribosomes, Golgi apparatus, lysosomes, mitochondria, and neurofibrils. We'll talk briefly about these components.

Endoplasmic Reticulum

Proteins are complex structures with very distinct and replicated folding patterns. Indeed, the folding of proteins is an important element of the "lock and key" aspect of proteins, allowing them to combine with other cellular components and to regulate metabolic functions (Gray, Bannister, Berry, & Williams, 1995; Standring, 2008). The folding is largely regulated by the **endoplasmic reticulum (ER)**, but misfolded protein can accumulate in the ER causing "ER stress" (Hetz & Mollereau, 2014, p. 233).

This metabolic dysfunction may be related to a number of neurodegenerative diseases. An accumulation of amyloid plaques and neurofibrillary

- Discuss the processes of propagation, inhibition, excitation, and summation.

- Recognize the relevance of the concept of feature detection to stimulus processing in the auditory system.

- Discuss the different ion channels and their relevance to conduction and propagation.

- Discuss the basic roles and functions of the different neurotransmitters, including glutamate, aspartate, gamma-

aminobutyric acid, glycine, acetylcholine, dopamine, norepinephrine, and adenosine triphosphate.

tangles characterizes Alzheimer's disease, and Lewy body accumulation accompanies Parkinson's disease. In amyotrophic lateral sclerosis (ALS), the accumulation of trans-activation response (TAR) deoxyribonucleic acid (DNA) binding protein is a characteristic of the familial version of that disease, and Creutzfelt–Jakob disease is characterized by misfolded prions. These diseases are now being characterized as "protein misfolding disorders," and pursuit of the misfolding mechanism is a major research focus for treatment and prevention of these devastating diseases.

Cellular Components of the Soma

The soma is the "heart" of the neuron: this is where proteins and enzymes are produced, energy is created, and waste removal processes are coordinated. The **nucleus** is a large, spherical structure found at the center of the soma. The nucleus contains the genetic information, DNA, which controls the synthesis of the proteins and enzymes in a cell. The nucleus will have at least one **nucleolus**, in which synthesis of ribosomal and ribonucleic acid (RNA) occurs. The **cytoplasm** within the nucleus has an aqueous form and contains sugar, amino acids, and proteins, as well as mitochondria,

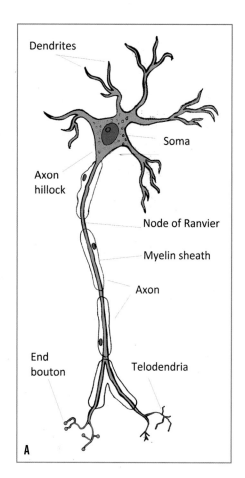

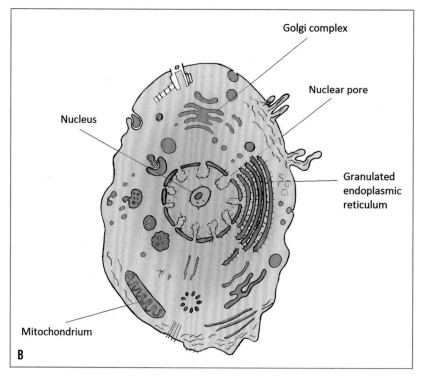

FIGURE 2–1.   **A.** The basic elements of neurons. Shown is a spinal motor neuron. **B.** Organelles within the soma of a typical neuron.

TABLE 2–1.	Basic Components of the Neuron
Component	**Function**
Dendrite	Receptor region
Soma	Contains organelles associated with metabolism
Axon	Transmits information from neuron
Hillock	Generator site for action potential
Myelin sheath	Insulator for axon
Schwann cells	Form myelin in PNS
Oligodendrocytes	Form myelin in CNS
Nodes of Ranvier	Permit saltatory conduction
Telodendria	Processes from axon
Terminal end boutons	Contain synaptic vesicles
Neurotransmitter	Substance that facilitates synapse
Synaptic cleft	Region between pre- and postsynaptic neurons

Source: Based on data of Seikel, Drumright, & King (2016).

critically important for energy generation. There are membranes in the cytoplasm that divide it into compartments, facilitating molecule transport and helping in the synthesis of lipids and proteins. One of these membranes is the ER. Proteins are critical building blocks of the cell, as we will see, and they are produced by the ER. ER is subdivided into rough (granular) and smooth (agranular) ER. Rough ER has an uneven surface due to the presence of ribosomes on its outer surface. These proteins will be exported from the cell. Smooth ER has far fewer ribosomes and includes enzymes that in special structures, such as the liver, are responsible for processing and eliminating toxic foreign substances. The smooth ER also synthesizes steroid hormones. The **ribosomes** are responsible for the production of proteins, which are critical actors in many cell functions. Proteins can be found in the cytoplasm, within other organelles, or on the membranes. The **Golgi apparatus** is involved in collecting, packaging and releasing proteins and lipids that are fabricated on the rough or smooth ER. Golgi complexes tend to group close to the nucleus, near the base of the dendrite, and opposite the axon hillock.

Enzymes are a class of protein that is critical to the function of cells, particularly neurons. Enzymes are contained within **lysosomes**, which arise from the Golgi apparatus (also known as the Golgi complex). Enzymes are responsible for breaking down and recycling other organelles.

All life requires energy, and **mitochondria** are the energy generators for the cell. As we will see in disorders such as traumatic brain injury and stroke, it is the failure of the energy generation system that ultimately results in cell death,

because cellular metabolism is critical for the proper function of neurons. The brain is only 2% of the total body weight of a person, but it uses 20% of its energy resources (Attwell & Laughlin, 2001). In order to accomplish this level of energy usage, there need to be very large numbers of mitochondria in neurons to produce the energy.

Mitochondria have a double membrane, consisting of an outer and an inner folded membrane, and the proteins necessary for metabolism are located on the inner membrane. Mitochondria are interconnected functionally with the nucleus because, even though they have their own genes, most of the genes responsible for cell metabolism are in the cell nucleus itself.

All of these organelles within the cell body must communicate. Communication among the various organelles in the cell body is accomplished by **neurofibrils**, which are threadlike structures located in the cytoplasm.

In summary, the smallest functional unit of the nervous system (NS) is the neuron, also known as the nerve cell.

- Each neuron consists of a soma (cell body) and cell processes.
- The soma includes all the organelles that are found in a typical animal cell, specifically the nucleus, nucleolus, cytoplasm, ER, ribosomes, Golgi apparatus, lysosomes, mitochondria, and neurofibrils.
- The nucleus contains the genetic information, deoxyribonucleic acid (DNA), which controls the synthesis of the proteins and enzymes in a cell. The nucleolus is where synthesis of ribosomal and ribonucleic acid (RNA) occurs.
- Endoplasmic reticulum (ER) is the site of production of proteins, which are critical building blocks of the cell.
- The Golgi apparatus is involved in collecting, packaging, and releasing proteins and lipids that are fabricated on the rough or smooth ER.
- Enzymes are responsible for breaking down and recycling other organelles.
- Mitochondria are the energy generators for the cell.

Gross Structure of the Neuron

The components of neurons are critical to understanding how a neuron functions, as well as how neurons function together. The major parts of the neuron are the soma, axon, and dendrite. Let's look at each of the components in some detail.

Soma

While the soma contains most of the organelles associated with cell metabolism, it also has landmarks related to neuronal function. The soma may be the site of both inhibitory and excitatory synapses, as will be discussed shortly. Areas of the soma that aren't involved in synapse are heavily overlaid with glial cell processes, specifically from astrocytes and oligodendrocytes.

Dendrites

Dendrites are the input system of the neuron (see Figure 2–1). They are highly branched or arborized and arise from the soma. The branching patterns likely arise from interaction with the environment through adhesive growth cones and the afferent processes of other neurons. Early in development there is a proliferation of dendritic processes, but these are pruned back if they are not stimulated through neural activity. Indeed, Ramon y Cajal was the first to realize that the more complex an organism is, the more complex is its dendritic tree (Ramon y Cajal, 1995). The branching patterns differ from neuron to neuron, but classes of neurons all have similar patterns. These patterns are very important for the given neuron because the length, frequency, and density of dendritic processes define the degree of integration of input to a neuron, as will be discussed.

Axons

The sole output of a neuron occurs at the axon. As with the dendrite, the axon arises from the soma. One of the most important sites on the axon is the **axon hillock**, which is the site of generation of the **action potential (AP)** (to be discussed). The first part of the axon hillock is the initial segment. At the **initial segment**, the cell membrane of the axon (termed the axolemma) at this location is the active site for action potential generation: it does not have myelin and often has inhibitory axo-axonal synapses from other neurons (the utility of this will become clear when we talk about synapses themselves). Axons may have a **myelin** coating, which greatly enhances conduction of impulses arising from the neuron. If the axon is myelinated, the coating will begin at the distal end of the initial segment. Myelin thickness increases with diameter of the axon (Noback, Demarest, & Strominger, 1991; Winans, Gilman, Manter, & Gatz, 2002).

Figure 2–1 shows the myelin sheath on the axon, and notice the prominent **node of Ranvier**. At the nodes the myelin is absent, and this permits saltatory conduction, a process that greatly increases the conduction rate of the axon. The nodes of Ranvier are specialized regions that have a high preponderance of sodium ion channels, which are the key element for that rapid conduction (Nolte, 1993).

The terminal region of the axon is highly specialized. At the end of the axon are the telodendria, processes that terminate in end *boutons* or "end buttons." The end *bouton* contains synaptic vesicles that hold neurotransmitter substance. This substance is the essence of communication between neurons. The terminal portion specializes, depending on whether the neuron is connecting with other neurons, muscle fibers, glands, or lymph tissue.

To summarize, the soma contains most of the organelles associated with cell metabolism and may be the site of both inhibitory and excitatory synapses.

- Dendrites are the input system of the neuron. They are highly branched or arborized, and arise from the soma.
- The sole output of a neuron occurs at the axon. The axon hillock is the site of generation of the AP.
- Axons may have a myelin coating, which greatly enhances conduction of impulses arising from the neuron.
- The nodes of Ranvier are locations where the myelin is absent, permitting saltatory conduction. Saltatory conduction allows discharge of the membrane to jump from node to node, thereby greatly speeding up axonal conduction.
- The terminal region of the axon is highly specialized. At the end of the axon are the telodendria, which terminate in end *boutons* or "end buttons." End *boutons* contain synaptic vesicles that hold neurotransmitter substance.

Neuronal Cell Types

The classification of neurons is complex and can take several different forms, all based on physical characteristics. This is not just a taxonomic exercise but rather a reflection of the fact that form follows function. A large dendritic "tree" will have an opportunity to take inputs from many different neurons, effectively summarizing their information into one input, whereas a dendrite with little arborization will average a much smaller set of inputs. We'll talk about classifying neurons based on: (a) the number of dendrites or axons, (b) the pattern of the dendritic tree, (c) axon length, and (d) the connections that the cell makes (function) (Figure 2–2).

Classification Based on Number of Dendrites

Neurons with one process extending from the body are called **unipolar** neurons. These neurons are predominantly made up of the axon and soma but have dendrites on one end. These are mostly found in insects, but many of our sensory cells start out developmentally as unipolar cells and transform into a more bipolar configuration called **pseudounipolar** neurons (see Figure 2–2). Neurons with two processes extending from the body (one dendrite and one axon) are called **bipolar**, and these can be found in our special senses, such as vision (retinal cells) and audition (vestibulocochlear nerve). Finally, neurons with many dendrites and one axon are called **multipolar** neurons. The majority of cells in the central nervous system (CNS) are multipolar because they need to integrate information from other neurons.

Classification Based on Dendrite Arborization

Dendrite arborization refers to the presence of "branches" leading to the dendrite. The more tendrils supplying the dendrite, the greater the degree of integration of information being input. You can think of this as a voting process: if 100 people vote in an election, the ability for one vote to sway the outcome is limited. If only five people vote, each of those votes

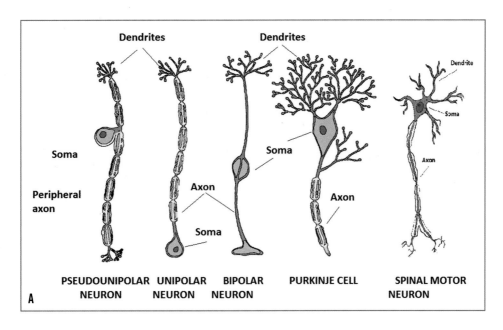

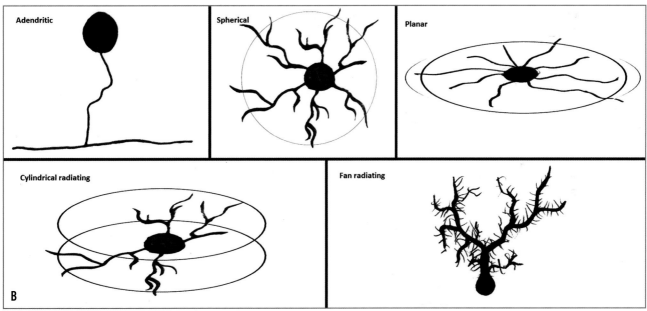

FIGURE 2–2.   **A.** Neuron types. *Source:* Adapted from Seikel, King, and Drumright (1997). **B.** Dendrite configurations. Note that there are sub-types within each of these categories. *Source:* Adapted from Filia, Spacek and Harris (2007).

takes on much greater power. So by analogy, if 100 neurons feed the input of a "downstream" neuron, those inputs all get summarized in the postsynaptic neuron. The importance of any one of those 100 input signals is muted and averaged with the others. On the other hand, if there are only five neurons feeding a postsynaptic neuron, the "value" of each of those five neurons' information is greatly increased. Dendrites are critical for processing information, since how they connect or synapse with other neurons determines how information is processed.

It can be useful to characterize neurons based on the pattern of their dendritic tree. As with all things neuronal, dendrites are small. For example, the average dendrite for human brain neurons in the globus pallidus from cell body to dendrite tip is 1000 μm (which is 1 mm, remembering that 25 mm is about 1 inch). The average dendrite diameter is only 4 μm at the soma, and around 0.3 μm at the tip (Filia, Spacek, & Harris, 2007). Over 100 years ago, Ramon y Cajal proposed the unipolar/bipolar/multipolar differentiation we've shown in Figure 2–2 as a way to start the discussion of neuron types, and the discussion continues today. Attempts at modeling and characterizing the three-dimensional structure of dendrites have shown promise (Baguear, 2011), but classifying dendrites based on visual representation remains the most widely accepted means of description. Some common dendrite configurations (see Figure 2–2B) include **adendritic** (in which the cell body only has axons), **spherical radiation** (as in stellate cells, in which dendrites radiate from all areas of the soma), **laminar radiation** (dendrites radiate away from the soma, but in a single plane, as in retinal cells, **cylindrical radiating** (dendrites in thick cylindrical pattern), and **spindle radiation** (dendrites emerge from opposite poles of the soma, seen in bipolar neurons of the cerebral cortex). Of great interest to us is the **fan radiation** that is seen in **Purkinje cells**. In this configuration there are only one or two dendrites arising from the soma, but those dendrites fan out into a broad tree.

These dendrite configurations have functional implications for information processing. **Stellate cells** have a star-like, spherical dendritic shape and have responsibility for integrating input from many different sources, particularly in the cerebellum. Purkinje cells have very striking arborizations, stereotypical for radiation, which, in the cerebellum, are responsible for taking inputs from parallel fibers in the cerebellum and translating that input into inhibitory output responses for fine motor control. While Purkinje cells are found throughout the nervous system, the cerebellum has the largest proportion of any area of the brain.

Classification Based on Axon Length

There are two types of neuronal cells classified based on their lengths of axons: **Golgi type I** and **Golgi type II**. Golgi type I neurons have long axons extending far beyond the soma, while Golgi type II neurons have short axons and their effects are apparent only in their nearest region. These two types of neurons have strikingly different roles. Golgi type I neurons are involved in communication between distant parts of the brain, such as different lobes of the cerebral cortex, or even communication between the cortex and spinal cord. In sharp contrast, Golgi type II neurons, also known as interneurons, have the important role of connecting neurons that are in close proximity (Stuart, Spruston, & Hausser, 2007).

Classification Based on Conduction Velocity

Conduction velocity refers to the rate at which information is conducted by neurons, and specifically by the axons of neurons. Conduction of the neural impulse depends largely on two factors: diameter of the axon and presence of myelin. Larger axons have a faster rate of conduction than smaller-diameter axons, and myelinated fibers have faster conduction than non-myelinated fibers.

Neurons are classified based on conduction velocity. **Class A and B fibers** are coated with myelin, and have subclasses as well. Class A fibers are broken down into alpha, beta, gamma, and delta fiber types (Table 2–2). **Alpha motor neurons** are the fastest neurons, conducting information up to 120 meters/second. Alpha motor neurons innervate most of the skeletal muscle of the body (extrafusal muscle fibers). **Gamma motor neurons** innervate the muscle component of the muscle spindle, the intrafusal muscle. **Sensory alpha fibers** are differentiated using Roman numerals and letters. Types Ia and Ib convey information about movement. **Type Ia neurons** are the afferent component of the muscle spindle. **Type Ib neurons** are the sensory component for Golgi tendon organs. Types II, III, and IV convey information about somatic sense. **Type II afferent fibers** convey touch and pressure information. **Type III** conduct pain, pressure, touch, and cool thermal sense and are delta class neurons. **Type IV** fibers convey pain and warm thermal sense.

Classification Based on Functional Connection

Neurons are classified as being **afferent** or **efferent**, based on their basic roles. Afferent neurons are those that transmit information to the central nervous system, such as those mediating visual, auditory, or taste information. The term "afferent" is generally synonymous with "sensory," although there are nuanced differences. In the same way, efferent neurons are those carrying information <u>from</u> the central nervous system to the periphery, and are generally synonymous with the term "motor neuron." **Interneurons** are by far the most common neuron in the nervous system. Interneurons provide communication between neurons.

In summary, classification of neurons can be discussed in terms of: (a) the number of dendrites or axons, (b) the pattern of the dendritic tree, (c) axon length, (d) conduction velocity, and (e) the connections the cell makes (function).

- Classification based on number of dendrites includes unipolar, bipolar, and multipolar neurons. Unipolar neurons have one process extending from the body, while bipolar neurons have two (one dendrite and one axon) and are found in our special senses. Neurons with many dendrites and one axon are called multipolar neurons, and these make up the majority of cells in the central nervous system (CNS).
- Classification based on pattern of the dendrite arborization would include adendritic (in which the cell body has only axons), spherical radiation (in which dendrites radiate from all areas of the soma), laminar radiation (dendrites radiate away from the soma in a single plane), and spindle radiation (dendrites emerge from opposite poles of the soma).
- Classification of neurons based on axon length results in two broad types of neuronal cells: Golgi type I and Golgi

TABLE 2–2.		**Classification of Sensory and Motor Fibers**		
Fiber class	Velocity (meters/sec)	Motor function		Sensory function
Class A				
Alpha (α)	50–120	Large alpha motor neurons innervating extrafusal muscle		
A-α Ia	120			Primary muscle spindle afferents
A-α Ib	120			Golgi tendon organs; touch and pressure receptors
A β (Beta)	70	Motor axons serving extrafusal and intrafusal fibers		
A β II				Secondary afferents of muscle spindles; secondary afferents for touch, pressure, vibration
A γ (Gamma)	40	Gamma motor neurons serving muscle spindles		
A Δ II (Delta)	15			Touch, pressure, pain, temperature sensation
Class B				
B	14	Unmyelinated pre-ganglion autonomic fibers		
Class C				
C	2	Unmyelinated, post-ganglion autonomic fibers		
C IV	2			Unmyelinated pain, temperature fibers

Source: Based on data of Seikel, Drumright, & King (2016).

type II. Golgi type I neurons have long axons extending far beyond the soma, while Golgi type II neurons have short axons and their effects are apparent only in their nearest region.

- Neurons are classified based on conduction velocity. Class A and B fibers have myelin. Class A fibers include alpha, beta, gamma, and delta fiber types. Alpha motor neurons innervate most of the skeletal muscle. Gamma motor neurons innervate the intrafusal muscle.
- Sensory alpha fibers are differentiated using Roman numerals and letters. Types Ia and Ib convey information about movement, and types II, III, and IV convey information about somatic sense. Type Ia neurons are employed in the muscle spindle, and type Ib neurons are found in Golgi tendon organs. Type II afferent fibers convey touch and pressure information, and type III conduct pain, pressure,

touch, and cool thermal sense, and are delta class neurons. Type IV fibers convey pain and warm thermal sense.
- Classification based on functional connection results in two broad classes. Neurons are afferent or efferent based on whether they receive information or transmit it.

GLIAL CELLS

Glial cells are the unsung heroes of the nervous system. They have traditionally been viewed as the physical and metabolic support system for neurons (the term "glia" means "glue"), but increasingly they are being seen as integral to the information transfer and storage function as well. Let's look at the "mighty glia!"

There are several different types of glial cells, each with their particular function (Figure 2–3 and Table 2–3). **Microglia** are **macrophages**, which are responsible for removing waste products (phage = mouth, so macrophages are "large mouthed"). Microglia provide the immune defense in the CNS through the release of cytokines (proteins, peptides, etc.) in inflammatory conditions such as infections, tumors, and trauma.

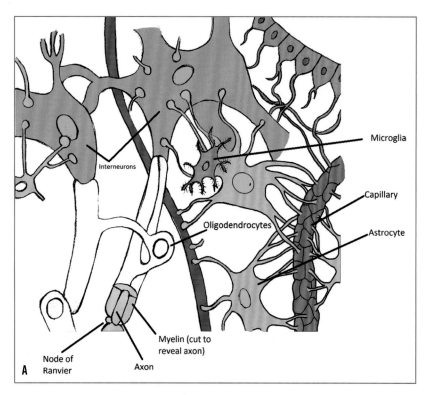

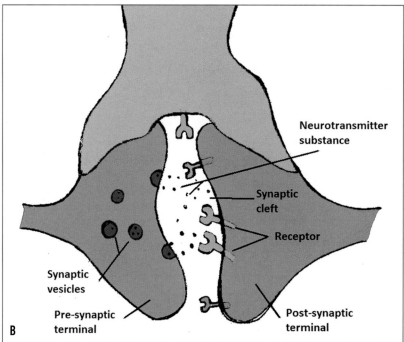

FIGURE 2–3.   **A.** Glial cells. **B.** Relationship of astrocyte to synapse. Note that the astrocyte is critical for recycling neurotransmitter released into the synapse.

TABLE 2–3.	Glial Cell Types and Functions	
Cell	**Location**	**Function**
Oligodendrocyte	CNS	Myelin generation for CNS axons
Schwann cells	Peripheral nervous sytem (PNS)	Myelin generation PNS axons; repair in PNS; phagocytosis in PNS
Astrocytes (astroglia)	CNS Protoplasmic astrocytes in gray matter; fibrous astrocytes found in myelinated fibers	Neurotransmitter uptake from synaptic cleft; repair in CNS; blood-brain barrier
Ependymal cells	CNS	Line spinal cord and ventricles; generation of cerebrospinal fluid; cilia support cerebrospinal fluid circulation
Radial glia	CNS	In neurogenesis, provide scaffold for neuron migration; in cerebellum regulate synaptic plasticity
Microglia	CNS	Macrophages in CNS
Satellite cells	PNS	Surround neurons in ganglia; regulate chemical environment

When Microphages Go Bad

One very important role of microglia is phagocytosis, which is the process of removing dead neural tissue from the nervous system. Microglia are sentinels residing in the parenchyma (space between cells) of the brain, watching for signs of sick and dead tissue. They make contact with the surface of the neuron and look for "eat me" signals, which are proteins called opsonins. Neurons also produce inhibitory "don't eat me" signals that block the phagocytosis (Brown & Neher, 2014, p. 209). Phagocytosis of sick and dying cells reduces inflammation of healthy neural tissue by eliminating toxins released by the dead or dying cells as they break down.

Sometimes things don't go as they're supposed to, though. Brown and Neher (2014) coined the term "phagoptosis," referring to the process of destroying neurons that are stressed but not ill. Stressing a neuron will cause the "eat me" signal to be exposed, but healthy neurons are supposed to inhibit this signal, avoiding phagocytosis. This is particularly apparent in cases of brain damage secondary to ischemia (blood flow being blocked to brain tissue). Ischemia typically damages neurons by depriving them of oxygen and nutrients, but it also creates inflammation in nearby neurons because of the toxins that are released by the dying neurons. It now appears that this inflammation can cause the slow phagocytosis of those healthy neurons by release of the excitotoxin glutamate. In experimental studies using non-humans, it has been shown that blocking the "eat me" signals or supporting maintenance of the "don't eat me" signals reduces cell damage after ischemia. Indeed, there is strong evidence that this loss of healthy neurons is part of the cascade of degeneration found in Alzheimer's disease and even in Parkinson's disease. For more on this topic, see the excellent article by Brown and Neher (2014).

Macroglia are diverse and numerous, consisting of astrocytes, oligodendrocytes, Schwann cells, radial glia, satellite cells, enteric glial cells, and ependymal cells. Let's look at each of these in turn.

Astrocytes (also known as astroglia) make up half the cells in the brain, filling the space between neurons. Their role is quite diverse, ranging from structural support to actual regulation of blood flow in the brain. A significant function of astrocytes is the regulation of ions and neurotransmitters within the space around neurons (extracellular space). Processes arising from the astrocytes encapsulate synapses and blood vessels, helping to regulate ions and neurotransmitters at the synapse (see Figure 2–3). This encapsulation provides a mechanism for nutrient transport, as well as a very important filter function known as the blood–brain barrier. The **blood–brain barrier** is a critical mechanism for selectively allowing specific substances to pass to the neuron, while selectively rejecting others (this selectivity appears to be based on size of the molecule, and thus those that are prohibited are termed macromolecules). The blood–brain barrier, for instance, is why it is fruitless to try to give a person with Parkinson's disease dopamine, since it will not pass the blood–brain barrier. Instead, the precursor to dopamine (levodopa) may be ingested, since it does cross the barrier.

Astrocytes are attached to capillary endothelial cells, which form tight junctions with the neurons. These tight junctions do not permit macromolecules to invade the brain but they do permit crucial molecules such as glucose and amino acids to pass through the barrier. The astrocytes transfer important metabolites from the blood to neurons and remove excess K+ from the interstitial fluid. During cerebral ischemia, the blood–brain barrier is disrupted and the circulating blood enters to the CNS, leading to a series of events such as the influx of ions and water into the brain.

The Critical Roles of the Astrocyte

Astrocytes are critical for regulation of synaptic functioning. First, they buffer K+ ions, which are released into the extracellular space during depolarization. Potassium ion channels in astrocytes allow the K+ to be absorbed by the astrocyte and then released in the area of the blood vessel away from the synapse. Astrocytes are able to sense the activity of neurons through this K+ absorption process and have ion channels for neurotransmitters released at the synapse. When stimulated, astrocytes release free Ca^{2+} into the intracellular space around other glial cells, which apparently helps regulate the release of nutrients and blood flow within the brain. (It is this blood flow that is the signal seen by functional magnetic resonance imaging [fMRI].) Astrocytes also absorb free radicals released during re-oxygenation of neural tissue after hypoxic trauma.

Astrocytes can also soak up water and Cl– ions. When a person has severe traumatic brain injury, this normally useful function can cause life-threatening brain swelling. Because of reduced metabolic function due to dysfunction of adenosine triphosphate (ATP) production in cells, intracranial pressure rises as cells are unable to clear fluid and ions. (For a review of the cascade of processes that cause intracranial edema, see Werner & Engelhard, 2007.)

Astrocytes are also buffers of neurotransmitters. They soak up glutamate from the synapse, which is converted to glutamine through enzyme processes and then moved to the neurons. This process is lifesaving, since in high concentrations glutamate is an **excitotoxin**, a neurotoxin that excites a neuron to death (for a review, see Michaelis, 1998).

Perhaps their most important function for our work in rehabilitation is their secretion of thrombospondins, which are responsible for development of new synapses. When neurons are damaged through cerebrovascular accident or trauma, astrocytes will pull away from the damaged neuron, releasing substances that promote and guide new neuron processes (neurotrophic factors) and new glial processes (gliotrophic factors). These factors promote development of new neural processes and synapses, and your rehabilitation therapy reinforces these synapses through use. You, the therapist, are literally rewiring the brain of a person who has suffered brain injury.

In the developing brain, astrocytes guide neurons to their destinations and regulate the formation of synapses and the production of new neurons. In the adult brain, astrocytes remove K+ from the extracellular space and neurotransmitter molecules from the synaptic cleft. They also **detoxify** free radicals, aid in synthesis of glutamate and γ-aminobutyrate neurotransmitters, support glucose storage, and maintain the integrity of the blood–brain barrier (Schwartz, Barres, & Goldman, 2010). Astrocytes also have a role in synaptic signaling that is still being revealed through research, but it is obvious that they are intimately involved in long-term memory (e.g., Bezzi & Volterra, 2011; Suzuki, Stern, Bozdagi, Huntley, Walker, Magistretti, & Alberini, 2011).

Oligodendrocytes and Schwann Cells

Myelin is a critical substance in both the CNS and the peripheral nervous system (PNS). Myelin serves as an insulator of axons, and importantly, myelin greatly enhances the conduction of impulses through the axon. In the central nervous system, **oligodendrocytes** generate the myelin, and **Schwann** cells have similar function in the PNS. In each case, the glial cell (oligodendrocyte or Schwann cell) produces myelin for a segment of the axon, wrapping the axon segment like a jelly roll. In the PNS, one Schwann cell serves exactly one segment, although oligodendrocytes in the CNS can provide myelin for multiple different axons, but still one segment at a time. As you can see in Figure 2–4, there is a gap between myelinated segments for both CNS and PNS myelin, and this is critical. That gap supports a process called **saltatory conduction**, in which an impulse essentially jumps from gap to gap in the myelin, much as trapeze artists swing from one trapeze to another. In this fanciful example, the trapeze is the space where there is no myelin (known as the node, or specifically, a node of Ranvier), and the performer is the impulse. This jumping saves a great deal of time in conduction, as we

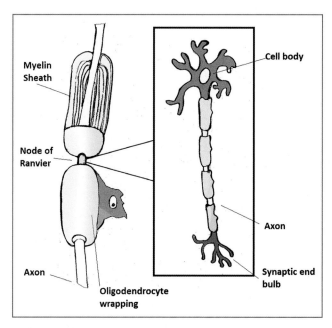

FIGURE 2–4. Configuration of myelin sheath and nodes of Ranvier on axon.

will see soon! There are many nodes on a single axon: in the femoral nerve in humans, which is about 0.5 meters long, there are between 300 and 500 nodes, which means that up to 500 Schwann cells were involved in myelinating that single axon (Schwartz, et al., 2010). If you do the math, you'll realize that each segment is less than 2 mm long, which is about the diameter of a number 2 pencil lead. If an axon is demyelinated through disease, conduction is either greatly slowed down or stops completely. We will talk more about this when we discuss demyelinating diseases.

Radial Glia

Radial glial cells are critical during development of the nervous system. They serve as scaffolds along which neurons migrate to their ultimate home (e.g., Noctor, Flint, Weissman, Dammerman, & Kriegstein, 2001). The radial glia have long processes that serve as a guidance system for migrating neurons during development and are critical for the development of the cerebral and cerebellar cortices. Disruption of these cells and this migration leads to severe cognitive and motor dysfunction (see Michaelis, 1990 for discussion of effects of prenatal alcohol exposure on these processes).

Satellite Cells and Enteric Glial Cells

Satellite cells appear to serve the PNS in a manner similar to astrocytes in the CNS. Satellite glial cells wrap peripheral neuron cell bodies of the sensory neurons of the somatic and

sympathetic nervous systems and apparently regulate ions in much the same way as astrocytes do. They have **receptors** for neurotransmitters and for K+ ions, but unlike astrocytes, satellite cells cover the entire PNS sensory neuron. They are likely very involved in buffering neurotransmitters and breaking them down after release at the synapse, as well as buffering and redistribution of ions (Hanani, 2010). Enteric glial cells are found in the autonomic nervous system of the digestive tract and are likely involved in neuroregulation.

Ependymal Cells

Ependymal cells (ependymocytes) are secreting glia found in the ventricles of the brain, making up the structure we'll talk about later, the choroid plexus. Ependymal cells secrete cerebrospinal fluid, which is important for protective buffering of the CNS structures.

To summarize, glial cells have traditionally been viewed as the physical and metabolic support system for neurons but are now seen as also critical for such important functions as long-term memory.

- There are several different types of glial cells. Microglia are macrophages that remove waste products and provide immune defense in the CNS. Macroglia include astrocytes, oligodendrocytes, Schwann cells, radial glia, satellite cells, enteric glial cells, and ependymal cells.
- Astrocytes (astroglia) provide structural support, regulation of blood flow, regulation of ions and neurotransmitters, and maintenance of the blood–brain barrier. Astrocytes guide neurons to their destinations in the developing nervous system and regulate the formation of synapses and the production of new neurons.
- Oligodendrocytes and Schwann cells are glial cells responsible for development of myelin in the central and peripheral nervous system, respectively.
- Radial glia provide the scaffold for migration of neurons during fetal development.
- Satellite cells wrap peripheral neuron cell bodies of sensory neurons of the somatic and sympathetic nervous systems, regulating ions. Enteric glial cells are found in the autonomic nervous system of the digestive tract, and are likely involved in neuroregulation.
- Ependymal cells secrete cerebrospinal fluid. They are found in the ventricles of the brain.

ACTION POTENTIAL

So far we've been talking about isolated parts, but it's now time to put those parts to use. The business of a neuron is to communicate, and the mechanism for communication is the synapse. The synapse is the "coin of the realm" of neural communication and is the product of many individual processes within and between neurons.

As we discussed in Chapter 1, the *synapse represents the point of communication between two neurons.* In reality, we also use it as a verb, as in "to synapse." We talk about the physical structure of a synapse but also about the process of making the connection. First, we'll describe the physical structure and then the process of communication. Because these processes are very complex, we'll put some of the supportive information into boxed notes in this section. Feel free to delve into that information to help you understand the underpinnings of this most complex and elegant process. The synapse is at the very heart of neurophysiology, because all neural function depends on intact, functional synapses.

The Physical Synapse

Synapses are the physical connections between neurons. We talk about **presynaptic** and **postsynaptic neurons** (Figure 2–5). The presynaptic neuron is the neuron that is sending information to the postsynaptic neuron. That is to say, the **presynapti**c neuron is upstream from the synapse between two neurons.

Remember that we talked about axons as the means by which information leaves a neuron. In Figure 2–5, notice that the dendrites of the postsynaptic neuron connect with the axon of the presynaptic neuron. The physical point of contact is the synapse (Kandel, Siegelbaum, & Schwartz, 1991).

Look at Figure 2–5 again for details of the synapse. This is a blow-up of the **end *bouton*** or end button, which is at the end of the **telodendria**. The end *bouton* contains **synaptic vesicles** that contain neurotransmitter, which is one of the most critical components of a synapse. As you look at these, notice also that some of these synaptic vesicles are at the edge of the end *bouton*, and neurotransmitter is being released. Mitochondria are essential elements for energy creation for use by the synapse, and they are found within the end *bouton* as well. Since synapses are the business parts of neurons, they are where most of the work is done and where energy is being most used in the neuron.

Now notice the gap between the end *bouton* and the **postsynaptic neuron**. This is referred to as the **synaptic cleft**. It is extremely small, on the order of 20 nm (20 billionths of a meter). Finally, if you look carefully at the postsynaptic neuron you'll see receptors. These receptors are sensitive to the neurotransmitter and will cause ion channels to open if they are stimulated. The receptors are very specific to the neurotransmitter and will ignore neurotransmitters that they aren't built to process. We now have the parts necessary to talk about communication between neurons.

Stimulation of a Neuron

Neurons are activated as a result of some outside stimulus that is sufficient and timely. Think of the neuron as a hibernating bear: if you tickle the bear with a feather, it might

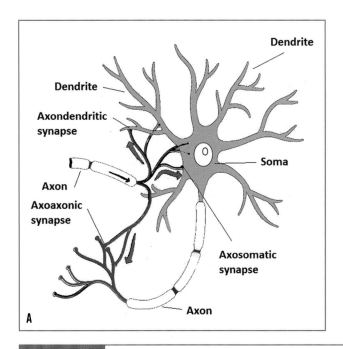

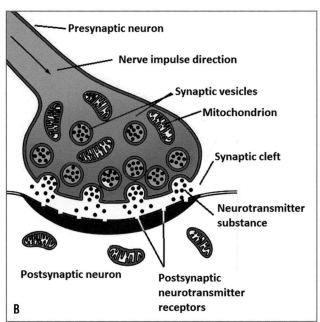

FIGURE 2–5.   **A.** Presynaptic and postsynaptic neurons and synaptic configurations. **B.** End *bouton* of telodendria. *Source:* Adapted from Seikel, Drumright, and King (2016).

rouse a little and go back to sleep. If you use two or three feathers at the same time, you might see an eye open. Twenty feathers at the same time, on the foot of the bear, will very likely send you running from the cave! There is a great deal of random "noise" in the nervous system, and neurons need a mechanism for rejecting the noise. Just like one feather on the sleeping bear's foot, a small, random stimulus is not going to be enough to cause it to respond. Even multiple stimuli, presented at different times, will likely not cause a neuron to take notice. If a neuron receives sufficient numbers of stimuli at about the same time (temporal proximity), the chance that the neuron will respond increases markedly. When you present an adequate stimulus in close temporal proximity, you are reaching the threshold of response for a neuron, and the neuron will respond. Let's look at the process of synapse in some detail, using tactile stimulation as a test case.

When a fly walks on your arm, you will likely feel it, but you may not feel a flea doing the same thing. The fly is heavy enough that it deflects one of your arm hairs, which stimulates a tactile receptor. The flea may not be a <u>sufficient stimulus</u> for the hair, since it is so small.

The movement of the hair causes the skin to move, which is sensed by Meissner's corpuscles residing in the epidermis (Gardner & Johnson, 2013), generating an action potential within the sensor. The sensor synapses with the dendrite of a spinal nerve, and the action potential arising from the sensor causes synaptic vesicles to migrate toward the synapse. Neurotransmitter within the vesicle is dumped into the synaptic cleft and makes contact with channel receptors on the spinal nerve dendrite. When these channel receptors are stimulated by the neurotransmitter, ion channels open up. It's really important to note something here: neurotransmitter does not enter the dendrite, but rather it serves as a stimulus to ion channels. The ion channels open up in response to the neurotransmitter, much like a key being put in a door lock. When the ion channels open, Na+ ions move into the cell. Because ions are electrically charged, movement of ions produces an electrical potential. At this tiny scale (opening up a few channels), the movement produces a **miniature postsynaptic potential** (**MPSP**). That is to say, it is miniature because there are just a few ions moving; it is postsynaptic because it is occurring in the neuron after (downstream from) the synapse, and it is an electrical potential.

The MPSP is the feather at the foot of the bear: a little stimulation will not be enough to make the neuron fire. A stimulus may not produce enough force to deform the skin of the bear's foot, or, if it does, it may not cause enough movement to generate an action potential. This threshold of stimulation is similar to what you've experienced when doing audiometric testing: there's an amount of pressure that is "**subliminal**" (below the "limen" or limit of sensation) and

will not generate an action potential. When we stimulate a neuron with sufficient input, we have reached the neuron's threshold, so it can respond. Of course, neurons can't raise their hands to tell us they've been stimulated, so let's see what a neuron does instead.[1]

As we said before, an MPSP is generated by movement of ions. This movement creates a small voltage that arises and then passes away, but the cell membrane is able to capitalize on that voltage if it is sufficiently large. We've been talking about ion channels being activated by neurotransmitter, but there's another group that are activated by presence of an electrical source, referred to as "electrical synapses." These **voltage-sensitive** ion channels open up in the presence of a voltage of sufficient strength, and when enough ion channels are opened up by the presence of neurotransmitter these voltage-sensitive channels sense the ion movement and open themselves up. Lateral excitation is the process by which one ion channel can stimulate an adjacent channel to open (Pereda, 2014).This starts a cascade of channel opening, with a wave of MPSP propagating down the dendrite, away from the initial point of activation. (In reality, it can propagate in any direction from its point of initiation, but only movement toward the soma does any good as far as communication is concerned.)

This MPSP wave of propagation will move across the dendrite membrane and across the soma until it reaches the axon hillock. You'll recall that the axon hillock is the "root" of the axon, where the axon arises from the soma. At the axon hillock, the AP is generated. The action potential is an all-or-nothing event that represents the output of the neuron. The action potential is the goal of all of the activities leading to this moment.

Electrical Synapses

By their nature, electrical synapses using voltage-sensitive ion channels have different response characteristics than those mediated by neurotransmitters. Electrical synapses work in conjunction with chemical synapses, but they lend a specific set of benefits to CNS function.

One of the most important benefits is synchronization. Because electrical synapses are much faster than chemical synapses, they are able to generate synchronous responses of a large number of neurons. Likewise, because they support lateral excitation, they are very useful in some spatial sensory systems, such as retinal cells. Electrical synapses are critical components in "escape circuits" that keep organisms out of trouble: if you sense

---

[1] It's really important to point out that hair cells of the cochlea are stimulated in a significantly different manner from neurons. Hair cells are so sensitive that the true threshold is that which exceeds the Brownian motion of molecules of air. See Hudspeth (2013) for a splendid review.

a lion about to eat you, rapid escape is a very good idea, and these channels mediate those circuits! Electrical synapses interact with chemical synapses during development, and are likely involved in early development of synaptic function in the brain.

The downside to these characteristics, however, is that high sensitivity and synchronous activity are also found in epileptic seizures, and it has been reported that electrical synapses may be the culprit in this disorder. Dysregulation of electrical synapses also has been proposed as a possible contributor to schizophrenia, Parkinson's disease, and autism spectrum disorder (Pereda, 2014).

Generating the Action Potential

The AP is a highly orchestrated and organized event that results in information being passed from one neuron to another neuron or to a muscle fiber. Let's look in detail at the process. We'll first talk about ion channels and gradients and then the action potential itself.

Ion Channels and Gradients

Ion channels are found throughout the body and are essentially gateways for positively and negatively charged particles (ions) to pass into and out of cells. There are two critical characteristics that make ion channels useful for communication. First, ion channels are very specific: each channel is "tuned" to a specific type or class of ions and is restrictive to the flow of other ions. Secondly, they can be triggered by electrical, chemical, or mechanical stimulation. These two characteristics mean that a specific stimulus (e.g., a neurotransmitter) will trigger an ion channel to allow a specific ion (e.g., positively charged potassium ions) to cross the membrane. As we mentioned earlier, when ions move, they are essentially creating a voltage. When an ion channel opens, it can pass up to 1,000,000 ions per second across the membrane, giving ion channels a tremendous edge over any other bodily function (Siegelbaum & Koester, 2012). Ion channels are regulated by a number of different events: they can sense a voltage (voltage-gated channels), they can sense neurochemistry (ligand-gated channels), or they can sense mechanical deformation (mechanically gated channels, such as those governed by the hair cell cilia). Some channels remain open, allowing specific ions to pass through them continually, and some have active pumping mechanisms to pump the ions into or out of the cell.

But what causes ions to move in the first place? To answer this, we're going to ask you to imagine a water tank on a hill. If you live in a city or town, water that you use is often stored in reservoirs or water tanks, and these are always in high places, for good reason. The reason a water tank is hoisted into the air on iron legs is to give gravity an opportunity to move the water from the tank to your tap. The elevated water tank or reservoir gives a gradient (high to low) that is directly analogous to the gradients that make ions move. There are two types of gradients at work with ions: electrical and chemical. If you have more positively charged particles on one side of a membrane than the other, ions will flow to equalize the charges between inside and outside the membrane. This is the electrical gradient, or ***membrane potential***. The "potential" part is that the ions have the "potential" to "run downhill" as a result of the gradient established. This is a force to be dealt with, just as the water from the tank has to be restrained by your water faucet.

The other gradient is a **chemical gradient**. The same concept holds, but we need a different analogy. Imagine that you have a glass of water and you put a drop of food coloring into it. Even if the water is still, you will see the food coloring disperse into the water, ultimately resulting in even distribution of the colorant. Essentially, when there is a concentration difference, molecules will flow to even out that difference. The chemical gradient is established when there are more of one molecule outside of the cell than inside or vice versa. Nature seeks rest.

These two analogies may help us see what's happening. There are three essential states of a neuron: polarized (resting), depolarized, and hyperpolarized.

Resting State

In the **resting state** of a neuron, the electrical potential within the cell is between −50 and −70 mV (millivolts) relative to the outside of the cell. The term "resting" is something of a misnomer. "Poised" might be a more apt term, since the state of polarization is one "poised" for depolarization! That is, there are more negative ions <u>in</u> the cell and more positive ions <u>outside</u> of the cell. Similarly, at rest there will be more K+ ions within the cell and more Na+ outside of the cell. At rest (resting potential), there are 30 times more K+ (positively charged potassium ions) on the inside of the cell than outside, while there are 10 times more Na+ ions outside than in. There are also markedly more negatively charged chloride ions (Cl−) outside the cell than within. This is a setup. When a cell is stimulated to depolarize, first the Na+ will be driven by the chemical gradient to leave the cell when a channel opens, and the K+ will be driven to enter the cell. In fact, the force is so great that K+ and Na− are leaking continually out of and into the cell, respectively. Sodium-potassium pumps work tirelessly to move these errant ions back where they belong to maintain the gradient, since the gradient is what will allow communication to happen. (Remember these pumps for a later discussion of brain injury, since it is the failure of our metabolism to fuel these pumps that can cause significant problems following trauma.) There is a chemical gradient, so that K+ "wants" to enter the cell to equalize the gradient, while Na− "wants" to leave the cell to equalize the gradient.

Stimulation

A postsynaptic ion channel needs adequate stimulation for an action potential to be generated. There are a couple of stages in this process. We've talked about neurotransmitter being dumped into the synapse to trigger the opening of the ion channels. You should realize that the nervous system is inherently leaky, so that neurotransmitter is being dumped in small quantities, randomly, all the time. Of course, it would not be useful for a neuron to respond every time a little neurotransmitter leaked out: neurons have a threshold system that keeps them from firing to random stimulation.

The **excitatory postsynaptic potential (EPSP)** is the depolarization of the membrane at the site of the synapse. An EPSP occurs as a result of an accumulation of **miniature excitatory postsynaptic potentials (mEPSPs)**, and this is nature's safeguard. A little leak will cause an mEPSP, but it takes many synaptic vesicles dumping into the synapse at about the same time to cause an EPSP. The EPSP is not an action potential, but it increases the likelihood of an AP. The EPSP causes a wave of depolarization away from the point of excitation, toward the soma, and ultimately toward the axon hillock. If that depolarization reaches the axon hillock, an AP will be triggered. Many mEPSPs will produce an EPSP, and the EPSP has a high probability of producing an AP. If this sounds a little "probabilistic" to you, you are right! Even though we refer to the AP as an "all-or-nothing" response, the events leading up to it are far from "all-or-nothing"!

Generation of the Action Potential

The cell at rest has a strong negative **intracellular** (within cell) **potential** of −70 mV. Stimulating an ion channel will cause ions to move across the membrane, but this movement may not be sufficient to trigger an AP. Most neurons have a threshold for the AP at about −55 mV. That is, opening one ion channel and allowing about 100,000 ions to pass through will not cause the intracellular potential to reach −55 mV. (Realize the scale of the ion channel activity: an ion channel will move about 100 million ions per second through its gates, so 1 ms of depolarization will allow "only" 100,000 ions to pass across the membrane in a single channel [Alberts, Johnson, Lewis, Raff, Roberts, & Walter, 2007].) In reality, the voltage-gated sodium channel is activated at around −55 mV and permits sodium to rush into the intracellular fluid, shifting the membrane potential from −70 mV to +30 mV before it closes. The voltage gated potassium channel is activated at around +30 mV and permits the potassium to rush out and restore the resting potential. However, if many channels are opened at about the same time, the intracellular potential will increase above that −55 mV level, and an action potential will be generated.

Generation of an action potential occurs in three stages, illustrated in Figure 2–6. The first stage is depolarization.

When the ion channel first opens, Na+ will rush into the cell, rapidly causing the **intracellular** (within–cell) potential to increase by 100 mV, reaching +30 mV (Figures 2–6 and 2–7). At the point marked "A" in the figure, the cell is at rest, and the intracellular potential is −70 mV. At point "B," a stimulus is received, causing a depolarizing mEPSP at the membrane. When the depolarization reaches the gate threshold at "C" (about −55 mV), an action potential is generated. Sodium ions now rush into the cell through the gates, raising the potential to +30 mV (a total of 100 mV change from resting state). The Na+ channels begin closing at "D," even as the K+ channels ("E") open, allowing potassium to leave the cell, thus driving the cell back to its resting level ("F"). Notice that the sodium-potassium pump is active here, reestablishing the ion balance of the cell. The cell is driven to its resting state and beyond by the addition of Cl− at "G," ultimately returning the polarized state at "H." Realize that "G" is the absolute refractory state, and the relative refractory state occurs as the neuron stabilizes to the point at "H."

This all happens quickly (see Figure 2–7). Na+ and K+ ions move across the membrane over the course of about 0.5 ms (a millisecond is 1/1000 of a second, so 0.5 ms is 5/10,000 of a second). The Cl− ions move into the cell, effectively clamping it strongly negative for another 0.5 ms. K+ and Na+ ion channels close and the sodium-potassium pump starts moving ions back across the membrane to reestablish that resting membrane potential. This brief period when a neuron cannot be stimulated to fire is termed the **absolute refractory period**. As the ions are moved back across the membrane, the neuron can once again depolarize, but the threshold is greater than during the resting state. This is the **relative refractory period**, during which a neuron can be stimulated, but it's more difficult than at resting membrane potential (RMP).

Propagation

The AP is generated at the axon hillock, which is the root of the axon. At this point, the wave propagates toward the distal parts of the axon in a very special way. Remember that ion movement causes a current in a cell. Just like the dendritic membrane, the axon has voltage-sensitive ion channels embedded in it. In the dendrite the channels are adjacent to each other, so the EPSP causes voltage-sensitive channels to open up sequentially, like dominoes falling one after the other. Many axons are covered with an insulating coat of lipid known as myelin: any ion channels that are covered by myelin are not stimulable. In axons, the myelin is configured so that there are gaps in the myelin coating, called **nodes**, and ion channels of the axon are located here. When the AP is generated, it causes this distant ion channel at the node to open, causing the membrane to depolarize. Depolarization causes the ion channel in the next node to open, creating another discharge. The neuron discharge initiated by the AP is passed from node to node in what is termed saltatory

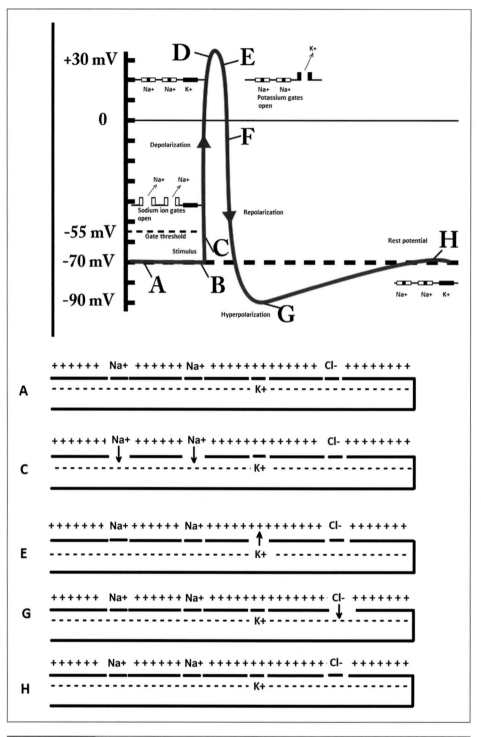

FIGURE 2–6. Stages of the action potential. **A.** Resting membrane potential of −70 mV. **B.** Neuron is stimulated, mEPSP is generated. **C.** Action potential threshold of −55 mV is reached and action potential is generated. Na+ gates open, allowing Na+ to flood cell. **D.** Approximately 1 ms post initiation, AP reaches its peak. **E.** Na+ gates close as K+ gates open, allowing K+ to flow out of neuron. **F.** Neuron begins process of repolarizing, returning toward resting membrane potential. Sodium-potassium pumps have been operational throughout and are restoring the cell to RMP. **G.** Cl− ions have entered cell, causing hyperpolarization, placing the cell in the absolute refractory period. **H.** Over 1 to 2 ms relative refractory period cell returns to RMP. *Source:* Adapted from C. R. Nave, Georgia State University.

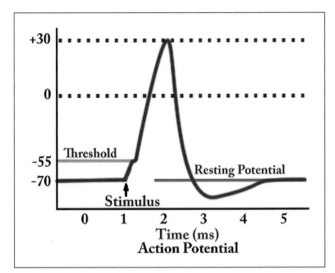

resting state. At resting state, the inside of the neuron is between −50 and −70 mV relative to the outside. At rest there are more negative ions in the cell and more positive ions outside of the cell. There are also more K+ ions in the cell and more Na+ and Cl− outside of the cell.

- Depolarization occurs when the ion channel first opens: Na+ rushes into the cell, rapidly causing the intracellular (within-cell) potential to increase by 100 mV, reaching +30 mV. When there is adequate stimulation, an action potential is generated. Secondly, sodium (Na+) ions rush into the cell, raising the potential to +30 mV. Potassium (K+) channels open, allowing potassium to leave the cell, driving the cell back to its resting level.
- The brief period when a neuron cannot be stimulated to fire is termed the absolute refractory period. During the relative refractory period, a neuron can be stimulated to fire, but it's more difficult than at resting state.

COMMUNICATION ACROSS THE SYNAPSE

While communication between neurons is the critical element that differentiates them from other cells, there is much more to neurons than simply transferring information. The complex processes that make up neurophysiology are found in the ways that the synapse occurs.

Excitation and Inhibition

So far we've been talking about exciting a neuron to activity, but there is another very important function that we need to discuss. Remember the EPSP generated at the dendrite as a result of stimulation? This EPSP is, by definition, excitatory: creation of an EPSP causes depolarization of the dendrite membrane, which will ultimately lead to the AP at the axon hillock. While excitation is important, it's equally important not to be excited. **Inhibitory postsynaptic potentials** (IPSP) are those dendritic responses that result in the membrane being hyperpolarized. That is to say, an IPSP clamps the membrane so it can't respond.

Both IPSP and EPSP have crucial roles in neuron interaction. For example, the auditory and visual systems have **feature detector** circuits that examine input for specific stimulus characteristics (e.g., horizontal line or steady-state tone: see Blakemore & Cooper, 1970). When the sensory system receives a stimulus to which this specific circuit responds, the feature detector becomes excited and passes that information up the nervous system. Importantly, it also inhibits other feature detectors adjacent to it (such as those sensing vertical lines or short-duration tones). This is considered to be a form of signal enhancement in that it not only strongly signals presence of a specific stimulus but inhibits any extraneous response that might make the information ambiguous.

conduction. Saltatory conduction greatly speeds up conduction of impulses through an axon. You'll want to remember this very important function of myelin when we talk about demyelinating diseases.

In summary, the synapse is the point of communication between two neurons. The physical synapse consists of pre- and postsynaptic neurons and their communicating elements, the end *bouton* of the presynaptic neuron and the receptor region of the postsynaptic neuron.

- Critical elements of the synapse include the telodendria, synaptic cleft, ion channels, synaptic vesicles, and neurotransmitter substance.
- Telodendria are terminal extensions of the presynaptic axon. The end *bouton* is the terminal point of the telodendria.
- Within the end *bouton* are synaptic vesicles, which hold the neurotransmitter substance. When the postsynaptic neuron is stimulated sufficiently, vesicles migrate to the margin of the end *bouton* and neurotransmitter substance is released into the synaptic cleft.
- Neurotransmitter stimulates the postsynaptic ion channels to open, initiating the physiological response of the mEPSP. If there are sufficient numbers of mEPSP, an AP will be initiated. The neuron is depolarized when an AP is initiated.
- Voltage-sensitive ion gates are stimulated by ion movement, thus supporting propagation of a wave of depolarization.
- Depolarization of a neuron (generation of the AP) occurs in three waves of activity that move the neuron from

As you can see, both excitatory and inhibitory functions are critically important: sometimes it's what you don't say that is really important!

Summation

When we talked about the EPSP, we discussed the miniature EPSP (mEPSP). Recall that many mEPSP will lead to EPSP. Neurons are accumulators of information, but again they need to guard against sending information forward that is really just random noise. To accomplish this they use two different methods: temporal and spatial summation. If enough mEPSP occur within a restricted span of time, the neuron accepts it as valid information and an EPSP occurs. If you have the same number of stimulations spread over a long period of time, the neuron interprets that as background chatter and ignores it. In the same way, if many synapses converge on one dendrite, the probability of activation of an EPSP is increased. Miniature IPSP and mEPSP will cancel each other out, but if there are more mEPSP, the result will be excitation. The total effect of all synaptic output is encoded as the frequency and intensity of nerve impulse generation and distributed to other cells (Moller, 2003).

Neurotransmitters

It's time to get a little more specific about neurotransmitters. Excitation or inhibition of the postsynaptic neuron is the result of the action of specific **neurotransmitters (NT)**. **Excitatory neurotransmitters** change the electrical charge and result in an action potential, while inhibitory neurotransmitters change the electrical charge away from an action potential. **Neurotransmitters** are attracted by receptor protein molecules on the cell membrane, and the NT will bind to a receptor that matches the shape of the NT. You can think of the neurotransmitter and ion channel as being a key and a lock: you can have many keys on your key ring, but only one of them opens your car door. This specificity gives your nervous system tremendous power to do the jobs it needs to do. We'll refer to neurotransmitters as "excitatory" or "inhibitory," but in reality they simply activate receptors, and the receptors either excite or inhibit neural response. In other words, the car key isn't the car!

In order to be classified as a neurotransmitter, a substance has to meet four criteria: (1) it must be synthesized in a presynaptic neuron, (2) there is sufficient NT in the presynaptic terminal to have an influence on the postsynaptic neuron, (3) it can be experimentally shown to act on a specific ion channel or pathway, and (4) there is a mechanism for removing it from the synaptic cleft (Schwartz & Javitch, 2013). This last element is a critical component, because removal of NT from the synapse is an important means of regulating neural function.

We've known about neurotransmitters since 1905, when John Langley first found them in the adrenal cortex (Schwartz & Javitch, 2013), but neurobiology has been able to greatly elaborate the types, roles, and nuances of these critical chemicals (Table 2–4). As we talk about neurotransmitters, you're going to see that hormones and neurotransmitters are quite similar and often overlap in function. The critical and defining difference is that neurotransmitters act on a neuron that is close to the point of release, whereas hormones act on more distant targets. The action elicited by neurotransmitters is typically short-lived (in the order of milliseconds), but the effect can be very long term (as in the brain change that occurs as a result of learning the cranial nerves). Please also realize that astrocytes can store and release neurotransmitters as well, a process that is believed to support long-term memory.

Neurotransmitters are generally classified as either small-molecule transmitters or nucleopeptides. Both are manufactured and housed in the vesicles, although vesicle size differs. Generally, acetylcholine, glutamate, gamma-aminobutyric acid (GABA), and glycine are considered small-molecule transmitters, and the catecholamines and serotonin are in the nucleopeptide class. We'll talk about these below.

Neurotransmitters are divided into four major classes: amino acids, acetylcholine, monoamines, and neuropeptides.

1. The major CNS neurotransmitters in mammals are made up of **amino acids**. Amino acids can be either excitatory or inhibitory. **Glutamate** and **aspartate** are excitatory amino acid neurotransmitters, while **gamma-aminobutyric acid (GABA)** and **glycine** are inhibitory neurotransmitters. Glutamate, aspartate, and GABA are all found in the brain and the spinal cord, but glycine is primarily active in the spinal cord.

    Glutamate is by far the most prevalent excitatory neurotransmitter in the nervous system, but excessive amounts of glutamate are toxic to the brain (termed excitotoxic) and can cause seizures. Aspartate stimulates some of the same receptors that glutamate does. GABA is the most prevalent inhibitory neurotransmitter in the CNS, and many sedatives act on the ion channels that are sensitive to GABA.

2. **Acetylcholine (ACH)** is a very important neurotransmitter, in that it is the means by which neurons activate muscles. As we'll discuss later, ACH is released into the junction between neuron and muscle fiber (the neuromuscular junctions), resulting in contraction of the muscle fiber. ACH is also present in other areas of the CNS, including the striatum and the nucleus basalis of Meynert at the base of the brain. ACH turns out to be critical to memory function and declines in association with the progression of Alzheimer's disease and other dementias. It is also a dominant neurotransmitter in the

TABLE 2–4.	Neurotransmitters and Dominant Function		
Neurotransmitter class	Neurotransmitter	Location	Function
Amino acids	Glutamate	Brain and spinal cord	Excitatory
	Aspartate	Brain and spinal cord	Excitatory
	Gamma aminobutyric acid (GABA)	Brain and spinal cord	Inhibitory
	Glycine	Spinal cord	Inhibitory
Acetylcholine		Motor end plate; striatum; parasympathetic nervous system; reticular activating system of brainstem	Memory function; motor activation; regulation of consciousness
Monoamines (catecholamine and serotonin)	Dopamine	CNS and PNS: hypothalamus, brainstem, basal ganglia (inhibition); cerebrum, substantia nigra, arcuate nucleus, solitary tract nucleus, ventral tegmentum, limbic area, cerebral cortex, amygdala, nucleus accumbens, olfactory tubercle	Attention; reward; emotion and affect; movement regulation and initiation
	Norepinephrine (noradrenaline)	CNS: amygdala, pons, and tegmentum of midbrain, cerebrum, cerebellum, hippocampus	Increases heart rate, fear-based vigilance; acute response to stress; sensory focus, attentional shift
Neuropeptides	Many peptides released by neurons: includes oxytocin, opioids, vasopressin, endorphins	CNS	Regulate emotion, social behavior

Source: Based on data of und Halbach, O. V. B., & Dermietzel, R. (2006). *Neurotransmitters and neuromodulators: Handbook of receptors and biological effects.* Hoboken, NJ: John Wiley & Sons.

parasympathetic nervous system. Importantly, it is the major neurotransmitter of the reticular activating system of the brainstem/thalamus, which is responsible for regulating consciousness, arousal, sleep, and wakefulness.

3. **Monoamines** include catecholamines (dopamine, norepinephrine/noradrenaline, and epinephrine) and **serotonin**. **Dopamine** (DA) is critically important and is a dominant neurotransmitter in the CNS. It is responsible for inhibition in the hypothalamus, brainstem, and basal ganglia. The substantia nigra projects DA to the basal ganglia, and a deficiency of DA there causes the primary signs of Parkinson's disease. Excesses of DA in the limbic system and DA insufficiency in the prefrontal cortex are seen in schizophrenia: the imbalance results in dysregulation of affect, emotion, attention, and motivation (Schwartz & Javitch, 2013). Reduction in DA is seen in attention deficit hyperactivity disorder (ADHD), and drugs such as cocaine and methamphetamine target the same receptors that DA stimulates. DA is involved in all aspects of the neural reward system, including important pathways associated with learning.

Norepinephrine (NE) (also known as **noradrenaline**) is both a hormone and a neurotransmitter, and receptors that respond to NE are termed noradrenergic. NE is termed a "stress hormone," as it is released under acute physical and/or psychological stress. NE causes an increase in heart rate, fear-based vigilance (by acting on the amygdala), and release of glucose in preparation for an acute response to threat. In the CNS, NE is generated in the locus coeruleus (in the pons) and the lateral tegmentum (in the midbrain) of the brainstem and has widespread effect throughout the nervous system. NE is active in the cerebrum, cerebellum, amygdala, and hippocampal areas, to name a few. NE appears to be a critical neurotransmitter involved in sensory focus and attentional shift. Audiologists and cognitive psychologists use the P300 evoked potential to examine a person's ability to recognize change in visual or auditory stimuli, and NE appears to mediate that important "oddball" response. NE is active in the orbitofrontal and anterior cingulate regions of the brain, both of which are related to reward and attention (for instance, these two areas are activated during meditation; see Hasenkamp & Barsalou, 2012).

Most of the serotonin in the body is produced in the intestine, but 10% is produced in the CNS. It appears to be important for regulation of mood and depression and is involved in regulation of appetite, memory, sleep, and learning. Medications known as selective serotonin reuptake inhibitors (SSRIs) are used to alleviate depression by allowing serotonin to remain in the nervous system longer.

4. **Neuropeptides.** Neuroactive peptides make up a large class of substances that includes both hormones and neurotransmitters. Within this class are opioids (sedatives), hormones that act on the pituitary (e.g., oxytocin), and insulin. Many of these also serve as neurotransmitters when they act on adjacent neurons. Neuropeptides are involved in sensory perception, emotion, pain, and stress responses.

We would be remiss if we didn't acknowledge the important role that **adenosine triphosphate (ATP) has** in neural communication. As a neurotransmitter, ATP is released when tissue is traumatized and is involved in transmitting the sense of pain from that trauma. Because of its role as the energy source for cellular metabolism, it is surprising to categorize it as a neurotransmitter, but it clearly fits the definition.

Dysarthria Caused by Medications

Neurotransmitter function is prone to intercession by specific medications. **Benzodiazepines** (anxiolytics: drugs that reduce anxiety) enhance the effect of the GABA neurotransmitter and may occasionally cause side effects that include slurred speech and ataxia. **Antiepileptics** such as phenytoin sodium and carbamazepine stabilize the inactivated state of the sodium channels and decrease electrical conductance among brain cells, and they can infrequently cause speech changes. Overdose of **lithium**, used to treat bipolar disorder, decreases norepinephrine release and increases serotonin synthesis, which may produce tremor, ataxia, and dysarthria.

Finally, one possible side effect of **dopamine receptor agonists** (antipsychotic drugs that activate dopamine receptors in the extrapyramidal system) is permanent tardive dyskinesia/orofacial dyskinesia and subsequent dysarthria. Orofacial dyskinesia (involuntary slow repetitive body movement) has a significant impact on communication.

Generally, antipsychotic and anxiolytic drugs have the greatest impact on speech by acting on the extrapyramidal system, producing hyperkinetic dysarthria. Other medications have far fewer speech-related side effects, and the dysarthria is typically transient, ending on termination of the medication. The significant caveat to this is that some medications taken in excess can have lasting effects due to neurotoxicity. We would be remiss if we failed to mention the neurotoxic effects of ethanol (alcohol). When taken in moderation, ethanol is reasonably benign with few subjective neurophysiological changes, but when taken in excess (as in chronic alcoholism), the effects on the nervous system can be devastating. For speech, these would result in ataxic dysarthria. Cognitive decline and dementia can be consequences of long-term excessive alcohol consumption.

In summary, neurons can be either excited or inhibited. EPSP are excitatory responses, while IPSP are those dendritic responses that result in the membrane being hyperpolarized.

- The process of summation is one in which the outputs of many neurons lead to a "summary response" by the nervous system. Temporal summation occurs when there are sufficient neural stimulations within a specific time frame for a stimulus to be considered relevant. Spatial summation occurs when a large enough area of the body is stimulated.
- There are many different neurotransmitters in the nervous system. Neurotransmitters are generally classified as either small-molecule transmitters or nucleopeptides. Acetylcholine, glutamate, gamma-aminobutyric acid, and glycine are considered small-molecule transmitters, and the catecholamines and serotonin are in the nucleopeptide class.
- Glutamate and aspartate are excitatory amino acid neurotransmitters, while GABA and glycine are inhibitory neurotransmitters. Glutamate is by far the most prevalent excitatory neurotransmitter in the nervous system, but excessive amounts of glutamate are toxic to the brain (termed excitotoxic), and can cause seizures. Aspartate stimulates some of the same receptors that glutamate does. GABA is the most prevalent inhibitory neurotransmitter in the CNS, and many sedatives act on the ion channels that are sensitive to GABA.
- Acetylcholine (ACH) is a very important neurotransmitter, in that it is the means by which neurons activate muscles. Monoamines include catecholamines (dopamine, norepinephrine/noradrenaline, and epinephrine) and

serotonin. Dopamine (DA) is responsible for inhibition in the hypothalamus and brainstem (substantia nigra and ventral tegmental area). Norepinephrine (NE) (also known as noradrenaline) is released under acute physical and/or psychological stress, causing an increase in heart rate, fear-based vigilance (by acting on the amygdala), and release of glucose in preparation for an acute response to threat.

- Neuropeptides include both hormones and neurotransmitters, including opioids (sedatives), hormones that act on the pituitary (e.g., oxytocin), and insulin.

CHAPTER SUMMARY

The smallest functional unit of the nervous system (NS) is the neuron, also known as the nerve cell. Each neuron consists of a soma (cell body) and cell processes. The soma includes all the organelles that are found in a typical animal cell, specifically the nucleus, nucleolus, cytoplasm, endoplasmic reticulum (ER), ribosomes, Golgi apparatus, lysosomes, mitochondria, and neurofibrils. The nucleus contains the genetic information, deoxyribonucleic acid (DNA), that controls the synthesis of the proteins and enzymes in a cell. The nucleolus is where synthesis of ribosomal and ribonucleic acid (RNA) occurs. Endoplasmic reticulum is the site of production of proteins, which are critical building blocks of the cell.

The Golgi apparatus is involved in collecting, packaging, and releasing proteins and lipids that are fabricated on the rough or smooth ER. Enzymes are responsible for breaking down and recycling other organelles. Mitochondria are the energy generators for the cell. The soma contains most of the organelles associated with cell metabolism and may be the site of both inhibitory and excitatory synapses. Dendrites are the input system of the neuron. They are highly branched or arborized and arise from the soma. The sole output of a neuron occurs at the axon. The axon hillock is the site of generation of the action potential. Axons may have a myelin coating, which greatly enhances conduction of impulses arising from the neuron. The nodes of Ranvier are locations where the myelin is absent, permitting saltatory conduction. Saltatory conduction allows discharge of the membrane to jump from node to node, thereby greatly speeding up axonal conduction. The terminal region of the axon is highly specialized. At the end of the axon are the telodendria that terminate in end *boutons* or "end buttons." End *boutons* contain synaptic vesicles that hold neurotransmitter substance. Classification of neurons can be discussed in terms of (a) the number of dendrites or axons, (b) the pattern of the dendritic tree, (c) axon length, and (d) the connections that the cell makes (function). Classification based on number of dendrites includes unipolar, bipolar, and multipolar neurons. Unipolar neurons have one process extend-

ing from the body, while bipolar neurons have two processes (one dendrite and one axon) and are found in our special senses. Neurons with many dendrites and one axon are called multipolar neurons, and these make up the majority of cells in the CNS. Classification based on pattern of the dendrite arborization includes adendritic (in which the cell body only has axons), spherical radiation (in which dendrites radiate from all areas of the soma), laminar radiation (dendrites radiate away from the soma in a single plane), and spindle radiation (dendrites emerge from opposite poles of the soma). Classification of neurons based on axon length results in two broad types of neuronal cells: Golgi type I and Golgi type II. Golgi type I neurons have long axons extending far beyond the soma, while Golgi type II neurons have short axons, and their effects are apparent only in their nearest region. Classification based on functional connection results in two broad classes. Neurons are afferent or efferent based on whether they receive information or transmit it. Neurons are also classified based on conduction velocity. Class A and B fibers have myelin. Class A fibers include alpha, beta, gamma, and delta fiber types. Alpha motor neurons innervate most of the skeletal muscle. Gamma motor neurons innervate the intrafusal muscle. Sensory alpha fibers are differentiated using Roman numerals and letters. Types Ia and Ib convey information about movement, and types II, III, and IV convey information about somatic sense. Type Ia neurons are employed in the muscle spindle and type Ib neurons are found in Golgi tendon organs. Type II afferent fibers convey touch and pressure information, and type III conduct pain, pressure, touch, and cool thermal sense, and are delta class neurons. Type IV fibers convey pain and warm thermal sense.

Glial cells have traditionally been viewed as the physical and metabolic support system for neurons but are now seen as also critical for such important functions as long-term memory. There are several different types of glial cells. Microglia are macrophages that remove waste products and provide immune defense in the CNS. Macroglia include astrocytes, oligodendrocytes, Schwann cells, radial glia, satellite cells, enteric glial cells, and ependymal cells. Astrocytes (astroglia) provide structural support, regulation of blood flow, regulation of ions and neurotransmitters, and maintenance of the blood–brain barrier. Astrocytes guide neurons to their destinations in the developing nervous system and regulate the formation of synapses and the production of new neurons. Oligodendrocytes and Schwann cells are glial cells responsible for development of myelin in the central and peripheral nervous systems, respectively. Radial glia provide the scaffold for migration of neurons during fetal development. Satellite cells wrap peripheral neuron cell bodies of sensory neurons of the somatic and sympathetic nervous systems, regulating ions. Enteric glial cells are found in the autonomic nervous system of the digestive tract and are likely involved in neuroregulation. Ependymal cells secrete cerebrospinal fluid and are found in the ventricles of the brain.

Synapse is the point of communication between two neurons. The physical synapse consists of pre- and postsynaptic neurons and their communicating elements, the end *bouton* of the presynaptic neuron, and the receptor region of the postsynaptic neuron. Critical elements of the synapse include the telodendria, synaptic cleft, ion channels, synaptic vesicles, and neurotransmitter substance. Telodendria are terminal extensions of the presynaptic axon. The end *bouton* is the terminal point of the telodendria. Within the end *bouton* are synaptic vesicles, which hold the neurotransmitter substance. When the postsynaptic neuron is stimulated sufficiently, vesicles migrate to the margin of the end *bouton*, and neurotransmitter substance is released into the synaptic cleft. Neurotransmitter stimulates the postsynaptic ion channels to open, initiating a physiological response known as the miniature excitatory postsynaptic potential (mEPSP). If there are sufficient numbers of mEPSP, an action potential (AP) will be initiated. The neuron is depolarized when an action potential is initiated. Voltage-sensitive ion gates are stimulated by ion movement, thus supporting propagation of a wave of depolarization. Depolarization of a neuron (generation of the action potential) occurs in three waves of activity that move the neuron from resting state. At resting state, the inside of the neuron is between −50 and −70 mV relative to the outside. At rest there are more negative ions in the cell and more positive ions outside of the cell. There are also more K+ ions in the cell and more Na+ and Cl− outside of the cell. Depolarization occurs when the ion channel first opens: Na+ rushes into the cell, rapidly causing the intracellular (within-cell) potential to increase by 100 mV, reaching +30 mV. When there is adequate stimulation, an action potential is generated. Secondly, sodium (Na+) ions rush into the cell, raising the potential to +30 mV. Potassium (K+) channels open, allowing potassium to leave the cell, driving the cell back to its resting level. The brief period when a neuron cannot be stimulated to fire is termed the absolute refractory period. During the relative refractory period a neuron can be stimulated, but it's more difficult than at resting state. Neu-

rons can be either excited or inhibited. EPSP are excitatory responses, while inhibitory postsynaptic potentials (IPSP) are those dendritic responses that result in the membrane being hyperpolarized. The process of summation is one in which the outputs of many neurons lead to a "summary response" by the nervous system. Temporal summation occurs when there are sufficient neural stimulations within a specific time frame for a stimulus to be considered relevant. Spatial summation occurs when a large enough area of the body is stimulated.

There are many different neurotransmitters in the nervous system. Neurotransmitters are generally classified as either small-molecule transmitters or nucleopeptides. Acetylcholine, glutamate, gamma-aminobutyric acid (GABA), and glycine are considered small-molecule transmitters, and the catecholamines and serotonin are in the nucleopeptide class. Glutamate and aspartate are excitatory amino acid neurotransmitters, while GABA and glycine are inhibitory neurotransmitters. Glutamate is by far the most prevalent excitatory neurotransmitter in the nervous system, but excessive amounts of glutamate are toxic to the brain (termed excitotoxic), and can cause seizures. Aspartate stimulates some of the same receptors that glutamate does. GABA is the most prevalent inhibitory neurotransmitter in the CNS, and many sedatives act on the ion channels that are sensitive to GABA. Acetylcholine (ACH) is a very important neurotransmitter, in that it is the means by which neurons activate muscles. Monoamines include catecholamines (dopamine, norepinephrine/noradrenaline, and epinephrine) and serotonin. Dopamine (DA) is responsible for inhibition in the hypothalamus and brainstem (substantia nigra and ventral tegmental area). Norepinephrine (NE) (also known as noradrenaline) is released under acute physical and/or psychological stress, causing an increase in heart rate, fear-based vigilance (by acting on the amygdala), and release of glucose in preparation for an acute response to threat. Neuropeptides include both hormones and neurotransmitters, including opioids (sedatives), hormones that act on the pituitary (e.g., oxytocin), and insulin.

CASE STUDY 2–1

Physician's Notes on Initial Physical Examination and History

This patient is a 37-year-old female (see Table 2–5 for terminology. Note that we are presenting the data of this case in chronological order to show the emerging speech and language signs and symptoms as the condition progresses). The patient's **DNA testing** revealed that **155 CTG repeats** were detected by the **Southern blot analysis**, confirming an autosomal dominant condi-

tion, with each offspring of this individual having a 50% risk of inheriting the **mutated allele**. Further, other family members were also considered to be at risk of having inherited this mutation. Genetic counseling was recommended. Her cardiac examination was satisfactory. She had no clinically significant **myotonia**, although she has mild facial weakness, and mild weakness in **finger abduction**, as well as **sternocleidomastoid (sternomastoid) wasting**. Her father had elevated glucose and it was not apparent whether or not she is a carrier. Her mother died

TABLE 2–5.	Terminology for Case Study 2–1
"c" score	Scoring on the Frenchay Dysarthria Assessment (FDA). See Table 2–7 for details of the *Frenchay Dysarthria Assessment* scoring.
Biceps	A muscle with two heads that lies on the upper arm between the shoulder and the elbow.
Bilevel positive airway pressure (BiPAP)	The BiPAP (also known as CPAP, continuous positive airway pressure) is a machine used for therapy for sleep apnea. BiPAP provides pressurized air through a mask to the patient's airway, preventing apnea.
CTG repeats	Sequences of three nucleotides repeated a number of times in tandem within a gene.
DAB classification system	Classification system for dysarthria, referring to the pioneering work of Darley, Aronson, and Brown at Mayo Clinic. For further information, see Darley, Aronson, & Brown (1969).
DNA testing	A means of determining the chromosomes in individual genes. Biochemical processes are used to identify the presence of genetic diseases, particularly forms in which there is a mutation in the genes.
Dysarthria	Motor speech disorder involving muscular weakness, dyscoordination, and alteration of muscle tone. It includes slow movement of the muscles used for speech production, including the lips, tongue, vocal folds, and/or muscles of respiration.
Electromyographic laboratory results	Results of laboratory testing technique to record the electrical activity of skeletal muscles.
Extension 4/5	See Table 2–6 concerning muscle testing.
Finger abduction and extension 4/5	See Table 2–6 concerning muscle testing.
Finger abduction	In this type of manual muscle testing, the fingers are given resistance on the distal phalanx, on the radial side of one finger, and the ulnar side of the adjacent finger.
Flaccid dysarthria	Dysarthria characterized by low muscle tone, paralysis or muscle weakness, and arising from lower motor neuron lesion.
Mutated allele	A mutated form of a gene.
Myopathy	Muscular weakness.
Myotonia	Prolonged contraction of skeletal muscles.
Myotonic dystrophy type I	A genetic disorder in which there is muscle loss and weakness. Often myotonic dystrophy is accompanied by heart problems. Myotonic dystrophy type I is inherited and is caused by mutations in the DMPK gene. In myotonic dystrophy type II, there is a mutation in the CNBP gene.
Nucleotides	These are organic molecules that form the DNA and RNA.
Pacemaker	Device placed in the chest to control abnormal heart rhythms of the heartbeat (arrhythmias). It uses low-energy electrical pulses to prompt the heart to beat at a normal rate.
Sarcoma	A malignant tumor of non-epithelial tissue.
Southern blot analysis	Method in molecular biology for the detection of DNA sequences in DNA samples.
Sternomastoid (sternocleidomastoid) wasting	Weakness of the sternomastoid muscle.
Tibialis anterior muscle (TA)	A long, narrow muscle in the anterior part of the lower leg.

in her early 50s from **sarcoma**. The **electromyographic laboratory** results showed significant findings of myotonia and **myopathy**, especially in the distal muscles (significant myotonic discharges in the **TA** and **biceps**). She was having regular physiotherapy as well as vitamin E therapy. She was scheduled for follow-up in four months.

4 Months Following Intake

At follow-up the patient reported difficulty in the upper limbs, tongue, and jaw. She reported frustration with her tongue function resulting in possible dysarthria. On examination, there was mild distal weakness in the upper limbs (finger abduction and **extension 4/5**; see Table 2–6 for definitions of muscle testing), mild facial weakness, and bulbar involvement. She presented with severe cardiac problems and was due to undergo neurophysiological evaluation for her heart condition. She was scheduled for follow-up in four months. She was to continue with magnesium, vitamin E, and Q-enzyme Q10.

Eight Months Following Intake

Four months later the patient was seen for follow-up. The patient had difficulties with her **pacemaker**, requiring replacement due to a misplaced wire. She told me that she had an episode with apnea at night and, as I discovered during the examination, she was not using the **BiPAP**. I recommended an evaluation from the pulmonologist again for a sleep study and, if necessary, for her to undergo a sleep study using the BiPAP at night. She was feeling worse neurologically, especially in distal parts of the upper limbs. On neurological examination I could not detect any significant difference other than the distal weakness previously seen, as well as the myotonia. She also appeared to present with mild dysarthria. I referred her to our speech therapist for an evaluation. She had lost significant weight and I told her that this is not a good sign for her muscle bulk. She was to be seen again in four months.

Medical Diagnosis

Myotonic dystrophy type I

1′0 Year Following Intake: Speech Examination

The *Frenchay Dysarthria Assessment* was administered to the patient. The results showed a moderate difficulty, with **"b-c" score**, revealing a **flaccid dysarthria** (see Table 2–7 for details of Frenchay scoring). The patient exhibits signs such as hypernasality, nasal emission, some imprecise consonants, and short phrases. This is consistent with the resonatory incompetence second cluster of the **DAB classification system**. More specifically:

1. Reflexes cough: Patient choked once during the day and sometimes had difficulty clearing phlegm from throat (c).
2. Reflexes swallow: Patient observed during drinking 1/2 cup of water and eating a cookie, with slowness during eating/drinking and pauses while drinking (b).
3. Respiration in speech: When asked to count from 1 to 20 as quickly as possible, the patient required up to four breaths to complete the task (c).
4. Palate fluids: Patient reports occasional difficulty of liquids going out of her nose (nasal regurgitation) once or twice per month (b).

TABLE 2–6.	Examining Muscle Strength

When examining a patient, identifying specific areas of muscular weakness helps to localize the site of lesion. Strength testing is completed for each muscle group, making sure that you test one side and then the next for each group, so you can compare strength for the two sides. Here is a muscle strength rating scale.

0/5	No contraction of muscle
1/5	Indication of muscle flicker, but no movement noted
2/5	Movement occurs, but not against gravity when tested in the horizontal plane
3/5	Movement occurs against, but not when there is resistance provided by the the examiner
4/5	Movement occurs against some resistance provided by the examiner
5/5	Normal strength

TABLE 2–7.	Frenchay Scoring Details

The *Frenchay Dysarthria Assessment* (FDA) utilizes a rating scale for all testing.

a score	Normal for age
b score	Mild abnormality noticeable to skilled observer
c score	Obvious abnormality but the patient can perform task/movements with reasonable approximation
d score	Some production of task but poor in quality, unable to sustain, inaccurate, or extremely labored
e score	Unable to undertake task/movement/sound

5. Palate maintenance: When patient was asked to say "ah-ah-ah" five times, the velum movement was found to be slightly asymmetrical, with maintenance of movement (b).

6. Palate in speech: When asked to say "/may pay/" and "/nay bay/," the patient showed moderate hypernasality and some nasal emission (c).

7. Laryngeal component: Sustained phonation for /a/ in 7 seconds (c).

8. Laryngeal component: Changes in volume when the patient counted from 1 to 5 revealed minimal difficulty; occasional numbers sounded similar (b).

9. Tongue component: Slow protrusion/retraction of the tongue (5 times in 5 seconds: b).

10. Tongue component: Slow movement (5 times in 7 seconds) in elevation of the tongue (b).

11. Tongue component: Diadochokinetic rate for the bisyllable /kala/ (repeated 10 times); one sound was well articulated, followed by deterioration of intelligibility as the number of repetitions increased (8 seconds) (c).

Speech-Language Diagnosis

Flaccid dysarthria

Questions Concerning This Case

1. What is the neuropathological basis of myotonic dystrophy?

2. How are the speech symptoms of flaccid dysarthria related to the general symptom of weakness?

Case provided by Dr. Kostas Konstantopoulos, European University Cyprus.

CHAPTER 2
STUDY QUESTIONS

1. _____ are a class of protein that are responsible for breaking down and recycling other organelles.

2. In the neuron, _____ are the energy generators for the cell.

3. _____ are the input system of a neuron.

4. _____ are the output system of the neuron.

5. The _____ _____ (location on the neuron) is the site of generation of the action potential.

6. _____ sheathing greatly enhances conduction of impulses arising from the neuron.

7. The _____ _____ _____ (portion of the axon) are locations where the myelin is absent, permitting saltatory conduction.

8. _____ conduction allows discharge of the membrane to jump from node to node, thereby greatly speeding up axonal conduction.

9. At the end of the axon are the telodendria that terminate in _____ _____.

10. _____ substance is found in synaptic vesicles in the end *boutons*.

11. _____ neurons have one process extending from the body.

12. _____ neurons have two processes extending from the body.

13. Neurons with many dendrites and one axon are called _____ neurons.

14. When classifying neurons based on axon length results, _____ _____ _____ neurons have long axons extending far beyond the soma.

15. When classifying neurons based on axon length, _____ _____ _____ neurons have short axons and their effects are apparent only in their nearest region.

16. _____ (type of glial cell) are responsible for removing waste products.

17. _____ (type of glial cell) provide the immune defense in the CNS through the release of cytokines (proteins, peptides, etc.) in inflammatory conditions such as infections, tumors, and trauma.

18. _____ (type of glial cell) aid in regulation of blood flow in the brain.

19. _____ (type of glial cell) aid in regulation of ions and neurotransmitters within the space around neurons (extracellular space).

20. _____ (type of glial cell) are involved in nutrient transport.

21. _____ (type of glial cell) are a critical component of the blood–brain barrier.

22. _____ (type of glial cell) detoxify free radicals, aid in synthesis of glutamate and γ-aminobutyrate neurotransmitters, support glucose storage, and maintain the integrity of the blood–brain barrier.

23. _____ (type of glial cell) detoxify free radicals from the neural space.

24. _____ (type of glial cell) generate myelin in the central nervous system.

25. _____ _____ (type of glial cell) generate myelin in the peripheral nervous system.

26. The term _____ _____ refers to the conduction process in which the impulse jumps from node to node in the axon.

27. _____ _____ (type of glial cell) serve as scaffolds along which neurons migrate to their final destination.

28. _____ _____ (type of glial cell) in the PNS regulate ions in much the same way as astrocytes do in the CNS.

29. _____ _____ (type of glial cell) are secreting glia found in the ventricles of the brain.

30. The _____ is the point of communication between two neurons.

31. On the figure to the right, please identify the structures and landmarks indicated.

a. _____

b. _____

c. _____ _____

d. _____ _____ _____

e. _____ (entire process)

f. _____ _____ (specific portion of process)

g. _____

h. _____ _____

32. On the figure to the right, please identify the structures and landmarks indicated.

    a. _____ _____

    b. _____ _____

    c. _____

    d. _____ _____

    e. _____ _____

    f. _____ _____ _____

33. The physical _____ consists of pre- and postsynaptic neurons and their communicating elements, the end *bouton* of the presynaptic neuron, and the receptor region of the postsynaptic neuron.

34. The _____ _____ of the telodendria is the terminal point.

35. _____ vesicles are found in the end *bouton*. These hold neurotransmitter substance.

36. When the postsynaptic neuron is stimulated sufficiently _____ _____ migrate to the margin of the end *bouton* and neurotransmitter substance is released into the synaptic cleft.

37. True or False: When ion channels are stimulated to open, neurotransmitter flows into the postsynaptic neuron.

38. When neurotransmitter stimulates the postsynaptic ion channels to open, a physiological response known as the miniature _____ _____ _____ _____ is initiated.

39. If there are sufficient numbers of mEPSP generated, an _____ potential will be initiated.

40. When we refer to a neuron as depolarized, we are saying that the _____ potential has occurred.

41. _____ sensitive ion gates are stimulated by ion movement.

42. In the _____ state of the neuron, the inside of the neuron is between −50 and −70 mV relative to the outside. There are more negative ions *in* the cell and more positive ions *outside* of the cell. There are also more K+ ions in the cell and more Na+and Cl− outside of the cell.

43. A neuron is depolarized when the _____ _____ opens.

44. The brief period when a neuron cannot be stimulated to fire is termed the _____ _____ period.

45. EPSP are termed excitatory/inhibitory (circle one) responses.

46. IPSP are termed excitatory/inhibitory (circle one) responses.

47. The term _____ refers to the condition in which the outputs of many neurons lead to a "summary response" by the nervous system.

48. _____ summation occurs when there are sufficient neural stimulations within a specific time frame for a stimulus to be considered relevant.

49. _____ summation occurs when a large enough area of the body is stimulated.

50. _____ are generally classified as either small-molecule transmitters or nucleopeptides. Acetylcholine, glutamate, gamma-aminobutyric acid (GABA), and glycine are considered small-molecule transmitters, and the catecholamines and serotonin are in the nucleopeptide class.

51. The neurotransmitter _____ is an excitatory amino acid neurotransmitter.

52. The neurotransmitter _____ is an inhibitory neurotransmitter.

53. The neurotransmitter _____ is the most prevalent excitatory neurotransmitter in the nervous system.

54. The neurotransmitter _____ is the most prevalent inhibitory neurotransmitter in the CNS.

55. The neurotransmitter _____ is the means by which neurons activate muscles.

56. The neurotransmitter _____ is responsible for inhibition in the hypothalamus and brainstem (substantia nigra and ventral tegmental area).

REFERENCES

Alberts, B., Johnson, A., Lewis, J., Raff, M., Roberts, K. & Walter, P. (2007). *Molecular biology of the cell* (5th ed.). New York, NY: Garland Science.

Attwell, D., & Laughlin, S. B. (2001). An energy budget for signaling in the grey matter of the brain. *Journal of Cerebral Blood Flow & Metabolism, 21*(10), 1133-1145.

Baguear, M. F. (2011). *Morphological study of dendritic spines* (Unpublished Master's thesis). Master's degree, Artificial Intelligence Research, Universidad Politecnica de Madrid.

Bezzi, P. & Volterra, A. (2011). Astrocytes: Powering memory. *Cell, 144*(5), 644–645.

Blakemore, C., & Cooper, G. F. (1970). Development of brain depends on the visual environment. *Nature, 228,* 477–478.

Brown, G. C., & Neher, J. J. (2014). Microglial phagocytosis of live neurons. *Nature Reviews Neuroscience, 15,* 209–216.

Darley, F. L., Aronson, A. E., & Brown, J. R. (1969). Clusters of deviant speech dimensions in the dysarthrias. *Journal of Speech and Hearing Research, 12*(3), 462–496.

Duffy, J. R. (2013). *Motor speech disorders-E-book: Substrates, differential diagnosis, and management.* St. Louis, MO: Elsevier Health Sciences.

Fiala, J. C., Spacek, J. & Harris, K. M. (2007). Dendrite structure. In G. Stuart, N. Spruston, & M. Hausser (Eds.). *Dendrites* (2nd ed., pp. 1–42). Oxford, UK: Oxford University Press.

Filskov, S. B., & Boll, T. J. (1981). *Handbook of clinical neuropsychology.* New York, NY: John Wiley & Sons.

Gardner, E. P., & Johnson, K. O. (2013). Touch. In E. R. Kandel, J. H. Schwartz, T. M. Jessell, S. A. Siegelbaum, & A. J. Hudspeth (Eds.), *Principles of neural science* (5th ed., pp. 498–529). New York, NY: McGraw-Hill.

Gray, H., Bannister, L. H., Berry, M. M., & Williams, P. L. (Eds.). (1995). *Gray's anatomy.* London, UK: Churchill Livingstone.

Hanani, M. (2010). Satellite glial cells in sympathetic and parasympathetic ganglia: In search of function. *Brain Research Reviews, 64*(2), 304–327.

Hasenkamp, W., & Barsalou, L. W. (2012). Effects of meditation experience on functional connectivity of distributed brain networks. *Frontiers in Human Neuroscience, 6,* 38.

Hetz, C., & Mollereau, B. (2014). Disturbance of endoplasmic reticulum proteostasis in neurodegenerative diseases. *Nature Reviews Neuroscience, 15*(4), 233.

Hudspeth, A. J. (2013). The inner ear. In E. R. Kandel, J. H. Schwartz, T. M. Jessell, S. A. Siegelbaum, & A. J. Hudspeth (Eds.), *Principles of neural science* (5th ed., pp. 654–681). New York, NY: McGraw-Hill.

Kandel, E. R., Siegelbaum, S. A., & Schwartz, J. H. (1991). Synaptic transmission. In E. R. Kandel, J. H. Schwartz, & T. M. Jessell (Eds.), *Principles of neural science* (3rd ed.). Norwalk, CT: Appleton & Lange.

Michaelis, E. K. (1990). Fetal alcohol exposure: Cellular toxicity and molecular events involved in toxicity. *Alcoholism, Clinical and Experimental Research, 14*(6), 819–826.

Michaelis, E. K. (1998). Molecular biology of glutamate receptors in the central nervous system and their role in excitotoxicity, oxidative stress and aging. *Progress in Neurobiology, 54*(4), 369–415.

Møller, A. R. (2003). *Sensory systems: Anatomy and physiology.* New York, NY: Academic Press.

Noback, C. R., Demarest, R. J., & Strominger, N. L. (1991). *The human nervous system.* Philadelphia, PA: Lea & Febiger.

Noctor, S., Flint, A., Weissman, T., Dammerman, R., & Kriegstein, A. (2001). Neurons derived from radial glial cells establish radial units in neocortex. *Nature, 409,* 714–720.

Nolte, J. (1993). *The human brain.* St. Louis, MO: Mosby Year Book.

Pakkenberg, B., & Gundersen, H. J. G. (1997). Neocortical neuron number in humans: Effect of sex and age. *Journal of Comparative Neurology, 384*(2), 312–320.

Pereda, A. E. (2014). Electrical synapses and their functional interactions with chemical synapses. *Nature Reviews Neuroscience, 15,* 250–263.

Ramon y Cajal, S. (1995). *Histology of the nervous system of man and vertebrates.* Oxford, UK: Oxford University Press.

Schwartz, J. H., Barres, B. A., & Goldman, J. E. (2010). The cells of the nervous system. In E. R. Kandel, J. H. Schwartz, T. M. Jessell, S. A. Siegelbaum, & A. J. Hudspeth (Eds.), *Principles of neural science* (5th ed., pp. 39–97). New York, NY: McGraw-Hill Medical.

Schwartz, J. H., & Javitch, J. A. (2013). Neurotransmitters. In E. R. Kandel, J. H. Schwartz, T. M. Jessell, S. A. Siegelbaum, & A. J. Hudspeth (Eds.), *Principles of neural science* (5th ed., pp. 289–306). New York, NY: McGraw-Hill Medical.

Seikel, J. A., Drumright, D. G., & King, D. W. (2016). *Anatomy & physiology for speech, language, and hearing* (5th ed.). Clifton Park, NY: Cengage Learning.

Seikel, J. A., King, D. W., & Drumright, D. G. (1997). *Anatomy & physiology for speech, language and hearing.* San Diego, CA: Singular

Siegelbaum, S. A., & Koester, J. (2012). Ion channels. In E. R. Kandel, J. H. Schwartz, T. M. Jessell, S. A. Siegelbaum, & A. J. Hudspeth (Eds.), *Principles of neural science* (5th ed., pp. 100–125). New York, NY: McGraw-Hill.

Standring, S. (2008). *Gray's Anatomy: The anatomical and clinical basis of practice* (40th ed.). London, UK: Churchill Livingstone.

Stuart, G., Spruston, N., & Hausser, M. (2007). *Dendrites* (2nd ed.). Oxford, UK: Oxford University Press.

Suzuki, A., Stern, S. A., Bozdagi, O., Huntley, G. W., Walker, R. H., Magistretti, P. J., & Alberini, C. M. (2011). Astrocyte-neuron lactate transport is required for long-term memory formation. *Cell, 144*(5), 810–823.

und Halbach, O. V. B., & Dermietzel, R. (2006). Neurotransmitters and neuromodulators: Handbook of receptors and biological effects. John Wiley & Sons.

Werner, C., & Engelhard, K. (2007). Pathophysiology of traumatic brain injury. *British Journal of Anaesthesia, 99*(1), 4–9.

Winans, S. S., Gilman, S., Manter, J. T., & Gatz, A. J. (2002). *Manter and Gatz's essentials of clinical neuroanatomy and neurophysiology* (10th ed.). Philadelphia, PA: F. A. Davis.

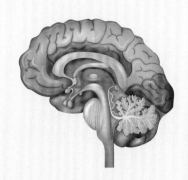

3 BASIC REFLEX AND SENSORY FUNCTION: HOW WE KNOW THE WORLD

INTRODUCTION

We have been discussing the cellular elements of the nervous system, which are the building blocks of sensation and action. Sensing the environment requires afferent nerves that mediate information coming from sensory receptors, such as the hair cells in hearing or touch receptors in the skin. The only way we, as organisms, can know the world is by paying attention to the sensory experiences we receive through these systems. (We'll have to enlarge the notion of "paying attention" when we start talking about this thing called "consciousness"!) Knowing our environment is one thing, but actually acting on that sensation requires motor function. This chapter introduces you to the basic level of sensory and motor integration: the reflex.

When we say "basic level," we mean *really* basic level. We are going to talk about the spinal reflex arc, which reflects the most basic level of stimulus-response in the nervous system. Reflexes at this level do not require anything resembling cognition, or even awareness. These reflexes are simply the organism's attempt to respond to a stimulus (usually in a protective fashion, or perhaps to acquire it for the purpose of eating it). Again, recognize that a reflex is the combination of a sensory experience and a motor response to that experience that is "hard wired" into your nervous system.

THE SPINAL REFLEX ARC

The most basic of reflexive systems in the body is the **spinal reflex arc**. The components of the spinal reflex arc are: (a) a receptor organ that senses some change in its environment, (b) a neuron that conveys that information to the spinal cord, (c) an interneuron, (d) a motor neuron to convey an impulse to muscle, and (e) a muscle fiber (Carpenter, 1991; Noback, Demarest, & Strominger, 1991).

This would be a good juncture to differentiate upper motor neuron (UMN) from lower motor neuron (LMN). As we discussed in Chapter 1, the nervous system is hierarchical, in that conscious thought and voluntary action are the specific domain of the cerebral cortex. When, for instance, you decide to flex your big toe, the signal to initiate this arises from the cerebral cortex. Impulses pass through the corticospinal tract through what are known as **upper motor neurons**.

- Differentiate encapsulated mechanoreceptors and the stimulus required for activation.

- Define the difference between low- and high-threshold receptors.

- Define nociception and silent nociception, and proprioception.

- Define the concepts of dermatome, myotome, and plexus.

- Define the special senses and describe the processes involved in activation of the sensation.

- Describe the elements of the visual system, including retinal

cells, the role of the retinal layers in visual processing, and graded potential in depolarization.

- Describe the major physical elements of the gustatory system, including taste receptors, chemoreceptors, papillae, microvilli, taste pores, filiform, foliate, and fungiform papillae.

- Describe the physical elements associated with audition and auditory transduction, including tip links, stereocilia, and physical differences between inner and outer hair cells.

- Describe the physiological processes of audition, including differences between outer and inner hair cell function, the process of depolarization of the hair cell, role of the spiral ganglion, and the activity of ions and neurotransmitters in the depolarization process.

- Discuss the elements of the vestibular system, including semicircular canals, ampulla, cupola, stereocilia, kinocilium, utricle, saccule, otolithic membrane, and otoliths.

At the end of this series of neurons is the final neuron that will activate the flexor of the big toe. This final neuron is termed the "**final common pathway**," or more typically, the **lower motor neuron**. Upper motor neurons are any neurons in the chain of activation except the last one, which is the lower motor neuron. Upper motor neurons can arise from many regions of the brain besides the cerebral cortex, but in all cases they exclude the final common pathway, the lower motor neuron. Please realize that this is not just a semantic discussion. The upper motor neurons undergo many other influences on their way to their target. The lower motor neuron may have a reflex in its circuit, as we are discussing here, and damage to the upper and lower motor neurons will have markedly different effects, depending on whether that reflex is affected. The reflex is left intact if the UMN is damaged, so the result is often **hyperactive reflexes**. In sharp contrast, if the LMN is damaged it is likely that there will be no intact reflexes associated with that neuron, making those reflexes absent or **hypoactive** (Nolte, 2002).

The basic reflex arc can be initiated by many different types of stimuli, such as pressure, heat and cold, or tendon stretching. In the following example, we'll be talking about the muscle spindle reflex where the sensation is a stretched muscle, the tendon, the sensor is a muscle spindle, and the response is muscle contraction.

The spinal reflex arc is perhaps most easily characterized by a reflex familiar to you, the patellar tendon response. When you go in for your physical examination, the physician may have you seated so your legs dangle, and then she may tap your knee with a hammer or the heel of her hand. When

she does this, if your reflexes are functioning correctly, your leg will kick in response. You didn't think, "Gee, I should kick when she does this." The response was purely reflexive, governed by a sensorimotor system that does not require conscious intervention or control (this is a good time to plant the seed of conscious control, though, since you could inhibit or at least modulate this response if you wanted to). Let's examine the components of this basic reflex arc.

Take a look at Figure 3–1 so we can identify the components of the reflex arc. First of all, there must be an adequate stimulus that stretches a **muscle spindle**. Muscle spindles are the workhorses of the anti-gravity muscles, because the purpose of the muscle spindle is to provide feedback to the muscle that it has been passively stretched. As an example, hold your arms out in front of you, with your eyes closed. As you hold your arms out, gravity is working to pull them back down, while you are working to hold them in place. Now open your eyes, and see that they are pretty much where you placed them in the first place, despite the forces trying to move them to the earth. How did you know, with your eyes closed, where your arms were supposed to be? The pull of gravity on your arms is considered "passive," in the sense that you are not actively contracting muscles to pull your arms down. Muscle spindles sense passive forces on your body and convey that information to the muscle that is opposed to that passive force. In this case, muscle spindles are telling your arm muscles that they need to contract a little more in order to resist gravity. The muscle spindle is designed to maintain a muscle posture (Bowman, 1971).

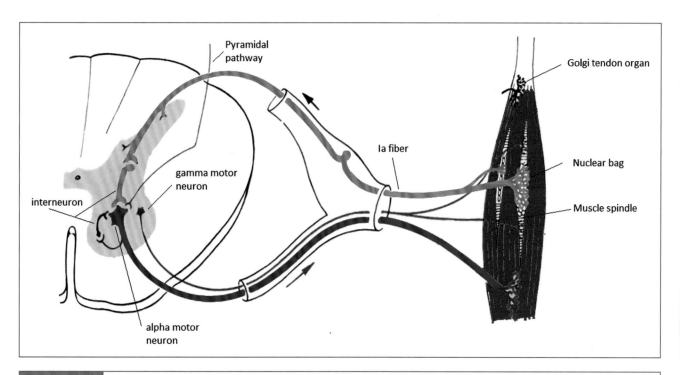

FIGURE 3–1. Muscle spindle and basic spinal reflex arc. Note that muscle length change is sensed by the nuclear bag fiber that runs parallel to intrafusal muscle fiber. That information is conveyed to the spinal cord via the afferent pathway and through the dorsal root ganglion. The afferent fiber synapses with a motor (efferent) neuron that contracts extrafusal muscle fiber to correct the length change. *Source:* Adapted from Baehr and Frotscher (2012).

Muscle spindles sense length changes in muscle fibers. Skeletal muscle is made up of **extrafusal** and **intrafusal fibers**. Extrafusal muscle fibers are the heavy hitters of the muscular system: they do all the work. Intrafusal muscle fibers are involved in the control of muscle posture through the muscle spindle, as we shall see. Intrafusal muscle fibers run parallel to extrafusal fibers, but intrafusal fibers have the important distinction of having muscle spindles attached to them.

There are two types of muscles spindles: **nuclear chain fibers** and **nuclear bag fibers**. Nuclear chain fibers are found near the end of the thin intrafusal (adjustment) fibers, and nuclear bag fibers are found on the thick intrafusal fibers, near the midpoint. The nuclear chain fibers convey information to the CNS about a static posture by means of either Group Ia or II fibers (i.e., holding your arm out against gravity), while the nuclear bag fibers relate information about passive movement of muscle by means of Group Ia nerve fibers. With these two pieces of information the brain can know the status of a muscle at any time.

The muscle spindle operates, then, as both a sensing unit and a means for maintaining a given posture. When the muscle is passively stretched, sensory information about that condition is conveyed to the central nervous system (CNS) by afferent fibers. When a muscle reaches a chosen posture, that information is conveyed to the CNS as well. In addition, the efferent innervation of the muscle spindle will activate the intrafusal muscle fiber, causing it to contract. In this way, the muscle spindle recalibrates to a newly established length so it is not continually trying to adjust muscle length to an earlier "setting."

Thus, as you move your arms or legs, the muscle spindle system is continually adapting to your new posture. Once that posture is held, the muscle spindle monitors any changes in length (that aren't caused by active contraction) and adjusts the muscle length to the "ideal setting" that you established when you reached a posture. You can see what an elegant solution this is to the problem of working against extraneous forces such as gravity, but you might also see the inherent problems if the system is damaged. If a person's nervous system cannot differentiate the passive movement from active movement, the result will be spasticity.

Now, if we return to the diagram in Figure 3–1, you can see the components in a new light. When extrafusal muscle is passively stretched, the muscle spindle sends this information to the CNS, where it activates a motor neuron that will cause gamma efferent fibers to contract in response to this change in posture. The contraction moves the muscle back to its original length, as defined by the muscle spindle and, more specifically, the intrafusal fiber. This is why it's so important for the intrafusal fiber to contract: it is the means by which the neuromotor system knows the posture your body is supposed to have at any given instant in time.

There is one more feature of this muscle spindle reflex system that is important to mention. We've talked a lot about activation, but there is an *inactivation* side to the muscle spindle as well. Muscles operate generally in opposition to other muscles. For example, when you raise your velum using the levator veli palatine, you are also working against the velar depressor, the *palatoglossus*. Muscles generally have antagonists to their action, so that any given movement caused by a muscle can be opposed by another muscle. This agonist-antagonist relationship allows us to have fine, graded movement, since I can contract the antagonist just a little to modulate the movement of an agonist, allowing me to, for instance, slow my hand's approach to my coffee cup so I don't knock it over. The muscle spindle is responsible not only for contracting the *agonist*, but also for graded inhibition of the *antagonist*, termed reciprocal inhibition (e.g., Yavuz, Negro, Diedrichs, Türker, & Farina, 2017).

This avoids co-contraction of musculature that works in opposition, a condition that would result in rigidity. When voluntary movement is initiated, both alpha and gamma systems are activated. There is speculation that the gamma system receives information from the cortex concerning the desired or *target* muscle length, and thus the gamma system provides feedback to the cortex when this length has been achieved (Pearson & Gordon, 2013). Thus, the gamma system may be a regulatory mechanism for voluntary movement, and damage to this system has devastating effects. Failure of the muscle spindle system can result in spasticity if it is left unchecked or in flaccidity if it is disabled through disease or trauma.

This inhibition typically occurs as a result of an inhibitory interneuron. When the extensor is activated, as in response to the muscle spindle, an interneuron in the circuit inhibits the flexor. In this way, muscle activation is not compromised by activation of muscles that counteract the intended movement. You may want to look at the note on the velum and spasticity for an idea of what can happen when that occurs as a result of cerebrovascular accident.

Spasticity and the Velum

You will recall the velum (or soft palate) from your speech and hearing science course. The velum is a critically important valve that closes off the nasopharynx from the oropharynx. This valve supports both speech and swallowing function, since closing the valve controls an important resonating chamber (nasal cavity) and helps the tongue create the important swallowing pressure that helps propel the bolus to the waiting esophagus.

When an individual has a cerebrovascular accident, the voluntary motor control system is often compromised and basic reflexes dominate the motor pattern. The muscles associated with the velum are endowed with muscle spindles, which maintain muscle position against the forces of gravity that would cause passive drift of those muscles. Clearly, the velum would drop open if you relaxed it, thanks to gravity's continual force, so the levator veli palatini is invested with muscle spindles to help maintain the velum's posture.

You'll also remember the genioglossus and palatoglossus. The genioglossus makes up the bulk of the tongue and, like the velum, is invested with muscle spindles to help it maintain its posture against gravity. The palatoglossus has muscle spindles as well. Now comes the drama.

When a person has reduced voluntary control, the muscle spindles can become hyperfunctional. In reality, their activity is typically inhibited by the voluntary control mechanism, and reflexes are always there, ready to act. When a person has a cerebrovascular accident, the muscle spindle system is free to act without restraint, and you will see the muscle spindles respond to passive movement as well as attempts at active movement. When a person attempts to elevate the velum, the muscle spindles of the genioglossus and palatoglossus are activated, pulling the velum down. At the same time, the spindles in the levator are activated, pulling the velum up. The result is a hypertonic velum that simply does not want to move. Moving the velum voluntarily requires a great deal of effort, since the person has a condition known as **spastic paralysis**. Spastic paralysis is the condition in which muscle contraction is made significantly more difficult as a result of the co-contraction of antagonist muscles due to loss of their inhibition.

Clinically, as you ask your client to produce, for instance, repeated "kuh" syllables (a diadochokinetic task), the tongue's repeated downward movement effectively "pumps up" the muscle spindle system of both the genioglossus and palatoglossus. The velum is pulled down and the tongue has a great deal of difficulty reaching the posterior hard palate for the /k/. As the string of "kuh" syllables proceeds, the tension increases to the point that it sounds like the person is choking on the speech. He or she isn't choking: it's the air escaping between the tongue and the hard palate that makes the sound you hear. Interestingly, the person's swallow may be quite functional if the pharyngeal reflex is intact, as it includes both excitatory and inhibitory elements that are outside of the voluntary system.

As you can see, the muscle spindle system has many functions, all of which help us to move about our environment. The muscle spindle responds to passive stretch, by contracting extrafusal muscle, adjusts intrafusal muscle to recalibrate the sensor, inhibits antagonist muscles during voluntary movement, and aids in graded motor responses.

GOLGI TENDON ORGANS

A sensor that is less well understood is the **Golgi tendon organ (GTO)**. One end of the GTO is attached to the origin or insertion of a muscle, and the other end is attached to the tendon connected to the muscle. When the muscle contracts, it places a strain on the GTO, which senses the tension between muscle and tendon. Passively stretching the muscle is not the primary stimulus for a GTO, and it actually takes a great deal of passive stretching to activate it (i.e., when you have stretched the muscle far enough that it places tension on the tendon). When a muscle is contracted, however, the GTO is quite responsive to the tension placed on it.

Apparently the GTO works closely with muscle spindle. When muscle is lengthened the muscle spindle is active, but the GTO senses the *tension* placed on the muscle rather than its length. If a muscle is tensed **isometrically** (that is, in a way that the structure that is supposed to move is anchored and immobile), the lengthening is minimal but the GTO will react to the tension placed on it by contraction. Similarly, passively stretching a muscle activates the muscle spindle, but the GTO remains silent.

OTHER SENSATION AND SENSORS

So far we have been talking only about the GTOs and muscle spindles. There are a many other receptors that deserve our attention. Remember, at the heart of this discussion is the notion that we are sentient organisms, and sensation is how we know our environment. Sensory receptors, including muscle spindles and GTOs, are nerve endings that have become specialized to **transduce** (change) energy from one form to another. We can broadly categorize sensors as *somatosensors* and *special sensors*. Special senses include the senses of vision, olfaction, taste, and hearing, and we'll deal with them separately.

Somatosensors

Somatosensory receptors are part of the system responsible for sensing general body information (somatic sense). You can further divide somatosensory receptors into **exteroceptors** and **interoceptors**. Exteroceptors are those that mediate senses that arise from the outside environment, such as cold, heat, pressure, and painful stimuli presented to the body (Moller, 2003). Interoceptors are those receptors that monitor the condition of your organs, as well as specific aspects of your physiology (such as amount of carbon dioxide in your blood). Taken together, exteroceptors and interoceptors provide your central nervous system with an exquisite data set concerning the current condition of your body (Table 3–1).

When one of these sensors is stimulated, information is conveyed to the CNS for processing. When you passively stretch a muscle, the nervous system hears about it, but that perception may not reach consciousness. At the microscopic level, there is also a critical threshold for even subconscious stimulation to trigger a response in the nervous system (if your body responded to <u>every</u> tiny stimulation, your nervous system would be overwhelmed). This **threshold** differs from sensor to sensor: the stimulus that can elicit a response from a given receptor is called the **adequate stimulus**. A given receptor converts excitatory energy, such as the pressure of touch, into electrochemical energy by the creation of a receptor potential that stimulates a neuron's dendrite. A strong stimulus generates a strong receptor potential, which increases the probability that your nervous system will respond to it. You can think about one of our favorite stimuli, sound. When that stimulus is introduced into the cochlea, we sense it thanks to the elegant organ of Corti and its hair cells. Louder sounds create a larger traveling wave, which is translated into greater deflection of the basilar membrane (and the perception of louder sound).

Exteroceptors are those somatic sensors that tell us about the world outside of our body. They can be further defined as **mechanoreceptors**, **thermoreceptors**, and **chemoreceptors**, depending on what causes them to respond. Mechanoreceptors respond to a stimulus that deforms them, such as pressure on the skin or, as in the muscle spindle, stretching. Thermoreceptors respond to changes in heat or cold, while chemoreceptors respond to the presence of some chemical stimulus. The only chemoreceptors that are exteroceptors are the special senses of taste and smell, although we have many interoceptors that are chemoreceptors. Skin receptors come in two basic designs: encapsulated and free (unencapsulated). Encapsulated sensors are those that are contained within a connective tissue capsule that translates the pressure or other sense to the nerve endings. Free or unencapsulated sensors do not have this capsule surrounding them, and therefore are directly stimulated by forces exerted on them. As we shall see, free receptors generally look the same but can have very different functions and they respond to very different stimuli.

There are four important encapsulated receptors: **Meissner's corpuscles**, sensing superficial epidermal stretch and light touch; **Merkel disk receptors**, sensing deep static pressure in the superficial epidermis; **Pacinian corpuscles**, sensing deep pressure and deep touch; and **Ruffini endings** (Ruffini's corpuscles), sensing deep stretch (Brodal, 2004). As you can see from Figure 3–2, these encapsulated receptors are

	TABLE 3–1.	Sensors and the Stimuli that Are Transduced		
Sense	**Class of sensation mediated**	**Sensor type**	**Stimulus**	**Pathway**
Pain	Superficial	Nerve ending	Aversive stimulation	Lateral spinothalamic and spinoreticular tracts
Temperature	Superficial	Thermosensor	Heat and cold	Lateral spinothalamic tract
Mechanical stimulation	Deep and superficial	Pacinian corpuscle; Golgi tendon organ, muscle spindle	Light and deep pressure; vibration; joint sense; muscle stretch	Dorsal and ventral spinocerebellar tracts
Kinesthetic sense	Deep	Labyrinthine (vestibular) hair cells	Motion of body	Medial longitudinal fasciculus, lateral vestibulospinal tract, medial vestibulospinal tract
Vision	Special	Photoreceptors	Light stimulation	Optric tract
Olfactory	Special	Chemoreceptors	Chemical stimulation	Olfactory tract
Gustation	Special	Chemoreceptors	Chemical stimulation	Thalamocortical pathway
Proprioception	Combined sensation	Golgi tendon organ; muscle spindle; labyrinthine; kinesthetic sense; *photoreceptors	Joint sense; muscle stretch; motion of body; *light stimulation	Dorsal column medial lemniscus pathways terminating at nucleus gracilis and cuneatus

*Visual stimulation has been added to this group because of the importance of visual information to knowledge of position in space.

Source: Adapted from Seikel, Drumright, & King (2016).

all very sensitive to force, so they are considered to be "low threshold" in that it doesn't take much force to activate them. Meissner's corpuscles are sensitive to movement or stretching of tissue and are found in the upper epidermal layer, particularly in the finger pads. Meissner's corpuscles give us that exquisite ability to sense things with our fingertips. Merkel receptors are found in the lips, and are sensitive to light pressure in the superficial epidermis. Ruffini's corpuscles are also low-threshold sensors, but they sense stretching of the skin (much like muscle spindles).

There are low-threshold free receptors (non-encapsulated receptors) that respond to mechanical forces as well. For instance, there are free receptors on the roots of hairs that are very sensitive to any movement (for instance, if a ladybug is walking on your arm, you feel it even though it only weighs about 0.2 gram). A difference in these low-threshold sensors is adaptation level: some sensors adapt quickly to stimulation, "turning off" after a short time, while others keep responding as long as stimulation is present. The sensors on the root of the hair that we just discussed are rapidly adapting sensors, so that once they are deformed and the ladybug stops walking they stop sending a message to the central nervous system (Bardoni et al., 2014).

Meissner's corpuscles, which mediate the highly sensitive pressure on your fingertips, are likewise rapidly adapting. They need to be continually responsive to change rather than static pressure, and they can sense the direction of force as well as the velocity of travel of objects on the skin (Brodal, 2004). Other receptors, such as Ruffini corpuscles and Merkel disk receptors, signal stretching of the skin and pressure, respectively. They keep signaling for longer periods after being deformed. Similarly, Pacinian corpuscles are very rapidly adapting and appear to be responsible for mediating higher-frequency vibratory sense (around 400 Hz), versus Meissner's corpuscles, which are responsive up to about 100 Hz (Brodal, 2004).

Another very important class of sensation is **pain sense**. Pain is an important part of life, even though we don't particularly like it! Pain provides us with a way of knowing our limits: touching a hot stove is not a good idea, so recoiling from it makes evolutionary sense. Pain sensors are called **nociceptors** (the Latin word "nocere" means "to do harm," so these are receptors that sense things that can hurt you). Nociceptors are actually myelinated fibers with free nerve endings. Nociceptors are considered to be high-threshold mechanoreceptors, since significant pressure (such as pinching) causes

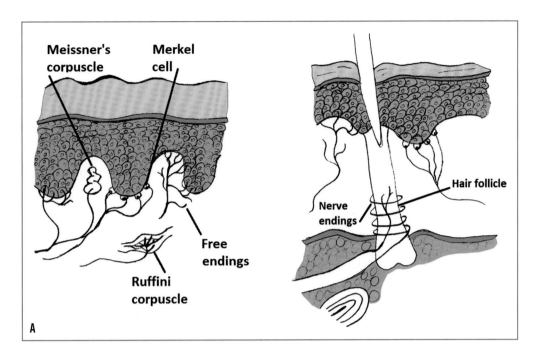

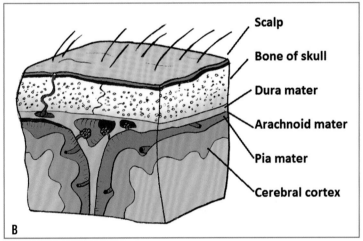

FIGURE 3–2.   Receptors within the epidermis. **A.** Meissner's corpuscles, Ruffini's corpuscles, Merkel cells, and free endings. *Source:* Adapted from Brodal (2004). **B.** Receptors *in situ* in epidermis of scalp. *Source:* Adapted from Seikel, Drumright, and King (2016).

the response. Some of these mechanoreceptors also mediate heat and cold or chemical changes in tissue caused by irritation and inflammation. These thermal receptors look the same as pain sensors under magnification but have the added properties of perceiving a range of stimulation. We sense the range of thermal experiences through cool, cold, warm, and hot sensors. Obviously, the painful stimuli are at the ends of the continuum (cold and hot), but the cool and warm sensors prepare us for those extremes so that we can avoid them. In contrast to other mechanoreceptors, nociceptors not only do not adapt to stimuli, but *they become more sensitive to the painful stimulus the longer you maintain it.*

You know this from your own experience, of course: walking with a rock in your boot doesn't get easier as you go along! Again, this is an appropriate response by your body, although it can lead to neurophysiological hypersensitization to pain, which increases the effects of these chronic conditions (Møller, 2003).

There is another group of mechanoreceptors that provide us with knowledge of how the joints of our bodies are oriented and moving. There are at least four types of sensors that reside within the joint capsule: some of them sense movement and rate of change of the joint, while others are similar to GTOs, in that they sense stretching of ligaments that bind the bones together. Studies on humans have revealed that stimulation of the sensors related to joint movement causes a person to perceive that the structure (in this case a finger) has moved. Thus, joint sense serves the subconscious proprioception function that helps us organize our navigation of space, but it also provides conscious knowledge of those movements as well (Dye, Vaupel, & Dye, 1998; Macefield, Gandevia, & Burke, 1990).

We would be remiss if we didn't mention proprioceptive sense. **Proprioception** refers to sensory perception related to the musculoskeletal system. The position sense of joints, tension on muscles, movement of the arms and legs, and so forth are all mediated by sensors within the muscle and skeletal systems. There are minute sensors within the joints, in the fascia, and, of course, in the muscles (muscle spindle) and tendons (Golgi tendon organs) that are informing me of my body "condition" at all times. Most of the sensation is related to stretching of tissue, and these are typically low-threshold sensors. "Silent nociceptors" are a group of pain sensors that mediate homeostasis. These sensors monitor the effluent of tissues that are damaged, such as cytokines released by the mucosa of the stomach in response to an assault on the tissue by bacteria or viruses. These sensors mediate the behaviors we know as "sickness," which serve to slow us down for the healing process (National Research Council. Committee on Recognition and Alleviation of Pain in Laboratory Animals, 2009).

In summary, muscle spindles are the mechanism for providing feedback to the neuromotor system concerning muscle length, tension, motion, and position.

- Muscle spindles run parallel to the intrafusal muscle fibers and provide information concerning change in length of muscle, whereas Golgi tendon organs sense muscle tension.
- Acceleration is sensed by means of nuclear bag fibers, which convey information concerning acceleration. Nuclear chain fibers respond to sustained lengthening.
- A segmental reflex is triggered when a muscle is passively stretched, and this activates the extrafusal muscles, which shorten the muscle.
- Tension of the muscle during contraction is sensed by the Golgi tendon organs, which mediate inhibition of antagonist muscles.
- Receptors transduce internal or external environment information into electrochemical impulses. Information from a receptor is sent to the CNS for processing.

REPRESENTATION OF THE SOMATIC SENSATION IN THE SPINAL CORD

The spinal cord receives sensory information from diverse sources, such as skin receptors for touch, temperature, and pain, as well as sensors in joints and muscles, as we will dis-

cuss. For the information to be useful in responding to the environment it has to enter the central nervous system. In our discussion of the muscle spindle response, the muscle spindle communicates with the spinal cord by means of a spinal nerve that enters the spinal cord segment. We also talked about multi-segment reflexes, which span more than one spinal cord segment.

Figure 3–3 shows a dermatome map for the human body. A **dermatome** is defined as an area of skin that is innervated by a single spinal nerve, and it represents the distribution of the cutaneous region served by the nerve (Barr, 1974). Sensory dermatomes are the receptive map for the body. Motor innervation arises from the ventral root of the spi-

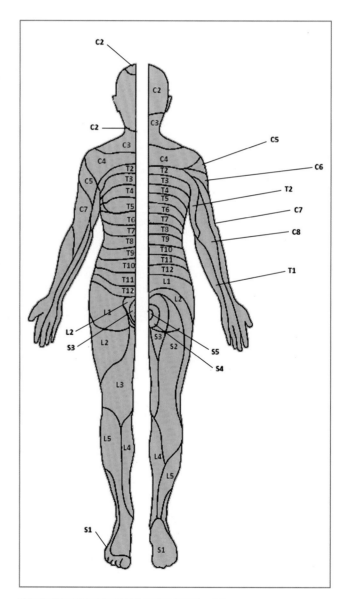

FIGURE 3–3. Dermatomes of the epidermal layer.

nal cord segment, and these nerves serve muscles of the legs, arms, thorax, and abdomen. Typically, efferent nerves combine to create **plexuses** (groups of nerves coming together for a common purpose; Table 3–2), and these plexuses give rise to the motor nerves that activate muscle. For example, cervical nerves C1, C2, C3, and C4 come together to form the cervical plexus, and this plexus gives rise to the phrenic nerve, which innervates the diaphragm. In contrast, the sensory nerves have specific territories or dermatomes that they serve. For instance, you can see that C2 and C3 have a sensory territory that serves the back of the neck and scalp. That is to say, if a mosquito bites you on your neck, the histamine that she introduces into your skin will cause an itch that will be mediated by C2 to the spinal cord. Neurologists can use this information to pinpoint lesions to the afferent nervous system. If, for instance, you have reduced or absent sensation below the level of your knees, the neurologist can infer that there is damage to the sensory component of the spinal cord in the lumbar and sacral regions.

Dermatomes actually overlap, so the correspondence is not as tight as one might guess from looking at the map. Although Herrington performed the first dermatome mapping, on monkeys, in 1898, the human dermatome map was developed through information gained from clinical evaluations of people with spinal cord injuries by Head in the 1920s (Brodal, 2004).

Dermatomes are important tools for the neurologist but also give clues as to site of lesion for the speech-language pathologist. That having been said, we will be much more interested in the cranial nerves that provide input about muscles and structures related to speech. We'll spend a whole chapter on those nerves!

SPECIAL SENSES

While somatic senses serve the broader needs of the body, including proprioception and homeostasis, some special senses have also evolved that are designed to mediate specific stimuli impinging on our bodies. This evolutionary process has taken quite some time, and we humans are the beneficiaries of these eons of development. Our cochlea is echoed in the lateral line organ of fish, and some form of an eye has evolved at least four times in history! Smell is so elemental that it is the only sense that doesn't enter the thalamus of the brain, and taste takes up a sizable portion of the cerebral cortex (the insula). Let's take a moment to examine these senses and a little of their mechanisms. Of course, for us, the sense of hearing is critical, but our work in swallowing as speech-language pathologists means that we need to have some knowledge of taste and olfaction as well.

Visual Sensation

Sensors for the visual system are both elegant and complex (Figure 3–4). Retinal cells of the eye are located in the posterior inner surface of the eye. Myelin is absent in the retinal sensors, which allows the structure of the retina to be essentially translucent (i.e., it allows light through). The paper-thin retina consists of eight layers. The outermost layer contains pigment cells that protect the retinal cells deep to them, as well as provide a bed for the photoreceptors. The photoreceptor layer includes rod and cone cells that are sensitive to light stimulation. The outer nuclear layer contains the nuclei of the photosensors, while the next five layers contain horizontal

TABLE 3–2.	**Nerve Plexuses of the Spinal Cord**	
Plexus	Nerve components	Function
Cervical	C1–C4	Motor fibers; innervate muscles of head, neck, and shoulders; interacts with X vagus and XI accessory; gives rise to phrenic nerve of diaphragm
Brachial	C4–C8, T1 and T2	Motor and sensory fibers; thorax, shoulders, arms, hands
Lumbar	L1–L4, T-12	Sensory and motor innervation; sensory innervation of pleurae and peritoneum; motor fibers; interacts with sacral plexus; motor innervation for abdomen, groin, thighs, knees, calves
Sacral	L4–S4	Sensory and motor innervation; interacts with lumbar plexus; gives rise to sciatic nerve; innervation of pelvis, buttocks, genitals, thighs, calves, feet
Coccygeal	S4, S5, coccygeal 1	Coccyx; sensation of skin in coccygeal region

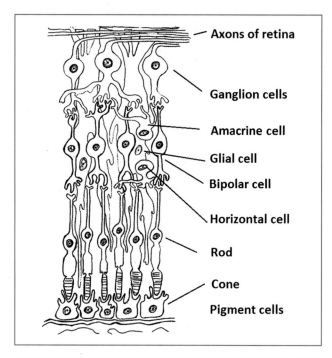

- Axons of retina
- Ganglion cells
- Amacrine cell
- Glial cell
- Bipolar cell
- Horizontal cell
- Rod
- Cone
- Pigment cells

FIGURE 3–4. Layers of the retina. The pigment layer is the most superficial layer, providing protection to the photoreceptors of the second layer. The outer nuclear layer includes cell bodies and axons of photoreceptors, while the outer plexiform, inner nuclear and inner plexiform layers include bipolar, Muller, and glial cells. The ganglion and nerve fiber layers are the beginning stages of the optic nerve.

bipolar cells and interneurons (amacrine cells), whose role is to sharpen the photoreceptor input through inhibition of non-target regions (see the box on Negative Afterimages). The deepest nerve fiber layer includes the axons of the ganglion cell layer, the final processing stage of the retina. The retina is particularly unique in that, despite being a sensory organ, it performs a great deal of pre-processing. By contrast, in the auditory system, that pre-processing primarily occurs in the brainstem.

Negative Afterimages and Feature Detection

Have you ever had the experience of briefly glancing at the sun and then quickly looking away? We all have experienced the blinding flash of that experience, but there's a secret embedded in the recovery process. Even after you look away, you can still see the image of the sun. The photoreceptors of your retina have been overstimulated and fatigued by the intensity of the light, similar to what you experience when you've heard a loud sound (temporary threshold shift). If you pay attention to this image, you'll see it change over time, reflecting the recovery of your visual system.

But there's more to that recovery than "meets the eye." Activation of rods and cones inhibits the spontaneous activity of adjacent neurons, a feature that enhances the image produced by making a stronger output difference between the activated cell and those around it. This is called edge enhancement. You can verify this effect by looking at a page that is solid black on half the page and white on the other: you'll see that the black edge appears even blacker than the field. Perceptual scientists have used these edge-effects to determine that the retinal neurons are actually feature detectors, capable of pre-processing basic visual features of the image being viewed. Hubel and Wiesel earned their Nobel Prize for work with visual neurophysiology, and some of their early work involved feature detection in the frog. They found there were feature detectors in the frog retina that sensed movement in an upwardly vertical direction, downwardly vertical direction, horizontal direction, etc., precisely mirroring the movements a fly would have in the visual field. Remarkably, these detectors were responsive <u>only</u> to one type of stimulus (e.g., upward vertical movement) and not to another stimulus. In fact, movement in that upward vertical dimension <u>inhibited</u> activity in the downward vertical detectors.

What does this have to do with negative afterimage? You can demonstrate the presence of feature detectors easily in your own visual system. Try this experiment. Stand in front of a cluttered shelf of your cupboard, or in front of a bookshelf with a variety of shapes and sizes, and then turn off the lights so it's good and dark. Let your eyes adapt to the dark for several minutes, and then flash your camera at the shelf and watch what happens. You will see the image during the flash instant, for sure, and then you will see it disappear and be replaced by a negative image, which will gradually decay. That negative afterimage is the product of the cells that are normally inhibited when viewing that image, but which were released from inhibition because of fatigue of the primary neurons. Want another example? Watch a blockbuster movie with credits that seem to go on forever. Pay close attention to the credits, without letting your eyes wander away from the screen. When you get to the very end of the credits, the scrolling stops on a final logo, and you will have the impression that the logo is moving in the opposite direction from the credits. You have fatigued feature detectors for movement in the vertical direction, going from top to bottom, and the detectors for the opposite direction are able to respond because of that fatiguing effect. Once you starting looking for the effect, you will see dozens of examples!

Unlike most other receptors, photoreceptors become hyperpolarized when stimulated. That is, they <u>turn off</u> when stimulated, but are depolarized or active in darkness. Another unique characteristic is that they produce a **graded potential** rather than an all-or-none action potential, so we can actually see shades of a color. Activation of retinal cells disinhibits bipolar cells, which produce action potentials that stimulate ganglion cells. We'll return to the visual system when we examine cranial nerves.

Olfactory Sensation

Olfaction refers to the sense of smell, and it is mediated by the first cranial nerve. Olfactory sense utilizes chemoreceptors, which respond to chemicals that impinge on the sensors. Olfaction and gustation are very important for speech-language pathologists because of our work in swallowing disorders. The sense of smell is not as well used in humans as in non-humans, such as dogs or cats, but its basic and important nature can be felt in the evocative nature of smells. The olfactory sense is tied closely to the hippocampus, which is the major memory element of the central nervous system. Smells can evoke memories for which there are no words because those memories were put in place before you had language. Smell is the most basic and oldest of our special senses.

Olfactory sensors are embedded in the olfactory epithelium, in the mucous membrane lining of the superior nasal cavity. The 10 million sensors take up very little space (about 1 cm^3) and undergo constant regeneration (Brodal, 2004).

Gustatory Sensation

Gustation (taste) is a very important process for speech-language pathologists because of its relationship with mastica-tion and deglutition. Taste is what keeps us eating to fulfill our nutritional requirements. Taste receptors (**taste buds**, or **taste cells**) are **chemoreceptors** that are found in the tongue epithelia within **papillae**. Taste pores within the papillae are openings that isolate a tasted substance. The material in the taste pore is held in place by small hair-like fibers called **microvilli**, which project from the taste cell into the **taste pore** (Figure 3–5).

We categorize tastes into five broad categories: sweet, salty, sour, bitter, and umami. The perception of taste arises from activation of taste sensors in varying combinations, so the taste of strawberries differs from that of chocolate because of the combinations of sensors that have been activated. You may have never run across the term *umami*. Umami is a basic "meaty" or protein-like flavor elicited by the spice monosodium glutamate. For over a century, we believed that taste receptors were restricted to zones of the tongue, with sweet tastes being sensed at the tip, salty at the sides in front, and sour at the sides in the back. Bitterness was thought to be sensed on the posterior tongue. The reality is that all the tastes can be sensed all over the tongue.

There are four basic forms that the papillae take. **Filiform papillae** dominate, but they aren't taste sensors at all. They look like small pink or gray threads on the dorsum of the tongue and have mechanoreceptors that give your tongue exquisite tactile sensory ability, permitting fine discrimination of the bolus characteristics. Bright red **fungiform papillae** are found among the filiform papillae on the tip and sides of the tongue. **Foliate papillae** populate the posterior lateral tongue and faucial pillars. A dozen or so **circumvallate** (or **vallate**) papillae are located on the posterior dorsal surface, arrayed in a V-formation.

Taste receptors (also known as taste buds; Figure 3–6) are chemosensors that work with saliva to do their job. Saliva

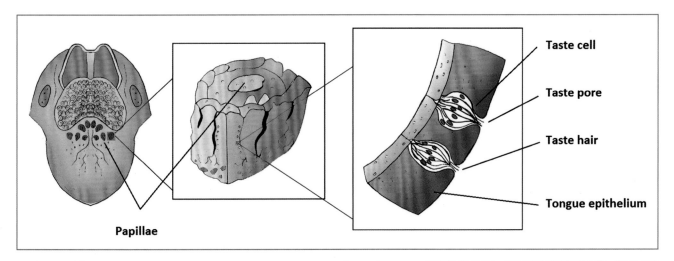

Papillae

Taste cell

Taste pore

Taste hair

Tongue epithelium

FIGURE 3–5. Taste buds of the tongue. Relationship among tongue, papillae, and taste buds. *Source:* Adapted from Seikel, Drumright, and King (2016).

is made of enzymes that dissolve materials you place in your mouth, putting the food into a format that your sensors can process. The taste buds are found throughout the tongue, but are concentrated on the lateral aspects of the anterior tongue, as well as the tongue dorsum. They are also found in the valleculae, on the velum, and even at the entrance of the larynx. There are even reports of taste sensors deep within the linings of the intestines (Bezencon, le Coutre, & Damak, 2006)!

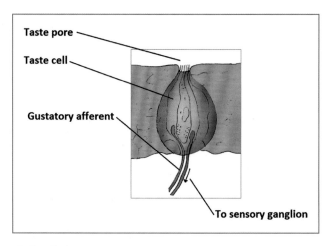

FIGURE 3–6. Fine structure of the taste bud, taste pore, and microvilli.

Auditory Sensation

Of course audition and vestibular function are bedrock processes for our professions. Acoustical information represents a disturbance in air that is translated to movement of the perilymph and, ultimately, endolymph fluids of the cochlea. Acoustic information is a mechanical stimulus that requires a mechanoreceptor, the hair cell. Hair cells have evolved into exquisite systems for sensing minute changes in air pressure, though we should humbly acknowledge that the auditory mechanism arises from the lateral line organ of fish.

There are two basic types of hair cells (Figure 3–7), inner and outer, with different structure and function. The **inner hair cells** are considered to be the primary mechanism for auditory discrimination of frequency, while the **outer hair cells** serve the critical role of sound amplification. There are about 3,500 inner hair cells (IHC) and 12,000 outer hair cells (OHC). Inner hair cells are arrayed in a single row along the basilar membrane, while outer hair cells are in three rows (Pickles, 2012).

Each hair cell has critically important **stereocilia** (also known as **cilia**) on the upper surface. On the IHC there are about 50 cilia, which are arrayed as a flattened "U," and on the OHC, about 150 cilia take the form of a "W." The cilia are very important to the transduction process. The cilia are graduated in length, but are all connected by means of tip links made up of fibrin molecules, which provide a rigid connection between the cilia. The cilia are thinner at the base than at the top, which means they are more prone to

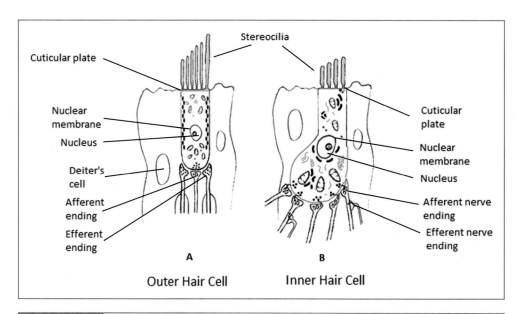

FIGURE 3–7. Hair cells of the cochlea. **A.** Outer hair cell of cochlea. Note that efferent endings of olivocochlear bundle synapse directly with cell body. **B.** Inner hair cell of cochlea. Note that efferent endings of olivocochlear bundle synapse with afferent component rather than cell body.

bending at the base. Because they are connected, when one cilium is deflected, all of the cilia will be deflected. Recall that movement of ions in a neuron results in the action potential. Movement of hair cell cilia causes ion channels to open up in the cilia tips, allowing potassium to enter the hair cell. Remember from your hearing science course that the traveling wave of the basilar membrane causes a maximal perturbation as the wave reaches its peak (see Hudspeth, 2014 for a remarkable review). This perturbation of the basilar membrane results in a shearing action between the tectorial membrane and the hair cell that causes the cilia to bend. Because the cilia are linked, even a small disturbance in the fluid can cause the discharge of the hair cell.

Similar to neurons, hair cells have a resting state. During that resting state, about 15% of the ion channels are open at any time. Depolarization of the hair cell happens when the cilia are deflected toward the tallest of the cilia, and the degree of deflection changes the degree of depolarization. This is a nice design, since it allows the auditory system to have a graded response to sound intensity. If the cilia are deflected in the opposite direction, the hair cell is hyperpolarized and cannot fire. The cilia are very sensitive to perturbation in the endolymph and can sense movement that is about 1/10,000 of the width of a human hair!

Tip links are like tiny springs, causing the ion channels to open rapidly. An area known as the active zone at the base of the hair cell releases glutamate as a result of depolarization of the hair cell.

The Stria Vascularis and Hair Cell Function

The stria vascularis has a critical role in maintaining ion balance within the scala media. When the cilia are deflected, potassium enters the hair cell, subsequently passing through the basilar membrane into the perilymph within the scala tympani. Potassium is taken up by the stria vascularis and re-cycled into the endolymph, maintaining the potassium-rich environment of the endolymph (Spicer & Schulte, 1996). The cross-membrane gradient between the endolymph and the superficial stria vascularis is created by ion pumps for Na+, Cl−, and K+. The superficial cells of the stria vascularis have K+ ion channels that allow osmotic movement into the endolymph, and it has been shown that mice genetically engineered without the ability to move potassium via the superficial cells have a demonstrable hearing loss (Casimiro, et al.). The ion gradient between the intermediate cells of the stria vascularis and the endolymph creates the +80 mV potential difference that drives hearing function (Wangemann, 2002). The hair cell, in contrast, has a negative potential of −70 mV, which produces a powerful 150 mV differential between the endolymph and the hair cell.

When ions enter the hair cell, they initiate the process of hair cell depolarization. Potassium ions cause the neurotransmitter glutamate to be released into the synaptic region between the hair cell and an VIII nerve fiber and this depolarizes the neuron, creating an action potential. This action potential is special to us in audiology and speech-language pathology because it represents sound impinging on the ear. The action potential generated by the depolarization is conducted out of the scala media to the spiral ganglion of the modiolus, and ultimately out of the inner ear into the brainstem. We talked earlier about "ganglia" being collections of nerves in the peripheral nervous system, and this "**spiral ganglion**" is the collection of VIII nerve cell bodies that create auditory transmission. The fibers will enter the CNS at the cochlear nucleus, the first nucleus of the brainstem auditory pathway (Musiek & Baran, 2007).

Depolarization of **outer hair cells** gives a different result. When outer hair cells depolarize, they shorten; when they hyperpolarize, they are at their resting length. Within the structure of the outer hair cell is the active element *prestin*. Prestin shortens when activated and is capable of contraction 100,000 times per second. In audition, the cycle of hair cell contraction is limited by the resistance of the basilar membrane/endolymph system (Hudspeth, 2014) and occurs in synchrony with the auditory stimulus. Each cycle of vibration gets a "kick" from the hair cell active element, essentially amplifying the sound.

Vestibular Sensors

The **vestibular system** is responsible for sensing changes in movement of the head, and by association, the body. It does this with a graceful array of mechanoreceptors, following the model of the cochlear hair cell. The three **semicircular canals** of the vestibular mechanism send information about position of the body in space to the CNS (see Figure 3–8). Each semicircular canal has an enlarged region known as the **ampulla**. Within the ampulla is the sensory mechanism, the crista ampularis. The crista ampularis is similar to the organ of Corti of the cochlea, in that it rests in fluid and has an overlying membrane, a cupola. Each of the receptor organs has about 6,000 hair cells, each with about 50 stereocilia. In contrast to cochlear hair cells, each hair cell has a kinocilium. Movement of a person's head in one semicircular canal plane is sensed by the cristae of that canal through cilia deflection.

The vestibular mechanism also has two otolithic organs, the **utricle** and **saccule**. In each of these there is a **macula**,

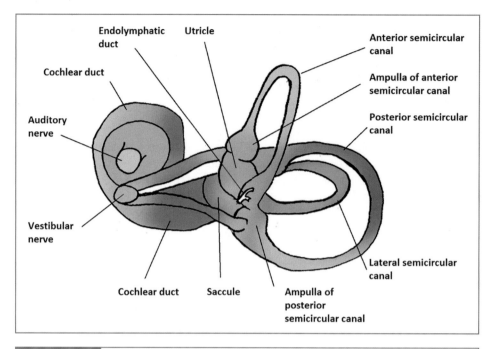

FIGURE 3–8. Semicircular canals of the vestibular mechanism.

the sensory organ endowed with hair cells and cilia, and the macula has an overlying otolithic membrane. The special feature of this sensor is that the otolithic membrane is invested with crystals known as **otoliths**. The otoliths serve as a mass that responds to inertial change arising from acceleration of the body.

In summary, special senses are utilized by the nervous system to provide information about specific classes of stimuli:

- Vision is mediated by retinal cells that uniquely hyperpolarize when stimulated. The 8 layers of the retina include pigment cells, which provide a bed for the photoreceptors. Photoreceptors include rod and cone cells which respond to light stimulation. The layers deep to the photoreceptors are made up of bipolar cells and interneurons which sharpen the image. The deepest nerve fiber layer includes the axons of the ganglion cell layer, the final processing stage of the retina.
- Olfaction refers to the sense of smell, mediated by the first cranial nerve. Chemoreceptors are embedded in the olfactory epithelium, in the mucous membrane lining of the superior nasal cavity, and sensation is transmitted to the hippocampus.
- Gustation (taste) receptors are chemoreceptor papillae of the tongue. Filiform papillae have mechanoreceptors that allow you to discriminate bolus characteristics. Fungiform papillae are found on the tip and sides of the tongue, and foliate papillae are on posterior lateral tongue and faucial

pillars. Cumvallate (vallate) papillae are located on the posterior dorsal surface.
- Auditory sensation arises from disturbance in air that is translated to movement of the perilymph and ultimately endolymph fluids of the cochlea. Hair cells are mechanoreceptors. The inner hair cells provide frequency discrimination and outer hair cells are sound amplifiers. Stereocilia (cilia) on the surface of the hair cell are connected by means of tip links, and movement of cilia causes ion channels to open up in the cilia tips, allowing potassium to enter the hair cell. An area known as the active zone at the base of the hair cell releases glutamate, causing depolarization of the postsynaptic VIII nerve fiber. Depolarization of outer hair cells causes the hair cell to shorten with each cycle of vibration, amplifying the sound.
- Vestibular sensation arises from two sensors, the crista ampularis of the ampulae and the otolithic organs. The crista ampularis senses movement in one of the planes of the semicircular canals, and the otolithic organs sense acceleration of the head.

CHAPTER SUMMARY

Sensors within the body give the CNS information about the world, while the spinal reflex arc is a basic response mechanism to stimulation. The spinal reflex arc consists of a sensory element, conduction of the sensory information to the CNS, and a response element. The muscle spindle reflex circuit includes a muscle spindle, which senses muscle length, as well as the afferent nerve that conveys that information to the spinal cord. The efferent component is responsible for contracting the extrafusal muscle to correct passive movement of the muscle. Nuclear chain fibers are found near the midpoint of the intrafusal fibers, and nuclear bag fibers are found on the thick intrafusal fibers. The nuclear chain fibers convey information about a static posture, and nuclear bag fibers relate information about passive movement. The Golgi tendon organ senses the degree of tension on the muscle. Dermatomes represent the distribution of cutaneous stimulation by spinal nerves. There is a great deal of overlap of the dermatomes, but they provide the neurologist with an indication of the site of spinal cord lesion. Sensors can be broadly categorized as somatosensors and special sensors. Somatosensors are those sensors that transduce information about body condition, while special sensors include vision, olfaction, taste, and hearing. Somatosensory receptors can be divided into exteroceptors and interoceptors. Exteroceptors mediate senses that arise from the outside environment (e.g., cold, heat, pressure, pain) and interoceptors monitor the condition of organs and physiology. Exteroceptors include mechanoreceptors, thermoreceptors, and chemoreceptors. Mechanoreceptors respond to a stimulus that deforms them, such as pressure on the skin. Thermoreceptors respond to changes in heat or cold, and chemoreceptors respond to some chemical stimulus. Skin receptors are either encapsulated or free (unencapsulated). Meissner's corpuscles sense superfi-cial epidermal stretch and light touch, Merkel disk receptors sense deep static pressure in the superficial epidermis, Pacinian corpuscles sense deep pressure and deep touch, and Ruffini endings sense deep stretch. Free receptors on the roots of hairs are sensitive to movement. Nociceptors are mechanoreceptors that sense painful stimuli, and some of them also sense hot and cold sensations. Silent nociceptors are a group of pain sensors that mediate homeostasis. These sensors monitor the effluent of tissues that are damaged, such as cytokines released by the mucosa of the stomach in response to an assault on the tissue by bacteria or viruses. These sensors mediate the behaviors we know as "sickness," which serve to slow us down for the healing process. Sensors that reside within the joint capsule transduce information about movement and rate of change of the joint and stretching of ligaments. Joint sense serves subconscious proprioception as well as conscious knowledge of movements. Proprioception refers to sensory perception related to the musculoskeletal system, including position sense of joints, tension on muscles, and movement of the arms and legs.

Special senses include vision, olfaction, gustation, and audition. Retinal cells are photoreceptors, sensing the presence of light and mediating the sense of vision. Olfactory sensors are chemoreceptors that respond to chemicals that reach the olfactory mucosa of the nose. Gustatory sense is mediated by taste receptors that receive chemicals that are held within taste pores. Auditory sensation is mediated by hair cells in the cochlea, while vestibular sensation is mediated by crista ampularis of the ampulla and the otolithic organs, the utricle and saccule.

CHAPTER 3
STUDY QUESTIONS

1. _____ spindles are the mechanism for providing feedback to the neuromotor system concerning muscle length, tension, motion, and position.

2. Muscle spindles run parallel to the _____ muscle fibers.

3. _____ _____ _____ sense muscle tension.

4. In the muscle spindle, _____ _____ fibers sense acceleration.

5. In the muscle spindle, _____ _____ fibers respond to sustained lengthening.

6. When a muscle is passively stretched, the muscle spindle is activated, resulting in contraction of the _____ muscle fibers, which shorten the muscle.

7. Tension of the muscle during contraction is sensed by the _____ _____ organs, which mediate inhibition of antagonist muscles.

8. On the figure below, please identify the components indicated.

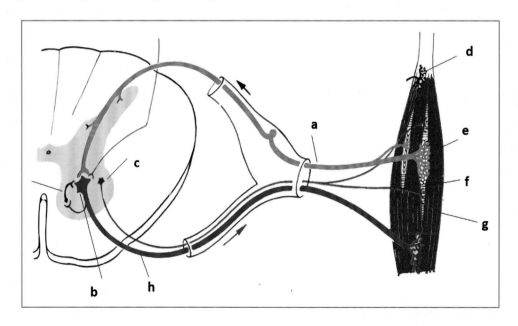

a. _____ fiber

b. _____ _____ neuron

c. _____ _____ neuron

d. _____ _____ organ

e. _____ _____ fiber   g. _____ muscle fiber

f. _____ _____   h. _____ fiber

9. _____ is defined as an area of skin that is innervated by a single spinal nerve, and it represents the distribution of the cutaneous region served by the nerve.

10. A _____ is a group of nerves coming together for a common purpose.

11. _____ cells of the eye sense light.

12. The outermost layer of the retina contains _____ cells that protect the retinal cells deep to them, as well as provide a bed for the photoreceptors.

13. True or False: Photosensors of the eye are found in the outer nuclear layer of the retina.

14. True or False: The patellar tendon reflex is an example of a spinal reflex arc.

15. Muscle spindles respond to passive/active (circle one) movement.

16. _____ muscle fiber makes up the bulk of a muscle.

17. When extrafusal muscle is passively stretched, the muscle spindle sends this information to the central nervous system where it activates a motor neuron that causes _____ efferent fibers to contract.

18. When a muscle contracts, it places a strain on the _____ _____ _____, which senses the tension between muscle and tendon.

19. The term for changing energy from one form to another is _____.

20. _____ (sensors) are part of the system responsible for sensing general body information (somatic sense).

21. Sensors that transduce sensations arising from the outside environment (e.g., heat, cold, pressure) are termed _____.

22. _____ are sensors that monitor the condition of your organs, as well as specific aspects of your physiology.

23. True or False: Muscle spindles would be considered interoceptors because they are embedded within muscle.

24. _____ This type of receptor responds to a stimulus that deforms it, such as pressure on the skin.

25. _____ (type of receptor) responds to changes in heat or cold.

26. _____ Taste sensors are an example of this type of receptor.

27. _____ _____ (type of encapsulated sensor) senses superficial epidermal stretch and light touch.

28. _____ _____ _____ (type of encapsulated sensor) sense deep static pressure in the superficial epidermis.

29. _____ _____ (type of encapsulated sensor) sense deep pressure and deep touch.

30. _____ _____ (type of encapsulated sensor) senses deep stretch.

31. Another name for pain sensor is _____.

32. _____ refers to sensory perception related to the musculoskeletal system and includes sensations related to position sense of joints, tension on muscles, movement of the arms and legs.

33. This figure is a representation of a _____ map.

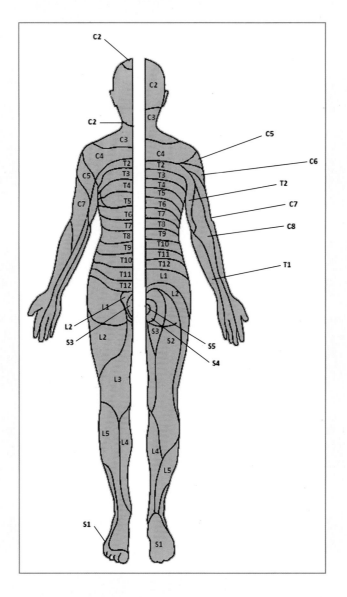

34. In the map of this image, the notation "C1" refers to the _____ _____ nerve.

35. _____ sense refers to the sense of smell.

36. _____ refers to the sense of taste.

37. Taste receptors are found within the _____ of the tongue epithelia.

38. _____ hair cells are considered to be the primary mechanism for auditory discrimination of frequency.

39. _____ hair cells serve the critical role of sound amplification.

40. There are approximately _____ (number of) inner hair cells.

41. There are approximately _____ (number of) outer hair cells.

42. _____ on each hair cell are deflected, causing ion flow into the hair cell.

43. Cilia on a given hair cell are connected by means of _____ _____.

44. Depolarization of _____ _____ _____ causes the hair cell to shorten, producing an impulse on the basilar membrane.

45. The _____ _____ is responsible for sensing changes in movement of the head.

46. The three _____ _____ of the vestibular mechanism send information about position of the body in space to the CNS.

47. The utricle and saccule respond to _____ of movement.

REFERENCES

Baehr, M., & Frotscher, M. (2012). *Duus' topical diagnosis in neurology: Anatomy, physiology, signs, symptoms,* (5th ed.) New York, NY: Thieme.

Bardoni, R., Tawfik, V. L., Wang, D., François, A., Solorzano, C., Shuster, S. A., . . . Scherrer, G. (2014). Delta opioid receptors presynaptically regulate cutaneous mechanoreceptory neuron input to the spinal cord dorsal horn. *Neuron, 81*(6), 1312–1327.

Barr, M. L. (1974). *The human nervous system* (2nd ed.). Hagerstown, MD: Harper and Row.

Bezençon, C., Le Coutre, J., & Damak, S. (2006). Taste-signaling proteins are coexpressed in solitary intestinal epithelial cells. *Chemical Senses, 32*(1), 41–49.

Bowman, J. P. (1971). *The muscle spindle and neural control of the tongue.* Springfield, IL: Charles C. Thomas.

Brodal, P. (2004). *The central nervous system* (3rd ed.). New York, NY: Oxford University Press.

Casimiro, C. C., Knollmann, B. C., Ebert, S. N., Vary, J. C., Greene, A. E., Franz, M. R., . . . Pfeifer, K. (2001). Targeted disruption of the Kcnq1 gene produces a mouse model of Jervell and Lange-Nielsen Syndrome. *Proceedings of the National Academy of Sciences USA, 98*(5), 2526–2531.

Carpenter, M. B. (1991). *Core text of neuroanatomy* (4th ed.). Baltimore, MD: Williams & Wilkins.

Dye, S. F., Vaupel, G. L., & Dye, C. C. (1998). Conscious neurosensory mapping of the internal structures of the human knee without intraarticular anesthesia. *American Journal of Sports Medicine, 26*(6), 773–777.

Hudspeth, A. J. (2014). Integrating the active process of hair cells with cochlear function. *Nature Reviews Neuroscience, 15*(9), 600–614.

Macefield, G., Gandevia, S. C., & Burke, D. (1990). Perceptual responses to microstimulation of single afferents innervating joints, muscles and skin of the human hand. *Journal of Physiology, 429*(1), 113–129.

Moller, A. R. (2003). *Sensory systems: Anatomy and physiology.* New York, NY: Academic Press.

Musiek, F. E., & Baran, J. A. (2007). *The auditory system: Anatomy, physiology and clinical correlates.* Boston, MA: Pearson.

National Research Council (US) Committee on Recognition and Alleviation of Pain in Laboratory Animals. (2009). *Recognition and alleviation of pain in laboratory animals.* Washington, DC: National Academies Press. Available from https://www.ncbi.nlm.nih.gov/books/NBK32658/ doi:10.17226/12526

Noback, C. R., Demarest, R. J., & Strominger, N. L. (1991). *The nervous system: Introduction and review.* Philadelphia, PA: Williams & Wilkins.

Nolte, J. (2002). *The human brain* (5th ed.). St. Louis, MO: Mosby Year Book.

Pearson, K. G., & Gordon, J. E. (2013). Spinal reflexes. In E. R. Kandel, J. H. Schwartz, T. M. Jessell, S. A. Siegelbaum, & A. J. Hudspeth (Eds.), *Principles of neural science* (5th ed., pp. 790–811). New York, NY: McGraw-Hill Medical.

Pickles, J. O. (2012). *An introduction to physiology of hearing* (4th ed.). Bingley, UK: Emerald Group.

Seikel, J. A., Drumright, D. G., & King, D. W. (2016). *Anatomy & physiology for speech, language and hearing* (5th ed.). Clifton Park, NY: Cengage Learning.

Spicer, S. S., & Schulte, B. A. (1996). The fine structure of spiral ligament cells relates to ion return to the stria and varies with place-frequency. *Hearing Research, 100*(1–2), 80–100.

Wangemann, P. (2002). K+ cycling and the endocochlear potential. *Hearing Research, 165*(1–2), 1–9.

Yavuz, U. S., Negro, F., Diedrichs, R., Türker, K. S., & Farina, D. (2017). Reflex circuitry originating from the muscle spindles to the tibialis anterior muscle. In *Converging clinical and engineering research on neurorehabilitation II* (pp. 177–181). Cham, Switzerland: Springer.

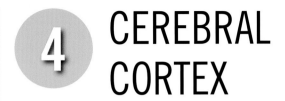

4 CEREBRAL CORTEX

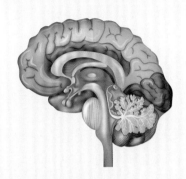

Learning Outcomes for Chapter 4

- Identify and define the larger functions of the lobes of the cerebrum, including frontal, parietal, occipital, temporal, and insular.

- Relate reflexive response to voluntary movement.

- Define the characteristics that differentiate the cerebral cortex from lower nervous system structures.

- Define the major differentiating structures of the cerebrum, including hemisphere, gyri, and sulci.

- Define and identify the specific gyri and sulci associated with speech, language, and hearing.

- Describe the physical elements and function of the meningeal linings.

- Describe the role of cerebrospinal fluid, its generation, and its circulation.

- Identify and describe the lateral, third, and fourth

INTRODUCTION

The cerebral cortex is the latest and highest evolutionary change in the human nervous system. The central nervous system is very hierarchical, and you can see the evolution within that hierarchy. We've alluded to this during our discussion of the spinal reflex arc, but it's time to put that into perspective. The spinal reflex arc is the basic sensorimotor communication system between the outside world and our bodies. A muscle stretches and the CNS causes it to return to its original length. Expand that to pain sensation, and painful stimulus causes a muscle to contract to protect the body (i.e., withdrawal from a hot stove). We can talk about pleasurable stimuli too, and how we move <u>toward</u> those.

We have fancier reflexes that cover multiple spinal cord segments, providing an even more complex response system. At the top of this spinal cord, an even more refined set of reflexes has evolved, housed in the brainstem (Figure 4–1). These reflexes mediate our interaction with the environment in complex ways, but at this level we still haven't reached a level of complexity that qualifies as "conscious." Even higher up in the CNS are the subcortical structures, particularly including the thalamus and basal ganglia. The thalamus is the major structure of the diencephalon (to be discussed in Chapter 5), and it is the last stop before the cerebral cortex for information that has come through senses from the spinal cord and brainstem sensory nerves. Put another way, the thalamus is the highest evolutionary sensory system that remains unconscious. In the same vein, the basal ganglia are a set of nuclei (to be discussed in Chapter 5) that are part of the highest non-conscious motor control system. These nuclei are close to consciousness and are capable of some very organized motor activity.

At the very top of this evolutionary pile is the cerebral cortex. The **cerebral cortex** is the place where consciousness arises and where voluntary action is initiated. Often we simply refer to "the cortex" rather than cerebral cortex because it is such a dominant force in our CNS. Realize that there are several other "cortices" (plural for cortex), since cortex simply means "bark," as in "bark of a tree."

So what is it that makes the cerebrum so special? It is the highest level of integration of all information that reaches the CNS, meaning that at this level sensory information from the eyes, ears, nose, skin, muscles, joints, and any other sense organs get integrated into one unified and organized whole (Craig, 2009). This is where our sense of self arises as a result of the interaction of some 17 billion neurons (Azevedo et al., 2009; Karlsen & Pakkenberg, 2011), because "self" is a concept that comes from weaving an image of what our senses tell us. Here's a number to boggle you: one cubic centimeter of the cerebral cortex (1 cm × 1 cm × 1 cm) contains about 44 million neurons (Pakkenberg & Gunderson, 1997), and each cubic centimeter of gray matter contains 90 billion synapses. The cerebral cortex has a volume of 1,000 cm^3 (0.4 cm thick and 2,500 sq. cm in surface area; Peters & Jones, 1984). This means that the average human brain ventricles and their means of communication.

- Describe the layers of the cerebral cortex, the dominant cell type by layer, and the general function of each layer in afferent and efferent processing.

- Identify the significant landmarks of the frontal lobe and their nominal roles, including superior frontal gyrus, middle frontal gyrus, inferior frontal gyrus, precentral gyrus, dorsolateral prefrontal cortex, supplementary motor area, premotor region, pars opercularis, pars orbitale, pars triangularis, and Broca's area

- Associate frontal lobe landmark and Brodmann area for BA 4, 6, 46/9, 44/45, and 11/10.

- Explain the significance of the motor homunculus.

- Identify the location and functional significance of the parietal landmarks, including the postcentral gyrus (SI), superior and inferior parietal lobules, intraparietal sulcus, postcentral sulcus, angular gyrus, supramarginal gyrus.

- Associate parietal lobe landmarks and Brodmann area for BA 1/2/3, 39, and 40.

- Identify the location and functional significance of the temporal lobe landmarks, including the superior, middle and inferior temporal gyri and sulci, Heschl's

gyrus, parahippocampal gyrus, Wernicke's area, and fusiform gyrus.

- Associate temporal lobe landmarks and Brodmann areas for BA 22, 41, 42, 21, and 20.

- Identify the location and functional significance of occipital lobe landmarks including preoccipital notch, parieto-occipital suture, calcarine sulcus, lingual gyrus, and cuneus, as well as their Brodmann areas (17, 19, 18).

- Associate insular cortex (BA 13, 14) and opercular components and their significance to speech, language, and cognition.

- Identify the components of the limbic system, including amygdala, hippocampus, cingulate gyrus, olfactory bulb and tract, and dentate gyrus.

- Identify the location and discuss the function of the medial cerebrum landmarks, including cingulate gyrus, corpus callosum, paracentral lobule, and precuneus.

- Identify the components of the corpus callosum and discuss the areas served by each component, including the genu, body, rostrum, anterior commissure, and splenium.

- Identify the components and discuss the functional significance of the inferior surface of the cerebrum, including the fusiform, lingual, and parahippocampal

gyri, temporal pole, gyrus rectus, olfactory sulcus, and hypophysis.

- Associate the regions of the inferior cortex with their Brodmann areas, including BA 37, 19, 27, 34, 38, 11, and 10.

- Describe the location and general function of projection, short and long association, and commissural fibers, as well as the significance of the corona radiata, and internal capsule.

- Describe the components and significance of the internal capsule, including the tracts of the posterior and anterior limbs, as well as the genu.

- Briefly differentiate the corticobulbar and corticospinal tracts, including origin, passage through the internal capsule, and broad function.

- Discuss the function of the specific long association fiber tracts, including the uncinate fasciculus, anterior and posterior cingulate cortex, superior longitudinal fasciculus, arcuate fasciculus, inferior longitudinal fasciculus, perpendicular fasciculus, occipitofrontal fasciculus, and fornix.

- Describe the functional differences between dominant and nondominant cerebral hemispheres, including functions for language, spatial processing, attention, handedness, skilled movement, analysis and synthesis, speed of processing, semantic processing differences, humor, idiom, sarcasm, and metaphor processing.

- Describe the functional differences found in parallel left and right hemisphere structures, including fusiform gyrus, dorsolateral prefrontal cortex, BA 44/45, and insular cortex.

- Describe the types of attention and their roles, including alerting, orienting, and executive attention.

- Explain the effects of hemispatial neglect and the hypothesized cause.

- Describe the types of misidentification syndromes and the common physical lesion sites for all of them.

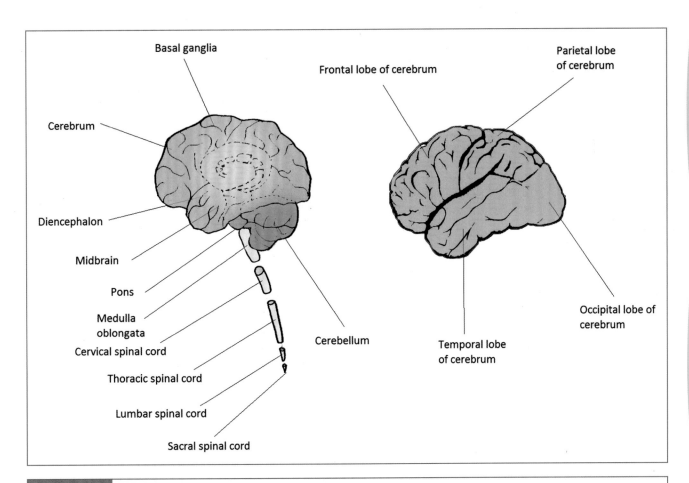

FIGURE 4–1.   Major components of the central nervous system.

of 17 billion neurons has over 90 trillion (90,000,000,000) synapses. If you were to count 1 synapse per second without stopping, you would be over 2,850 years old before you finished!

In the same vein, the cerebral cortex is where we are able to voluntarily respond or act on the environment. At the spinal cord and brainstem levels, we're simply <u>reacting</u> to stimuli, but the cerebral cortex allows us to <u>respond</u> to stim-

uli based on reasoned decision making. We are consciously aware at the level of the cortex, and we make conscious decisions to act from there, and this is critically important to us as therapists. The ability to reflect on our actions and make change is essential for success in any endeavor. We are conscious because of the complexity of the cerebral cortex, and we can make sense of our sensory universe and make decisions about how to respond to it. Pretty heady stuff!

Confabulation

Confabulation is a process of creating an unreal representation of reality based on missing components of memory. This is not the same as lying, which is a deliberate attempt to misrepresent yourself or other information. You can think of reality as a "connect the dots" picture: the dots are our sensations and our memory of how those sensations connect with other information. I smell bread cooking, see sunlight coming in the window, and hear birds singing: my cognitive processes connect these sensory perceptions with memories of their occurrence in the past, so that I have a percept that binds them together and very likely elicits a strong positive emotional response. I think about the times I've sat at the kitchen table, eating freshly baked bread, listening to the beautiful sounds of the day. We weave the fabric of reality from these perceptions and memory of them having occurred in the past, either together or separately (for instance, I have smelled bread baking in a bakery, and have heard birds at the park). Because we have amazingly powerful memories and multiple, multiple sensory inputs at any instant, this reality we weave looks and feels "solid" and immutable. Enter brain damage.

A client of ours had suffered brain damage from a cardiac event that left her anoxic for several minutes. The brain damage was diffuse, ultimately thinning her cerebral cortex. As she emerged from her coma it was apparent that she had numerous deficits and yet had a very intact language and speech system, as well as an excellent sense of humor. Essentially, she had lost a great deal of her memory and her "gnosis," or knowledge, of objects (tactile agnosia is the inability to "know" what something is when perceived through the touch modality). She had tactile agnosia, some auditory agnosia, visual agnosia, and cortical blindness (cortical blindness occurs when the pathways for vision are intact but a lesion to the cerebral cortex causes one to be unable to see).

Our client had all the components necessary to demonstrate exquisite confabulation. Her memory, sensation, and cognitive processes had significant holes, so the "dots" in her connect-the-dots picture were much farther spaced apart than ours. With her intact language and speech system, she simply wove the parts she did have into a fabric that made sense to her. Her mind "wanted" an intact reality, and she wove that reality out of the content she had available. She had the memory of flying in a small plane, and one of spending a fun weekend in Reno, and wove that into a story of piloting a small plane to Reno for a weekend at the blackjack tables.

But what is it that gives such super-powers to the cerebral cortex? All of that neural density and complexity leads to a level of self-organization that we are only just now dreaming of in the computer science and artificial intelligence worlds. The brain is the most complex and highly evolved structure in the known universe, and the very nature of that complexity and that neural density gives it the possibility for creating this most complex of the cognitive processes, consciousness. We need to acknowledge, as we lay out a framework of structures and their functions, that the whole is very much greater than the sum of the parts! Since the cerebral cortex reflects something of the pinnacle of this entire neurophysiological process, let's look at it in detail.

Cerebrovascular Accident Due to Arteriosclerosis

Cerebrovascular accident (CVA), also known as stroke, is a condition arising from loss of oxygen and nutrients to the brain. CVA can occur from one of two broad etiologies: ischemia or hemorrhage. **Ischemia** refers to loss or reduction of blood flow due to some blockage, such as a clot or a narrowing of an artery, while **hemorrhage** is blood being released out of the blood vessel into the surrounding area. These two phenomena are often related. **Arteriosclerosis** is a category of diseases in which there is a thickening of an artery wall that results in stenosis (narrowing) of the artery. The artery wall loses elasticity, which contributes to increased blood pressure (**hypertension**). **Atherosclerosis** is a form of arteriosclerosis in which the white blood cells and smooth muscle cells combine to occlude the artery. Because many of the white blood cells are still functional, inflammation occurs at the site. Other cells, including cholesterol and triglycerides, contribute to the occlusion. The accumulated cells crystallize on the inner surface, and if they break loose from the blockage, they enter the bloodstream as a floating clot known as an **embolus**. An **embolism** is the condition in which an embolus becomes lodged in a location.

Both arteriosclerotic plaque and embolus can cause a CVA, as either can starve an organ of blood. A common site of occlusion is the bifurcation of the common carotid artery into the internal and external carotid arteries. If an embolus is sufficiently large to block the internal carotid artery, all of the speech and language areas will be affected due to ischemia involving the middle cerebral artery.

GENERAL STRUCTURES AND LANDMARKS OF THE CEREBRAL CORTEX

The cerebral cortex consists of a number of important landmarks that all coalesce into this marvelously functioning structure. Let's start with some basic concepts.

The cerebral cortex is a voluminous structure that, on gross examination, has two mirror-image halves (**cerebral hemispheres**), a number of outfoldings and infoldings, and large separations or fissures. The larger components of the central nervous system are separated by three **meningeal linings** that protect and support the structure of the brain.

The cortex itself is a 4-mm thick layer of gray matter (neuron cell bodies) that overlies a mass of white matter fibers. This layer folds in on itself in many locations, forming **gyri** (plural of gyrus) as outfoldings, and **sulci** (plural of sulcus), which are infoldings.

Major Sulci and Fissures

As shown in Figure 4–2, there are numerous major landmarks that help us navigate the cerebral cortex. The cerebral cortex is divided into left and right hemispheres, separated by the **superior longitudinal fissure**. Each hemisphere has a significant **precentral gyrus**, which is the boundary between the frontal and parietal lobes (to be discussed later). On each side is the temporal lobe, separated from the frontal and parietal lobes by the **lateral fissure** (or **lateral sulcus** or **Sylvian fissure**).

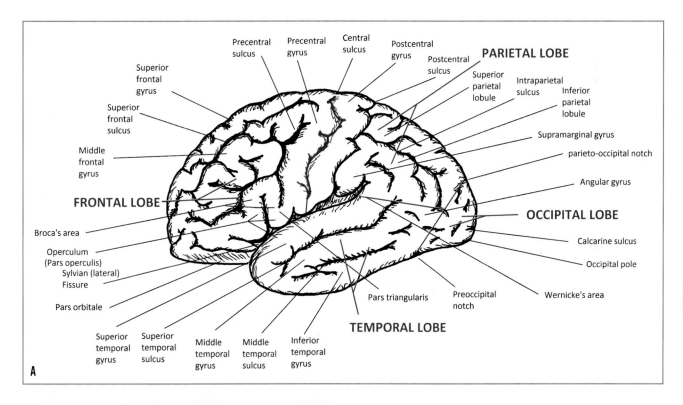

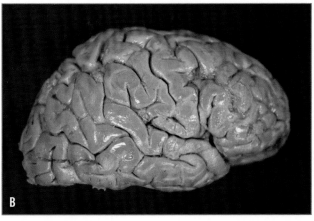

FIGURE 4–2. **A.** Lateral surface of the left hemisphere and **B.** photograph of lateral cortex. *continues*

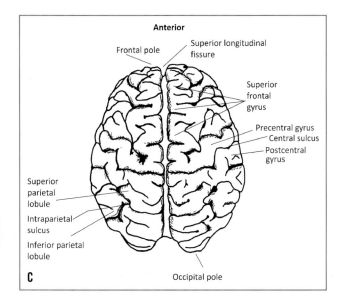

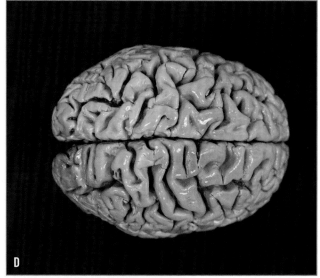

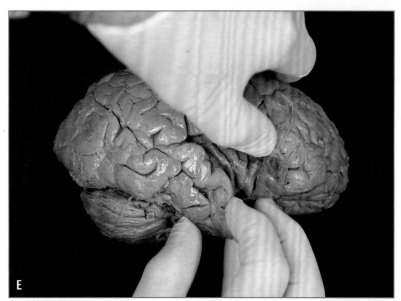

FIGURE 4–2. *continued* **C.** Superior surface of the cerebral cortex and **D.** photograph of superior cortex. **E.** Deflection of the operculum to reveal insular cortex. *continues*

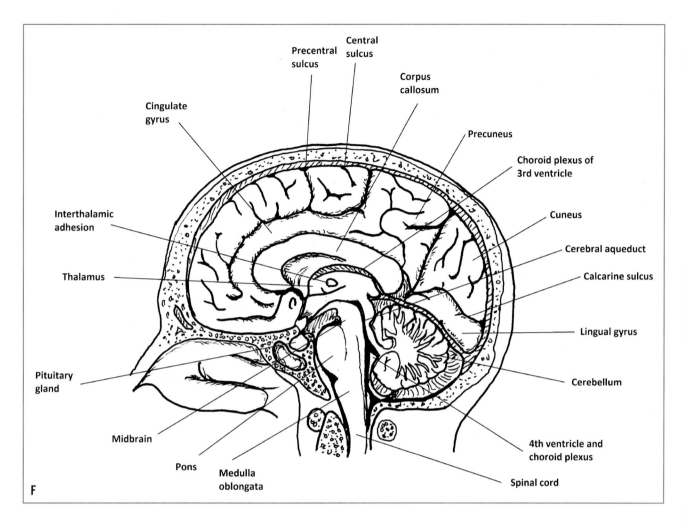

Precentral sulcus

Central sulcus

Corpus callosum

Cingulate gyrus

Precuneus

Choroid plexus of 3rd ventricle

Interthalamic adhesion

Cuneus

Cerebral aqueduct

Thalamus

Calcarine sulcus

Lingual gyrus

Pituitary gland

Cerebellum

Midbrain

4th ventricle and choroid plexus

Pons

Medulla oblongata

Spinal cord

F

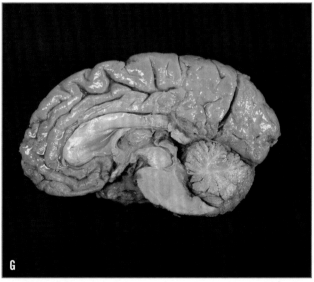

G

FIGURE 4–2. *continued* **F.** Medial surface of cerebral cortex and **G.** photograph of medial surface.

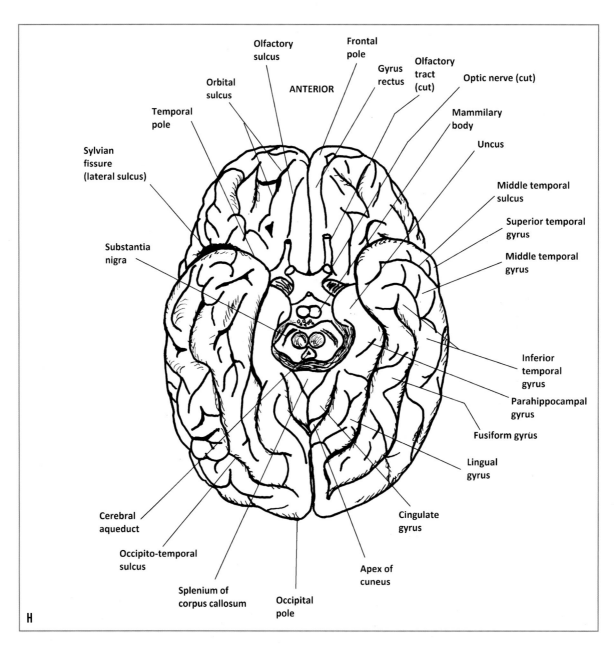

Olfactory sulcus

Frontal pole

Orbital sulcus

Gyrus rectus

ANTERIOR

Olfactory tract (cut)

Optic nerve (cut)

Temporal pole

Mammilary body

Sylvian fissure (lateral sulcus)

Uncus

Middle temporal sulcus

Superior temporal gyrus

Middle temporal gyrus

Substantia nigra

Inferior temporal gyrus

Parahippocampal gyrus

Fusiform gyrus

Lingual gyrus

Cerebral aqueduct

Cingulate gyrus

Occipito-temporal sulcus

Apex of cuneus

Splenium of corpus callosum

Occipital pole

H

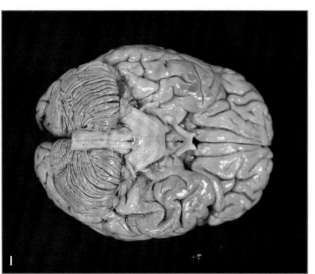

I

FIGURE 4–2. *continued* **H.** Inferior surface of cerebrum and **I.** photograph of inferior surface.

Meningeal Linings

The entire CNS is wrapped with a triple-layer meningeal lining that protects and provides nutrients to the neurons and glial cells. There are three meningeal coverings: the dura mater, the arachnoid mater, and the pia mater (Figure 4–3). The **dura mater** (*dura* = tough; *mater* = mother) is the outermost layer of the meninges and is composed of two layers of tough connective tissue that are tightly bound together. The outer layer is more inelastic than the inner layer, and the space between them is termed the epidural space. The **arachnoid mater** is a spider-like covering (arachnoid = spider; *mater* = mother) that lies beneath the dura mater and through which many blood vessels of the brain pass. It is a lacey, filamentous lining, spider-like in structure, and is easily disrupted during dissection. The innermost layer is the **pia mater** (*pia* = pious; *mater* = mother), which delicately envelopes all of the sulci and gyri of the CNS. It contains the major blood vessels that serve the surface of the cerebrum (Baehr & Frotscher, 2012).

The role of the meninges is to protect the brain. The dura mater has firm attachment to the skull, keeping the two hemispheres and lesser structures from moving very much during acceleration, thereby protecting the brain from trauma associated with movement of the brain within the brain case.

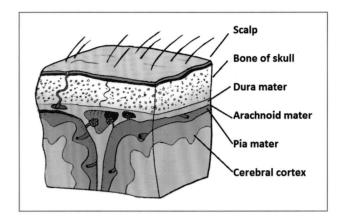

FIGURE 4–3. Layers of meningeal linings, as related to the superficial bone of the skull and the deep tissue of the brain. Note that the dura mater is superficial to the arachnoid mater, with the pia mater being the deepest of the meningeal linings, through which much of the cerebrovascular supply of the superficial brain courses.

Subdural Hematoma

A **hematoma** is an accumulation of blood outside of the vascular system, typically arising from hemorrhage. A **subdural hematoma** (SDH) is an accumulation of blood below the dura mater of the brain. Hemorrhage can arise from two major causes: trauma and aneurysm.

Trauma-induced subdural hematomas frequently arise from traumatic brain injury. An SDH may arise from trauma or from a penetrating, fracturing wound to the skull, but the result is that blood vessels within the meningeal linings rupture (Mori & Maeda, 2001). In both cases, the SDH arises from a response to an acceleration injury. Blood accumulates into the area beneath the dura mater (superficial to the brain) and exerts increasingly greater pressure on brain structures. On imaging, the brain structures will appear asymmetrical, with midline structures being pushed away from the hematoma. If the pressure is not alleviated, the brainstem may herniate through the foramen magnum, compressing nuclei and pathways essential for life. This is obviously a life-threatening situation, and the patient is in grave danger of death. In days before improved imaging, patients with subdural hematoma were often referred to as "talk and die" patients because they would be admitted to the emergency room for treatment of traumatic brain injury and would be lucid and talking, but would slip into a coma. The hemorrhage would produce the pressure discussed above, causing irreversible damage to the brainstem. Fortunately, modern imaging techniques have made it possible to visualize such injuries in a timely (and often lifesaving) manner.

Chronic subdural hematoma (CSDH) is defined as bleeding in the brain that occurs following the original injury by many days or weeks. Males are more likely to suffer from these than females, and those in their sixth and seventh decade of life are much more likely to develop the condition. The etiology of CSDHs is less obvious, as they can occur spontaneously. Certainly hypertension is a risk factor, as is chronic alcohol use or prior neurosurgery. The highest risk factor for CSDH is prior mild head injury (Mori & Maeda, 2001).

The dura mater has four infoldings that support and surround major structures of the brain. The two cerebral hemispheres are separated by the **falx cerebri**, which is attached to the anterior and posterior inner brain case (Figures 4–4A and 4–5). The falx cerebri is perpendicular to the primary dural lining and separates the left and right cerebral hemispheres down to the level of the corpus callosum (to be discussed). The **falx cerebelli** is a similar vertical shelf that separates the two cerebellar hemispheres, while the **tentorium cerebelli** is a horizontal dural shelf that separates the cranium into superior (cerebral) and inferior (cerebellar) regions (see Figure 4–5). A final dural subdivision is the **diaphragma sellae**, which encases the hypophysis (pituitary

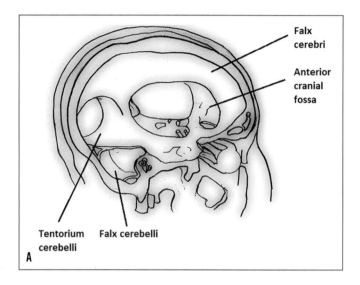

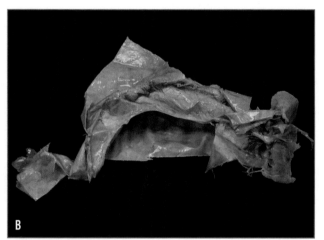

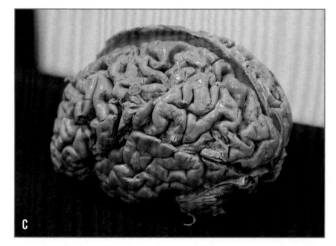

FIGURE 4–4. Dura mater components. **A.** Note that the falx cerebri separates left and right cerebral hemispheres, while the falx cerebelli separates the cerebellar hemispheres. The tentorium cerebelli separates the cerebrum above from the cerebellum, below. The diaphragma sellae is not shown. **B.** Photograph of portion of dura mater removed from cerebrum. **C.** Falx cerebri in situ.

gland), a pedunculated structure that arises from the base of the brain. The diaphragma sellae forms a boundary between the pituitary gland and the hypothalamus and optic chiasm. The dura mater also encircles the cranial nerves as they exit the brainstem (Figure 4–6). The **tentorium cerebelli** has a very important role in that it supports the cerebrum and keeps its mass from compressing the cerebellum and brainstem, which would most certainly happen if the dural lining were absent.

Problems arise from the dural shelves, however, during acceleration trauma, as in vehicular accidents. A **subdural hematoma** occurs when a cerebral blood vessel is ruptured. The pressure from the hematoma can push against the dural shelf, causing a shift in the brain that can be life-threatening and most likely will cause brain damage. Subdural hematoma

may also cause herniation of the brainstem into the foramen magnum of the skull, an acutely life-threatening condition.

Taken as a whole, the meningeal linings provide a significant protection for the structures of the CNS. The tough dura mater separates delicate neural tissue from bone. The pia mater supports the nutritive function of the vascular supply by encasing the blood vessels serving the brain. Cerebrospinal fluid courses through the arachnoid mater (as well as superficial to the dura mater).

The Ventricles and Cerebrospinal Fluid

Cerebrospinal fluid (CSF) bathes the CNS, providing a cushion for the neural tissue, some nutrient delivery, and an important waste removal process that occurs during sleep

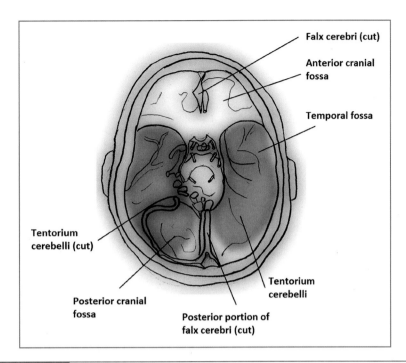

FIGURE 4–5. Superior view of dura mater. Note that the tentorium cerebelli forms the resting place for the cerebrum, with cavities defined by the dura holding the laterally placed temporal lobes, anterior frontal lobe (anterior cranial fossa), and the parietal and occipital lobes. The cerebellum will reside beneath the tentorium cerebelli within the posterior cranial fossa.

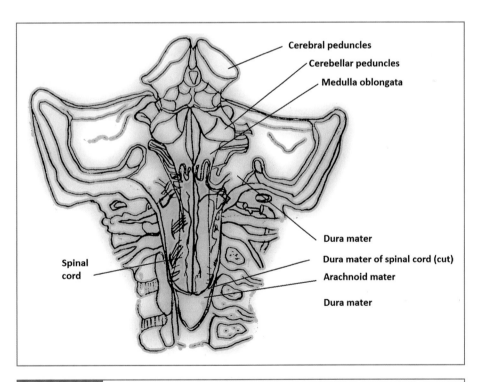

FIGURE 4–6. Meningeal linings of the brainstem and spinal cord. Note that the dura mater of the brainstem region would encase the cerebellum (removed), and that the tentorium cerebellum is found at the level of the midbrain in the brain stem. Cranial nerves transit the dura mater on the way to exit or enter the braincase.

(Xie et al., 2013). The ventricles of the CNS are the product of flexing the neural tube during embryonic development, and CSF is generated within these spaces. The system of ventricles consists of four cavities: the right lateral ventricle, the left lateral ventricle, the third ventricle, and the fourth ventricle (Figure 4–7). Within each ventricle is a choroid plexus that produces CSF. While all ventricles produce CSF, the **choroid plexuses** of the lateral ventricles produce the bulk of the fluid. CSF encases the cerebral cortex, providing a cushion that protects against sudden acceleration, and the presence of CSF in the ventricles further supports this protective function.

The two **lateral ventricles** are the largest of the ventricles. They consist of four spaces that extend into each of the lobes of the cerebral cortex and are shaped somewhat like a horse-shoe opened toward the front of the brain. The **anterior horn** of the lateral ventricles projects into the frontal lobes to the genu of the corpus callosum. The medial wall of the lateral ventricles is the **septum pellucidum**, a thin membrane separating the left and right lateral ventricles. The inferior margin is the head of the caudate nucleus, to be discussed. The central portion of the lateral ventricles is located within the parietal lobe and includes the region between the interventricular foramen of Monro (the means of communication between the lateral and third ventricles) and the splenium. The superior boundary of the lateral ventricles is the corpus callosum, and the inferior is part of the caudate nucleus of the basal ganglia. The **posterior** or **occipital horn** extends

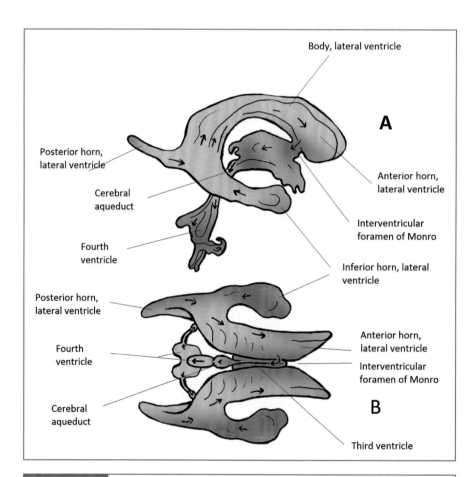

FIGURE 4–7.   Ventricles of the cerebrum, showing lateral, third, and fourth ventricles. **A.** Lateral view of ventricles. Note that the anterior horn resides within the frontal lobe, while the body spans portions of the posterior frontal lobe and the anterior parietal lobe. The inferior horn resides within the temporal lobe, while the posterior horn is within the occipital lobe. The third ventricle communicates with the lateral ventricles by means of the interventricular foramen of Monro, and with the fourth ventricle by means of the cerebral aqueduct. Arrows indicate direction of flow of cerebrospinal fluid. **B.** Superior view of ventricular system, showing relationship among ventricles.

into the occipital lobe to a tapered end, with its superior and lateral surfaces being the corpus callosum. The inferior horn is housed in the temporal lobe, curving down behind the thalamus and terminating behind the temporal pole. The hippocampus is the lower margin of the inferior horn.

The **third ventricle** rests between the left and right thalami and hypothalami and is connected with the lateral ventricles by means of the **interventricular foramen of Monro**. The roof of the third ventricle is the **tela choroidea**, a part of the pia mater of the ventricle. The ventricle extends inferiorly to the level of the optic chiasm. The **interthalamic adhesion** (*massa intermedia* or intermediate mass) crosses the third ventricle, connecting the left and right thalami. The CSF of the lateral ventricle passes into the third ventricle by means of left and right interventricular foramina.

The **fourth ventricle** resides between the cerebellum and the brainstem, specifically spanning the regions of the medulla and pons. CSF flows from the third ventricle to the fourth ventricle by means of the **cerebral aqueduct**, a tiny and vulnerable passageway (Figure 4–8). In order to see the fourth ventricle, you must remove the cerebellum. The floor of the fourth ventricle is the junction of the pons and medulla, and the cerebellum forms the roof of the fourth ventricle. The fourth ventricle has three openings: the paired **left and right lateral apertures** (foramina of Luschka) and the **median aperture** (foramen of Magendie) conduct CSF to the subarachnoid space behind the brainstem and beneath the cerebellum.

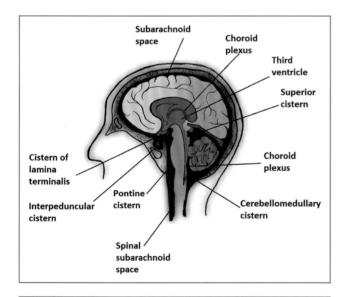

FIGURE 4–8. Diagram showing cisterns of the meninges. Cisterns are openings within the pia and arachnoid mater through which cerebrospinal fluid flows. Note the choroid plexus of the third and fourth ventricles, which create cerebrospinal fluid (lateral ventricle choroid plexus is not shown).

Circulation of CSF

Approximately 500 mL of CSF is created by the choroid plexuses of the ventricles every 24 hours, with about 125 mL being in the ventricular system at any time. CSF is under constant pressure, flowing out of the ventricles and into the periventricular space, ultimately being absorbed into the venous drainage system. This circulation of CSF provides critical waste removal from the intercellular spaces of the brain. Circulation of the CSF begins at the most distal point in the ventricular system, the lateral ventricles. From there, CSF courses through the interventricular foramina of Monro to the third ventricle, and then via the cerebral aqueduct to the fourth ventricle. From there the CSF enters the circulation around the brain structures by means of the three foramina (the paired foramina of Luschka and the medially placed foramen of Magendie), entering the cerebellomedullary cistern beneath the cerebellum. CSF then flows through around the periphery of the cerebellum and cerebrum, to exit through the dural arachnoid granulations of the venous system. The CSF may also course from the fourth ventricle through the subarachnoid space surrounding the spinal cord.

To summarize, the cerebral cortex is protected by cerebrospinal fluid and the meningeal linings, dura mater, pia mater, and arachnoid mater.

- The meningeal linings give support for delicate neural and vascular tissue. The dura mater divides into segments that correspond to the regions of the brain supported, including the falx cerebri, falx cerebelli, tentorium cerebelli, and diaphragma sellae. The spinal meningeal linings similarly protect the spinal cord from movement trauma.
- Two lateral ventricles are connected with the third ventricle by means of the interventricular foramen of Monro. The third and fourth ventricles communicate by means of the cerebral aqueduct. CSF flows from lateral ventricles to third and then fourth ventricles and exits the brain through the foramina of Luschka and foramen of Magendie at the level of the cerebellum. CSF courses around the brain and spinal cord, exiting the cranial space through the arachnoid granulations, into the venous drainage system.

Cell Types of the Cerebral Cortex

The cerebral cortex is approximately 4 mm thick and is made up of six cell layers. The cellular layers of the cerebral cortex bear a functional relationship to the primary activity of a brain region, as we'll see (Figure 4–9). The layers of the cerebral cortex consist of both pyramidal and non-pyramidal cells (Peters & Jones, 1984). **Pyramidal cells** are large, pyramid-shaped cells involved in initiation of motor function. The pyramidal cells orient so their axons project medially away

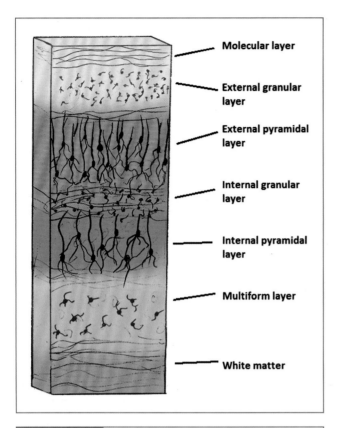

Molecular layer

External granular layer

External pyramidal layer

Internal granular layer

Internal pyramidal layer

Multiform layer

White matter

FIGURE 4–9. Layers of the cerebral cortex. The outer surface of the cerebrum (cortex) is about 4 mm thick, and is made up of six layers of cell bodies. Note that the white matter is deep to the cortex, and consists of the axons of neurons found within the cortex.

Layers of the Cerebral Cortex

The cerebral cortex consists of six layers: (1) the outermost molecular layer, (2) the external granular layer, (3) the external pyramidal layer, (4) the internal granular layer, (5) the internal pyramidal layer, and (6) the multiform layer. The **outermost molecular layer** consists mostly of glial cells and axons from neurons of succeeding layers. The second (**external granular**) and third (**external pyramidal**) layers consist of small and large pyramidal cells, respectively, and are very involved in motor function. The fourth (**internal granular**) layer receives sensory input from the thalamus and is made up of non-pyramidal cells. The fifth (**internal pyramidal**) layer is made up of large pyramidal cells that project to motor centers beyond the cerebral cortex (basal ganglia, brainstem, spinal cord). This layer is the origin of some of the tracts and fibers that connect the cortex with the subcortex, to be discussed. The sixth (**multiform**) layer consists of pyramidal cells that project to the thalamus (Briggs & Usrey, 2008).

The dominant function of an area of the cortex determines the prevalent type of neuron in that region. As an example, the pyramidal layers are thickest in areas of the cerebral cortex responsible for motor function, so you will see layers 3 and 5 with the greatest representation of cells. In areas that receive a great deal of sensory information, you will see a preponderance of stellate cells, so layers 2 and 4 will be most richly represented. The precentral gyrus or motor strip (to be discussed) is the region of primary motor output, and it has extremely rich representation of the fifth layer and only a thin fourth layer. In contrast, the somatosensory receptive region of the postcentral gyrus has a rich fourth layer with few cells in the pyramidal layers. Areas that associate sensory and motor functions will have representation of both sensory and motor layers.

We owe a significant debt of gratitude to Korbinian Brodmann, who, in the early part of the twentieth century, developed a regional classification scheme of the brain based on the dominant cellular representation that he identified through light microscopy (Brodmann & Garey, 2007; Kandel & Hudspeth, 2013). His microscopic analysis showed that localized areas of the brain were dominated by specific cell types, and his "map" of the brain (the **Brodmann brain map**) has become a standard means of navigating and discussing brain function. Figure 4–10A–C will provide a reference point for our discussion of structure and function of the cerebral cortex. We'll talk about both the lateral and medial cerebral cortex, and finally the inferior surface of the cerebral cortex. You might also want to refer to Tables 4–1 and 4–2 as you go through this section.

from the cortical layer. One apical pyramidal cell dendrite typically projects to the outer layer of the cortex, with many basal dendrites projecting horizontally through the layer in which the cell body resides. The pyramidal cell axons project into the white matter beneath the cortex or beyond the cortex as projection fibers. They will also typically have axon branches within the cortex as well.

Non-pyramidal cells are small and are often star-shaped (**stellate**). They are involved in sensory function or associative intercommunication among brain regions. Their axons usually project only a short distance, typically staying within the same layer or to an adjacent layer. Non-pyramidal cells typically connect regions within the cerebral cortex, whereas pyramidal cells will typically project to more distant regions.

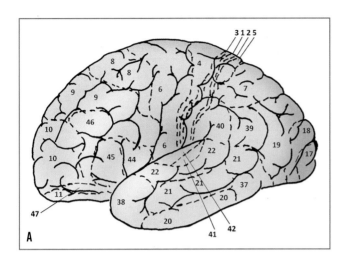

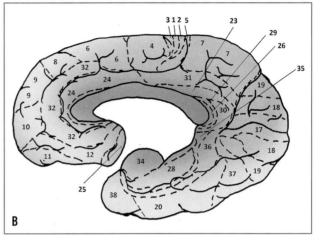

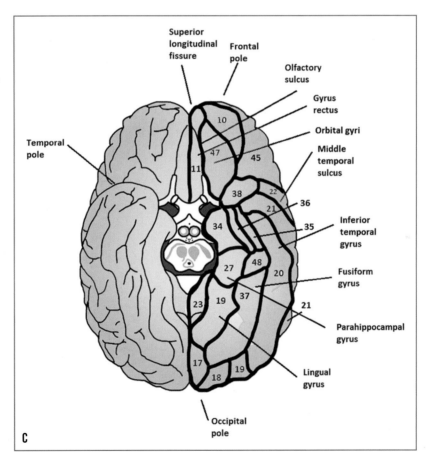

TABLE 4-1.	Locations Associated with Brodmann Areas	

Brodmann Number	Name and putative function	Location
3	Rostral postcentral gyrus (somatic sense reception area; a.k.a. *area posctentralis oralis*)	Rostral postcentral gyrus
1	Intermediate postcentral gyrus (somatic sense integration; a.k.a. *area postcentralis intermedia*)	Postcentral gyrus
2	Caudal postcentral gyrus (somatic sense integration; a.k.a. *area postcentralis caudalis*)	Caudal postcentral gyrus
4	Precentral gyrus (motor strip or primary motor cortex; a.k.a. gigantopyramidal; *area gigantopyramidalis*)	Precentral gyrus
5	Preparietal (a.k.a. *area praeparietalis*)	Dorsal parietal lobe; part of superior parietal lobule
6	Premotor cortex (premotor area; a.k.a. agranular frontal; *area frontalis agranularis*)	Anterior to precentral gyrus in frontal lobe
7	Superior parietal (a.k.a. *area parietalis superior*)	Part of superior parietal lobule and some of precuneus in medial cerebral surface
8	Intermedial frontal (a.k.a. *frontalis intermedia*)	Part of superior frontal gyrus, with extension into cingulate gyrus; functionally part of frontal eye field controlling conjugate eye movement
9	Granular frontal area (part of dorsolateral prefrontal cortex DLPFC or DLPC; a.k.a. granular frontal; *area frontalis granularis*)	Superior frontal gyrus and middle frontal gyrus
10	Anterior prefrontal cortex (a.k.a. frontal pole; frontopolar region; *area frontopolaris*)	Anterior-most frontal lobe
11	Straight gyrus (part of prefrontal cortex; a.k.a. orbitofrontal cortex; *area praefrontalis*)	Anterior-inferior frontal pole
12	Prefrontal area; part of orbitofrontal cortex (a.k.a. *area praefrontalis*)	Anterior-inferior medial cortex
13	Insular cortex	Deep to operculum (BA 44, 45)
15	Anterior Insular cortex (not originally identified by Brodmann in humans, but subsequently identified in humans by Fischer, Andersson, Furmark, & Fredrikson, 1998)	Deep to operculum (BA 44, 45)
16	Posterior Insular cortex (not defined in humans by Brodmann)	Deep to operculum (BA 44, 45)
17	Striate cortex (a.k.a., calcarine sulcus; *area striata*; primary visual cortex)	Posterior aspect of occipital lobe, bounded by calcarine sulcus
18	Parastriate area (higher order processing area for visual cortex: sometimes called secondary visual cortex; a.k.a. *area parastriata*)	On medial cortex, in posterior aspect including parts of the cuneus and lingual gyrus; on lateral cortex, includes areas surrounding striate cortex
19	Lingual gyrus (higher order processing area for visual cortex; a.k.a. *area parastriata*)	On inferior surface of cortex, medial to fusiform gyrus
20	Inferior temporal gyrus (a.k.a. *area temporalis inferior*)	Visible on lateral and inferior surface of temporal lobe
21	Middle temporal gyrus (a.k.a. *area temporalis media*)	Immediately superior to inferior temporal gyrus
22	Superior temporal gyrus (includes Wernicke's area in posterior aspect; a.k.a., *area temporalis superior*)	Forms superior lateral margin of temporal lobe

TABLE 4–1.   *continued*

Brodmann Number	Name and putative function	Location
23	Ventral posterior cingulate gyrus (a.k.a. ventral posterior cingulate; posterior cingulate cortex, PCC; *area cingulate posterior ventralis*)	Visible on medial view in posterior, adjacent to BA 17; visible as medial most aspect in posterior-inferior cerebrum
24	Ventral anterior cingulate gyrus (a.k.a. anterior cingulate cortex, ACC; *area cingularis anterior ventralis*)	Anterior aspect of cingulate gyrus, visible on medial view only
25	Subgenual area (portion of ventral prefrontal cortex; subgenal area, referring to genu of corpus callosum; a.k.a. *area subgenualis*)	Inferior cerebrum, in medial view, beneath genu of corpus callosum
26	Ectosplenial area (a.k.a. *area ectosplenialis*)	Posterior-most aspect of cingulate gyrus
27	Parahippocampal gyrus	On inferior surface, medial-most structure that is immediately lateral cerebral peduncles
28	Entorhinal area (a.k.a. *area entorhinalis*)	On medial surface, inferior to uncus
29	Granular retrolimbic (a.k.a., *area retrolimbica granularis*)	In medial view, posterior to cingulate gyrus
30	Agranular retrolimbic (a.k.a. *area retrolimbica granularis*)	In medial view, posterior to cingulate gyrus
31	Dorsal posterior cingulate (a.k.a. *area cingularis posterior dorsalis*)	In medial view, posterior-superior cingulate cortex
32	Dorsal anterior cingulate (a.k.a. *area cingularis anterior dorsalis*)	In medial view, anterior aspect of cingulate gyrus
33	Pregenual (a.k.a. *area praegenualis*)	Anterior-inferior aspect of cingulate gyrus
34	Dorsal entorhinal (a.k.a. uncus; *area entorhinalis dorsalis*)	Inferior surface, anterior to parahippocampal gyrus and lateral to cerebral peduncles
35	Perirhinal (a.k.a. *area perirhinalis*)	In posterior medial view, posterior to uncus and anterior to visual reception area
36	Ectorhinal (a.k.a. *area ectorhinalis*)	In posterior medial view, anterior to visual association areas 18 and 19
37	Occipitotemporal (a.k.a. fusiform gyrus, *area occipitotemporalis*)	On inferior surface, lateral to lingual gyrus, extending to lateral surface of temporal lobe
38	Temporopolar (a.k.a. *area temporopoloris*)	On inferior surface, lateral and anterior surfaces, anterior-most region of temporal lobe
39	Angular gyrus (a.k.a. *area angularis*)	On lateral cortex, posterior to superior temporal gyrus in parietal lobe
40	Supramargingal gyrus (*area supramarginalis*)	On inferior-lateral surface of parietal lobe, bordering temporal lobe
41	Heschl's gyrus (a.k.a. anterior transverse temporal; *area temporalis transversa anterior*)	On medial surfaces of temporal lobe, within lateral sulcus at mid-anterior region of temporal lobe
42	Higher order processing area for audition (part of belt) (a.k.a. posterior transverse temporal, *area temporalis transversa posterior*)	Region in lateral sulcus anterior to Heschl's gyrus
43	Subcentral (a.k.a. *area subcentralis*)	Inferior-lateral cerebrum in post-central gyrus
44	Pars operculum (a.k.a. opercular; *area opercularis)*; with BA 45, makes up Broca's area	On inferior-lateral surface of cerebrum, posterior to precentral gyrus

continues

TABLE 4–1.   *continued*

Brodmann Number	Name and putative function	Location
45	Pars triangularis (a.k.a. *area triangularis*); with BA 44, makes up Broca's area	On inferior-lateral surface of cerebrum, adjacent to pars operculum
46	Middle frontal gyrus; (part of dorsolateral prefrontal cortex; a.k.a. middle frontal gyrus; *area frontalis media*)	On lateral surface, superior to pars triangularis (BA 45)
47	Orbital area (a.k.a. *area orbitalis*)	On lateral-inferior surface in anterior cortex, and medial aspect of inferior surface.
52	Parainsular cortex (a.k.a. *area parainsularis*)	Located in lateral sulcus, superior aspect of temporal lobe

Note. If an area does not have a specific name, it is referred to in parentheses. Alternate names are also given in parentheses. Note that there are gaps in the numbering (for instance, BA 48 is missing). These gaps reflect the presence of Brodmann areas in non-humans, but absent in humans.

Sources for nomenclature: Brodmann, K., & Garey, L. J. (2007). *Brodmann's: Localisation in the Cerebral Cortex.* New York, NY: Springer. Kaiser, D. A. (2010). Cortical cartography. *Association of Applied Psychophysiology and Biofeedback, 38*(1), 9–12. NeuroNames Ontologies (BrainInfo (1991–present), National Primate Research Center, University of Washington, http://www.braininfo.org.); Mark Durban, Ph.D., University of Colorado; http://spot.colorado.edu/~dubin/talks/brodmann/neuronames.html

TABLE 4–2.   Major Landmarks of the Cerebral Cortex and Evident Functions

Region or lobe	Landmark	Primary function
Cerebral hemisphere	Superior longitudinal fissure	Separates cerebral hemisphere
Cerebral hemisphere	Sylvian fissure	Separates frontal and parietal lobes from temporal lobe
Cerebral hemisphere	Central sulcus	Separates frontal and parietal lobes
Frontal, temporal, parietal, occipital lobes	Lateral ventricle	Creation and circulation of CSF
(between thalami and hypothalamus: not in cerebrum)	Third ventricle	Creation and circulation of CSF
(between pons/medulla and cerebellum: not in cerebrum)	Fourth ventricle	Creation and circulation of CSF
Frontal lobe (dominant hemisphere)	Pars triangularis: Broca's area	Expressive language
Frontal lobe	Dorsolateral prefrontal cortex	Executive function
Frontal lobe	Precentral gyrus	Primary motor cortex (MI) motor execution; source of corticobulbar and corticospinal tracts
Frontal lobe	Premotor gyrus	Motor planning; execution of complex motor acts
Frontal lobe	Supplementary motor area (SMA)	Motor planning
Frontal lobe	Pars opercularis	Overlies insula
Frontal lobe	Pars orbitales	Limbic association area: memory, emotion, motor inhibition, processing of reward and punishment, and intellect

TABLE 4–2. *continued*

Region or lobe	Landmark	Primary function
Parietal lobe	Postcentral gyrus	Primary sensory cortex (SI); receives somatic sensation
Parietal lobe	Intraparietal sulcus of superior parietal lobule	Part of dorsal visual "where" stream; guidance for hand movement and acquisition of target
Parietal lobe	Angular gyrus	Reading comprehension, mathematical calculation, semantic processing
Parietal lobe	Supramarginal gyrus	Phonological processing
Temporal lobe	Wernicke's area	Language comprehension
Temporal lobe	Superior temporal sulcus	Language comprehension
Temporal lobe	Heschl's gyrus (core)	Auditory reception
Temporal lobe	Belt	Auditory signal differentiation
Temporal lobe	Parabelt	Auditory information processing
Temporal lobe	Inferior temporal gyrus	Part of ventral "what" visual stream; integration of visual information for identification of source
Occipital lobe	Calcarine sulcus	Primary reception of visual information (VI)
Occipital lobe	Lingual gyrus	Higher order visual processing
Occipital lobe	Cuneus	Higher order visual processing and sense of agency
Insular cortex	Anterior gyri, circular sulcus, central sulcus	Emotion processing; sense of self, insight, awareness; gustation; in dominant hemisphere, speech praxis
Limbic system (shared between cortical and subcortical structures)	Uncus (amygdala), parahippocampal gyrus (hippocampus), cingulate gyrus, olfactory bulb, dentate gyrus	Emotion processing and regulation
Medial cerebral cortex	Corpus callosum	Fibers connecting specific areas of one hemisphere with other hemisphere
Frontal and parietal lobe, medial cerebral cortex	Paracentral lobule (parietal lobe)	In frontal lobe, part of SMA; in parietal lobe, sensory and motor integration concerning urination and defecation
Parietal lobe, medial cerebral cortex	Precuneus (parietal lobe)	Visuospatial processing, episodic memory, sense of agency
Medial cerebral cortex	Cingulate gyrus	Emotional assessment and regulation, attention
Inferior occipital lobe	Fusiform gyrus	Identification of facial features (dominant hemisphere) and face identity (non-dominant hemisphere
Inferior occipital lobe	Lingual gyrus	Higher order processing for vision
Inferior temporal lobe	Parahippocampal gyrus and hippocampus	Memory function and olfaction
Inferior temporal lobe	Uncus (amygdala)	Fear processing and response; part of olfactory system
Inferior temporal lobe	Temporal pole	Emotion processing, face recognition, integration of emotion, autobiographical memory
Inferior frontal lobe	Gyrus rectus	Mediation of emotion, memory retrieval

Cortical Folding

We've talked about gyri and sulci, but how do they develop? Clearly, having gyri (outfoldings) and sulci (infoldings) allows the brain to have more surface area. If you wad up a piece of paper, you haven't changed the surface area of the paper, but you've made the overall "package" more compact. That having been said, the gyri and sulci are pretty well organized, since we can identify many specific functions and cell types related to specific gyri, such as the precentral gyrus. How do they get there?

Cortical tissue contains cells known as "**progenitors**," which are predetermined to become a specific cell type. As the brain develops, it receives afferent stimulation through contact with the environment. This stimulation mediates development of gyri. When stimulation is blocked through damage to the sensory system (e.g., vision), the gyri are malformed, and even distant gyri are altered due to lack of stimulation (Sun & Hevner, 2014). It may be that stimulation causes increased activity and synaptic development in a region, thus increasing volume within that cortical zone, resulting in a gyrus. Other gyri develop as a result of the pressures of the cerebrospinal fluid in ventricles,

although even this gyrus development, which appears to be caused by mechanical force of CSF pressure, appears to have genetically programmed progenitor cells that guide **gyrogenesis** (Sun & Hevner, 2014).

There are several conditions that correspond to breakdown in gyrogenesis. **Lissencephaly** is absence of gyri in the brain, seemingly caused by interference with cell migration during development. **Polymicrogyria** is characterized by many small gyri, typically caused by viral infection or hypoxia (loss of oxygenation of the brain tissue). People with Down syndrome have a narrow superior temporal gyrus, an area critical for language development, and maldevelopment of gyri around the Sylvian fissure has been associated with deficient language development generally (Galaburda & Geschwind, 1981). Albert Einstein, one of the most brilliant individuals of the twentieth century, was known to have reduced and late language development but exceptionally strong visuospatial and mathematical abilities. Post-mortem examination of his brain revealed absent gyrification in the right parietal opercular region overlying the right insula and reduced Sylvian fissure size, but highly developed right inferior parietal lobule (Sun & Hevner, 2014).

LOBES OF THE CEREBRAL CORTEX

The cerebral cortex is divided by the **cerebral longitudinal fissure** (also known as the superior longitudinal fissure or the interhemispheric fissure) into mirror-image left and right cerebral hemispheres (see Figure 4–2C). As you will remember, the falx cerebri runs through this space between the two hemispheres. The cerebral longitudinal fissure separates the hemispheres down to the level of the corpus callosum, the major group of fibers that provides communication between the two hemispheres.

The surface of the brain is quite convoluted, marked by outfoldings (gyri) and infoldings (sulci) that arise from early development. The brain begins development as a smooth monolith, but as it grows, it folds in on itself, creating the gyri and sulci. The result of this is greatly increased surface area of the cortex, one of the things that give the cerebral cortex its power.

The cerebral cortex is divided into five lobes (see Figure 4–2A). Four of these lobes are reasonably easy to identify and share names with the bones that overlie them: frontal, parietal, occipital, and temporal lobes. The fifth lobe (the insular lobe) requires you to pull part of the frontal lobe back to reveal it, so it is more difficult to find.

Look at the cerebral cortex in Figure 4–2A again, and find the **lateral sulcus** (also known as the **Sylvian fissure**).

This fissure completely separates the temporal lobe from the frontal and parietal lobes. Now find the **central sulcus**, dividing the cerebral cortex into front and back halves. This is the dividing line between the frontal lobe (anterior to the sulcus) and the parietal lobe (posterior to the sulcus). (You may also run across the term **Rolandic fissure** or **Rolandic sulcus** referring to the central sulcus.) If you look at the medial view of the cerebral cortex you will see that the central sulcus does not actually extend down that medial surface, but rather the **precentral gyrus** (anterior to the sulcus) reflects around to become the **postcentral gyrus** (posterior to the sulcus). When you are looking at a specimen, this feature helps you identify the central sulcus.

Frontal Lobe

The frontal lobe is the largest of the lobes and has great responsibility in terms of cognition and language. It houses the centers associated with planning events, initiation and execution of movement, and other important cognitive and metacognitive functions. It also contains the center associated with expressive language, Broca's area. The posterior boundary of the frontal lobe is the central sulcus, and the medial boundary is the superior longitudinal fissure.

There are a number of important frontal lobe landmarks to discuss. The frontal lobe can be divided into four major gyri: the **superior frontal gyrus**, **middle frontal gyrus**, **infe-**

rior frontal gyrus, and **precentral gyrus**. This would be a good time to compare Figures 4–2A and 4–10A so we can refer to Brodmann areas related to these gyri.

Brodmann's areas (BA) 46 and 9 are collectively referred to as the **dorsolateral prefrontal cortex** (DLPC or DLPFC). While this region has slightly different functions between the left and right hemispheres, the general role of the DLPFC is to direct the actions of the cerebral cortex. It tends to be active any time you willfully perform an action and is a critically important component of executive functions. **Executive functions** are metacognitive functions that use the cognitive processes to accomplish goals, such as directing attention, communication, planning, goal setting, etc.

Aphasia

Aphasia is a loss or reduction in comprehension and/or production of language arising from brain damage. The inability or reduced ability for naming (**anomia**) is the most prominent sign and is present in all aphasias. Naming of an object involves a series of stages, such as visual processing/recognition of the object, semantic processing, selection of an abstract representation, and finally the execution of the motor action for naming.

In visual processing and recognition of an object, occipito-parietal activation (referred to as the dorsal visual stream) ensures object localization and attention, while occipito-temporal activation (ventral visual stream) ensures subject recognition. Reception and recognition of a familiar object takes place in the occipito-temporal fusiform region. Patients with a lesion in this region area may demonstrate **apperceptive visual agnosia**, which involves being able to copy or describe an object but being unable to recognize it when it is presented. The lack of recognition leads to a lack of naming. **Progressive visuoperceptual deficit** is a symptom in diseases such as **posterior cortical atrophy** (PCA) and **Alzheimer's disease** (AD). In both conditions, there may be a disruption of dorsal (occipito-parietal) or ventral (occipito-temporal) networks. Bilateral involvement of occipito-temporal lesions may also be seen in infectious diseases such as **encephalitis** or vascular diseases such as **top-of-the-basilar syndrome** (Gleichgerrcht, Fridriksson, & Bonilha, 2015).

The semantic processing of the meaning of an object (either as general conceptual knowledge or as specific features of the object) takes place in anterior temporal lobes, more prominently in the left hemisphere. The patient with a lesion in such areas may present semantic paraphasias and circumlocutions. The superior gyrus of the left posterior temporal cortex is also responsible for semantic errors (Gleichgerrcht et al., 2015).

The selection of an abstract mental representation of an object takes place in areas such as the posterior portions of the temporal cortex and angular and inferior frontal gyri, including Broca's area. One study (Hebb & Ojemann, 2013) proposed including the thalamus in the network involving these areas. Numerous disease states can cause loss of this mental representation. Vascular lesions such as CVA (stroke), degeneration such as **logopenic primary progressive aphasia** (an aphasia characterized by impairments of naming and repetition), AD, and temporal lobe epilepsy lead to anomia and word retrieval symptomatology (Gleichgerrcht et al., 2015).

The execution of object naming takes place in processing areas such as the inferior frontal gyrus, the motor cortex, and the insula. A number of studies (Hickok, 2012; Hickok & Poeppel, 2007) proposed a dorsal pathway of processing information that transforms the mental into articulatory motor sound representations. This is in contrast to a proposed ventral pathway that is responsible for processing information for comprehension. The latter connects the temporal lobes with the temporoparietal junction. The agrammatic nonfluent forms of primary progressive aphasia, Broca's aphasia, and/or Wernicke's aphasia rarely arise from lesions in the inferior frontal gyrus or insula, unlike nonfluent aphasia from infarct.

The **precentral gyrus** (predominantly BA 4) is responsible for direct voluntary activation of the muscles of the body. You will remember the important reflexes that cause muscles to contract. The precentral gyrus provides the volitional function that is parallel to reflexive response, in that skilled motor function arises from activation of this region of the brain. It is time to introduce the important concept of **spatiotopic representation**. You are likely already familiar with tonotopic representation of sound in the cochlea, where high frequencies are analyzed at the basal end of the cochlea, while low frequencies are processed at the apex. The physical body is arrayed in a very similar fashion on the precentral and postcentral gyrus. Figure 4–11 is a view of the cerebrum along the precentral gyrus and postcentral gyrus, essentially representing a coronal section through the brain. This view is termed the **homunculus**, which means "little body." Study this for a minute. The right side of the image represents the location of the precentral gyrus (also known as the motor strip) at which activation of the musculature associated with the image occurs. Realize that our knowledge of this mapping reflects many years of work by early neuroscientists in mapping the brain through direct brain stimulation (Penfield & Roberts, 1959; Schaltenbrand & Woolsey, 1964). Notice that the lower leg and foot are tucked into the superior longitudinal fissure, on the medial surface of the cerebrum. The knee, upper leg, arm, and hand are represented at the superior and

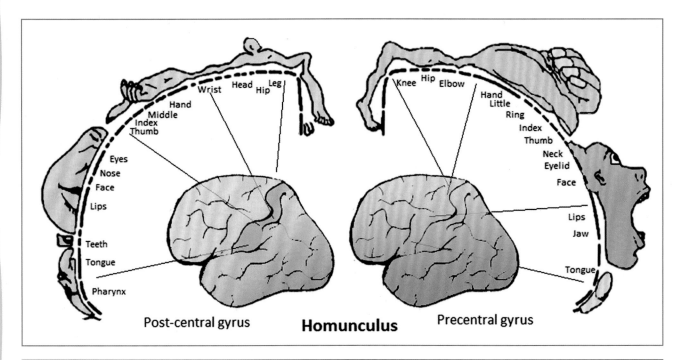

Post-central gyrus   **Homunculus**   Precentral gyrus

FIGURE 4–11. Sensory and motor homunculus of the human cerebral cortex. Note that the size of the homunculus parts reflects the magnitude of the components dedicated to that particular structure.

superior-lateral aspects of the precentral gyrus. Structures of the head and mouth are located on the lateral surface.

One more important aspect of the homunculus is the fact that the relative size of the structure reflects the density of the cortical neurons that serve that area. The lower leg has relatively few cortical neurons serving it, but the fingers are very well represented. The more neurons there are to activate a structure, the higher the degree of specificity is available. Basically, having more neurons gives you the ability to make highly refined movements: there's a reason you don't play a violin with your feet! We are going to see this spatiotopic array repeated in other areas as well, as it reflects an organizational principle of the nervous system: inputs to the cerebral cortex are spatially organized.

The **supplementary motor area (SMA)** is a region that includes parts of the superior and middle frontal gyrus, abutting the precentral gyrus. As you can see from the Brodmann map, BA 6 traverses the entire medial cerebral cortex, and the superior aspect of this encompassing the superior and middle frontal gyri are considered to be the SMA. BA 6 is termed the **premotor region**, and it can be thought of as a motor preparation and planning region. The SMA is specifically involved in motor rehearsal and perhaps in inhibition of motor response. Axons arising from the precentral gyrus, the premotor region, and the SMA give rise to the corticospinal and corticobulbar tracts, the major motor tracts of voluntary

movement on the side of the body opposite to the area of the cortex giving the command. We will talk more about how this "contralateral innervation" occurs when we discuss pathways of the brain.

Now look at the inferior frontal gyrus in Figures 4–10A and 4–2A. This gyrus is home to three important regions, the **pars opercularis**, **pars orbitale**, and **pars triangularis**. The pars opercularis ("opercular part" or "frontal operculum"; operculum means "lips") is the region overlying the "hidden lobes" of the insular cortex, to be discussed. BA 44 and 45 of the frontal operculum are considered to be the critically important **Broca's area**, an extremely important region for speech motor planning within the dominant hemisphere. The pars orbitale (orbitofrontal cortex, OFC) is BA 11, the portion of the inferior frontal lobe overlying the eyes. BA 11 and 10 are often considered to be part of the **limbic association area**, to be discussed. As such, the pars orbitale is associated with memory, emotion, motor inhibition, processing of reward and punishment, and intellect (Kringelbach & Rolls, 2004). The orbitofrontal cortex is apparently involved in normalization of traumatic events, and a dysfunction of the OFC is seen in posttraumatic stress disorder (PTSD) (Dileo, Brewer, Hopwood, Anderson, & Creamer, 2008). It is also involved in the reward system for learning (De Young, 2010), as well as behavioral inhibition and smell recognition (Malloy, Bihrle, & Duffy, 1993).

Upper Motor Neuron Dysarthria

Dysarthria is a motor speech disorder characterized by muscular weakness, dyscoordination, and deficit in muscle tone. The site of lesion determines the specific dysarthria characteristics. Lesions of the left dorsal corticobulbar tract have been associated with dysarthria and oromotor impairment, as have lesions of the ventral corticobulbar tract in the right hemisphere (Kwon, Lee, & Jang, 2016; Liégeois, Tournier, Pigdon, Connelly, & Morgan, 2013). Dysarthria may arise from a lesion in any region of the brain involved in motor execution, which includes the motor cortex of the cerebrum, the internal capsule, the basal ganglia, the brainstem, and the cerebellum. While we'll discuss the other causes of dysarthria as we study those subcortical areas, the dominant dysarthria arising from lesion to the cerebral cortex is spastic dysarthria.

An upper motor neuron (UMN) lesion can occur at the level of the cortex or anywhere along the upper motor neuron pathway, prior to termination at the lower motor neuron. Upper motor neurons are defined as any motor neurons in a chain that lead to the final neuron in the path, which is termed the lower motor neuron (LMN). The LMN often has a reflex associated with it, such as the patellar tendon reflex, which you may be familiar with. If the LMN is damaged, the reflex is often lost. If the UMN is damaged, the reflex can become hyperactive. A particularly damaging lesion can occur at the internal capsule. Because the internal capsule is a point at which many fibers condense into a very compact space, a relatively small infarct (loss of blood supply to a region of the brain) at the internal capsule can affect a large number of efferent fibers. For example, **lacunar infarcts** are micro-hemorrhages arising often from hypertension, and this type of infarct in the internal capsule produces weakness of the face, arm, and/or leg, or a pure motor stroke with signs such as hyperreflexia and spasticity.

The effect of a UMN lesion is **spasticity**, **hypertonia**, and **hyperreflexia**, which translate to muscular weakness, altered speaking rate, and imprecise articulation in the patient for whom there is cranial nerve involvement. The term used to describe the effects of UMN lesion on speech is **spastic dysarthria**.

Spastic dysarthria is found to involve bilateral patterns of white matter volume loss in the area underlying the motor cortex (BA 4), the frontoparietal operculum (BA 43), and a possible involvement of the projection fibers that connect the cortex with the basal ganglia (corticofugal projection fibers) (Clark, Duffy, Whitwell, Ahlskog, Sorenson, & Josephs, 2014). Additional areas of white matter loss include the premotor cortex (BA 6) and the posterior prefrontal cortex, as well as areas in the corpus callosum and anterior brainstem, particularly the genu of the cerebral peduncle. If you recall the homunculus, you'll remember that the dorsal areas of the sensorimotor cortex are specialized to arm reaching and hand function, while the dorsolateral sensorimotor cortex is specialized to speech articulation and involves the corticobulbar tract in the orofacial nuclei, articulatory muscles, and connections with anterior cingulate and supplementary motor area, basal ganglia, and cerebellum. Some researchers have proposed that in humans (as opposed to non-human primates) there is an additional direct system of activation that consists of the larynx area in the motor cortex and proceeds to the nucleus ambiguus innervating the laryngeal muscles. This direct activation system could be considered a pathway specialized to speech (Conant, Bouchard, & Chang, 2014).

Frontotemporal Dementia

Frontotemporal dementia (FD) is a disorder with a progressive nerve cell loss in the frontal or temporal lobes of the brain affecting adults typically between 45 and 65 years of age. FD includes three clinical variants, with the last two of them especially important to the speech-language pathologist: behavioral or frontal variant FD, semantic dementia, and progressive nonfluent aphasia.

The patient with the **behavioral variant FD** exhibits an insidious onset of changes in personality and social conduct, such as apathy, loss of insight, early disinhibition, change in food preferences, and lack of empathy. The early recognition of these signs helps in the differential diagnosis between FD and Alzheimer's disease. The patient with **semantic dementia** exhibits difficulty in naming and describing objects as well as word-finding behavior. These difficulties progress to difficulties in comprehension, matching an object with its written word, and matching objects that belong to the same semantic category. The patient with **progressive nonfluent aphasia** exhibits difficulties in word-finding, produces short sentences that degenerate over time to monosyllabic words, and may ultimately be mute. The language of patients with semantic dementia is often characterized by circumlocution, while the language of patients with progressive nonfluent aphasia is often characterized by long pauses.

Frontotemporal dementia has another side to it that must give the therapist pause (Cavallera, Giudici, & Tommasi, 2012). You have perhaps heard the amazing music of Maurice Ravel, composer of *Bolero* and other pieces. Miller, Cummings, Mishkin, Boone, Prince, Ponton, and Cotman (1998) have shown that presence of frontotemporal dementia appears to allow right hemisphere creative processes to dominate, and there are numerous cases of individuals developing Pick's disease (frontotemporal dementia) and showing an artistic side even as speech and language degenerate.

Parietal Lobe

The parietal lobe is the area posterior to the central sulcus, with its posterior border being a line drawn from the parieto-occipital sulcus to the preoccipital notch (see Figure 4–2A). The inferior boundary is the lateral sulcus. The parietal lobe has primary responsibility for reception and processing of somatic (body) sense and for integrating that sense with other senses.

The parietal lobe is divided into three large areas: the postcentral gyrus, the superior parietal lobule, and the inferior parietal lobule. Immediately posterior to the central sulcus is the **postcentral gyrus**. Posterior to that gyrus are the **superior parietal lobule** and **inferior parietal lobules**, separated from each other by the **intraparietal sulcus**. All of these structures have significant roles and implications for motor function and visuomotor integration.

The postcentral gyrus (BA 1, 2, 3, and perhaps 5) is the primary site of somatosensory reception, and the first level of sensory integration of that information. Take another look at the homunculus in Figure 4–11, and you will see that the entire ventral surface of the human body is projected onto the postcentral gyrus, similar to how control of those components is governed by the precentral gyrus. You can also see that certain areas are very highly represented with dense sensory information, indicated by the size of the structure. As with the precentral gyrus, the face and mouth have disproportionately greater representation, relative to the rest of the homunculus, indicating the number of neurons serving those areas. This means that these areas have significantly greater sensory receptor density, so you have much finer sensory discrimination in these regions. For instance, you can discriminate between two points on the tongue much more finely than two points on your back. Take two cotton-tipped applicators and touch your friend's tongue with the stick end of those applicators at two locations about 1 cm apart at the same time. With her eyes closed, she will be able to tell you that it is two contacts as opposed to one. If you do the same thing in the middle of her back, she will probably say that you're only touching one location. This is because the number of receptors for tactile sensation is much more dense on the tongue than on the back. These receptors help you form a bolus of food or help you identify something stuck in your teeth, but you don't do that much fine work with the surface of your back!

The **postcentral sulcus** divides the postcentral gyrus from the superior and inferior parietal lobules. The superior parietal lobule and the intraparietal sulcus are part of the dorsal visual stream, also known as the "where" stream. At the intraparietal sulcus, visual information about the location of an object in space is integrated with body sense (i.e., where the body is in space), and that information is transmitted to the precentral gyrus to guide the process of grasping for the object.

The inferior parietal lobule is an important higher order processing area of the cerebral cortex that integrates vision, audition, and somatic sense. The angular gyrus is primarily responsible for processing of written language, while the supramarginal gyrus is involved in phonetic processing.

The **angular gyrus** (BA 39) is located posterior to Wernicke's area, the critical language processing area of the temporal lobe. This association is not only relevant, but highly important. The angular gyrus is essential for comprehension of written material. The angular gyrus processes information from visual, auditory, and somatosensory centers and is involved in mathematical calculation and some aspects of cognitive function. Difficulty writing language (**agraphia**), difficulty with reading language (**alexia**), and problems understanding word meaning (**semantic processing deficits**) can arise from lesions to the left angular gyrus. A lesion to the right angular gyrus can cause a disorder that disconnects an action from the agent performing the action (i.e., I would not comprehend that I am the person completing an action; Farrer, Frey, Van Horn, Tunik, Turk, Inati, & Grafton, 2007). The angular gyrus apparently works with the supramarginal gyrus in reading and rhyming activity and may be involved in development of phonology during childhood (Church, Coalson, Lugar, Petersen, & Schlaggar, 2008). The **supramarginal gyrus** (BA 40) is intimately involved in processing of phonological information (Sugiura, Ojima, Matsuba-Kurita, Dan, Tsuzuki, Katura, & Hagiwara, 2011).

Temporal Lobe

The temporal lobe is one of the later evolutionary components of the cerebrum, and it houses some very important regions for the disciplines of speech-language pathology and audiology. It is the site of auditory reception, integration of vision with audition for identification of speakers, memory function, auditory comprehension, and even face recognition. The temporal lobe is bordered by the lateral sulcus medially and projects back to the parietal and occipital lobes posteriorly. Important landmarks of the temporal lobe include the **superior**, **middle**, and **inferior temporal gyri** (and associated sulci) of the lateral temporal lobe; **Heschl's gyrus** on the superior and medial surface of the posterior temporal lobe; and the **parahippocampal gyrus**.

Take a look at the **superior temporal gyrus** (BA 22) in Figure 4–10A. In the posterior aspect of BA 22 is the area known as **Wernicke's area**. Damage to this area of the dominant hemisphere (the left hemisphere in right-handed peo-

ple) can cause a profound receptive aphasia, particularly if the damage extends into the middle temporal gyrus.

Anterior to Wernicke's area is **Heschl's gyrus** (BA 41) and the higher order processing area associated with it, BA 42. Heschl's gyrus is the core region for reception of auditory information (Kaas, & Hackett, 2000), and this gyrus extends into the lateral sulcus on the medial surface of the temporal lobe. BA 42 is considered to be part of a belt around the core, involved in processing information received at BA 41 (Figure 4–12).

The **middle temporal gyrus** (BA 21) and **inferior temporal gyrus** (BA 20) are important for auditory processing

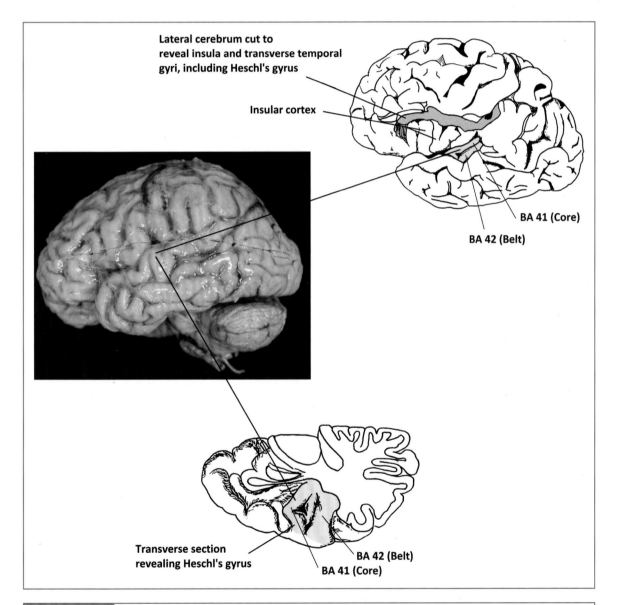

FIGURE 4–12. Detail of Heschl's gyrus (BA 41) of the temporal lobe. Note that BA 42 would be considered part of the belt region. *Source:* Redrawn from photograph by John A. Beal, PhD, Department of Cellular Biology and Anatomy, Louisiana State University Health Sciences Center Shreveport, LA.

and auditory-visual integration of information (the ventral visual stream) used to identify an auditory or visual stimulus (i.e., answering the question, "What is it?").

Recent meta-analysis (Ardila, Bernal, & Rosselli, 2016) reveals how these areas interact for language function through two functional networks. The first network involves Wernicke's area, BA 21 (middle temporal gyrus), BA 22 (superior temporal gyrus), and the primary auditory association cortex (BA 41 and BA 42), which work together for auditory processing of language. The second network appears to include BA 20 (inferior temporal area), BA 37 (fusiform gyrus), BA 38 (temporopolar area), BA 39 (angular gyrus), and BA 40 (supramarginal gyrus) as part of the greater "language association area," an extended system of Wernicke's area (Ardila et al., 2016).

The inferior temporal lobe has two very important regions. The **parahippocampal gyrus** (BA 34) marks the location of the hippocampal formation deep within the cerebrum. The hippocampus is an important structure involved in placing memory into long-term storage, navigation in space, and the sense of smell. The **fusiform gyrus** is lateral to the parahippocampal gyrus, and is important for face recognition.

Occipital Lobe

Take a look at the occipital lobe in Figures 4–2A and 4–10A. This is the most posterior of the cerebral structures, marked by the **preoccipital notch** in the inferior aspect and the **parieto-occipital suture** in the superior aspect. Visual information that reaches consciousness arrives at the **calcarine sulcus** (BA 17) of the occipital lobe, which is visible on the lateral posterior surface of the cerebrum, although most of the sulcus is found through inspection of the medial surface. The **lingual gyrus** (BA 19 of inferior cerebrum) is also visible on medial view, as is the **cuneus** (BA 18, 19). We will examine the inferior surface shortly, but recognize that there is a large area, the fusiform gyrus, that is responsible for face recognition. While the calcarine sulcus is the primary reception area for vision, the cuneus and the lingual gyrus are both involved in higher order processing, as we'll discuss later. You might remember our discussion of the homunculus earlier and how that represented a recurring theme of spatiotopic (or in the case of the cochlea, tonotopic) representation. The calcarine sulcus has a similar array representing the visual fields, although it is not quite as straightforward: the image from the retinas is inverted (upside-down) and reversed, so that the left hemisphere receives the right visual field. This left-for-right representation is another constant in nature, by the way, and is the product of decussation of the efferent and afferent pathways. Decussation of tracts is pervasive throughout the nervous system, as you will see in later chapters.

Insula or Insular Cortex

The **insular cortex** (BA 13, 14), or insula (insula means "island"; the original name for the insula was the island of Reil), is an area that is hidden under the **operculum** of the cerebral cortex (operculum means "covering" in Latin). The operculum consists of three parts: the **frontal operculum** (BA 45), the **frontoparietal operculum** (BA 44 and inferior 1, 2, 3, and 40), and the **temporal operculum** (medial temporal lobe BA 38, 41, 4). If you look at the lower portion of Figure 4–2A, you'll see that part of the cerebral cortex has been pulled back to reveal the insula. To see it, you must deflect the temporal lobe laterally and lift up the parietal and frontal operculum. You'll see a **circular sulcus** that separates the insula from the rest of the cortex. The insula is actually just a pouch-like continuation of the cerebral cortex, hidden from view, but continuous with the rest of the cortex. The insula consists of four gyri separated by three sulci. The **central sulcus of the insula** separates the posterior long gyrus of the insula from two short gyri in the anterior aspect. The two anterior short gyri appear to be involved in processing of emotional states (Dalgleish, 2004) and in the right (nondominant) hemisphere are particularly related to development of your perception of self (Craig, 2009). The insula in the left (dominant) hemisphere is involved in planning the articulation of speech, and a lesion there will produce a condition known as verbal apraxia (Dronkers, 1996). Its primary function is most likely gustation (the perception of taste; Kobayashi, Kennedy, & Halpern, 2006), but many more functions have likely been added as we evolved.

Apraxia of Speech

Apraxia of speech (AOS) is a motor planning disorder that is characterized by inconsistent articulatory errors, articulatory groping, and loss of articulatory fluency in the absence of muscular weakness. Studies that differentiate the neuroanatomical basis of apraxia of speech are separated into two types. Patients who experience apraxia of speech in combination with aphasia tend to have a lesion of the left anterior insular cortex, Broca's area (BA 44/45), and the precentral/premotor region (BA 4/6) (Dronkers, 1996; Hillis, Work, Barker, Jacobs, Breese, & Maurer, 2004; Richardson, Fillmore, Rorden, LaPointe, & Fridriksson, 2012). If they exhibit apraxia without aphasia, the lesions tend to be in the left premotor and motor cortices (BA 4/6) (Graff-Radford, Jones, Strand, Rabinstein, Duffy, & Josephs, 2014).

Apraxia of speech can be a particularly frustrating disorder to an individual. Often individuals with AOS will also have a nonfluent aphasia because of the proximity of Broca's area to the insular cortex. These individuals often have good language comprehension and are typically quite conscious of the speech difficulty of AOS, making the halting and groping speech of AOS difficult to tolerate.

Limbic System

The limbic system is not an anatomically distinct structure, but rather a group of structures that mediates some very complex processes, including motivation, emotional behavior, affect, and sexual drive. The limbic system includes the **uncus**, which is formed by the **amygdaloid body** or **amygdala**, the **parahippocampal gyrus** (including the hippocampal formation), the **cingulate gyrus**, the **olfactory bulb** and tract, and the **dentate gyrus**. The limbic system is almost entirely hidden: the cingulate gyrus is visible in medial view (BA 24, 23, 31, and 30), and you can see the uncus (BA 34) from that view as well.

In summary, the lateral cerebral cortex consists of a number of important landmarks on the two mirror-image hemispheres.

- The frontal lobe is involved in cognition and executive function, expressive language function, and emotional regulation.
- The parietal lobe receives somatic input representing body sense (postcentral gyrus) and integrates this with motor function (superior parietal lobule and intraparietal sulcus), and visual (angular gyrus) and auditory information (supramarginal gyrus). The angular gyrus is critical to the language process of reading, and the supramarginal gyrus is involved in phonetic processing.
- The occipital lobe receives all visual input that reaches consciousness at the calcarine sulcus.
- The temporal lobe has three major gyri. The superior temporal gyrus includes the lateral aspect of Heschl's gyrus as well as Wernicke's area. The posterior aspect of the middle temporal gyrus works with Wernicke's area in language processing, as do more diverse structures such as the supramarginal gyrus and angular gyrus. The inferior temporal gyrus is involved in visual-auditory integration. The parahippocampal gyrus is found on the inferior temporal lobe, and the fusiform gyrus is part of the inferior occipital lobe of the cerebrum.
- The insular cortex has been shown to be important for language programming, and is strongly implicated in apraxia of speech in the left hemisphere, and self-perception and empathy insight in the right hemisphere.
- The limbic system is composed of many cortical parts, including the amygdala, dentate gyrus, hippocampus, cingulate gyrus, and olfactory bulb and tract. It is important for emotional processes, sex drive, and motivation.

MEDIAL SURFACE OF THE CEREBRAL CORTEX

The medial surface of the cerebral cortex is the surface that separates the two cerebral hemispheres. Structurally, the medial faces are mirror images, but we will see some significant differences when we discuss function. You will want to refer to Figures 4–2F and 4–10B as we discuss this surface.

The medial surface is hidden from view until the two hemispheres are separated. First, recognize that the postcentral and precentral gyri extend into the medial surface. If you recall the homunculus, you'll remember that the medial surface is responsible for activation of the lower leg and foot and that sensory information from the leg and foot arrive in that region as well. When we talk about the cerebrovascular supply, we'll recognize that damage to this medial surface can cause loss of motor function for those regions served (paraplegia), but more on that later! (This does underscore, however, the importance of our knowledge of the nervous system in serving our clients and patients.)

Figure 4–2F also shows the **corpus callosum**, which has been severed to permit this view. The corpus callosum is a collection of what are called commissural fibers, connecting the two cerebral hemispheres and allowing communication between them. The corpus callosum allows each region of the cerebral cortex (e.g., BA 44 of the right hemisphere and BA 44 of the left hemisphere) to communicate by means of myelinated fibers, allowing each hemisphere to be influenced by the other. The corpus callosum is the floor of the superior longitudinal fissure.

The corpus callosum is made up of over 400 million fibers (Catherine, 1994) and is divided into four major regions: rostrum, genu, body, and splenium. Each reflects the areas of the cerebral cortex being served.

Fibers that course through **genu** of the corpus callosum allow the anterior frontal lobes to communicate. The posterior frontal lobes and parietal lobes communicate by means of fibers that run through the **body** (also known as the **trunk**) of the corpus callosum. The temporal and occipital lobes are served by the **splenium** of the corpus callosum. Immediately inferior to the genu is the **rostrum**, which provides communication between the left and right orbital regions, as well as some of the premotor regions. Immediately below the corpus callosum, you can see the **anterior commissure**. The anterior commissure serves as the means of communication between the right and left olfactory areas as well as portions of the inferior and middle temporal gyri.

If you look at the superior aspect of the medial surface, you'll see that the postcentral and precentral gyri are continuous. This reflection is termed the **paracentral lobule**. Just posterior to this is the **precuneus**, an often-overlooked structure of the parietal lobe. The precuneus is involved in visuospatial processing, episodic memory function, and the sense of agency in action. Similar to the insular cortex, the precuneus appears to support the concept of self-awareness of an individual (Cavanna & Trimble, 2006). Posterior to the precuneus is the cuneus (BA 17), a gyrus in the occipital lobe that is involved in visual information processing, but also apparently in impulse control (Crockford, Goodyear, Edwards, Quickfall, & el-Guebaly, 2005). The paracentral lobule spans the frontal and parietal lobes. The frontal component is part of the supplementary motor area, while the posterior paracentral lobule is involved in integration of sensory and motor integration for the lower body, including control of defecation and urination.

The prominent medial structure immediately superior to the corpus callosum is the **cingulate gyrus** (BA 23, 24, 25, 29, 30, 31, 33). This is a very diverse region with responsibilities focused on emotional assessment, regulation, and response. We discuss its function under association fibers, below.

INFERIOR SURFACE OF THE CEREBRAL CORTEX

As you can see in Figure 4–2H, the inferior (or ventral) surface of the cerebral cortex has numerous structures and landmarks, with functions related to the lobes within which they reside. The bulk of the posterior-inferior cerebrum composed of the temporal and occipital lobes, with less representation of the inferior frontal lobe.

Posterior-Inferior (Ventral) Cerebral Cortex

The largest functional area of the posterior cerebral cortex is the **fusiform gyrus** (BA 37), lateral and adjacent to the **lingual** (BA 19) and **parahippocampal gyri** (BA 27). The fusiform and lingual gyri are part of the occipital lobe, while the parahippocampal gyrus is in the inferior temporal lobe. These three areas work closely together: you will remember that we discussed the calcarine sulcus (BA 17) when we talked about the occipital lobe; you can see it at the bottom of Figure 4-2H. Adjacent and anterior to that is the lingual gyrus, which is termed a "higher order processing region" for vision: visual information enters the cerebral cortex at the calcarine sulcus, and then analysis of that information begins with the lingual gyrus (Stern et al., 1996). Lateral to the lingual gyrus is the fusiform gyrus, which, in the right hemisphere, is responsible for face recognition (Kanwisher, McDermott, & Chun, 1997), while the left fusiform gyrus is responsible for identification of components of faces (McCandliss, Cohen, & Dehaene, 2003). Immediately anterior to the lingual gyrus is the parahippocampal gyrus, which houses the hippocampus, a critical structure for placing information into long-term memory, as well as for learning and memory of place or location (White & Gaskin, 2006). Anterior and slightly medial, the parahippocampal gyrus is the uncus (BA 34), the external

representation of the amygdaloid body (or amygdala). The uncus combines with the lateral olfactory stria to make up the primary olfactory cortex, also known as the **pyriform lobe**. This is a major generator of the fear emotion, which is an adaptive response to phenomena that pose a danger to us. So, your calcarine sulcus sees a face, your fusiform gyrus identifies its characteristics, your hippocampus helps you recall where and when you've seen it before, and your amygdala is called into action when you realize it's a ferocious tiger! (By the way, your frontal lobe is then called in to calm you down when you realize it's just a movie!)

Anterior-Inferior Cerebral Cortex

From the view in Figure 4–2H, you can see the **temporal pole** (BA 38), the anterior-most aspect of the temporal lobe. The temporal pole is one of the later evolutionary products of our brain development, and it has apparent roles in emotion processing, face recognition, and perhaps integrating emotion with perception (Olson, Plotzker, & Ezzyat, 2007). It is also involved in autobiographical memory (Dupont, 2002), and auditory discrimination (Zatorre, 1988).

Looking at the inferior view of the cerebral cortex found in Figure 4–2H, find the gyrus rectus immediately adjacent to the superior longitudinal fissure. The **gyrus rectus** (BA 11, a.k.a. straight gyrus) is functionally related to the cingulate gyrus and the **orbital gyri** (BA 10), all of which are involved in mediation of emotion. The **olfactory sulcus** is an indentation in the cerebral cortex that holds the olfactory tract as it courses from its origin on the medial surface of the ethmoid cribriform plate. (We'll talk more about the olfactory tract when we discuss cranial nerves.) The orbital region and the gyrus rectus are considered to be components associated with emotional regulation and have been found to become reduced in volume in people with clinical depression (Ballmaier et al., 2004). This region may also be involved in retrieval of old memories (Kroll, Markowitsch, Knight, & von Cramon, 1997).

Also visible in this inferior view is the corpus callosum and the stalk or base of the hypophysis (the stalk is known as the **tuber cinereum**, and the hypophysis is also known as the pituitary gland). As we discussed earlier, the corpus callosum provides communication between the two cerebral hemispheres, while the hypophysis is important for autonomic regulation that is mediated by the hypothalamus. You can see the stalk of the hypophysis situated just behind the *optic chiasm*, a prominent landmark. While it is not part of the cerebral cortex, the optic chiasm is the juncture of the optic tract and optic nerve and is the point where information from the left visual field crosses to the right hemisphere. If you look a little lower in this image, you'll see a dark area known as the **substantia nigra**. This "black substance" is a group of nuclei that produce dopamine to be used by the basal ganglia and play a critical role in regulation of movement. The substantia nigra resides in the cerebral peduncles, the major pathway for information passing to and from the cerebrum.

In summary, the medial and inferior surfaces of the cerebral cortex have many landmarks that are critical to function. The medial surface of the cerebral cortex is the surface that separates the two cerebral hemispheres.

- The postcentral and precentral gyri extend into the medial surface, with the areas in the medial surface being associated with activation and sensation of the lower leg and foot.
- The corpus callosum is a collection of commissural fibers connecting the two cerebral hemispheres and allowing communication between them. The corpus callosum is composed of four major regions: rostrum, genu, body, and splenium, and they reflect the areas of the cerebral cortex being served.
- The body (trunk) of the corpus callosum connects the posterior frontal lobes and parietal lobes, while the splenium connects the temporal and occipital lobes. The rostrum allows the orbital regions of the frontal lobe and part of the premotor region to communicate. Fibers that course through genu of the corpus callosum allow the anterior frontal lobes to communicate.
- The paracentral lobule is the point of reflection of the precentral and postcentral gyri on the medial surface, and the precuneus of the parietal lobe is involved in visuospatial processing, episodic memory function, and the sense of agency in action. The cuneus of the occipital lobe is involved in visual information processing as well as impulse control.
- The cingulate gyrus is important for emotional regulation.
- The inferior surface of the cerebral cortex includes the fusiform gyrus (face recognition), the lingual gyrus (visual processing), and the parahippocampal gyri (memory). The uncus overlies the amygdaloid body that generates fear responses.
- On the anterior-inferior surface is the temporal pole of the temporal lobe (responsible for autobiographical memory),

and the gyrus rectus and orbital gyri, which are involved in emotional regulation and mediation.
- The olfactory sulcus is an indentation in the cerebral cortex that holds the olfactory tract, and the splenium of the corpus callosum can be seen in the posterior aspect. The stalk of the hypophysis (pituitary gland) can be seen in the mid regions.

MYELINATED FIBERS

We have just reviewed many critical gyri and sulci of the cerebral cortex, but they would be irrelevant without the ability to communicate with the rest of the brain and the external world. This communication comes by means of **myelinated fibers**. The cerebral cortex itself is made up of the cell bodies of neurons, which appear gray in color (a.k.a., gray matter). The axons of those fibers and of other neurons in the cerebrum are white due to the presence of myelin (discussed in Chapter 2), and this "white matter" provides the critical communication among parts of the cerebral cortex.

There are three types of communicating fibers: projection fibers, association fibers, and commissural fibers.

Projection Fibers

Projection fibers make up the efferent and afferent tracts between the cortex and the brainstem or the spinal cord. These projection fibers connect the cortex with distant locations. Take a look at Figure 4–13. In this image, we have removed the cerebral cortex so you can see only the white matter. Notice that the fibers look like they are radiating upward toward the cerebral cortex: this is termed the **corona radiata,** a mass of projection fibers running from

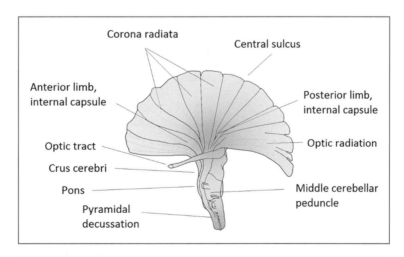

FIGURE 4–13. Corona radiata. *Source:* After view of Carpenter (1966).

and to the cortex. The corona radiata condenses as it courses down, forming an "L" shape (visible in transverse section) as it reaches a location known as the **internal capsule** (Figure 4–14). The internal capsule represents something of a central hub for fibers leaving or entering the cerebrum, as almost all of them pass through this very small location. As you can see in Figure 4–14, the anterior aspect of the internal capsule (anterior limb) serves the frontal lobe and separates two structures known as the caudate nucleus and putamen. The posterior limb includes the **optic radiation**, a group of fibers projecting to the calcarine sulcus for vision. Notice the reference to the thalamic radiations in both anterior and posterior limbs: we'll talk about the thalamus shortly, but almost all of the *afferent* fibers entering the cerebrum arise from the thalamus. The thalamus is important to language. A lesion in the thalamus, such as an infarct, may produce aphasia with intact or minimally impaired repetition and lexical processing. Auditory comprehension is impaired and the language is characterized by semantic paraphasias due to the inability

of the patient to bind a concept to its lexical representation (Crosson, 2013).

Take a look at the genu and posterior limb, and you will see indications for the corticospinal and corticobulbar tract. These are major projection fibers that arise from the cerebrum and pass through the internal capsule to activate muscles in the body.

Corticobulbar and Corticospinal Tracts

Projection fibers arise from the V layer of the cerebral cortex in areas such as the precentral gyrus, premotor region, and supplementary motor area (SMA). Projection fibers, by definition, continue beyond the cerebrum and include fibers that activate musculature of the skeleton. The cerebral cortex is the origin of the major motor tracts that project to the subcortical regions, brainstem, and spinal cord. The large pyramidal cells of the cortex send their axons (projection fibers) to specific targets outside of the cortex. The **corticospinal**

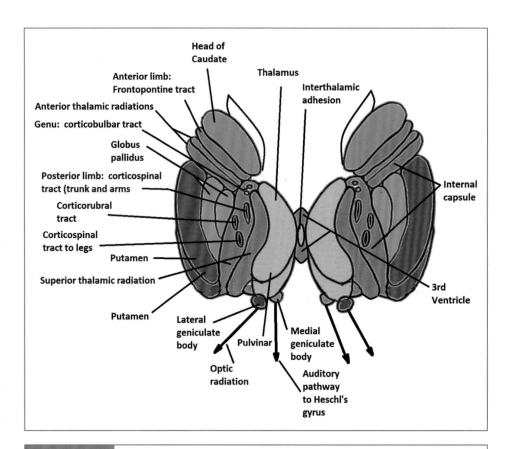

FIGURE 4–14. Internal capsule, showing major tracts. Note that the internal capsule is divided into three parts. The anterior limb serves the frontopontine tract and the anterior thalamic radiation. The posterior limb serves the posterior thalamic radiation and corticospinal tract. The genu serves the corticobulbar tract. *Source:* After view of Carpenter (1978).

and **corticobulbar tracts** as well as the **corticopontine fibers** pass through the internal capsule.

Corticobulbar Tract

The lateral portion of the primary motor area (BA 4) is the origin of the corticobulbar tract. The axons project ipsilaterally through the internal capsule (genu) into the cerebral peduncle, the pons (basis pontis), and the medulla. At the level of the midbrain, pons, and medulla, the axons project to the nuclei of the cranial nerves both ipsilaterally and contralaterally. Exceptions are the nuclei of the facial (VII) and hypoglossal (XII) nerves, which receive mainly contralateral projections, and the nucleus of the spinal accessory nerve, which receives mainly ipsilateral projections. The corticobulbar tract innervates the nuclei of the cranial nerves trigeminal (V), facial (VII), glossopharyngeal (IX), vagus (X), accessory (XI), and hypoglossal (XII). In the nucleus ambiguus, the tract contributes to the motor region of the vagus nerve. We will discuss the cranial nerves in detail in Chapter 7.

Corticospinal Tract

The **corticospinal tract**, like the corticobulbar tract, originates in neurons of the primary motor cortex, the supplemental motor area, and premotor cortex. The axons project to the posterior portion of the internal capsule, the medial portion of the cerebral peduncle, the pons, and the pyramids of medulla (ipsilaterally). Approximately 80% of the fibers cross the midline at the decussation of pyramids. These fibers descend to the spinal cord as the lateral corticospinal tract, while those fibers remaining ipsilateral will descend as the anterior corticospinal tract. Fibers of the anterior corticospinal tract will ultimately decussate immediately prior to synapse with the alpha and gamma lower motor neuron. All lateral corticospinal tract axons are accompanied by the fibers of the rubrospinal tract, a component of the extrapyramidal system that is involved in skillful movements of hands and fingers. Widespread lesions the length of the corticospinal tract involving areas such as the internal capsule, cerebral peduncle, and pons will result in spastic hemiplegia, hyperreflexia, and hypertonia.

Association Fibers

Association fibers make up the second group of white matter fibers in the cerebrum (Figure 4–15). These are classified as either short or long association fibers: short association fibers connect one gyrus with an adjacent gyrus, but long association fibers provide communication between distant locations of the cerebrum. We'll talk about eight of these: the uncinate fasciculus, cingulate gyrus, superior longitudinal fasciculus, arcuate fasciculus, inferior longitudinal fasciculus, perpendicular fasciculus, occipitofrontal fasciculus, and fornix.

Because of their significance in spanning the cerebrum, long association pathways have been carefully studied. The **uncinate fasciculus** connects the orbital portion, inferior, and middle frontal gyri with the anterior temporal lobe, and it appears to be part of the limbic system, being important

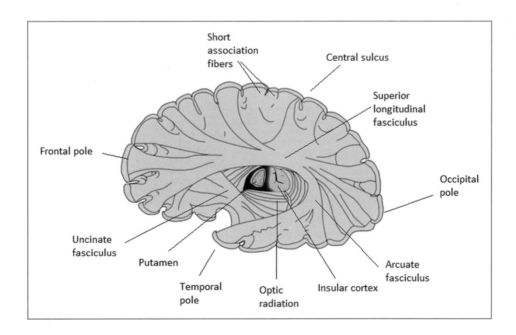

FIGURE 4–15. Tracts of the cortical white matter. *Source:* After view of Carpenter (1978).

for object name retrieval (Papagno et al., 2010) and emotion (Gaffan & Wilson, 2008).

One of the most significant structures of the medial cerebral cortex is the **cingulate gyrus** (BA 23, 24, 25, 29, 30, 31, 33), discussed briefly above. It is often seen as a bridge between the limbic system, which is involved in emotional responses, and the frontal lobe, which is involved in cognitive responses. Thus, the cingulate gyrus appears to be responsible for regulation of emotional activity (Posner, Rothbart, Sheese, & Tang, 2007). The cingulate gyrus is typically divided into anterior (**anterior cingulate cortex**, ACC) and posterior parts (**posterior cingulate cortex**, PCC). The anterior cingulate cortex (BA 24, 25) is involved in emotional response and regulation, impulse control, empathy, and cognitive processes. It is seen as the "executive" component of the cingulate gyrus and has regions that are involved in both visceral and skeletal muscle control (Vogt, Finch, & Olson, 1992). In addition, BA 24 of the ACC regulates maternal behavior; stimulation of this area in non-humans releases oxytocin (Beyer, Anguinano, & Mena, 1961), and stimulation to the upper part of area 24 in cats causes defensive gestures, including hissing, flattened ears, and arched back (Skultety, 1963). BA 25 projects to the brainstem solitary tract nucleus and ultimately the laryngeal muscles and is seen as essential for vocalized emotional response (Wyss & Sripanidkulchai, 1984). In humans, the posterior aspect of the ACC is active during periods of sustained attention (e.g., Grant, Courtemanche, Duerden, Duncan, & Rainville, 2010). The ACC is involved in some autonomic regulation, including blood pressure and heart rate regulation, but is also activated during error correction and other cognitive functions (Bush, Luu, & Posner, 2000). The PCC (BA 29, 30, 23, and 31) is activated during eye movement, memory, and spatial orientation (Vogt et al., 1992). The PCC has connections with the hippocampus and appears to be involved in autobiographical memory (Maddock, Garrett, & Buonocore, 2001). While the ACC is involved in more cognitive activity related to emotional regulation, the PCC seems to take on an evaluative function related to its activity in the spatial environment. Taken together, the cingulate gyrus assesses sensory input and modifies cortical activity related to painful or fearful stimuli.

The **superior longitudinal fasciculus** (SLF) includes four subgroups of fibers: SLF I, SLF II, SLF III, and the arcuate fasciculus (Makris, Kennedy, McInerney, Sorensen, Wang, Caviness, & Pandya, 2005). SLF I fibers connect superior parietal lobule and precuneus (lateral and medial BA 7) with the premotor and eye regions of the frontal lobe (BA 6, 8, 9). SLF II fibers connect the temporo-occipito-parietal region (BA 19), the angular gyrus (BA 39), the supramarginal gyrus (BA 40), and the postcentral gyrus (BA 1, 2, 3) with the dorsolateral prefrontal cortex (BA 6, 46). SLF III connects the supramarginal gyrus (BA 40) with the inferior parietal lobe (BA 43), the postcentral gyrus higher order processing region (BA 3 and 2), the precentral gyrus (BA 4), the premotor region (BA 6), and Broca's area (BA 44). Researchers have suggested a relationship of SLFIII to phonemic and articulatory aspects of language in humans (Schmahmann, Smith, Eichler, & Filley, 2008). It appears to be an important region in monitoring orofacial and hand actions in primates. The **arcuate fasciculus** connects the supramarginal gyrus (BA 40), Wernicke's area (posterior BA 22), and the temporo-occipital region (BA 19: Makris et al., 2005; Martino, Hamer, Berger, Lawton, Arnold, de Lucas, & Duffau, 2013). The arcuate fasciculus has classically been viewed as playing a critical role in connecting the temporal lobe language areas, including Wernicke's area, with the phonetic processing area of the parietal lobe (the supramarginal gyrus) and the expressive language region of the frontal lobe (Broca's area). Some authors maintain that the arcuate fasciculus is the primary pathway between frontal motor planning areas and Wernicke's area (Bernal & Ardila, 2009), and electrical stimulation of this pathway in awake individuals will produce aphasic signs (Duffau, Gatignol, Moritz-Gasser, & Mandonnet, 2009). Improved visualization techniques using diffusor tensor imaging have shown that the arcuate fasciculus does indeed connect Wernicke's area with the supramarginal gyrus, but the connection with Broca's areas is completed by means of SLF III. It appears that the arcuate fasciculus is important for the recognition of acoustic stimuli and the auditory processing of information, and thus, a lesion to it may lead to conduction aphasia (Schmahmann et al., 2008). Disruption of the arcuate fasciculus has been interpreted as the cause of conduction aphasia through disconnection of the two language centers, but it may also arise from disruption of the phonetic processing function of the supramarginal gyrus (Bernal & Ardila, 2009). Some have suggested that the extreme capsule, located between the claustrum and the orbital frontal cortex, may also have an important role in language by connecting Broca's and Wernicke's areas (Schmahmann et al., 2008).

The **inferior longitudinal fasciculus** connects the temporal pole with the occipital lobe, making up the ventral stream for visual processing. The **perpendicular fasciculus** appears to connect the fusiform gyrus (BA 37) with the superior parietal lobule (BA 5 and 7 of dorsal cortex), while the **occipitofrontal fasciculus** provides communication between the occipital lobe and frontal lobe (Kier, Staib, Davis, & Bronen, 2004). The **fornix** connects the hippocampus with the thalamus and mammillary bodies and may be involved in memory function (Hamani et al., 2008).

Commissural Fibers

The final group of fibers are those that connect the two hemispheres of the brain. The major set is the corpus callosum, but the anterior commissure also consists of commissural fibers.

Cortical Myelin Disorders

Speech or language symptomatology associated with white matter loss has been found in a number of genetic diseases. X-linked adrenoleukodystrophy (X-ALD) is a genetic disease characterized by malfunction of the adrenal cortex/myelin in the nervous system and a consequent severe inflammatory demyelination in 20% of patients. In this form of the disease, the individual has symptomatology that includes impaired speed of information processing, cognitive impairment (including memory and executive function), and language impairment correlated with the degree of involvement (Edwin, Speedie, Kohler, Naidu, Kruse, & Moser, 1996).

Mitochondrial encephalopathy with lactic acidosis and stroke-like episodes (MELAS) is another genetic disease characterized by seizures, hemiparesis, and cortical blindness. Patients with this disease show areas of white matter and cortical infarction as well as cerebral edema. They also show atrophy of the cerebral and cerebellar cortices, which is believed to be the cause of the disease. Symptoms include headaches, confusion, aphasia and apraxia, temper outbursts, and aggressive and paranoid behavior (Thommeer, Verhoeven, van de Vlasakker, & Klompenhouwer, 1998).

Inhalation of heated heroin vapor causes a progressive spongiform leukoencephalopathy that affects the white matter. Symptoms include cerebellar dysarthria, bradykinesia, rigidity, and hypophonia progressing to pseudobulbar palsy, akinetic mutism, and spastic quadraparesis (Offiah & Hall, 2008).

In summary, myelinated fibers are axons of neurons arising from the cortex itself. There are three types of communicating fibers: projection fibers, association fibers, and commissural fibers.

- Projection fibers make up the tracts that connect the cortex, the brainstem, and the spinal cord.
- The corona radiata condenses to form the internal capsule, a central hub for fibers leaving or entering the cerebral cortex. The anterior aspect of the internal capsule (anterior limb) serves the frontal lobe and separates the caudate nucleus and putamen. The posterior limb includes the optic radiation, a group of fibers projecting to the calcarine sulcus for vision. The genu and posterior limbs carry the corticospinal and corticobulbar tract.
- Association fibers can be either short or long. Short association fibers connect one gyrus with an adjacent gyrus, but long association fibers provide communication between distant locations of the cerebral cortex.

- The uncinate fasciculus connects the orbital portion and inferior and middle frontal gyri with the anterior temporal lobe and is part of the limbic system. The cingulate gyrus is divided into anterior cingulate cortex (ACC) and posterior cingulate cortex (PCC). The anterior cingulate cortex is involved in emotional response and regulation, impulse control, empathy, and cognitive processes.
- The superior longitudinal fasciculus (SLF) is a massive set of association fibers divided into four groups. SLF I connects the superior parietal lobule and precuneus with the premotor and eye regions of the frontal lobe. SLF II connects the temporo-occipito-parietal region, angular gyrus, supramarginal gyrus, and postcentral gyrus with the dorsolateral prefrontal cortex. SLF III connects the supramarginal gyrus with the inferior parietal lobe, the postcentral gyrus, the precentral gyrus, the premotor region, and Broca's area. The arcuate fasciculus connects the supramarginal gyrus, Wernicke's area, and the temporo-occipital region. Language comprehension and expression are most likely linked through the arcuate fasciculus and the fibers of SLF III.
- The inferior longitudinal fasciculus connects the temporal pole with the occipital lobe, making up the ventral stream for visual processing. The perpendicular fasciculus connects the fusiform gyrus with the superior parietal lobule. The occipitofrontal fasciculus provides communication between the occipital lobe and frontal lobe. The fornix connects the hippocampus with the thalamus and mammillary bodies.
- The middle longitudinal fasciculus is located in the white matter of the inferior parietal lobule caudally and proceeds into the superior temporal gyrus by connecting some association and paralimbic cortical areas. This fiber tract may be important in language by sending information about spatial organization, memory, and motivation to linguistic processing.
- Commissural fibers make up the final group of association fibers. The corpus callosum is the primary set of commissural fibers, but the anterior commissure connects olfactory regions from both hemispheres.

THE OTHER HALF: HEMISPHERIC SPECIALIZATION

Hemispheric specialization (HS) refers to the differential specialization for a task by one cerebral hemisphere over the other. We will very often refer to the left hemisphere as the **dominant hemisphere**, but this is actually just shorthand for "dominant for language." Because language function is so vital to our existence as humans, we have become very accustomed to downplaying the role of the right hemisphere (called the **nondominant hemisphere**), while giving deference to the left hemisphere. In reality, it's not quite that clear cut. Let's start by looking at handedness (Table 4–3).

Handedness is the most obvious manifestation of hemispheric specialization. Approximately 90% of humans are right-handed. This reflects left-hemisphere dominance for skilled motor acts (Taylor & Heilman, 1980). When motor acts don't require much skill, both hemispheres are entrained equally, but as skill, speed, and accuracy increase, the left hemisphere becomes the dominant hemisphere. You have demonstrated this to yourself inevitably when you've attempted to write with your left hand (if you're right-handed). The nondominant hand is able to perform fairly gross acts well, but when you need refinement you have to return to the dominant hand. Right-handed people most always have language and other analytic functions in their left hemispheres. Left-handed people may well have these language and analytic functions in their right hemispheres, but they may also have mixed laterality. **Mixed laterality** is the case in which functions, such as language, are shared between the two hemispheres. As we discuss hemispheric specialization, we are using left and right hemisphere as proxies for dominant and nondominant hemispheres, although we acknowledge that people who are left-handed very likely have a significantly different configuration. It is worth remembering that if your client is pre-morbidly left-handed, then the probability is that the right hemisphere is dominant.

The left hemisphere is very detail oriented, sequential, and fast. The right hemisphere takes the details and places them into context, or creates a whole from them. The left hemisphere has a very powerful judgment system, so that it can compare two items and identify whether they are the same or different, or whether one has a better quality than the other. The right hemisphere will provide the context upon which the judgments can be placed but is not very involved in the judgment itself. The left hemisphere can organize stimuli, but the right hemisphere can see how the items in categories fit into a whole. The left hemisphere is particularly well suited for analysis, with its attention to detail and rapid, sequential processing. The left hemisphere processes brief auditory stimuli, while the right hemisphere processes auditory stimuli of longer duration. In contrast, the right hemisphere is much more involved in synthesizing the details into one coherent whole.

The reality is that the left and right hemispheres operate very well together, and the functions that are lateralized to one or the other hemisphere serve as complements to functions of the other hemisphere. Face recognition is an excellent example of this concept (Lochy, de Heering, & Rossion, 2017). A face that is presented visually to the left hemisphere is analyzed into its component parts: the left fusiform gyrus will identify lips, eyes, eyebrows, nose, and so forth, but it will stop there. The same information presented to the right fusiform gyrus will result in putting the face together and identifying who it is. The left hemisphere sees the parts, while the right hemisphere sees the whole; the left hemisphere analyzes and the right synthesizes.

Another striking asymmetry between the two hemispheres is found in the amygdaloid body (amygdala). The amygdala of the limbic system is responsible for helping us recognize and respond to fearful stimuli and is an important

TABLE 4–3.	Functional Differences Between the Cerebral Hemispheres
Left hemisphere	Right hemisphere
Grammar, including morphology, syntax, and phonology	Context of language, suprasegmental aspects of language
Detail oriented, insensitive to context	Places detail in context
Strong judgment and categorization capacity (Aron, Robbins, & Poldrack, 2004)	Non-judgment but gives context for judgment via bilateral DLPFC (Aron, Robbins, & Poldrack, 2004)
Organization based on categorization	Views elements outside of categories and how they fit together as a whole
Rapid response	Slow response
Impulsive	Reflective
Analysis	Synthesis
Significant pathology of left hemisphere: aphasia	Significant pathology of right hemisphere: left hemispatial neglect

structure for emotion processing. Psychopaths are individuals who do not empathize, and they have smaller amygdalae on the right side than the normal population. In contrast, altruists have larger right-side amygdalae (Marsh, Finger, Schechter, Jurkowitz, Reid, & Blair, 2011; Marsh, Stoycos, Brethel-Haurwitz, Robinson, VanMeter, & Cardinale, 2014). The working hypothesis is that the deactivation of the amygdala in the psychopath relates to failure to recognize the suffering of others, while the activation of the right amygdala relates to the extreme empathy and compassion of the altruist. The right amygdala is more active and appears to increase in volume in people engaged in compassion training (Valk et al., 2017).

We have already talked about the critical left hemisphere language components: Broca's area for syntax, the left insular cortex for planning the articulatory configuration, the left supramarginal gyrus for phonetic processing, and the left posterior superior temporal gyrus (Wernicke's area) for language comprehension. These areas represent the cornerstone of classical language representation in the brain. In contrast, the right hemisphere seems at first glance to have been left out of the language picture entirely. This is far from the reality of the situation. Remember that language consists of form (syntax, morphology, phonology), content (semantics), and use (pragmatics). The left hemisphere is certainly dominant for form, but what about content and use?

Some of the more striking differences between the hemispheres have emerged from lesion studies in which people have undergone **right hemisphere damage** (RHD) (Ferré & Joanette, 2016). People with RHD will typically have intact form and, at first glance, intact content. They will be able to form complete and coherent sentences that don't have fillers or paraphasias, as seen in left hemisphere lesions. What becomes apparent on close examination is that people with RHD have a more concrete and inflexible vocabulary. When presented, for instance, with the sentence, "The fan is running" and a picture of a baseball fan (fanatic) running across a field, the person with RHD will likely say that the picture is wrong. If presented with a window fan designed to cool a room, the person with RHD will agree that it's now the correct picture. It appears that the left hemisphere maintains the portion of the semantic base that includes what we call **denotative meaning**, or the dictionary meaning. This is the first meaning you think of when you hear a word. In the example of "the fan is running," the denotative meaning is that image of the window fan. When that definition doesn't work, apparently the right hemisphere is called into action, looking for alternatives. It is able to come up with the **connotative meaning**, or the alternative meaning that fits the image presented. Researchers haven't determined if the connotative meanings are held in the right hemisphere or if there is simply a deficit in being able to identify the need to find alternate meanings. It may be a failure to inhibit that first response, coupled with some rigidity about considering alter-

natives. Whatever the cause, the right hemisphere has a very important role in processing complex, ambiguous semantic information and providing disambiguating solutions. The left hemisphere quickly identifies the meaning and stops there if the right hemisphere has been disabled. The left hemisphere seems much more concrete and literal, while the right hemisphere appears to be more flexible and figurative (Lundgren & Brownell, 2016).

This semantic dichotomy is found in humor as well. If you examine virtually any cartoon, you will see that it contains two components. The first component is the "given" part, where the content makes perfect sense at first impression. The second component is the twist that an added piece of information gives, which changes the original meaning completely. It is this second, paradoxical information that tickles you and makes the cartoon funny. A person with RHD will not recognize the humor, because he or she has difficulty disambiguating paradoxical information. Similarly, when presented with idioms such as "he has a heavy heart" or "she has a good eye," a person with RHD may well interpret these literally (Tompkins, Boada, & McGarry, 1992). Idioms and metaphors will not make sense (Giora, Zaidel, Soroker, Batori, & Kasher, 2000).

Sarcasm and humor presented orally are very often problematic for people with RHD as well. Sarcasm depends on exaggerated intonation and, for instance, eye rolling. Intonation is largely the domain of the right hemisphere (e.g., Lalande, Braun, Charlebois, & Whitaker, 1992; Rodriguez, 2009), and seeing the nuance of eye rolling as conveying emotional content is beyond the capacity of the left hemisphere. The sarcastic comment, "Weren't YOU the life of the party?" may well be interpreted literally, and the message will clearly not be delivered. The right hemisphere interprets the face and voice (Costanzo et al., 2015) for emotion, allowing interpretation or "connotation."

One other striking difference between left and right hemispheres has to do with pragmatics. As members of human society, we follow sets of rules, often laid down culturally, about behavior in context. These rules include issues related to speech and language as well, including turn-taking, recognizing cues that a person wants to change topic, making inferences, etc. The right hemisphere is critically important for social processing (Blake, 2009; Minga, 2016; Pobric, Lambon Ralph, & Zahn, 2016;). A person with RHD may have difficulty identifying the appropriate response for a given environment. Clearly, going into a church and going into a bar will have two very different social and cultural responses, but a person who has difficulty identifying context may not select the correct response for a given environment. This same person may not recognize that a conversation partner is bored with the topic and wants to change it or wants to take a conversational turn. Similarly, the humor deficit that is seen in many people with RHD makes them seem aloof and distant and can isolate them from social contact. The language deficit in RHD runs deep but is not immediately apparent in an individual with the disorder (Beeman & Chiarello, 1998).

There are some remarkable differences between the two hemispheres for localized function as well, one of which is directly involved in what is arguably the most frequent deficit in RHD. You will recall that there are basic cognitive functions, including memory, attention, perception, visuospatial processes, and linguistic processes. Attention is a critically important function, in that it allows us to focus our resources on a problem in order to solve it, and this is the domain of the right hemisphere (Wang, Buckner, & Liu, 2014).

There are three large categories of attention: alerting, orienting, and executive (Raz & Buhle, 2006). You are in a room and you sense movement in your peripheral vision. You have been alerted to the stimulus. Having been alerted, you turn to the stimulus, which is orienting attention. The third and most powerful form of attention is executive attention, which allows you to direct your resources to accomplish a task. In this case, you see a friend and you say "hello," or you see a rhinoceros and you climb a tree! Your executive attention brings your cognitive capacity into focus for the purpose of analyzing, clarifying, and acting. Let's look at the neural substrate of these types of attention.

Alerting attention is the basic attention set in preparation for a stimulus. It also includes phenomena such as vigilance and is related to the physiological state of arousal. While waiting for a stimulus, the thalamus, brainstem, and right anterior cingulate gyrus are active. Physiological arousal depends heavily on the reticular formation of the brainstem and the intralaminar nuclei of the thalamus, which make up the reticular formation. Alerting attention also brings into play the tegmentum of the brainstem, right anterior cingulate cortex, right parietal lobe, and right dorsolateral prefrontal cortex (Mottaghy, Willmes, Horwitz, Müller, Krause, & Sturm, 2006).

Orienting attention is the process of bringing attention to a specific stimulus. You can orient to a physical stimulus (the sound of a twig being broken when something steps on it) or an internally generated stimulus (the thought of a project that is due tomorrow). In either case, you bring your attention to a stimulus, in preparation for action. The network involved in this appears to be the sensory system being activated (i.e., visual, auditory, tactile), the pulvinar of the

thalamus (an auditory/language relay), the superior colliculus (a visual relay of the brainstem), and the right superior parietal lobe, temporoparietal juncture (TPJ: intersection of temporal and parietal lobes), and superior temporal gyrus (Raz & Buhle, 2006).

Executive attention is perhaps the most important form of attention for active use of cognitive processes. This form of attention allows us to act on our perceptions and is a critically important component of executive function. You will recall that executive function is the ability to use cognitive processes to accomplish goals. Executive attention focuses our ability to complete these tasks. The critical anatomical sites of activation in executive attention are the right DLPFC, right TPJ, and right ACC.

The common feature here is the right hemisphere. All of the forms of attention strongly arise from right hemisphere activation, and this leads to the strongest hypothesis about RHD. Many researchers feel that damage to the right hemisphere attentional network, specifically the right DLPFC and right TPJ, is the key to the dysfunction that characterizes the disorder. The most common deficit seen in RHD is **hemispatial neglect** and **visual neglect**, which involve failure to attend to stimuli within the left field of perception (Bartolomeo, Thiebaut de Schotten, & Doricchi, 2007; Lunven & Bartolomeo, 2017).

In **left visual neglect**, persons fail to attend to images in their left visual field, which results in simply not knowing that something is going on in that visual field until they are alerted to attend to it. People with left neglect will eat the food on the right side of their plates, copy the right side of an image, and read only the right side of a written passage. It is not that they cannot see the material, but rather they fail to attend to it. You can bring the material to their attention and they will recognize it, but they will quickly lose attention to the left field.

Left hemispatial neglect includes not being aware of the left side of the body, so that self-care will not include shaving the left side of your face, brushing your left teeth, or washing the left side of your body. People with hemispatial neglect will often bump into doorways with the left side of their bodies because they simply are not aware of the left doorway and the left side of the body. (See the boxed note on misidentification syndromes.)

Misidentification Syndromes

The right hemisphere is the keeper of empathy and compassion, theory of mind, and understanding of insights and awareness. Fragmentation of the right hemisphere results in fragmentation of that which is my identity. Misidentification syndromes are the heart of this dissociation of the person. Hemispatial neglect

is seen by many as a misidentification syndrome, and hemispatial neglect is as common in RHD as aphasia is in LHD.

Let's look briefly at these disorders which can occur as part of RHD. The discussion below is based on the lesion identification work of Feinberg and colleagues (2013; Feinberg, Venneri, Simone, Fan, & Northoff, 2010).

Asomatognosia refers to unawareness of ownership of half of the body or of a limb (typically of the left arm). This is a confusion about ownership, but a therapist can improve the patient's awareness by providing tactile stimulation to the arm and tracing it to the patient's body. This appears to be a condition of confused dissociation, and treatment can alleviate the symptoms.

Somatoparaphrenia is also a misidentification of a body part (e.g., an arm), as belonging to someone else, but includes delusions and confabulations about to whom the arm belongs. This person is resistant to any information to the contrary and will likely not be convinced otherwise. The individual with somatoparaphrenia may create elaborate stories to explain where the body part came from (Vallar & Ronchi, 2009). A severe form of this disorder (body integrity disorder: Blom, Hennekam, & Denys, 2012) may lead to the compulsion to have a body part amputated.

Capgras syndrome is the belief that a close relative or friend, or even a building, has been replaced by an imposter. The person might be in her own home and insist that it looks like her home but it really isn't. The patient may feel that her spouse has been replaced by an imposter. This delusion is considered a psychiatric condition and is often treated with antipsychotic medications. It can be found in people who have suffered right hemisphere stroke.

Anosognosia refers to a lack of acknowledgment of a disease. This may accompany hemispatial neglect, in that the person doesn't acknowledge that there is paralysis despite clear evidence. This disorder poses significant problems, both at the acute stage following stroke and during recovery and treatment. People with right hemisphere stroke may suffer anasognosia and deny that they've had a stroke. If they don't have paralysis caused by damage to the motor pathway, they won't have the frequent signs of stroke (slurred speech, broken syntax, jargon), so they may go untreated. Failure to get early treatment for ischemic stroke greatly reduces the degree of recovery. Later, during therapy, the individual will still deny a problem. It is very difficult to convince someone to work on an issue in therapy if he or she doesn't feel there is a problem to be worked on.

All of these syndromes involve right hemisphere lesions. In the RHD population, the causes of misidentification syndromes seem to revolve around size and location of lesion. Lesions to the right insular cortex, claustrum, precuneus, cuneus, and orbitofrontal cortex reduce the sense of self and self-image. The claustrum coordinates the disparate parts of the cerebrum to orchestrate a wholeness of person, and dyssynchrony of the claustrum function could well result in loss of the solid sense of self. Similarly, damage to the temporoparietal juncture (TPJ) and dorsolateral prefrontal cortex (DLPFC) are common to all misidentification syndromes, and it is intrinsic to the executive attention network. Failure of this network results in an inability to focus attention on relevant stimuli. TPJ lesion is a constant in hemispatial neglect.

It is helpful to look at the spectrum of misidentification syndromes from a lesion standpoint. Feinberg examined lesion sites along a continuum from paralysis to somatoparaphrenia and found that the greater the lesion space, the more significant is the misidentification syndrome. Somatoparaphrenia, with neglect, delusion, and confabulation, has the largest right hemisphere lesion, with paralysis alone being the least. Somatoparaphrenia has lesions that include the cingulate gyrus, parietal lobe, and frontal lobe. Lesions causing hemispatial neglect are smaller in volume. All disorders include the right temporoparietal juncture, and most also include the DLPFC.

Hemispatial and visual neglect appear to arise from a failure of the attention network in the right hemisphere, but the failure has many more implications than not seeing the left visual field or being aware of your left arm. When the attentional network is not activated, the right hemisphere is, in essence, muted (Koch, Bonni, Giacobbe, Bucchi, Basile, Lupo, Versace, Bozzali, & Caltagirone, 2012). The left hemisphere becomes hyperresponsive, while the right hemisphere reduces activation. The critical function of the right hemisphere in providing context and synthesis is either muted or disabled because of inactivation, so people reading only the right side of a written passage will not only make that reading error, but will not recognize that they made that error. They can say the words and understand the words, but they don't put the passage together so that they recognize that it doesn't make sense.

There are even deeper implications. We remember that the left BA 44, 45 is Broca's area, the critically important language area of the frontal lobe. BA 44, 45 of the right hemisphere is <u>not</u> language related, but rather is responsible for inhibiting the impulsive responses of the left DLPFC (Aron, Robbins, & Poldrack, 2004). When the right hemisphere is deactivated, the left DLPFC is able to perform impulsive actions. The left DLPFC is more active in impulsive, risk-taking individuals, while the right DLPFC is more active in reflective, cautious individuals (Chokron, Dupierrix, Tabert, & Bartolomeo, 2007).

There is an even deeper problem associated with deactivation of the right hemisphere. The left insular cortex is critically important for speech production, and damage to this area seen in apraxia of speech, a significant inability to organize the articulators for speech production. The right insular cortex has no function in speech or language, but is rather the seat of insight and perception of self (Craig, 2002, 2009). The right insular cortex appears to be the center for empathy and compassion, insight (the "aha" moment), and that feeling of well-being that you have when you finally figure out your personal agency and "place in the universe." Practices that are designed to increase compassion actually cause the right insula to increase in volume (Valk et al., 2017), and the insula is always active during compassionate meditation. Empathy is the acknowledgment of the suffering of others, while compassion is the desire to change or ameliorate that suffering. Consider now the impact of disabling the center associated with compassion and its impact on interpersonal interactions. Remember, the damage is not <u>to</u> the right insular cortex, but rather the problem very likely arises from failure to activate the right insula.

Thus, the right hemisphere and right subcortex appear to be critically important for the function of the whole person. Loss of right hemisphere function is not simply loss of, for instance, the left visual field, but is potentially a profound alteration of an individual's personality. In many ways, LHD can cause loss of critical language and analytic functions, but RHD can result in loss of many of those elements that are the glue of society and social interaction, including humor, pragmatics, the capacity for compassion, and empathy. Please realize that the right hemisphere is "quiet" and not involved in the high structure of language, but it is really an extraordinarily important participant in making a person whole.

CHAPTER SUMMARY

The cerebral cortex is made up of two grossly identical but mirror-image hemispheres that are connected by means of the corpus callosum and separated by the superior longitudinal fissure. The frontal lobe is involved in cognition and executive function, expressive language function, and emotional regulation.

The parietal lobe receives somatic input representing body sense (postcentral gyrus) and integrates this with motor function (superior parietal lobule and intraparietal sulcus), and visual (angular gyrus) and auditory information (supramarginal gyrus). The angular gyrus of the parietal lobe is critical to the language process of reading, and the supramarginal gyrus is involved in phonetic processing.

The occipital lobe receives all visual input that reaches consciousness at the calcarine sulcus. The temporal lobe has three major gyri. The superior temporal gyrus includes the lateral aspect of Heschl's gyrus as well as Wernicke's area. The posterior aspect of the middle temporal gyrus works with Wernicke's area in language processing. The inferior temporal gyrus is involved in visual-auditory integration. The parahippocampal gyrus is found on the inferior temporal lobe. The limbic system is composed of many cortical parts, including the amygdala, dentate gyrus, hippocampus, cingulate gyrus, and olfactory bulb and tract. It is important for emotional processes, sex drive, and motivation.

The medial surface of the cerebrum is the surface that separates the two cerebral hemispheres. The postcentral and precentral gyri extend into the medial surface, with the areas in the medial surface being associated with activation and sensation of the lower leg and foot. The corpus callosum is a collection of commissural fibers connecting the two cerebral hemispheres and allowing communication between them. The corpus callosum is composed of four major regions: rostrum, genu, body, and splenium, and they reflect the areas of the cerebral cortex being served. The body (trunk) connects the posterior frontal lobes and parietal lobes, while the splenium connects the temporal and occipital lobes. The rostrum allows the orbital regions of the frontal lobe and part of the premotor region to communicate. Fibers that course through genu of the corpus callosum allow the anterior frontal lobes to communicate. The paracentral lobule is the point of reflection of the precentral and postcentral gyri on the medial surface, and the precuneus of the parietal lobe is involved in visuospatial processing, episodic memory function, and the sense of agency in action. The cuneus of the occipital lobe is involved in visual information processing as well as impulse control. The cingulate gyrus is important for emotional regulation.

The inferior surface of the cerebral cortex includes the fusiform gyrus (face recognition), the lingual gyrus (visual processing), and the parahippocampal gyri (memory). The uncus overlies the amygdaloid body, which generates fear responses. On the anterior-inferior surface is the temporal pole of the temporal lobe (autobiographical memory) and the gyrus rectus and orbital gyri, which are involved in emotional regulation and mediation. The olfactory sulcus is an indentation in the cerebral cortex that holds the olfactory tract, and the splenium of the corpus callosum can be seen in the posterior aspect. The stalk of the hypophysis (pituitary gland) can be seen in the mid regions.

The lateral portion of the primary motor area gives rise to the corticobulbar tract, which controls the muscles associated with speech. The axons project through the genu of the internal capsule, terminating in the brainstem. At this level, the axons project to the nuclei of the cranial nerves both ipsilaterally and contralaterally. The corticobulbar tract innervates the nuclei of the cranial nerves trigeminal (V), facial (VII), glossopharyngeal (IX), vagus (X), accessory (XI), and hypoglossal (XII). In the nucleus ambiguus, the tract contributes to the motor region of the vagus nerve. The corticospinal tract originates in the primary motor cortex, the supplemental motor area, and premotor region. The axons project to the posterior internal capsule and the medial portion of the cerebral peduncle. At the medulla, approximately 80% of the fibers cross the midline at the decussation of pyramids and descend through the spinal cord as the lateral corticospinal tract. Those fibers remaining ipsilateral will descend as the anterior corticospinal tract.

Myelinated fibers are axons of neurons arising from the cortex itself. There are three types of communicating fibers:

projection fibers, association fibers, and commissural fibers. Projection fibers make up the tracts that connect the cortex, brainstem, and spinal cord, as well as the fibers carrying afferent information to the cortex. The corona radiata condenses to form the internal capsule, a central hub for projection fibers leaving or entering the cerebrum. The anterior aspect of the internal capsule (anterior limb) serves the frontal lobe and separates the caudate nucleus and putamen. The posterior limb of the internal capsule includes the optic radiation, a group of fibers projecting to the calcarine sulcus for vision. The genu and posterior limbs carry the corticospinal and corticobulbar tract. Association fibers can be either short or long. Short association fibers connect one gyrus with an adjacent gyrus, but long association fibers provide communication between distant locations of the cerebral cortex. There are many identified groups of long association fibers. The uncinate fasciculus connects the orbital portion and inferior and middle frontal gyri with the anterior temporal lobe and is part of the limbic system. The cingulate gyrus is divided into anterior cingulate cortex (ACC) and posterior cingulate cortex (PCC). The anterior cingulate cortex is involved in emotional response and regulation, impulse control, empathy, and cognitive processes. The PCC appears to take on an evaluative function related to its activity in the spatial environment. The superior longitudinal fasciculus (SLF) is a massive set of association fibers divided into four groups. SLF I connects the superior parietal lobule and precuneus with the premotor and eye regions of the frontal lobe. SLF II connects the temporo-occipito-parietal region, angular gyrus, supramarginal gyrus, and postcentral gyrus with the dorsolateral prefrontal cortex. SLF III connects the supramarginal gyrus with the inferior parietal lobe, the postcentral gyrus, the precentral gyrus, the premotor region, and Broca's area. The arcuate fasciculus connects the supramarginal gyrus, Wernicke's area, and the temporo-occipital region. Language comprehension and expression are most likely linked through the arcuate fasciculus and the fibers of SLF III. The inferior longitudinal fasciculus connects the temporal pole with the occipital lobe, making up the ventral stream for visual processing. The perpendicular fasciculus connects the fusiform gyrus with the superior parietal lobule. The occipitofrontal fasciculus provides communication between the occipital lobe and frontal lobe. The fornix connects the hippocampus with the thalamus and mammillary bodies. Commissural fibers make up the final group of association fibers. The corpus callosum is the primary set of commissural fibers, but the anterior commissure connects olfactory regions from both hemispheres.

Hemispheric specialization (HS) refers to the differential specialization for a task by one cerebral hemisphere over the other. In 90% of the population, the left hemisphere is dominant for language. The right hemisphere is considered to be the nondominant hemisphere. The left hemisphere is analytical, detail oriented, rapid, impulsive, and judgmental. It processes information in a sequential fashion. The right hemisphere is more reflective, synthesizing, and slower to respond. It places information into context. The left amygdala is larger in people who are altruistic and smaller in people who are psychopathic. People with right hemisphere damage may have difficulties with nonliteral meanings of words, humor, pragmatics, sarcasm, and idioms. People with right hemisphere dysfunction will often demonstrate left hemispatial neglect. This deficit seems to be related to a deficit in attention. Three types of attention are: alerting, orienting, and executive. Alerting attention is the basic attention set in preparation for a stimulus. Orienting attention is the process of bringing attention to a specific stimulus. Executive attention allows us to act on our perceptions and is a critically important component of executive function. In left visual neglect, persons fail to attend to images in their left visual field, which results in simply not knowing that something is going on in that visual field until they are alerted to attend to it. In people with right hemisphere dysfunction, lack of activation of BA 44, 45 of the right hemisphere may cause them to have impulsive responses due to lack of inhibition of the left DLPFC. The right insular cortex is the seat for compassion, insight, and empathy, and it is possible that this area is not as active in people with right hemisphere dysfunction as a result of reduced hemispheric activation.

CASE STUDY 4–1

Physician's Notes on Initial Physical Examination and History

This 83-year-old male patient was admitted at the neurosurgical clinic regarding visual defects and speech disorders. The patient underwent a thorough examination and a lesion was diagnosed consistent with high-grade glioma, affecting parts of left primary visual cortex, calcarine sulcus, and areas responsible for the integration of sensory input in language (Figures 4–16 and 4–17).

The patient presented with right unilateral **hemianopsic defect** (see Table 4–4 for terminology. Note that we are presenting the data of this case in chronological order to show the emerging speech and language signs and symptoms as the condition progresses) with retained central vision. Written and spoken language disturbances were also noted.

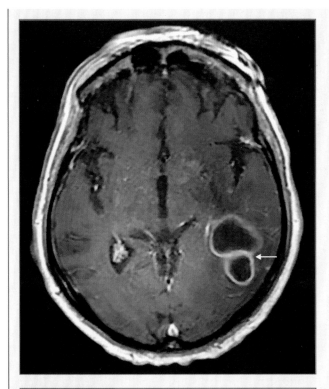

FIGURE 4–16. Contrast-enhanced T1 -weighted MRI, transverse view. Note arrows indicate lesion site. Axial view of the brain demonstrates a mass with peripheral enhancement consistent with High grade glioma (*white arrow*) adjacent to the left temporo-occipital region. *Source:* Figure courtesy of Dr. Kyriakos Paraskeva, MD, Resident of Neurosurgery, Nicosia General Hospital, Cyprus.

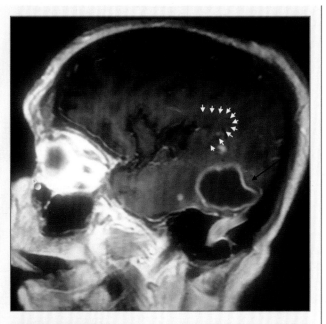

FIGURE 4–17. Contrast-enhanced T1-weighted MRI. Sagittal view of brain parenchyma displays intact angular gyrus (*white arrows*) and lesion of primary visual cortex (*black arrow*). *Source:* Figure courtesy of Dr. Kyriakos Paraskeva, MD, Resident of Neurosurgery, Nicosia General Hospital, Cyprus.

The patient was unable to comprehend words and letters or to retrieve and recognize objects and familiar faces respectively, despite having them projected onto a whiteboard. He was unable to perceive simple written symbols or to understand the meaning of written sentences. The patient also demonstrated anomia.

Associate disorders included **alexia** (incomprehensible written language), **paralexia** (distortion, poor syntax, and inability to recognize the difference between similar written words), **paragraphia** (associated with damage of angular gyrus, not presented in this case), and **alexia without paragraphia** (intact angular gyrus in subcortical lesions preserving associative areas). The location of the lesion was found to be Brodmann's areas 17, 18, 19.

Medical Diagnosis

Glioma affecting occipital lobe.

TABLE 4–4.	Terminology for Case Study 4–1
Hemianopsic defect	Visual field loss.
Alexia	Deficit of comprehension of written language.
Paralexia	Reading disturbance that includes reversals, distortions, transpositions of letters, words, and syllables.
Paragraphia	Writing letters other than those intended.
Alexia without paragraphia	Inability to read in absence of paragraphia.

Treatment

Maximum safe microsurgical resection of the lesion assisted by neuronavigation and intraoperative neuromonitoring. Postoperatively, the patient fared well with moderately restored language and vision. He was transferred to the oncology department for further management.

Speech-Language Considerations

The lesion involved the calcarine cortex (BA 17) as well as association areas BA 18 and 19, cuneate gyrus and lingual gyri). While the affected area involved only the visual cortex and the immediately surrounding region, the effect was far-ranging, including loss of comprehension of written information, difficulty with face recognition (a function of the fusiform gyrus, also adjacent to the calcarine sulcus), and difficulty with writing (perhaps because of the visual perception difficulties arising from the lesion).

Questions Concerning This Case

1. The lesion nominally involved only the region of the calcarine sulcus, lingual gyrus, and cuneate gyrus. What would account for the difficulties with face recognition and expressive writing problems?
2. The cuneate gyrus has been implicated in establishment of one's self-efficacy (i.e., knowledge of self). Do you see indications of confusion concerning the patient's self-perception?

From the case book of Dr. Kyriakos Paraskeva, MD, Resident of Neurosurgery, Nicosia General Hospital, Cyprus.

CASE STUDY 4–2

Physician's Notes on Initial Physical Examination and History

This 92-year-old male was admitted at the neurosurgical clinic regarding right motor weakness, sudden onset of severe headache, impaired consciousness, and speech difficulties. An urgent **MRI** scan of the brain was obtained. A space-occupying lesion with malignant findings was revealed, spanning the left inferior frontal gyrus, temporal pole, frontal operculum, anterior insula, portion of basal ganglia, occipitofrontal and uncinate fasciculus (Figures 4–18 and 4–19).

The patient's **gait disturbances** were the most prominent sign, accompanied by **dysarthria** (see Table 4–5 for terminology). The individual's speech was slurred and confused. Verbal responses were sluggish, while syntax and phrase structure were substantially impaired. **Agrammatism** and **dysprosody** resulted in "telegraphing speech." Intonation was almost absent, with bad sentence articulation and consecutive word omission. In contrast, speech perception was intact with preserved word repetition ability.

Associate disorders included **nonfluent aphasia** (**expressive aphasia; Broca's aphasia**), and **conduction aphasia** (ruled out in this case). The location of the lesion included Brodmann's areas 6, 43, 44, 45, 38, 21, and 22, which involved Broca's area, the anterior left insula, a portion of auditory cortex, and temporal pole.

Medical Diagnosis

Malignant tumor of left lateral cortex

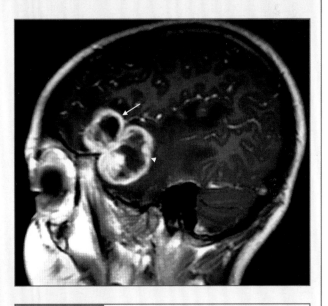

FIGURE 4–18. Contrast-enhanced T1-weighted MR. Sagittal view of the brain illustrates Broca's area (*white arrow*) and portion of temporal pole (*white arrowhead*) infiltration. *Source:* Figure courtesy of Dr. Kyriakos Paraskeva, MD, Resident of Neurosurgery, Nicosia General Hospital, Cyprus.

Treatment

Maximum safe microsurgical resection of the lesion assisted by neuronavigation and **intraoperative neuromonitoring**. The patient was referred to the oncology department for further treatment.

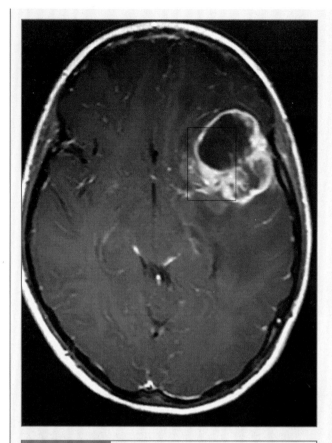

FIGURE 4–19. Contrast-enhanced T1-weighted MR. Axial (transverse) view depicts left anterior insula (*area confined by black square*) infiltration. *Source:* Figure courtesy of Dr. Kyriakos Paraskeva, MD, Resident of Neurosurgery, Nicosia General Hospital, Cyprus.

Speech-Language Considerations

The magnitude of the affected left hemisphere left the individual with significant speech and language impairment. BA 6 includes portions of the precentral gyrus and premotor gyrus, while BA 44, 45 are Broca's area. BA 38 is the inferior aspect of the temporal pole, while BA 21 is the middle temporal gyrus. BA 22 is the superior temporal gyrus. Taken together, the superior and middle temporal gyri are involved in receptive language processing and include Wernicke's area. Broca's area involvement would result in nonfluent aphasia, while Wernicke's area lesion would result in fluent aphasia. Motor strip involvement in the lateral cortex would potentially result in paralysis of muscles of speech. Involvement of the left insular cortex would result in apraxia of speech. This constellation of lesions in the dominant hemisphere represents near total involvement of the speech and language systems.

TABLE 4–5.	Terminology for Case Study 4–2
Agrammatism	Speech of nonfluent (Broca's) aphasia, consisting of predominantly content words.
Broca's aphasia (nonfluent aphasia)	Aphasia affecting language expression, resulting from lesion to BA 44, 45 and associated white matter.
Conduction aphasia	Aphasia resulting from lesion to the arcuate fasciculus. The primary differential characteristic of conduction aphasia is relatively spared expression and comprehension but deficit in repetition.
Dysarthria	Motor speech disorder involving muscular weakness, dyscoordination, and alteration of muscle tone.
Dysprosody	Deficit in the prosodic component of speech, predominantly involving elements of stress arising from intonation and vocal intensity variation.
Nonfluent aphasia	Broca's aphasia (expressive aphasia).
Fluent aphasia (a.k.a. Wernicke's aphasia; receptive aphasia)	Language deficit arising from neurological etiology and resulting in loss of comprehension of language. Typical site of lesion is the posterior superior temporal gyrus and posterior middle temporal gyrus in the dominant hemisphere.
Gait disturbances	Gait described as abnormal, unsteady, staggering, and uncoordinated.
Intonation	Variation in vocal fundamental frequency.
Intraoperative neuromonitoring	Monitoring for brain function during neurosurgical procedures, including electroencephalography (EEG), electromyography (EMG), and evoked responses (such as auditory evoked brainstem responses).
MRI (magnetic resonance imaging)	Diagnostic technique that uses magnetic fields to show an image of the body's soft tissue and bones.

Questions Concerning This Case

1. The tumor was in the left hemisphere, and involved many of the speech and language areas of the brain. Which area would account for the apraxic signs?
2. Intonation refers to the use of fluctuations in fundamental frequency for the purpose of conveying suprasegmental meaning. We think of the nondominant hemisphere (typically right hemisphere) as mediating both perception and production of intonation (see the final section of this chapter entitled "The Other Half" for further discussion of the nondominant hemisphere). Given that this individual's left hemisphere speech areas were affected, why would there be loss of intonational variation (hint: the speech was halting and telegraphic).

From the case book of Dr. Kyriakos Paraskeva, MD,
Resident of Neurosurgery, Nicosia General Hospital, Cyprus.

CASE STUDY 4–3

Physician's Notes on Initial Physical Examination and History

This 68-year-old male was referred from Nicosia General Hospital Neurosurgical Department regarding behavioral changes, progressive unsteadiness, and urine **incontinence**. Radiographic presentation revealed an intraventricular tumor projecting more to the left lateral ventricle, causing occlusion of the foramen of Monro and dilatation of the ventricular system (Figures 4–20 and 4–21). **Semiology** and radiographic findings such as were consistent with the diagnosis of **obstructive hydrocephalus** (see Table 4–6 for terminology. Note that we are presenting the data of this case in chronological order to show the emerging speech and language signs and symptoms as the condition progresses).

The patient suffered from **left tactile agnosia**, left sided **dyspraxia**, **pseudohemianopsia**, **anomia for smell**, impaired spatial synthesis of the right hand resulting in difficulty copying complex figures, short-term memory defi-

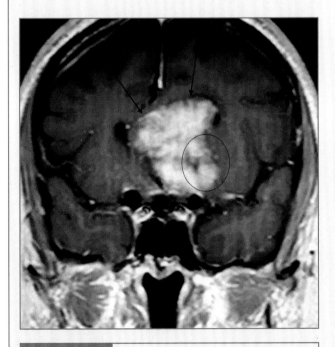

FIGURE 4–20. FLAIR-weighted MRI. Coronal view of the brain indicates tumor with intraventricular extension (*black arrows*) and hypothalamic infiltration (*area confined by black circle*). *Source:* Figure courtesy of Dr. Kyriakos Paraskeva, MD, Resident of Neurosurgery, Nicosia General Hospital, Cyprus.

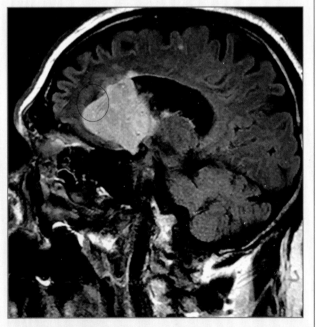

FIGURE 4–21. FLAIR-weighted MRI. Sagittal view of the brain exposes genu of corpus callosum compromise (*area confined by black circle*). *Source:* Figure courtesy of Dr. Kyriakos Paraskeva, MD, Resident of Neurosurgery, Nicosia General Hospital, Cyprus.

TABLE 4–6.	Terminology for Case Study 4–3
Anomia for smell	Inability to identify names to describe smells.
Incontinence	Loss of control of urine release from the bladder.
Left-sided dyspraxia	Inability to plan a motor act in absence of muscular weakness (in this case, inability to plan a motor act using the left side of the body).
Pseudohemianopsia	Condition wherein a stimulus is seen accurately until the nasal visual field of one eye and the temporal visual field of the other eye are simultaneously stimulated, one field will be found to be blind.
Tactile agnosia	Inability to recognize an object presented through the tactile sensation.
Semiology	Study of signs.
Obstructive hydrocephalus (ex-vacuo hydrocephalus)	Hydrocephalus arising from trauma that prohibits flow of cerebrospinal fluid, causing increased cerebrospinal fluid pressure within the brain.

cits, decreased spontaneity of speech, and incontinence. Associate disorders included disconnection syndrome and obstructive hydrocephalus.

The location of the tumor included the ventricular system, fornix, cavum septum pellucidum, caudate nucleus, genu of corpus callosum, lateral portion and roof of the third ventricle, foramen of Monro, choroid plexus, portion of the thalamus, and portion of the hypothalamus.

Medical Diagnosis

Tumor in left hemisphere, impinging on ventricles.

Treatment

Maximum safe microsurgical resection of the tumor assisted by intraoperative neuronavigation and neuromonitoring. Histopathology results were consistent with the diagnosis of central neurocytoma. Patient's speech disorder never resolved in a two-year follow-up.

Speech-Language Considerations

This tumor would have had a significant impact on the speech of the individual, beyond the effects of hydrocephalus. The hydrocephalus would arise from obstruction of the foramen of Monro, implying that the major impact would be within the left lateral ventricle, since CSF would not be able to pass from the lateral ventricle to the third ventricle. Compression of the left frontal, parietal, and temporal lobes would result from this obstruction. In addition to the compression of the cortex, the tumor involved the genu of the corpus callosum, roof of the third ventricle (inferior corpus callosum), thalamus, and hypothalamus. One would predict difficulty with interhemispheric interaction as a result of partial severing of the corpus callosum, with damage to the genu causing likely auditory difficulties. Damage to the thalamus and hypothalamus, either from the tumor or from surgical removal, would result in deficits related to processing sensory information (thalamus) and regulation of bodily metabolic function (hypothalamus). This tumor would have the potential of profound impact on speech and language, considering compression of the left hemisphere and loss of thalamus input (including audition).

Questions Concerning This Case

1. Given what you know about damage to the left hemisphere, what dysfunction would you predict with compression of the left frontal, parietal, occipital, and temporal lobes, secondary to hydrocephalus?

From the case book of Dr. Kyriakos Paraskeva, MD, Resident of Neurosurgery, Nicosia General Hospital, Cyprus.

CASE STUDY 4–4

Physician's Notes on Initial Physical Examination and History

This male patient was admitted at the neurosurgical clinic regarding memory deficits and speech and gait disturbances. An MRI scan of the brain was obtained. An occupying lesion consistent with **craniopharyngioma** (tumor that develops from residual cells of Rathke's pouch) arising from the anterior superior margin of the pituitary gland with some extension into the third ventricle was visualized (Figures 4–22, 4–23, and 4–24).

The patient presented with hypoadrenalism and hypothyroidism. He was complaining about fluctuations between somnolence and insomnia. There was reduced sensation of thirst (anterior osmoreceptors) and difficulty in independent ambulation (due to **CSF hydrodynamics** alteration and potential obstructive hydrocephalus). The patient's speech was comprehensible, though sluggish and slurred. He was able to understand written tasks and obey oral and/or written commands. Spatial synthesis and orientation to place and time was normal. Writing ability remained intact. Deep and superficial sensation, smell, and deep tendon reflexes were preserved. No cranial nerve abnormalities or cerebellar dysfunction was noted during clinical examination. Mini Mental State Examination (MMSE) was also employed in order to define memory and perception deficits. Associated disorders included diabetes insipidus, hypothalamic disturbances, and obstructive hydrocephalus.

Medical Diagnosis

Craniopharyngioma at the anterior superior margin of the pituitary gland, extending into the third ventricle. Location of the lesion included the pituitary gland and stalk, third ventricle, hypothalamus, mammillary bodies, lamina

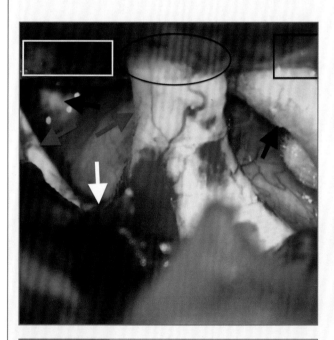

FIGURE 4–22. Intraoperative image of craniopharyngioma microsurgical resection. Optic nerves (*red arrows*), optic chiasm (*white arrow*), optic foramen of sphenoid bone (*area confined by black circle*), ipsilateral and contralateral Internal carotid arteries (*black arrows*), part of planum sphenoidale (*area confined by white rectangle*), and portion of anterior clinoid process (*area confined by black square*). *Source:* Figure courtesy of Dr. Kyriakos Paraskeva, MD, Resident of Neurosurgery, Nicosia General Hospital, Cyprus.

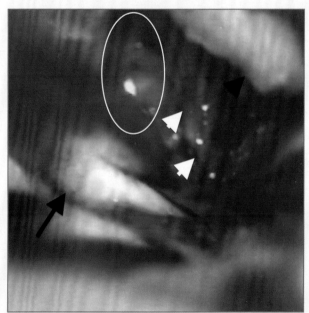

FIGURE 4–23. Intraoperative image of craniopharyngioma microsurgical resection pituitary stalk (*white arrowheads*), optic nerve (*black arrow*), internal carotid artery (*black arrowhead*), and portion of craniopharyngioma (*area confined by white circle*). *Source:* Figure courtesy of Dr. Kyriakos Paraskeva, MD, Resident of Neurosurgery, Nicosia General Hospital, Cyprus.

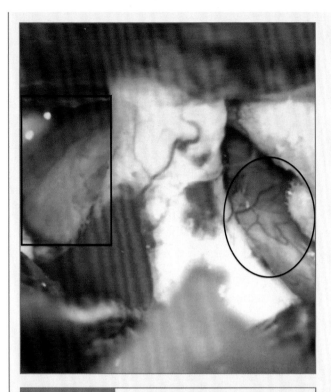

FIGURE 4–24.   Intraoperative image of craniopharyngioma microsurgical resection. Subchiasmatic and retrochiasmatic projection of the grayish tumor (*area confined by black rectangle*), and opticocarotid projection of craniopharyngioma (*area confined by black circle*). *Source:* Figure courtesy of Dr. Kyriakos Paraskeva, MD, Resident of Neurosurgery, Nicosia General Hospital, Cyprus.

TABLE 4–7.	Terminology for Case Study 4–4
ACA	Anterior carotid artery.
a-comm	Anterior communicating artery.
Craniopharyngioma	Tumor typically arising from pituitary gland, and often involving optic nerve and chiasm.
Frontotemporal incision	Incision at the pterion.
ICA	Internal carotid artery.
Intraoperative neuromonitoring	Monitoring for brain function during neurosurgical procedures, including electroencephalography (EEG), electromyography (EMG), and evoked responses (such as auditory evoked brainstem responses).
Microsurgical resection	Surgery using microsurgical techniques.
p-comm	Posterior communicating artery.
Pterional craniotomy	Surgically opening the skull at the pterion. The pterion is the point at which frontal, parietal, temporal, and sphenoid bones communicate, on the lateral aspect of the skull.
Semiology	The study of signs.
Transylvian approach	Surgical approach through the Sylvian fissure.

terminalis, optic nerve and chiasm, and anterior perforated substance, with small feeders from **p-comm**, **ICA**, **ACA**, and **a-comm** (see Table 4–7 for terminology. Note that we are presenting the data of this case in chronological order to show the emerging speech and language signs and symptoms as the condition progresses.).

Treatment

The patient underwent a large right frontotemporal incision, and head was positioned with slight lateral rotation. A combined subfrontal/**pterional craniotomy** was performed assisted by intraoperative neuromonitoring. Tumor was reached via transylvian approach, and gross total microsurgical resection was accomplished from several corridors such as subchiasmatic, opticocarotid, lamina terminalis, and lateral to carotid artery. Tumor biopsy was performed of what pathologically proved to be a craniopharyngioma.

The patient was discharged on the eleventh postoperative day. (See Neuroquest software for a video of the surgery.)

One Year Post Surgery

On one-year follow-up with several MRI scans there was no recurrence, though slurred speech, endocrine dysfunction, and hypothalamic semiology overshadowed the aforementioned positive surgical result.

Speech-Language-Hearing Considerations

This patient presented with dysarthria prior to surgery. The primary site of involvement was the pituitary gland and the third ventricle, so it is reasonable to assume that there was compression of the thalamus as a result of the tumor, and perhaps damage to the inputs to the thalamus as a result of surgery. The thalamus receives input from almost all sensory systems of the body and is intimately related to speech, language, and hearing. The pulvinar is associated with language function, while the medial geniculate body is the last auditory relay before the cerebral cortex. If these nuclei were involved, one would predict both language and auditory consequences. Further, if the motor nuclei of the thalamus were damaged through either tumor or surgical procedure, speech involvement could be predicted. Based on the fact that the patient was admitted with dysarthria that did not remit following treatment, it is likely that the damage to the thalamus arose from the tumor itself, and removal of the tumor did not alleviate the effects of compression.

Questions Concerning This Case

1. Remember that the pituitary gland is at the base of the brain and that the optic chiasm crosses around it. What would you predict would occur to the patient's visual ability as a result of this tumor and/or its removal?

2. Knowing what you do about the structures superior to the pituitary gland (i.e., those on either side of the pituitary on the inferior cortex), could you envision any other possible consequences of compression? You might want to review Figure 4–2H as you think about this.

From the case book of Dr. Kyriakos Paraskeva, MD, Resident of Neurosurgery, Nicosia General Hospital, Cyprus.

CHAPTER 4
STUDY QUESTIONS

1. The term _____ actually refers to bark, as in bark of a tree.

2. Outfoldings of the cerebral cortex are known as _____.

3. Infoldings of the cerebral cortex are known as _____.

4. Please identify the structures and landmarks indicated on this figure.

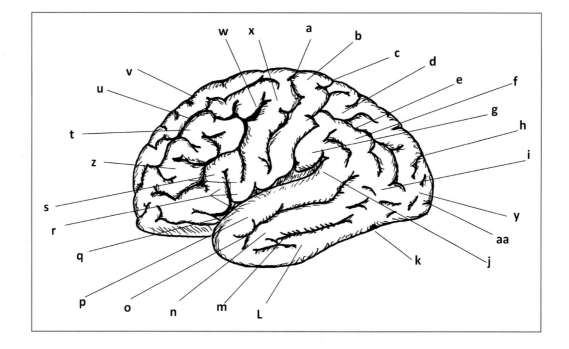

a. _____ sulcus

b. _____ gyrus

c. _____ sulcus

d. _____ _____ lobule

e. _____ sulcus

f. _____ _____ lobule

g. _____ gyrus

h. _____ notch

i. _____ gyrus

j. _____ area

k. _____ notch

l. _____ _____ gyrus

m. _____ _____ sulcus

n. _____ _____ gyrus

o. _____ _____ sulcus

v. _____ _____ gyrus

p. _____ _____ gyrus

w. _____ sulcus

q. _____ fissure

x. _____ gyrus

r. _____ (area overlying insula)

y. _____ sulcus

s. _____ area

z. _____ lobe

t. _____ _____ gyrus

aa. _____ pole

u. _____ _____ sulcus

5. The _____ gyrus is also known as the motor strip.

6. Somatosensory information arrives at the _____ gyrus.

7. The _____ _____ fissure completely separates the left and right cerebral hemispheres.

8. The _____ _____ separates the temporal lobe from the frontal and parietal lobes.

9. The outermost meningeal lining is the _____ _____.

10. The innermost meningeal lining is the _____ _____.

11. The _____ mater is the intermediate meningeal lining.

12. The _____ _____ is the dural component that separates the two cerebral hemispheres.

13. The _____ _____ is the dural component that separates the two cerebellar hemispheres.

14. The _____ _____ is the dural shelf that separates the cerebrum from the cerebellum.

15. The _____ _____ is the dural component that encases the hypophysis (pituitary gland).

16. _____ _____ bathes the CNS, providing a cushion for the neural tissue.

17. Cerebrospinal fluid is generated within the ventricles, specifically by secreting epithelial structures called the _____ plexus.

18. The _____ horn of the lateral ventricles projects into the frontal lobe.

19. The _____ horn of the lateral ventricles projects into the occipital lobe.

20. The _____ ventricle is between the left and right thalamus.

21. The _____ _____ of _____ connects the lateral and third ventricles.

22. The _____ _____ crosses the third ventricle, connecting the left and right thalami.

23. The _____ ventricle resides between the cerebellum and the brainstem.

24. The _____ _____ connects the third and fourth ventricles.

25. Please identify landmarks of the ventricular system from the figure.

    a. _____ ventricle

    b. _____ ventricle

    c. _____ horn

    d. _____ foramen of _____

    e. _____ horn

    f. _____ ventricle

    g. _____ aqueduct

    h. _____ horn

26. Please match each layer of the cerebral cortex with its dominant descriptor.

    _____ external pyramidal layer

    _____ outermost molecular layer

    _____ external granular layer

    _____ multiform layer

    _____ internal pyramidal layer

    _____ internal granular layer

    a. consists mostly of glial cells and axons from neurons of succeeding layers

    b. small pyramidal cells

    c. large pyramidal cells

    d. non-pyramidal cells

    e. large pyramidal cells that project to motor centers beyond the cerebral cortex

    f. pyramidal cells that project to the thalamus

27. The _____ sulcus divides the parietal and frontal lobes.

28. Please identify the lobe in which the following landmarks or functions reside, using the indicated letter.

a. frontal lobe

b. parietal lobe

c. occipital lobe

d. temporal lobe

e. insular lobe

_____ seat of cognitive function   _____ dorsolateral prefrontal cortex

_____ visual reception   _____ Heschl's gyrus

_____ auditory reception   _____ precentral gyrus

_____ somatic sense reception   _____ postcentral gyrus

_____ intraparietal sulcus   _____ supplementary motor area

_____ supramarginal gyrus   _____ superior temporal gyrus

_____ angular gyrus   _____ hippocampus

_____ calcarine sulcus   _____ fusiform gyrus

_____ Wernicke's area   _____ parahippocampal gyrus

_____ Broca's area

29. Please provide Brodmann numbers for the following areas.

_____ precentral gyrus   _____ premotor region

_____ _____ Broca's area   _____ orbitofrontal cortx

_____ Wernicke's area   _____ _____ _____ somatosensory cortex (postcentral gyrus)

_____ angular gyrus   _____ Heschl's gyrus

_____ supramarginal gyrus   _____ parahippocampal gyrus

_____ _____ dorsolateral prefrontal cortex   _____ calcarine sulcus

_____ supplementary motor area (SMA)   _____ _____ insular cortex

30. The area overlying the insula is termed the _____.

31. Executive function is the process of utilizing cognitive capacity to accomplish goals. The _____ _____ _____ (BA 46/9) is the site for control of executive functions.

32. The _____ gyrus is responsible for direct activation of muscles.

33. True or False: The view of the homunculus shows distorted size of the structures, so that, for instance, the fingers of the hand are large and the foot is small. This representation reflects the amount of innervation that a specific region receives.

34. True or False: On the homunculus, structures related to speech (articulators, larynx) are on the lateral aspect, while structures of the lower body (e.g., legs) are on the superior and medial aspect.

35. True or False: The supplementary motor area (SMA) is considered a premotor region that is involved in motor preparation.

36. _____ area is considered the expressive language area of the cortex.

37. _____ area is considered the area where language comprehension occurs.

38. The _____ cortex (BA 10, 11) is involved in emotion regulation, normalization of traumatic events, and behavioral inhibition. It is in the anterior-inferior frontal lobe.

39. True or False: The intraparietal sulcus is part of the "where" visual stream (dorsal visual stream).

40. True or False: The angular gyrus is responsible for motor planning and execution.

41. True or False: The supramarginal gyrus is involved in phonetic processing.

42. The site of auditory reception in the cortex (BA 41) is termed _____ gyrus.

43. The _____ sulcus is the site of visual reception in the cortex.

44. The left _____ cortex is the site of motor planning for articulation of speech.

45. The _____ _____ is the site of processing the sense of taste in the cortex.

46. The _____ _____ is a set of commissural fibers that connect left and right hemispheres.

47. Visible in the medial view of the cerebrum, the _____ gyrus is involved in emotion regulation.

48. Visible on the inferior surface of the cortex, the _____ gyrus is involved in face recognition.

49. Visible on the inferior surface of the cortex, the _____ gyrus is the location of the hippocampus.

50. The corticobulbar tract is made up of _____ fibers.

51. The _____ _____ is the "radiating crown" of myelinated fibers projecting to and arising from the cerebral cortex. These fibers condense to form the internal capsule.

52. The _____ limb of the internal capsule includes the corticospinal tract.

53. The _____ of the internal capsule includes the corticobulbar tract.

54. The corticospinal and corticobulbar tracts arise from the _____ gyrus of the cerebral cortex.

55. The corticospinal tract decussates at the level of the _____ in the brainstem.

56. _____ association fibers connect two adjacent gyri.

57. _____ association fibers connect distant gyri in the same hemisphere.

58. _____ fibers connect homologous regions of the left and right cerebral hemispheres.

59. The _____ gyrus is a set of long association fibers that connect the limbic system with the prefrontal cortex. It is largely responsible for emotion regulations.

REFERENCES

Ardila, A., Bernal, B., & Rosselli, M. (2016). How extended is Wernicke's area? Meta-analytic connectivity study of BA20 and integrative proposal. *Neuroscience Journal*. http://dx.doi:10.1155/2016/4962562

Aron A. R. , Robbins, T. W., & Poldrack, R. A. (2004). Inhibition and the right inferior frontal cortex. *Trends in Cognitive Sciences, (4)*, 170–177.

Azevedo, F. A., Carvalho, L. R., Grinberg, L. T., Farfel, J. M., Ferretti, Aron, A. R., Robbins, T. W., & Poldrack, R. A. (2004). Inhibition and the right inferior frontal cortex. *Trends in Cognitive Sciences*, *8*(4), 170–177.

Baehr, M., & Frotscher, M. (2012). *Duus' topical diagnosis in neurology: Anatomy, physiology, signs, symptoms* (5th ed.). New York, NY: Thieme.

Ballmaier, M., Toga, A. W., Blanton, R. E., Sowell, E. R., Lavretsky, H., Peterson, J., . . . Kumar, A. (2004). Anterior cingulate, gyrus rectus, and orbitofrontal abnormalities in elderly depressed patients: An MRI-based parcellation of the prefrontal cortex. *American Journal of Psychiatry*, *161*(1), 99–108.

Bartolomeo, P., Thiebaut de Schotten, M., & Doricchi, F. (2007). Left unilateral neglect as a disconnection syndrome. *Cerebral Cortex*, *17*(11), 2479–2490.

Beeman, M. J., & Chiarello, C. (1998). Complementary right-and left-hemisphere language comprehension. *Current Directions in Psychological Science*, *7*(1), 2–8.

Bernal, B., & Ardila, A. (2009). The role of the arcuate fasciculus in conduction aphasia. *Brain*, *132*(9), 2309–2316.

Beyer, C., Anguiano, G., & Mena, F. (1961). Oxytocin release in response to stimulation of cingulate gyrus. *American Journal of Physiology—Legacy Content*, *200*(3), 625–627.

Blake, M. L. (2009). Inferencing processes after right hemisphere brain damage: Maintenance of inferences. *Journal of Speech, Language, and Hearing Research*, *52*(2), 359–372.

Blom, R. M., Hennekam, R. C., & Denys, D. (2012). Body integrity identity disorder. *PLoS One*, *7*(4), e34702.

Briggs, F., & Usrey, W. M. (2008). Emerging views of corticothalamic function. *Current Opinion in Neurobiology*, *18*, 403–407.

Brodmann, K., & Garey, L. J. (2007). *Brodmann's: Localisation in the cerebral cortex*. New York, NY: Springer.

Bush, G., Luu, P., & Posner, M. I. (2000). Cognitive and emotional influences in anterior cingulate cortex. *Trends in Cognitive Sciences*, *4*(6), 215–222.

Carpenter, M. B. (1978). *Core text of neuroanatomy*. Baltimore, MD: Williams & Wilkins.

Catherine, A. (1994). Quantitative morphology of the corpus callosum in attention deficit hyperactivity disorder. *American Journal of Psychiatry*, *151*, 665–669.

Cavallera, G. M., Giudici, S., & Tommasi, L. (2012). Shadows and darkness in the brain of a genius: Aspects of the neuropsychological literature about the final illness of Maurice Ravel (1875–1937). *Medical Science Monitor: International Medical Journal of Experimental and Clinical Research*, *18*(10), MH1.

Cavanna, A. E., & Trimble, M. R. (2006). The precuneus: A review of its functional anatomy and behavioural correlates. *Brain*, *129*(3), 564–583.

Chokron, S., Dupierrix, E., Tabert, M., & Bartolomeo, P. (2007). Experimental remission of unilateral spatial neglect. *Neuropsychologia*, *45*(14), 3127–3148.

Church, J. A., Coalson, R. S., Lugar, H. M., Petersen, S. E., & Schlaggar, B. L. (2008). A developmental fMRI study of reading and repetition reveals changes in phonological and visual mechanisms over age. *Cerebral Cortex*, *18*(9), 2054–2065.

Clark, H. M., Duffy, J. R., Whitwell, J. L., Ahlskog, J. E., Sorenson, E. J., & Josephs, K. A. (2014). Clinical and imaging characterization of progressive spastic dysarthria. *European Journal of Neurology*, *21*(3), 368–376.

Conant, D., Bouchard, K. E., & Chang, E. F. (2014). Speech map in the human ventral sensory-motor cortex. *Current Opinion in Neurobiology*, *24*(1), 63–67.

Costanzo, E. Y., Villarreal, M., Drucaroff, L. J., Ortiz-Villafañe, M., Castro, M. N., Goldschmidt, M., . . . Camprodon, J. A. (2015). Hemispheric specialization in affective responses, cerebral dominance for language, and handedness: Lateralization of emotion, language, and dexterity. *Behavioural Brain Research*, *288*, 11–19.

Craig, A. D. (2002). How do you feel? Interoception: The sense of the physiological condition of the body. *Nature Reviews Neuroscience*, *3*(8), 655–666.

Craig, A. D. (2009). How do you feel—now? The anterior insula and human awareness. *Nature Reviews Neuroscience*, (10), 59–70.

Crockford, D. N., Goodyear, B., Edwards, J., Quickfall, J., & el-Guebaly, N. (2005). Cue-induced brain activity in pathological gamblers. *Biological Psychiatry*, *58*(10), 787–795.

Crosson, B. (2013). Thalamic mechanisms in language: A reconsideration based on recent findings and concepts. *Brain and Language*, *126*(1), 73–88.

Dalgleish, T. (2004). The emotional brain. *Nature Reviews Neuroscience*, *5*(7), 583.

DeYoung, C. G. (2010). Personality neuroscience and the biology of traits. *Social and Personality Psychology Compass*, *4*(12), 1165–1180.

Dileo, J. F., Brewer, W. J., Hopwood, M., Anderson, V., & Creamer, M. (2008). Olfactory identification dysfunction, aggression and impulsivity in war veterans with post-traumatic stress disorder. *Psychological Medicine*, *38*, 523–531.

Dronkers, N. F. (1996). A new brain region for coordinating speech articulation. *Nature*, *384*(6605), 159–161.

Duffau, H., Gatignol, P., Moritz-Gasser, S., & Mandonnet, E. (2009). Is the left uncinate fasciculus essential for language? *Journal of Neurology*, *256*(3), 382–389.

Dupont, S. (2002). Investigating temporal pole function by functional imaging. *Epileptic Disorders: International Epilepsy Journal with Videotape*, *4*, S17–S22.

Edwin, D., Speedie, L. J., Kohler, W., Naidu, S., Kruse, B., & Moser, H. W. (1996). Cognitive and brain magnetic resonance imaging findings in adrenomyeloneuropathy. *Annals of Neurology*, *40*, 675–678.

Farrer, C., Frey, S. H., Van Horn, J. D., Tunik, E., Turk, D., Inati, S., & Grafton, S. T. (2008). The angular gyrus computes action awareness representations. *Cerebral Cortex*, *18*(2), 254–261.

Feinberg, T. E. (2013). Neuropathologies of the self and the right hemisphere: A window into productive personal pathologies. *Frontiers in Human Neuroscience*, *7*, 472.

Feinberg, T. E., Venneri, A., Simone, A. M., Fan, Y., & Northoff, G. (2010). The neuroanatomy of asomatognosia and somatoparaphrenia. *Journal of Neurology, Neurosurgery & Psychiatry*, *81*(3), 276–281.

Ferré, P., & Joanette, Y. (2016). Communication abilities following right hemisphere damage: Prevalence, evaluation, and profiles. *Perspectives of the ASHA Special Interest Groups*, *1*(2), 106–115.

Fischer, H., Andersson, J. L., Furmark, T., & Fredrikson, M. (1998). Brain correlates of an unexpected panic attack: A human positron emission tomographic study. *Neuroscience Letters*, *251*(2), 137–140.

Gaffan, D., & Wilson, C. R. (2008). Medial temporal and prefrontal function: Recent behavioural disconnection studies in the macaque monkey. *Cortex*, *44*(8), 928–935.

Galaburda, A. M., & Geschwind, N. (1981). Anatomical asymmetries in the adult and developing brain and their implications for function. *Advances in Pediatrics*, *28*, 271–292.

Giora, R., Zaidel, E., Soroker, N., Batori, G., & Kasher, A. (2000). Differential effects of right-and left-hemisphere damage on understanding sarcasm and metaphor. *Metaphor and Symbol*, *15*(1–2), 63–83.

Gleichgerrcht, E., Fridriksson, J., & Bonilha, L. (2015). Neuroanatomical foundations of naming impairments across different neurologic conditions. *Neurology*, *85*, 284–292.

Graff-Radford, J., Jones, D. T., Strand, E. A., Rabinstein, A. A., Duffy, J. R., & Josephs, K. A. (2014). The neuroanatomy of pure apraxia of speech in stroke. *Brain and Language*, *129*, 43–46.

Grant, J. A., Courtemanche, J., Duerden, E. G., Duncan, G. H., & Rainville, P. (2010). Cortical thickness and pain sensitivity in zen meditators. *Emotion*, *10*(1), 43.

Hamani, C., McAndrews, M. P., Cohn, M., Oh, M., Zumsteg, D., Shapiro, C., . . . Lozano, A. M. (2008). Memory enhancement induced by hypothalamic/fornix deep brain stimulation. *Annals of Neurology*, *63*(1), 119–123.

Hebb, A. O., & Ojemann, G. A. (2013). The thalamus and language revisited. *Brain and Language*, *126*, 99–108.

Hickok, G. (2012). Computational neuroanatomy of speech production. *Nature Reviews Neuroscience*, *13*, 135–145.

Hickok, G., & Poeppel, D. (2007). The cortical organization of speech processing. *Nature Reviews Neuroscience*, *8*, 393–402.

Hillis, A. E., Work, M., Barker, P. B., Jacobs, M. A., Breese, E. L., & Maurer, K. (2004). Re-examining the brain regions crucial for orchestrating speech articulation. *Brain*, *127*(7), 1479–1487.

Kaas, J. H., & Hackett, T. A. (2000). Subdivisions of auditory cortex and processing streams in primates. *Proceedings of the National Academy of Sciences*, *97*(22), 11793–11799.

Kandel, E. R., & Hudspeth, A. J. (2013). The brain and behavior. In E. R. Kandel, J. H. Schwartz, T. M. Jessell, S. A. Siegelbaum, & A. J. Hudspeth (Eds.), *Principles of neural science* (5th ed., pp. 5–21). New York, NY: McGraw-Hill.

Kanwisher, N., McDermott, J., & Chun, M. M. (1997). The fusiform face area: A module in human extrastriate cortex specialized for face perception. *The Journal of Neuroscience*, *17*(11), 4302–4311.

Karlsen, A. S., & Pakkenberg, B. (2011). Total numbers of neurons and glial cells in cortex and basal ganglia of aged brains with Down syndrome—a stereological study. *Cerebral Cortex*, *21*(11), 2519–2524.

Kier, E. L., Staib, L. H., Davis, L. M., & Bronen, R. A. (2004). MR imaging of the temporal stem: Anatomic dissection tractography of the uncinate fasciculus, inferior occipitofrontal fasciculus, and Meyer's loop of the optic radiation. *American Journal of Neuroradiology*, *25*(5), 677–691.

Koch, G., Bonni, S., Giacobbe, V., Bucchi, G., Basile, B., Lupo, F., Versace, V., Bozzali, M. & Caltagirone, C. (2012). Theta-burst stimulation of the left hemisphere accelerates recovery of hemispatial neglect. *Neurology*, *78*(1), 24–30.

Kobayashi, C., Kennedy, L. M., & Halpern, B. P. (2006). Experience-induced changes in taste identification of monosodium glutamate (MSG) are reversible. *Chemical Senses*, *31*(4), 301–306.

Kringelbach, M. L., & Rolls, E. T. (2004). The functional neuroanatomy of the human orbitofrontal cortex: evidence from neuroimaging and neuropsychology. *Progress in Neurobiology*, *72*(5), 341–372.

Kroll, N. E., Markowitsch, H. J., Knight, R. T., & von Cramon, D. Y. (1997). Retrieval of old memories: The temporofrontal hypothesis. *Brain*, *120*(8), 1377–1399.

Kwon, H. G., Lee, J., & Jang, S. H. (2016). Injury of the corticobulbar tract in patients with dysarthria following cerebral infarct: Diffusion tensor tractography study. *International Journal of Neuroscience*, *126*(4), 361–365.

Lalande, S., Braun, C. M. J., Charlebois, N., & Whitaker, H. A. (1992). Effects of right and left hemisphere cerebrovascular lesions on discrimination of prosodic and semantic aspects of affect in sentences. *Brain and Language, 42*(2), 165–186.

Liégeois, F., Tournier, J., Pigdon, L., Connelly, A., & Morgan, A. T. (2013). Corticobulbar tract changes as predictors of dysarthria in childhood brain injury. *Neurology, 80*(10), 926–932.

Lochy, A., de Heering, A., & Rossion, B. (2017). The non-linear development of the right hemispheric specialization for human face perception. *bioRxiv*. https://doi.org/10.1101/122002

Lundgren, K., & Brownell, H. (2016). Figurative language deficits associated with right hemisphere disorder. *Perspectives of the ASHA Special Interest Groups, 1*(2), 66–81.

Lunven, M., & Bartolomeo, P. (2017). Attention and spatial cognition: Neural and anatomical substrates of visual neglect. *Annals of Physical and Rehabilitation Medicine, 60*(3), 124–129.

Maddock, R. J., Garrett, A. S., & Buonocore, M. H. (2001). Remembering familiar people: The posterior cingulate cortex and autobiographical memory retrieval. *Neuroscience, 104*(3), 667–676.

Makris, N., Kennedy, D. N., McInerney, S., Sorensen, A. G., Wang, R., Caviness, V. S., & Pandya, D. N. (2005). Segmentation of subcomponents within the superior longitudinal fascicle in humans: A quantitative, in vivo, DT-MRI study. *Cerebral Cortex, 15*(6), 854–869.

Malloy, P., Bihrle, A., & Duffy, J. (1993). The orbitomedial frontal syndrome. *Archives of Clinical Neuropsychology, 8*, 185–201.

Marsh, A. A., Finger, E. C., Schechter, J. C., Jurkowitz, I. T., Reid, M. E., & Blair, R. J. R. (2011). Adolescents with psychopathic traits report reductions in physiological responses to fear. *Journal of Child Psychology and Psychiatry, 52*(8), 834–841.

Marsh, A. A., Stoycos, S. A., Brethel-Haurwitz, K. M., Robinson, P., VanMeter, J. W., & Cardinale, E. M. (2014). Neural and cognitive characteristics of extraordinary altruists. *Proceedings of the National Academy of Sciences, 111*(42), 15036–15041.

Martino, J., Hamer, P. C. D. W., Berger, M. S., Lawton, M. T., Arnold, C. M., de Lucas, E. M., & Duffau, H. (2013). Analysis of the subcomponents and cortical terminations of the perisylvian superior longitudinal fasciculus: A fiber dissection and DTI tractography study. *Brain Structure and Function, 218*(1), 105–121.

McCandliss, B. D., Cohen, L., & Dehaene, S. (2003). The visual word form area: Expertise for reading in the fusiform gyrus. *Trends in Cognitive Sciences, 7*(7), 293–299.

Miller, B. L., Cummings, J., Mishkin, F., Boone, K., Prince, F., Ponton, M., & Cotman, C. (1998). Emergence of artistic talent in frontotemporal dementia. *Neurology, 51*(4), 978–982.

Minga, J. (2016). Discourse production and right hemisphere disorder. *Perspectives of the ASHA Special Interest Groups, 1*(2), 96–105.

Mori, K., & Maeda, M. (2001). Surgical treatment of chronic subdural hematoma in 500 consecutive cases: Clinical characteristics, surgical outcome, complications, and recurrence rate. *Neurologia Medico-Chirurgica, 41*(8), 371–381.

Mottaghy, F. M., Willmes, K., Horwitz, B., Müller, H. W., Krause, B. J., & Sturm, W. (2006). Systems level modeling of a neuronal network subserving intrinsic alertness. *Neuroimage, 29*(1), 225–233.

Offiah, C., & Hall, E. (2008). Heroin-induced leukoencephalopathy: Characterization using MRI, diffusion-weighted imaging, and MR spectroscopy. *Clinical Radiology, 63*, 146–152.

Olson, I. R., Plotzker, A., & Ezzyat, Y. (2007). The enigmatic temporal pole: A review of findings on social and emotional processing. *Brain, 130*(7), 1718–1731.

Pakkenberg, B., & Gundersen, H. J. G. (1997). Neocortical neuron number in humans: Effect of sex and age. *Journal of Comparative Neurology, 384*(2), 312–320.

Papagno, C., Miracapillo, C., Casarotti, A., Lauro, L. J. R., Castellano, A., Falini, A., . . . Bello, L. (2010). What is the role of the uncinate fasciculus? Surgical removal and proper name retrieval. *Brain, 134*, 405–414.

Penfield, W., & Roberts, L. (1959). *Speech and brain mechanisms*. London, UK: The Princeton University Press.

Peters, A. L. A. N., & Jones, E. G. (1984). Classification of cortical neurons. *Cerebral Cortex, 1*, 107–121.

Pobric, G., Lambon Ralph, M. A., & Zahn, R. (2016). Hemispheric specialization within the superior anterior temporal cortex for social and nonsocial concepts. *Journal of Cognitive Neuroscience, 28*(3), 351–360.

Posner, M. I., Rothbart, M. K., Sheese, B. E., & Tang, Y. (2007). The anterior cingulate gyrus and the mechanism of self-regulation. *Cognitive, Affective, & Behavioral Neuroscience, 7*(4), 391–395.

Raz, A., & Buhle, J. (2006). Typologies of attentional networks. *Nature Reviews Neuroscience, 7*(5), 367–379.

Richardson, J. D., Fillmore, P., Rorden, C., LaPointe, L. L., & Fridriksson, J. (2012). Re-establishing Broca's initial findings. *Brain and Language, 123*(2), 125–130.

Rodriguez, A. D. (2009). Aprosodia secondary to right hemisphere damage. *SIG 2 Perspectives on Neurophysiology and Neurogenic Speech and Language Disorders, 19*(3), 71–76.

Schaltenbrand, G., & Woolsey, C. N. (1964). *Cerebral localization and organization*. Madison, WI: The University of Wisconsin Press.

Schmahmann, J. D., Smith, E. E., Eichler, F. S., & Filley, C. M. (2008). Cerebral white matter: Neuroanatomy, clinical neurology, and neurobehavioral correlates. *Annals of the New York Academy of Sciences, 1142*, 266–309.

Seikel, J. A., Drumright, D. G., & King, D. W. (2016). *Anatomy & physiology for speech, language and hearing* 5th Ed. Clifton Park, NY: Cengage Learning.

Skultety, F. M. (1963). Stimulation of periaqueductal gray and hypothalamus. *Archives of Neurology, 8*(6), 608–620.

Stern, C. E., Corkin, S., Gonzalez, R. G., Guimaraes, A. R., Baker, J. R., Jennings, P. J., . . . Rosen, B. R. (1996). The hippocampal formation participates in novel picture encoding: Evidence from functional magnetic resonance imaging. *Proceedings of the National Academy of Sciences, 93*(16), 8660–8665.

Sugiura, L., Ojima, S., Matsuba-Kurita, H., Dan, I., Tsuzuki, D., Katura, T., & Hagiwara, H. (2011). Sound to language: Different cortical processing for first and second languages in elementary school children as revealed by a large-scale study using fNIRS. *Cerebral Cortex, 21*(10), 2374–2393.

Sun, T., & Hevner, R. F. (2014). Growth and folding of the mammalian cerebral cortex: From molecules to malformations. *Nature Reviews Neuroscience, 15*, 217–232.

Taylor, H. G., & Heilman, K. M. (1980). Left-hemisphere motor dominance in righthanders. *Cortex, 16*(4), 587–603.

Thomeer, E. C., Verhoeven, W. M., van de Vlasakker, C. J., & Klompenhouwer, J. L. (1998). Psychiatric symptoms in MELAS: A case report. *Journal of Neurology, Neurosurgery and Psychiatry, 64*, 692–693.

Tompkins, C. A., Boada, R., & McGarry, K. (1992). The access and processing of familiar idioms by brain-damaged and normally aging adults. *Journal of Speech, Language, and Hearing Research, 35*(3), 626–637.

Valk, S. L., Bernhardt, B. C., Trautwein, F. M., Böckler, A., Kanske, P., Guizard, N., . . . Singer, T. (2017). Structural plasticity of the social brain: Differential change after socio-affective and cognitive mental training. *Science Advances, 3*(10), e1700489.

Vallar, G., & Ronchi, R. (2009). Somatoparaphrenia: A body delusion. A review of the neuropsychological literature. *Experimental Brain Research, 192*(3), 533–551.

Vogt, B. A., Finch, D. M., & Olson, C. R. (1992). Functional heterogeneity in cingulate cortex: The anterior executive and posterior evaluative regions. *Cerebral Cortex, 2*(6), 435–443.

Wang, D., Buckner, R. L., & Liu, H. (2014). Functional specialization in the human brain estimated by intrinsic hemispheric interaction. *Journal of Neuroscience, 34*(37), 12341–12352.

White, N. M., & Gaskin, S. (2006). Dorsal hippocampus function in learning and expressing a spatial discrimination. *Learning & Memory, 13*(2), 119–122.

Wyss, J. M., & Sripanidkulchai, K. (1984). The topography of the mesencephalic and pontine projections from the cingulate cortex of the rat. *Brain Research, 293*(1), 1–15.

Xie, L., Kang, H., Xu, Q., Chen, M. J., Liao, Y., Thiyagarajan, M., . . . Nedergaard, M. (2013). Sleep drives metabolite clearance from the adult brain. *Science, 342*(6156), 373–377.

Zatorre, R. J. (1988). Pitch perception of complex tones and human temporal-lobe function. *Journal of the Acoustical Society of America, 84*(2), 566–572.

5 ANATOMY OF THE SUBCORTEX

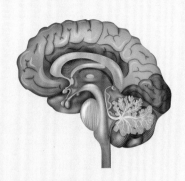

Learning Outcomes for Chapter 5

- Discuss the components of the basal ganglia and their function in motor control and activation.

- Recognize visually the components of the basal ganglia as related to the internal capsule when presented in transverse section.

- Recognize the etiologic relationship between the basal ganglia function and the hyperkinesias and hypokinesia as related to neurotransmitter imbalance.

- Discuss the importance of the hippocampal formation, and identify the components.

- Describe the components and function of the diencephalon.

- Identify the role of the nuclei of the thalamus as related to speech and hearing, including the pulvinar, lateral and medial geniculate bodies, and intralaminar nuclei.

- Identify the dominant pathology related to the subthalamus.

- Discuss the role of the hypothalamus.

INTRODUCTION

While the cerebral cortex is extraordinarily important, it does not work alone. There are many highly organized subsystems that undergird the work of the cerebrum. Let's examine the structures of the subcortex.

The subcortex consists of nuclei and pathways that lie inferior and deep to the cerebrum and include the structures of the basal ganglia, diencephalon, brainstem, and cerebellum (Table 5–1). Each of these subsystems is responsible for significant control of afferent and/or efferent information: a lesion to any of these systems can have a devastating effect on sensory or motor function, and in some cases, on cognition and language. We will discuss the cerebellum in Chapter 8.

BASAL GANGLIA

The **basal ganglia** (also known as the basal nuclei) are a group of nuclei deeply involved in motor control. The nuclei of the basal ganglia include the **caudate nucleus**, the **putamen**, and the **globus pallidus**. Some authors also include the **amygdala (amygdaloid body)**, **claustrum**, **subthalamic nucleus,** and **substantia nigra** as components of the basal ganglia.

First, let's orient to the location of the basal ganglia. Figure 5–1 shows the ascending and descending fibers of the cortex as they pass through the internal capsule. If you look closely at Figures 5–1 and 5–2A, you will see that the **internal capsule** passes between the globus pallidus and the caudate nucleus. Just lateral to the globus pallidus is the putamen. The caudate nucleus and putamen are sometimes characterized as the **striate body** (**corpus striatum**) because the nuclei take a striped appearance as the descending and ascending fibers of the internal capsule pass through spaces between the nuclei. Likewise, the globus pallidus and putamen taken together are referred to as the **lentiform** or **lenticular nucleus** because they look lens-shaped. The close relationship between the nuclei of the basal ganglia and the ascending and descending pathways underscores their importance for motor function.

The caudate nucleus is shaped like a horseshoe, or perhaps a croissant, with its head in the anterior aspect and the tail curving down in the posterior aspect. We already crossed the amygdala in our discussion of the inferior cerebrum. You'll remember the uncus in the medial cortex and the fact that the amygdala is the structure underlying the landmark.

The caudate consists of **head**, **body**, and **tail**, and the head of the caudate protrudes into the anterior horn of the lateral ventricle (Figure 5–2C). The body comprises the floor of that ventricle, and the lateral part of the body is adjacent to the thalamus. The amygdala can be found in the roof of the inferior horn of the lateral ventricle. The globus pallidus is divided into internal and external portions (*globus pallidus interna* and *globus pallidus externa*).

TABLE 5–1.	Major Structures of Subcortex	
Structure	Components	Primary function
Basal ganglia	Caudate nucleus; head, body, tail	Influence voluntary motor activity
	Putamen	Influence voluntary motor activity
	Globus pallidus	Influence voluntary motor activity
	(Subthalamic nucleus)*	Produces glutamate; inhibits muscular responses
	(Substantia nigra)*	Provides dopamine for basal ganglia
	Striate body (corpus striatum)	Combination of caudate and putamen; receives input broadly
	Lentiform nucleus	Combination of globus pallidus and putamen
Internal capsule	Anterior, posterior, genu	Contains pathways for fibers passing to and from cerebral cortex
Claustrum	Internal and external capsules	Reciprocal communication among insula, premotor gyrus, precentral gyrus, occipital and temporal lobes; perhaps synchronization of cortex to create seamless temporal image of activities
Hippocampal formation	Hippocampus is within the temporal lobe, but included here because of associated nuclei: dentate gyrus, entorhinal cortex, pes hippocampus, fimbria, fornix, indusium griseum	Processing of olfactory information; processing of short-term memory information
	Entorhinal cortex	Receives olfactory input
	Dentate gyrus	Receives olfactory input from entorhinal cortex
Thalamus	Includes 26 pairs of nuclei, including pulvinar, intralaminar nuclei, medial and lateral geniculate bodies	All sensation exception olfaction is received at thalamus
	Pulvinar	Relay associated with language
	Intralaminar nuclei	Relay associated with reticular activating system
	Medial geniculate body	Relay associated with auditory function
	Lateral geniculate body	Relay associated with visual function
Epithalamus	Includes pineal body, habenular nuclei and commissure, striae medullaris, and posterior commissure	Secretion of regulatory chemicals
Subthalamus	Subthalamic nucleus	Projects to thalamus and receives input from basal ganglia
Hypothalamus	Consists of multiple nuclei, including supraoptic, paraventricular, anterior and lateral hypothalamic areas, dorsomedial, ventromedial, arcuate and lateral hypothalamic nuclei	Organizational structure of limbic system; interacts with amygdala, septum, parahippocampal formation, cingulum; regulates desire and satiation, reproductive physiology, response to environmental temperature
Cerebellum	Anterior, posterior lobes, flocculonodular lobes, vermis, nuclei (dentate, fastigial, emboliform, globose)	Responsible for coordination of sensation and motor activity; receives somatic and vestibular sense and coordinates with motor commands from cortex for control of graded movement

*Considered by some to be part of basal ganglia.

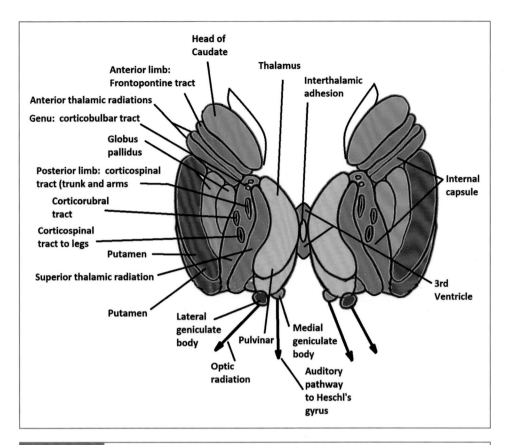

FIGURE 5–1. Components of basal ganglia as related to internal capsule. *Source:* After view of Carpenter (1978).

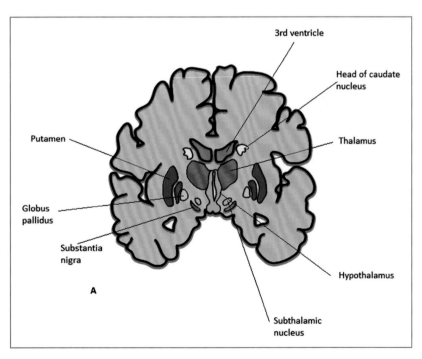

FIGURE 5–2. **A.** Coronal section revealing components of basal ganglia.

continues

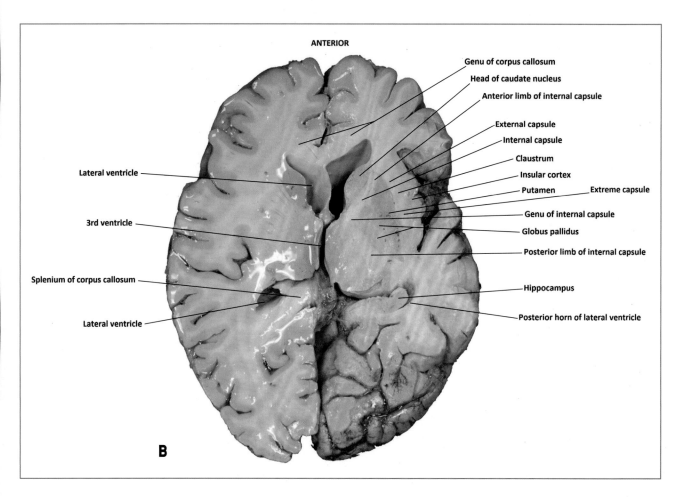

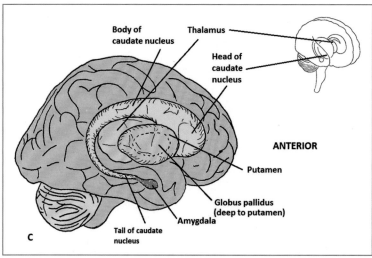

FIGURE 5–2. *continued* **B.** Photograph of transverse view of cerebrum showing structures of basal ganglia, internal and external capsule, and claustrum. **C.** View of basal ganglia in context of cerebral cortex. *continues*

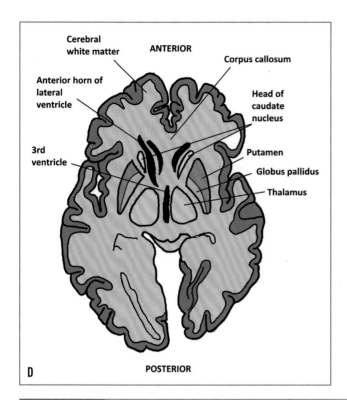

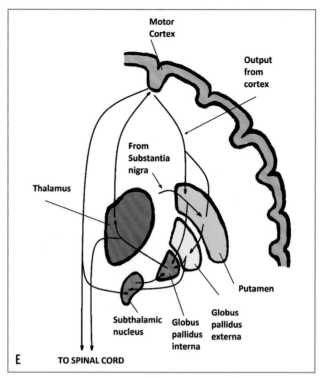

FIGURE 5–2. *continued* **D.** Drawing of transverse section showing structures of basal ganglia. **E.** Input-output circuit of basal ganglia. Note that input from the motor cortex is fed to the putamen, where it is passed to direct and indirect pathways. The direct pathway leads to the globus pallidus *interna*, while the indirect pathway leads to the globus pallidus *externa* and subsequently the subthalamic nucleus. Output of the globus pallidus *interna* is directed to the thalamus, which sends feedback to the motor cortex as well as to the spinal cord via the pedunculopontine nucleus.

Huntington's Disease

Hyperkinesias are disorders characterized by extraneous, uncontrolled movement. Because the basal ganglia are involved in the control of movement, and particularly of stereotyped or repetitive movements, hyperkinetic disorders focus on lesions to this system.

Huntington's disease (HD) is an autosomal dominant disorder that always results in extraneous movement known as **chorea**. Degeneration of the basal ganglia and concomitant atrophy of the cerebral cortex (particularly of the frontal lobes) result in large, uncontrollable movement of arms, head, trunk, and legs. The speech of an individual with HD is characterized by interruption caused by uncontrolled movement of the structures associated with it. Functions affected include uncontrolled adduction and abduction of the vocal folds, inspiration and expiration, contraction and relaxation of abdominal musculature, and protrusion and retraction of the tongue. The cortical degeneration results in a decline of cognitive function that co-occurs with the onset of the movement disorder. As with many progressive neuromuscular diseases, death of the patient typically occurs secondary to pneumonia, since the respiratory system is compromised by the movement disorder. Unfortunately, suicide is a significant cause of death, perhaps due to the psychiatric problems arising from the cortical degeneration in this disease.

The **claustrum** is an extremely thin layer of gray matter residing lateral to the putamen and medial to the insular cortex (see Figure 5–2B). It is located between the **external** and **extreme capsules**, which are white matter projection pathways. It has reciprocal communication with the precentral gyrus, premotor gyrus, occipital lobe, and temporal lobe, and specifically with the insular cortex. It appears that the claustrum associates with virtually the entire cortex, perhaps connecting the insula with all motor and sensory function (Crick & Koch, 2005). The external and extreme capsules are association fibers that connect a wide range of cortical structures, which is an apparent role of the claustrum as well. Crick and Koch liken the claustrum to the director of an orchestra, in that it appears to provide synchronization of your experiences with your consciousness and is perhaps involved in cross-modal interaction (Ettlinger & Wilson, 1990). You may recall our discussion of the essential role of the insula in integrating your sense of self and development of empathy and compassion. The claustrum likely plays an important role in establishing the essential connectivity to support these developments. Indeed, Yin, Terhune, Smythies, and Meck (2016) hypothesize that the claustrum synchronizes the temporal activities of the cortex, thereby supporting the integration of body sense for the purposes of consciousness. Bamiou, Musiek, and Luxon (2003) reviewed the role of the insula and claustrum in auditory processing disorder, finding that damage to these two structures may result in auditory agnosia.

The basal ganglia work together in a very complex fashion to initiate, facilitate, and terminate movement. They also have circuitry supporting stereotyped movements. For those going into speech-language pathology, the basal ganglia take on particular importance as the source of numerous **hyperkinesias** (conditions in which there is extraneous movement), since these typically arise from lesion of the basal ganglia or imbalance in neurotransmitters.

Our understanding of the circuit for the basal ganglia is quite well established (Figure 5–2E). In 1912, Wilson first realized the relevance of the basal ganglia to a genetic syndrome (hepatolenticular degeneration, also known as Wilson's disease) that resulted in a "wing-beating" tremor, an involuntary, rhythmic movement of the arms. Since then, numerous diseases and conditions have been linked to lesions within this system that cause either hyperkinesia (extraneous movements) or hypokinesia (reduction in movement, ending in muscular rigidity).

The function of the basal ganglia circuit depends on the delicate balance among three neurotransmitters (you will recall our discussion of neurotransmitters in Chapter 2). There are three neurotransmitters acting on the basal ganglia: dopamine (DA), gamma-aminobutyric acid (GABA), and glutamate (GL). Remember that DA and GL are excitatory, while GABA is inhibitory. The striate body (putamen and caudate) serves as the input for the basal ganglia, while the globus pallidus and subthalamic nuclei serve as the output system. There are two basic circuits at the level of the basal ganglia. The first circuit is the **direct pathway**, which is involved in initiation of action. GABA, the inhibitory neurotransmitter, is the agent for direct activation: the inhibition process *allows* motor activity to occur. That is, the excitatory state for output is non-action. The second circuit is termed the **indirect pathway**, which is responsible for inhibiting

output of the motor system. So, the direct pathway facilitates movement through GABA, while the indirect pathway inhibits movement through GABA and GL. A critical player we haven't mentioned is DA, which is produced at the substantia nigra. DA activates the striate body, which allows both direct and indirect pathways to function. Without DA, there is no initiation of movement and no inhibition of movement. This will translate into the rigidity that is seen in Parkinson's disease (DeLong & Wichmann, 2007; Kreitzer & Malenka, 2008; Redgrave et al., 2010; Wichmann & DeLong, 2013).

In summary, the basal ganglia include the caudate nucleus, the putamen, the globus pallidus, and sometimes the amygdala.

- The basal ganglia are intimately involved in motor function.
- The internal capsule passes between the globus pallidus and the caudate nucleus (the striate body or corpus striatum). The globus pallidus and putamen together are termed the lentiform or lenticular nucleus. The globus pallidus is divided into internal and external portions.
- The head of the caudate protrudes into the anterior horn of the lateral ventricle, the body comprises the floor of the ventricle, and the body is adjacent to the thalamus.
- The basal ganglia work together in a very complex fashion to initiate, facilitate, and terminate movement. The basal ganglia are the source of numerous hyperkinesias arising from lesion or imbalance in neurotransmitters.
- The function of the basal ganglia circuit depends on the delicate balance among dopamine, GABA, and glutamate. Dopamine and glutamate are excitatory, while GABA is inhibitory. The striate body (putamen and caudate) is the input for the basal ganglia, and the globus pallidus and subthalamic nuclei are the output.
- There are two circuits in the basal ganglia. The direct pathway is involved in initiation of action through inhibition performed by GABA, since the default mode of the basal ganglia is excitation. The indirect pathway inhibits output of the motor system. The substantia nigra produces dopamine, which promotes direct and indirect pathways to function.

Parkinson's Disease

Parkinson's disease (PD) was first identified by James Parkinson in 1817 and was originally termed "shaking palsy" (the term **palsy** means paralysis). Parkinson's disease is caused by degeneration of the substantia nigra, the small mass of cells within the cerebral peduncles that creates dopamine for use by the basal ganglia. The loss of dopamine results in the signs and symptoms of PD, which include a global reduction in range of movement and reduced ability to exert force with musculature. The patient with PD will walk with a festinating gate (short, shuffling steps); will have reduced extrapyramidal function (including reduced arm swing, adjustment of posture when sitting, trunk rotation during turning while walking); and a characteristic "pill rolling" tremor of the hands. Speech in PD is characterized by reduced vocal intensity, reduced articulator range of motion, and frequently (paradoxically) increased diadochokinetic rate.

The progression of the disease results in increasing co-contraction of agonist and antagonist muscles, resulting in muscular rigidity. In later stages of PD, there is cognitive decline as well. Death from PD typically arises from pneumonia, as the lungs become compromised by global immobility and reduced respiratory movement.

HIPPOCAMPUS

The hippocampus is critically involved in many functions, but memory is perhaps its most important role. While it is not technically a subcortical structure, since it is embedded within the temporal lobe, it is such an intrinsic component of the limbic system that we include it in this chapter. As part of the limbic system, it communicates with the hypothalamus and temporal lobe (Figure 5–3). You may recall that we discussed the parahippocampal gyrus earlier in reference to the inferior cerebrum.

The parahippocampal gyrus (BA 27) is the outer manifestation of the critically important hippocampus within. The hippocampus is unique in the central nervous system in its design and function. Structurally, the hippocampus itself is broken into major parts: CA1, CA2, CA3, subiculum, presubiculum, and parasubiculum (see Figure 5–3B). The **hippocampal formation** consists of the hippocampus, the **dentate gyrus**, and the **entorhinal cortex** (Andersen, Morris, Amaral, Bliss, & O'Keefe, 2007). The gross structure of the hippocampus includes the **pes hippocampus** ("foot of the hippocampus"), which is the anterior projection of the hippocampus, and the **fimbria** of the hippocampus, which is a medial layer of white fibers continuous with the fornix. The **fornix** is a group of commissural fibers that gives communication between the hippocampus and the hypothalamus. The fibers of the fornix terminate in the mammillary body. The **dentate gyrus** provides an intimate connection with the cingulate gyrus, by means of the **indusium griseum**.

Functions of the hippocampus are diverse and critical (Amaral & Lavenex, 2007; Andersen et al., 2007). The hippocampal formation is intrinsic to memory function, emotion, attention, and physical navigation through space. Let's examine the components of the hippocampal formation.

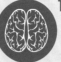

The Case of HM

The hippocampus is one of the most important structures in memory function, being responsible for at least some of our ability to navigate our spatial world, as well as the ability to place memories into long-term storage.

Henry Molaison (known as HM in the literature) was born in 1926 and suffered a bicycle accident as a child that left him with intractable epileptic seizures. Seizure disorders frequently involve the temporal lobe and often include uncontrolled interhemispheric activation of brain structures. In this case, the physician in charge of Molaison's treatment identified the temporal lobes as the likely site of activity and performed bilateral **ablation** (destruction) of the hippocampi.

The result of the surgical procedure produced a profound and irreversible memory dysfunction in Molaison, in which his short-term memory was preserved, but he was left with no ability to place any information into long-term storage. The result was that Molaison was always aware of what was going on around him and could remember interactions for a short while, but he was only able to remember past events that occurred up to his surgery in 1953. That is to say, Molaison was unable to recognize the progression of time beyond the day of his surgery, as no new memories could be placed in storage to mark that time. To him, every day was September 1, 1953. Molaison's working memory and **procedural memory** remained functional, so that he could briefly remember interactions and perform motor functions (procedures) such as eating, opening doors, operating home equipment, etc.

Molaison was one of the most studied individuals in the history of neuroscience, and you can read about his life and the research performed on him in numerous sources. (For a very readable account, see Corkin, 2013.)

In coronal section, the hippocampus has the appearance of a seahorse, which led to its name (hippo = horse in Greek). The parahippocampal gyrus is the floor of the inferior horn of the lateral ventricle, and lateral to this is the fusiform gyrus. The physical location of the hippocampus is adjacent to the fusiform face area (fusiform gyrus), which is specialized for face recognition in the right hemisphere and recognition of the parts of the face in the left hemisphere (Tsao, Freiwald, Tootell, & Livingstone, 2006).

The **entorhinal cortex** receives input from the olfactory stria as well as from cortical regions (insula, cingulate gyrus, superior temporal gyrus, and orbitofrontal cortex). Information from the entorhinal cortex projects to the dentate gyrus (via the perforant pathway), then to the pyramidal cells of

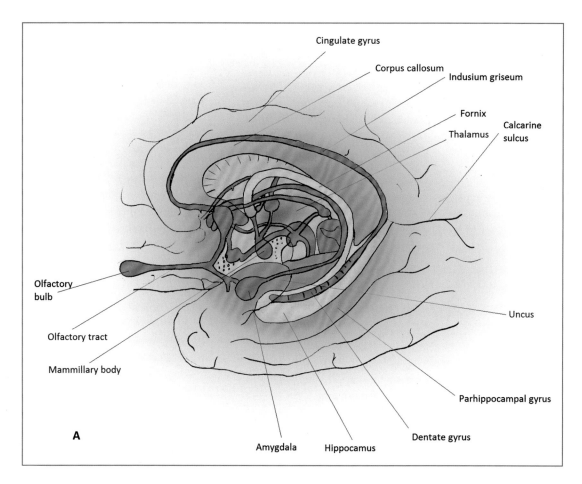

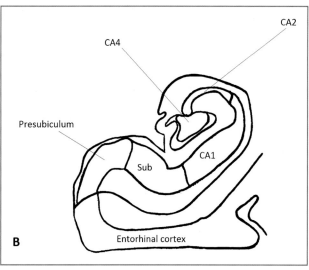

FIGURE 5–3. Hippocampal formation. **A.** Hippocampus in context of limbic system structures. *Source:* After view of Seikel, King, and Drumright (1997). **B.** Cross-section through hippocampus showing subnuclei. *Source:* After view of Andersen et al. (2007).

CA3 in the hippocampus, and from there to the pyramidal cells of CA1. The entorhinal cortex information that goes to the hippocampus is not returned to the cortex until it reaches the CA1 level, when it is reciprocated to the entorhinal cortex. A typical model for sensory input to the cerebrum involves reciprocal innervation. For instance, information about

body state that arises in the thalamus projects to the cerebral cortex, and then the same location in the cortex projects its state back to the thalamus. This is <u>not</u> the case for these early inputs to the hippocampus.

In summary, the hippocampal formation is critically involved in many functions.

- The hippocampus is involved in memory function, emotion, attention, and physical navigation through space. Although not technically a subcortical structure, it is an intrinsic component of the limbic system and communicates with the hypothalamus and temporal lobe. The hippocampus is adjacent to the fusiform face area.
- The hippocampal formation consists of the hippocampus, the dentate gyrus, entorhinal cortex, pes hippocampus, fimbria, and fornix. The fibers of the fornix terminate in the mammillary body, while the dentate gyrus provides communication with the cingulate gyrus by means of the indusium griseum.
- The hippocampus is divided into CA1, CA2, CA3, subiculum, presubiculum, and parasubiculum. The entorhinal cortex receives input from the olfactory stria, insula, cingulate gyrus, superior temporal gyrus, and orbitofrontal cortex, and this information projects to the dentate gyrus, and then to CA3, and subsequently to CA1.

DIENCEPHALON

The diencephalon consists of the thalamus, epithalamus, hypothalamus, and subthalamus. This area is small but mighty.

Thalamus

There is a left and right **thalamus**, and the paired thalami provide the final relay for sensory information directed toward the cerebral cortex. The thalamus is the medialmost structure of the subcortex (Figure 5–4). It is found medial to the basal ganglia (see Figure 5–2C) and precisely lateral to the third ventricle (it forms the lateral walls of this ventricle, as shown in Figure 5–1). With the exception of olfaction, all body sensation passes through the thalamus, making it a very important brain region. While still the subject of debate, apparently only pain and temperature sense are consciously perceived at the thalamus. That having been said, you can't localize pain without the cerebral cortex, even though you can be aware of it. Each nucleus of the thalamus that communicates with a cortical region also receives efferent, corticothalamic projections from the same region, known as reciprocal communication. The thalami are separated from the globus pallidus and putamen by the internal capsule. Thalamic efferents project to the cerebral cortex by means of the internal capsule and the corona radiata. The thalamus is composed of 26 functionally different nuclei in three regions that are defined by the internal medullary lamina (see Figure 5–4B). The thalamus is the communication link between the cerebellum and globus pallidus with the motor portion of the cerebral cortex, as shown in Figure 5–4C.

There are some very important nuclei in the thalamus for those of us in the fields of audiology and speech-language

pathology. The **pulvinar** is related to language function: a lesion to this nucleus can cause aphasia. The **lateral geniculate body** (LGB) serves as a visual relay, while the **medial geniculate body** (MGB) is the correlate for hearing. These two regions are likely involved in integration of visual with auditory information (for instance, visually locating the source of a sound), although the inferior colliculus of the brainstem is clearly involved in that function as well.

One of the most important functional regions of the thalamus consists of the paired intralaminar nuclei. The intralaminar nuclei are the functional heart of the **reticular activating system (RAS)**. The RAS is responsible for arousing the cerebral cortex and may be involved in focusing cortical regions to heightened awareness. If you examine, for instance, the stages of awakening or arousal of a person who has suffered a traumatic brain injury, you can see the manifestations of the RAS in that process of emerging from coma. (This explains the critical nature of damage to the thalamic region as well as the brainstem regions that also make up the RAS.)

Epithalamus

The **epithalamus** is a collection of nuclei that connect the limbic system with other brain components and are involved in secretion of regulatory chemicals (Figure 5–5). The epithalamus includes the pineal body (a gland that is involved with development of the gonads), the habenular nuclei and commissure, the striae medullaris, and the posterior commissure (Noback, Demarest, & Strominger, 1991).

Subthalamus

The **subthalamus** is an important motor regulatory nucleus situated beneath the thalamus. The subthalamic nucleus is a lens-shaped structure within the internal capsule: it projects to the thalamus and receives input from the globus pallidus and motor cortex. The subthalamus is remarkable for the occurrence of **ballism** (a hyperkinesia characterized by very large muscular movements of arms and legs) as a result of lesion.

Hypothalamus

The **hypothalamus** is found on the floor of the third ventricle and is composed of numerous nuclei. It is considered to be the organizational structure of the limbic system, interacting with the cingulate gyrus, septal area, parahippocampal gyrus, amygdala, and hippocampal formation to regulate reproductive physiology, desire and satiation relative to food and drink, control of digestion, and certain metabolic functions. Remarkably, damage to the hypothalamus can result in loss of heart rate acceleration and sweating, loss of shivering when cold, and failure to move to warm areas when cold. A person

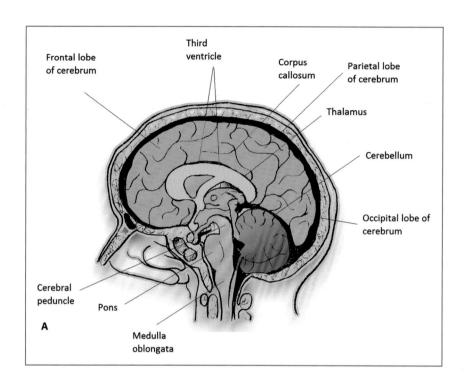

Frontal lobe
of cerebrum

Third
ventricle

Corpus
callosum

Parietal lobe
of cerebrum

Thalamus

Cerebellum

Occipital lobe of
cerebrum

Cerebral
peduncle

Pons

Medulla
oblongata

A

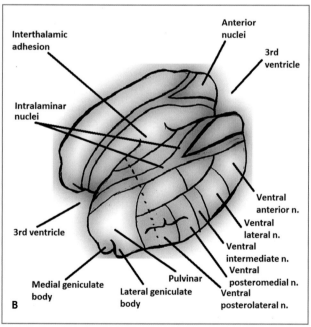

Interthalamic
adhesion

Anterior
nuclei

3rd
ventricle

Intralaminar
nuclei

3rd ventricle

Medial geniculate
body

Lateral geniculate
body

Pulvinar

Ventral
anterior n.

Ventral
lateral n.

Ventral
intermediate n.

Ventral
posteromedial n.

Ventral
posterolateral n.

B

FIGURE 5–4. Thalamus. **A.** Medial view of cerebral cortex and subcortical structures, showing location of thalamus. **B.** Nuclei of thalamus. *Source:* After view of Netter (1983). *continues*

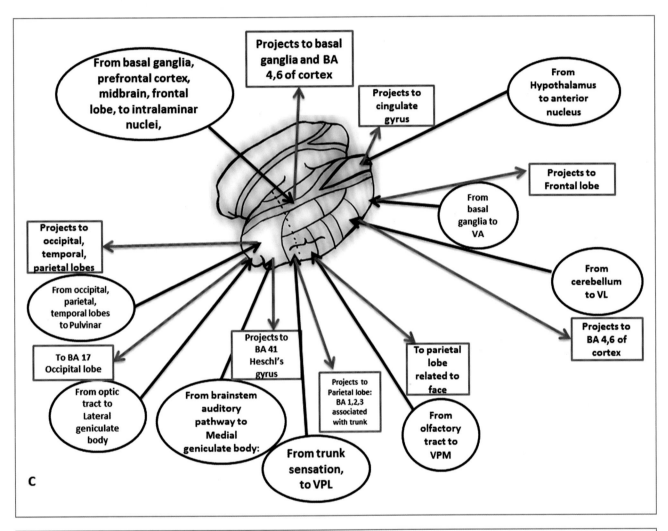

FIGURE 5–4. *continued* **C.** Schematic showing inputs to (*black*) and projections from (*red*) thalamus. *Source:* After view of Seikel, Drumright, and King (2016). VA = ventral anterior nucleus; VL = ventral lateral nucleus; VP = ventral posterior nucleus; VI = ventral intermediate nucleus; LD = lateral dorsal nucleus; LP = lateral posterior nucleus; VPM = ventral posteromedial nucleus; VPL = ventral posterolateral nucleus; LGB = lateral geniculate body; MGB = medial geniculate body.

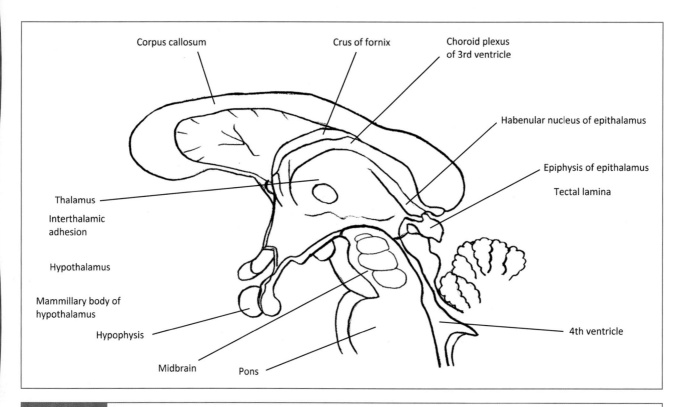

FIGURE 5–5.   Sagittal view, showing hypothalamus, epithalamus, and subthalamus. *Source:* After view of Netter (1983) and Baehr and Frotscher (2012).

with a lesion to the satiety center may engage in voracious eating, and damage to the feeding center may result in starvation and/or dehydration. The hypothalamus is involved with the physical manifestations of emotion, including eye-watering, heart rate acceleration, sweating, goosebumps, flushing, and dry mouth (Horn, & Swanson, 2012).

In summary, many structures beneath the cerebral cortex are involved in modifying information received by the cortex, as well as in modifying the commands arising from it.

- The diencephalon consists of the thalamus, epithalamus, hypothalamus, and subthalamus. The left and right thalami provide the final relay for sensory information directed toward the cerebral cortex. The thalamus is medial to the basal ganglia and precisely lateral to the third ventricle. The thalami are separated from the globus pallidus and putamen by the internal capsule. All body sensation except olfaction passes through the thalamus. Thalamic efferents project to the cerebral cortex by means of the internal capsule and the corona radiata. The thalamus is the communication link between the cerebellum and globus pallidus with the motor portion of the cerebral cortex.
- The thalamus is composed of 26 functionally different nuclei. The pulvinar is related to language function, and a lesion to the pulvinar can cause aphasia. The lateral geniculate body is a visual relay, and the medial geniculate body

is an auditory relay. The intralaminar nuclei are major components of the reticular activating system, which is responsible for arousing the cerebral cortex and perhaps focusing cortical regions to heightened awareness.
- The epithalamus connects the limbic system with other brain components. It is involved in secretion of regulatory chemicals. The epithalamus includes the pineal body, the habenular nuclei and commissure, the striae medullaris, and the posterior commissure.
- The subthalamus projects to the thalamus and receives input from the globus pallidus and motor cortex and works with the basal ganglia to control movement.
- The hypothalamus is considered to be the organizational structure of the limbic system. It interacts with the cingulate gyrus, septal area, parahippocampal gyrus, amygdala, and hippocampal formation to regulate reproductive physiology, desire and satiation relative to food and drink, control of digestion, and certain metabolic functions.

CHAPTER SUMMARY

The basal ganglia are intimately involved in motor function. The basal ganglia include the caudate nucleus, the putamen, the globus pallidus, and sometimes the amygdala. The internal capsule passes between the globus pallidus and the caudate nucleus. The globus pallidus and caudate are termed the striate body or corpus striatum. The globus pallidus and putamen together are termed the lentiform or lenticular nucleus.

The head of the caudate protrudes into the anterior horn of the lateral ventricle, while the body comprises the floor of the ventricle and is adjacent to the thalamus. The basal ganglia work together in a very complex fashion to initiate, facilitate, and terminate movement. The basal ganglia are the source of numerous hyperkinesias arising from lesion or imbalance in neurotransmitters. The striate body is the input for the basal ganglia, and the globus pallidus and subthalamic nuclei are the output. There are two circuits in the basal ganglia. The direct pathway is involved in initiation of action, while the indirect pathway inhibits output of the motor system. The substantia nigra produces dopamine, which promotes direct and indirect pathways to function.

While not technically a subcortical structure, the hippocampal formation is included because of its role in the limbic system. It is involved in memory function, emotion, attention, and physical navigation through space, and consists of the hippocampus, the dentate gyrus, entorhinal cortex, pes hippocampus, fimbria, and fornix. The fibers of the fornix terminate in the mammillary body, while the dentate gyrus provides communication with the cingulate gyrus by means of the indusium griseum.

The hippocampus is divided into CA1, CA2, CA3, subiculum, presubiculum, and parasubiculum. The entorhinal cortex receives input from the olfactory stria, insula, cingulate gyrus, superior temporal gyrus, and orbitofrontal cortex, and this information projects to the dentate gyrus, and then to CA3, and subsequently to CA1.

The diencephalon consists of the thalamus, epithalamus, hypothalamus, and subthalamus. The thalamus provides the final relay for sensory information directed toward the cerebral cortex. The thalami are separated from the globus pallidus and putamen by the internal capsule. All body sensation except olfaction passes through the thalamus. Thalamic efferents project to the cerebral cortex by means of the internal capsule and the corona radiata. The thalamus is the communication link between the cerebellum and globus pallidus with the motor portion of the cerebral cortex. A lesion to the pulvinar of the thalamus can cause aphasia. The lateral geniculate body is a visual relay and the medial geniculate body is an auditory relay. The intralaminar nuclei are major components of the reticular activating system, which is responsible for arousing the cerebral cortex and perhaps focusing cortical regions to heightened awareness.

The epithalamus connects the limbic system with other brain components. It is involved in secretion of regulatory chemicals. The epithalamus includes the pineal body, the habenular nuclei and commissure, the striae medullaris, and the posterior commissure.

The subthalamus projects to the thalamus and receives input from the globus pallidus and motor cortex and works with the basal ganglia to control movement. The hypothalamus is considered to be the organizational structure of the limbic system. It interacts with the cingulate gyrus, septal area, parahippocampal gyrus, amygdala, and hippocampal formation to regulate reproductive physiology, desire and satiation relative to food and drink, control of digestion, and certain metabolic functions.

CASE STUDY 5–1

Physician's Notes on Initial Physical Examination and History

This is a 57-year-old female who reported **orolingual choreic movements** five years ago (see Table 5–2 for terminology. Note that we are presenting the data of this case in chronological order to show the emerging speech and language signs and symptoms as the condition progresses.). The upper and lower limbs and trunk were affected progressively. Her husband reported that there was also a change in her behavior characterized by impatience and aggression. The patient has no family history of hereditary neurological disease. During examination, the patient was alert with some difficulties in orientation to space. The **Mini Mental State Examination (MMSE)** was 23/30 (increased difficulty in concentration). The examination of the cranial nerves was normal. Muscle strength was full in all four extremities (see Table 5–3 for definitions of muscle

testing), with normal muscle tone and bulk. The **deep tendon reflexes** were symmetrically brisk in the upper and lower limbs and the **plantar response** was extension on the left. The sensory examination for light touch, **pinprick**, and **vibration sense** was normal. There was disturbance of the joint position sense on the left. **Finger-to-nose** and **heel-to-shin examinations** were normal and **Romberg** was normal. There were significant involuntary movements in all four extremities, trunk, and mouth. The patient's symptomatology progressively developed over a few years. Blood examinations for **FBC, biochemistry, neuroacanthocytosis**, serum ceruloplasmin, copper, **immunological assay**, and **genetic testing** for neurological disease were scheduled.

Three Months After Intake

The genetic testing revealed detection of two **alleles** of 17[+/−1] and 44 [+/−3] CAG repeats. The conclusion of

TABLE 5–2.	Terminology for Case Study 5–1
"c" or "d" scores	Scoring on the *Frenchay Dysarthria Assessment* (FDA). See Table 5–4 for details.
2-1-0	Shorthand meaning the time of day that the patient needs to take a medication. In this example, the patient needs to take 2 tablets in the morning, 1 tablet in the afternoon, and none in the evening.
Alleles	Alleles represent two forms of a gene, a dominant and a recessive one. If an organism has one allele, then the dominant trait is expressed.
Biochemistry	Biochemical analysis is a set of methods that analyze the substances of organisms and their chemical reactions.
Botox (botulinum toxin, BOTOX) injection	Botulinum toxin is a neurotoxic protein that does not allow the release of the neurotransmitter acetylcholine. There are 8 types of botulinum toxin. Types A and B have a medical use to produce flaccidity in various spasms and hyperkinesias that exist in different neurological diseases.
Ceruloplasmin	The major copper-carrying protein in the blood, and plays a role in iron metabolism.
Clonazepam (active ingredient), Klonopin (brand name) 0.5 mg	An anticonvulsant medication used in seizures and panic attacks. It belongs to a class of drugs known as benzodiazepines.
Coenzyme Q10 100 mg	Coenzyme is an antioxidant that is used to protect the cells from chemicals (radicals) by helping specific proteins (enzymes) to speed up the rate of chemical reactions in the body.
Deep tendon reflexes	Reflexes mediated by muscle spindle receptors, including patellar and Achilles tendon reflexes.
Dysarthria	Motor speech disorder involving muscular weakness, dyscoordination, and alteration of muscle tone. It includes slow movement of the muscles used for speech production, including the lips, tongue, vocal folds, and/or muscles of respiration.
Dystonic posture	A posture in the body that is the result of the neurological movement disorder known as dystonia. Dystonia is characterized by unpredictable and uncontrollable contraction of a muscle group. Contraction is sustained for a period before relaxing. Dystonia can be spontaneous or induced by action of a muscle of a muscle group.
Finger-to-nose examination	Medical examination that measures coordination. It is a part of examination for the cerebellar function. In this exam, the doctor asks the patient to fully extend the arm and then touch the nose.
Frenchay Dysarthria Assessment (FDA)	A standardized test to assess nonspeech and speech movements of lips, jaw, tongue, phonation, intelligibility, etc. (see Table 5–4 for details concerning scoring of the FDA.)
Full blood count (FBC)	Laboratory testing of blood.
Genetic testing (DNA testing)	This studies chromosomes in individual genes and uses biochemical testing to identify the presence of genetic diseases, particularly the forms in which there is a mutation in the genes.
Heel-to-shin examinations	Medical examination that measures coordination. It is a part of the examination for cerebellar function. In this exam, the doctor asks the patient to run the heel of one foot down the contralateral shin (equivalent to the finger-to-nose test).
Huntington's disease (Huntington's chorea)	An inherited neurodegenerative disease exhibiting symptomatology that includes lack of coordination, unsteadiness in gait, and uncontrollable and unpredictable movement in specific parts of the body. The disease will result in dysarthria, dysphagia, and dementia.
Hyperkinetic dysarthria of chorea	A type of dysarthria that is characterized by strained-strangled phonation, intermittent hypernasality, articulatory distortions irregular diadochokinesis, and quick, involuntary movements of the articulators that affect speech prosody and intelligibility.
Immunological assay	This tests for the presence of antigens (foreign substances attached to proteins or lipids).

TABLE 5–2.   *continued*

Klonopin	See clonazepam.
Mini Mental State Examination (MMSE)	A short worldwide screening cognitive test that measures attention, orientation, working memory, recall, language, and the ability to follow commands.
Neuroacanthocytosis	In this condition, the blood contains cells called acanthocytes. Acanthocytes are misformed red blood cells found in many inherited neurological diseases, including those resulting in chorea.
Orolingual choreic movements	Quick movements of the face and tongue that are abnormal and involuntary in nature and characterized as chorea.
Pinprick sense	Sensation of pinprick on the skin, mediated by the spinothalamic pathway.
Plantar response	The plantar reflex in infants is stimulated by rubbing a blunt object on the sole of the foot with moderate force. The normal plantar response includes extension (dorsiflexion) of the big toe and abduction or fanning of the other toes. This reflex is inhibited by cortical control around 6 months of age and is seen in only pathological conditions in adults.
Romberg	Test used to assess balance. In this test, the patient stands with feet together, eyes open, and hands by the sides and then closes the eyes while the examiner observes him/her.
Tetrabenazine (active ingredient), Xenazine (brand name)	Medication used to alleviate and decrease the uncontrollable movements in the body (chorea) caused by Huntington's disease. The medication decreases the levels of neurotransmitters such as dopamine, serotonin, and norepinephrine.
Vibration sense	Medical testing that involves the application of a vibrating tuning fork to the great toe of a patient. Then, the doctor asks the patient to describe the sensation.
Wilson's disease	A genetic disorder caused by the mutation of the ATP7B gene. In this disease, copper levels increase in the liver and brain. Its symptoms involve fatigue, pain in the abdomen, uncontrollable movements, muscle stiffness, dysarthria, dysphagia, etc.
Xenazine	See tetrabenazine.

TABLE 5–3.	**Examining Muscle Strength**

When examining a patient, identifying specific areas of muscular weakness helps to localize the site of lesion. Strength testing is completed for each muscle group, making sure that you test one side and then the next for each group, so you can compare strength for the two sides. Here is a muscle strength rating scale.

0/5	No contraction of muscle
1/5	Indication of muscle flicker, but no movement noted
2/5	Movement occurs, but not against gravity when tested in the horizontal plane
3/5	Movement occurs against, but not when there is resistance provided by the the examiner
4/5	Movement occurs against some resistance provided by the examiner
5/5	Normal strength

the testing showed that one allele (17[+/−1] CAG repeats) was within normal range (<36 CAG repeats), but the other allele (44 [+/−3] CAG repeats) was expanded into the **Huntington's** disease (HD) causing range (>35 CAG repeats), thus confirming the diagnosis of HD. Other family members are also at risk of having inherited the mutation. Each offspring of this individual has a 50% risk of inheriting the mutation. Genetic counseling was recommended.

Nine Months After Intake

The patient presented with advanced stage of the disease with involuntary movements of the upper and lower limbs and trunk. She also presented orolingual involuntary movements with **dystonic posture**, which impaired her ability to speak and eat. She was on treatment with **tetrabenazine** (25 mg, three times per day), vitamin E (400 units once daily), and **coenzyme Q10** (100 mg **2-1-0**). At examination, she was alert and oriented to place, but due to the dystonic posture of the face, she was not able to speak. She appeared to follow conversation with eye movements and body language. The patient was referred for routine blood analysis and started treatment with **clonazepam** 0.5 mg with gradual increase to one tablet twice a day in an attempt to resolve the dystonic posture of the face and orolingual function, in order to improve her ability to speak and eat. Her husband agreed to inform us of the progression, and in case of no improvement, the patient was to be scheduled for **Botox injection**.

Nine Months After Intake: Speech Examination (Hyperkinetic Dysarthria)

The patient was alert, and when asked about familiar topics she was eager to answer questions. Her speech during dialogue was characterized perceptually by slow rate, imprecise consonants, vowel prolongations, prolonged intervals, and inappropriate silences. The speech diagnosis is **hyperkinetic dysarthria of chorea**. When counting to 10, the patient was able to produce two or three numbers per breath accurately.

The *Frenchay Dysarthria Assessment* (FDA) was administered to the patient. The results correlated with the neurologist's impression for primarily hyperkinetic involvement in this patient. There was found moderate to severe difficulty, resulting in **"c" or "d" scores** in most of the domains assessed (see Table 5–4 for details of Frenchay scoring). More specifically:

- Reflexes (swallow): Patient exhibited slow eating of a cookie and choked once during drinking of water via a cup (c).
- Respiration in speech: Speech was very shallow (only 2–3 words per exhalation produced) (d).

TABLE 5–4.	Frenchay Scoring Details
The *Frenchay Dysarthria Assessment* (FDA) utilizes a rating scale for all testing.	
a score	Normal for age
b score	Mild abnormality noticeable to skilled observer
c score	Obvious abnormality but the patient can perform task/movements with reasonable approximation
d score	Some production of task but poor in quality, unable to sustain, inaccurate, or extremely labored
e score	Unable to undertake task/movement/sound

- Lips seal: Patient able to attempt closure when saying /p/ 10 times but unable to maintain it (d).
- Lips alternate: Shapes for the repeated production of "oo ee" (10 times) recognized as different (d).
- Lips in speech: Consistently poor movements acoustically represented as explosive with many omissions of labial shaping.
- Laryngeal component time: Sustained phonation for /a/ in 9 seconds (c).
- Laryngeal component pitch: Minimal change in pitch—shows difference between high and low during singing of a scale for 6 notes (d).
- Laryngeal component volume: Only limited change in volume and great difficulty in control during counting from 1 to 5 with increasing volume on each number (d).
- Laryngeal component during speech: Voice production is inappropriate in most situations, exhibiting paralinguistic features with intonation (d). However, no breathiness, hoarseness, or harshness was observed.
- Tongue component (protrusion): Patient was able to protrude/retract tongue to lip (5 times in 7 seconds) (d). The movement was irregular and accompanied by facial grimace.
- Tongue component elevation: Gross movement of the tongue when the patient tried to elevate it (5 times) (d).
- Tongue component lateral: Labored lateral tongue movement (5 times) produced in 7 seconds.
- Tongue component diadochokinetic rate: The word /kala/ was produced (10 times) with tongue changes in position and imprecise consonants/distorted vowels present (d). Time to complete: 13 seconds.
- Tongue during speech: There was grossly distorted articulation, with distorted vowels and frequently omitted consonants (d).

- Intelligibility: During the production of 10 cards with written words the patient was intelligible in only 3 words (d).

Medical Diagnosis

Huntington's disease (HD)

Speech-Language Diagnosis

Hyperkinetic dysarthria

Questions Concerning This Case

1. What brain regions are affected to cause the excessive movements seen in hyperkinesia?
2. Dementia will be an eventual outcome of this disease. What brain regions are affected to cause the cognitive deficit in Huntington's disease?

Case provided by Dr. Kostas Konstantopoulos, European University Cyprus.

CASE STUDY 5–2

Physician's Notes on Initial Physical Examination and History

This is a 68-year-old male who had noticed **micrographia** a year ago and consulted a private neurologist who prescribed **pramipexole** and **levodopa** (see Table 5–5 for terminology. Note that we are presenting the data of this case in chronological order to show the emerging speech and language signs and symptoms as the condition progresses.). The patient reported mild improvement in his symptoms with medication. Lately, he has developed the same difficulty in singing in church due to **hypophonia,** and he reported vivid dreams as well. The MRI scan of the brain revealed evidence of multiple focal **white matter hyperintensities** involving the frontal and parietal lobes as well as minimal **periventricular hyperintensities** compatible with long-standing white matter changes due to **small vessel disease**. There was dilatation of the lateral ventricles and **extra-axial CSF** spaces compatible with the patient's age. Past medical history involved **hypertension (Norvasc 5 mg, atenolol 50 mg od, HCTZ 50 mg od**, aspirin 75 mg od, **enalapril 10 mg 2 tabs bid**, and **Aldactone 25 mg od**). The social history involves no use of alcohol or smoking. The patient is married and has two healthy children.

The patient was alert with a normal mental status. He presented mild **dysarthria** and hypophonia. The gag reflex was reduced. When walking, the patient leaned to the left with mildly reduced right arm swing. There was mild **bradykinesia** and **rigidity** in the right hand. There was also no muscle weakness, the **DTRs** were symmetric, and **plantar response** was flexor bilaterally (see Table 5–3 for definitions of muscle testing). There was no sensory deficit, and cerebellar function was normal. Current medication is 2,1 tabs **Mirapexin ER od** and **Sinemet tabs 100/25 tds**. With his current medication, the patient presents minimal disability.

Current Medical Examination: Six Months Following Intake

The patient complained of bradykinesia and difficulty walking. He also reported sleepiness in the morning hours and mild swallowing dysfunction. On examination, there was dysarthria, **hypomimia**, and **shuffling gait with flexed posture**. Medication involves Sinemet 100/25 7-11-3-4-7 (denotes the time of day to take the medication) and **citalopram 20 mg od.** Referral to speech therapist for evaluation.

Speech Examination: Six Months Following Intake

Dysphagia assessment using **VFSS** showed effective but slow mastication; reduced lingual control allowing liquid to prematurely escape to the level of the valleculae prior to swallow response (oral phase), mild delay in swallow response, **laryngeal penetration** of thin liquids, but no aspiration noted. There was minimal bolus residue in the valleculae, but otherwise the pharyngeal swallow was functional for all consistencies. In the esophageal phase of the swallow, there were primary and secondary peristaltic waves functional for clearance of liquid; however, there was delayed emptying of pureed and solid bolus from distal esophagus above the level of **LES**. Mild distal esophageal spasm was noted. The impression was of mild oropharyngeal dysphagia. Recommendations for thin liquids with aspiration precautions and soft solids.

His speech during dialogue was characterized perceptually by **monopitch**, **monoloudness**, and a harsh voice quality. The *Frenchay Dysarthria Assessment* (FDA) showed mild **"b" score to "c" score** (see Table 5–4 for details of Frenchay scoring):

- Respiration in speech: There were very occasional breaks in fluency due to poor respiratory control. The patient reported occasionally having to stop to take a deep breath during speech (b).
- Lip seal: Lip seal not consistent for plosion on each sound /p/ /p/ 10 times (b).
- Lips alternate: Patient able to articulate "oo ee" in 15 seconds but the rhythm of production was faltering with variability in rounding or spreading the lips (b).
- Lips in speech: The speech shows some weakness or briskness and occasional omissions in plosives (b).

TABLE 5–5. **Terminology for Case Study 5–2**

"b-c" score	Scoring on the *Frenchay Dysarthria Assessment* (FDA). See Table 5–4 for details of the Frenchay scoring.
Aldactone	See spironolactone.
Amlodipine (active ingredient), Norvasc (brand name) 5 mg	A medication used in decreasing the level of hypertension by widening blood vessels and improving blood flow.
Aquazide	See hydrochlorothiazide.
Atenolol (active ingredient), Tenormin (brand name) 50 mg	A medication used to lower high blood pressure and provide a relief for chest pain.
bid	Twice a day.
Bradykinesia	Slowness of movement. It is one of the main features for the diagnosis of Parkinson's disease.
Carbidopa and levodopa (active ingredients), Sinemet (brand name) 100/25	A medication used to treat Parkinson's disease. It includes a combination of two substances, carbidopa and levodopa.
Celexa	See citalopram.
Citalopram (active ingredient), Celexa (brand name) 20 mg	This belongs to a class of drugs known as selective serotonin reuptake inhibitors (SSRIs), used for the treatment of depression.
Deep tendon reflexes (DTRs)	Reflexes mediated by muscle spindle receptors, including patellar and Achilles tendon reflexes.
Dysarthria	Motor speech disorder involving muscular weakness, dyscoordination, and alteration of muscle tone. It includes slow or or sometimes quick (with reduced range in the case of Parkinson's disease) movement of the muscles used for speech production, including the lips, tongue, vocal folds, and/or muscles of respiration.
Enalapril (active ingredient), Vasotec (brand name) 10 mg 2 tabs	Used to treat high blood pressure (hypertension) and congestive heart failure (by decreasing the rate of blood pumping by the heart).
Vasotec	See enalapril.
Extra-axial CSF	It denotes areas such as sulci, fissures, basal cisterns, and ventricles of cerebrospinal fluid (CSF).
Hydrochlorothiazide (HCTZ) (active ingredient), Aquazide (brand name) 50 mg	Medication used to lower hypertension.
Hypertension	Blood pressure that is higher than 140 (systolic) over 90 (diastolic) millimeters of mercury (mmHg). The systolic blood pressure is the pressure that the heart pumps blood, while the diastolic blood pressure is the pressure associated with relaxation of the heart muscle as the heart refills with blood.
Hypomimia	Also called "masked face"; denotes a reduced facial expression. It is a sign of Parkinson's disease.
Hypophonia	Low vocal intensity. It is a sign of Parkinson's disease.
Laryngeal penetration	Passage of food or liquid into the larynx but not past the vocal folds. It is distinguished from aspiration, in which the passage of food or liquids goes beyond the level of the vocal folds.

TABLE 5–5. *continued*

Levodopa (active ingredient)	The primary medication used to increase the level of dopamine in the basal ganglia to alleviate the signs of Parkinson's disease.
Lower esophageal sphincter (LES)	This includes muscles in the lower esophagus used to close the esophageal opening and prevent the acid content of the stomach from entering the esophagus.
Micrographia	It involves writing with small cramped letters and is frequently present in Parkinson's disease.
Mirapexin	See pramipexole dihydrochloride monohydrate.
Monoloudness	Voice lacking normal variations of intensity.
Monopitch	Voice lacking normal fundamental frequency variation.
Norvasc	See amlodipine.
od	Medical shorthand for "every day."
Parkinson's disease	A degenerative movement disorder caused by the lack of production of the neurotransmitter dopamine by the substantia nigra. Signs of Parkinson's disease include tremor (hands, arms, legs), bradykinesia (slowness of movement), rigidity (stiffness in the limbs), postural instability (impaired balance), and hypokinetic dysarthria.
Periventricular hyperintensities	"Periventricular" refers to areas adjacent to the lateral ventricles. "Hyperintensities" refers to areas shown by the MRI, specifically areas that reflect lesions produced by axonal loss and demyelination.
Plantar response	The plantar reflex in infants is stimulated by rubbing a blunt object on the sole of the foot with moderate force. Normal plantar response includes extension (dorsiflexion) of the big toe and abduction or fanning of the other toes. This reflex is inhibited by cortical control around 6 months of age and is seen in only pathological conditions in adults.
Pramipexole dihydrochloride monohydrate (active ingredient), Mirapexin ER (brand name)	This medication is used to treat stiffness, tremor, and muscle spasms and is prescribed in Parkinson's disease.
Rigidity	Muscle stiffness. It is one of the main features of Parkinson's disease.
Shuffling gait with flexed posture	The gait is characterized by small shuffling steps and a flexed body posture.
Sinemet	See carbidopa and levodopa.
Small vessel disease (coronary microvascular disease)	A disease in which there is damage in the walls of the small arteries.
Spironolactone (active ingredient), Aldactone (brand name) 25 mg	A medication used to lower high blood pressure and heart failure.
tds	3 times a day.
Tenormin	See atenolol.
Videofluoroscopy (VFSS)	Test used for the assessment of swallowing dysfunction through radiography.
White matter hyperintensities	Signal in the MRI that shows lesions due to axonal loss in the brain.

- Laryngeal component time: Sustained phonation for /a/ was 5 seconds (c).
- Laryngeal component pitch: Patient was able to represent four distinct pitch changes with uneven progression when singing a scale (c).
- Laryngeal component volume: Patient accurately demonstrated changes in volume while counting from 1 to 5 with a noticeably uneven progression (c).
- Laryngeal component during speech: Voice production required effort and attention; voice deteriorated unpredictably. There were difficulties with modulation, clarity of phonation, or pitch variation, but patient was able to control these on occasion (c).
- Tongue component (protrusion): Patient was able to protrude and retract tongue (5 times in 5 seconds) (b). The task was slow but otherwise normal.
- Tongue component (elevation): Patient was able to point the tongue toward the nose and then toward the chin slowly (5 times in 6 seconds) (b).
- Tongue component (lateral): Slow movement of the tongue side to side (5 times), produced in 6 seconds.
- Tongue component: Diadochokinetic rate of the word /kala/ (10 times) with one sound well articulated but the other poorly presented; the task deteriorated with time. Task took 10 seconds to complete (c).

Medical Diagnosis

Parkinson's disease.

Speech-Language Diagnosis

Hypokinetic dysarthria.

Questions Concerning This Case

1. The neurologist recognized hypophonia as one of this patient's signs. How does hypophonia relate to the tongue and larynx information derived from the FDA?
2. The speech-language pathologist diagnosed hypokinetic dysarthria. This dysarthria is characterized by paucity of movement of the muscles involved in speech. How does this relate to the micrographia identified by the physician?

Case provided by Dr. Kostas Konstantopoulos, European University Cyprus.

CASE STUDY 5–3

Physician's Notes on Initial Physical Examination and History

This was a 41-year-old female who exhibited tremor in her right limbs. The brain MRI revealed a solitary lesion of 9 mm diameter, possibly **inflammatory**, within the right **centrum semiovale** (see Table 5–6 for terminology. Note that we are presenting the data of this case in chronological order to show the emerging speech and language signs and symptoms as the condition progresses). Due to her **postural tremor** of right limbs, I tried administering **gabapentin 300 mg tds** (I did not give **Inderal** due to **orthostatic hypotension**).

Four Days Following Intake

The patient developed nausea and headaches with gabapentin after three days use and so I asked her to stop this medication and consider an alternative (**Trileptal**) for the following week.

Four Months Following Intake

The history for the **EEG** report shows **fainting episodes** and a single demyelinating lesion in the patient's brain. The findings of the EEG study showed that hyperventilation induced an episode without electrographic correlate. This is a normal EEG recorded in wakefulness. During hyperventilation, there was reproduction of the patient's symptoms without an electrographic correlate.

Two Years, 7 Months Following Intake

The patient came for a follow-up for involuntary movements of the right upper and lower limbs. The patient reported that her muscle strength and bulk were worsening over the past months but the involuntary movements have improved with the use of **Lyrica** (see Table 5–3 for definitions of muscle testing). She also reported episodes with fainting in the last few months.

On examination there was weakness of the right lower limb together with decreased **pinprick sensation**. In addition, there was action-induced (intention) tremor of the upper and lower limbs. Continued with Lyrica and she will be seen again in four months time.

Three Years, 8 Months Following Intake

A new brain MRI was performed. The results showed a demyelinating **T2 lesion** of high density in the right corona

TABLE 5–6.   Terminology for Case Study 5–3

"c" or "d" scores	Scoring on the *Frenchay Dysarthria Assessment* (FDA). See Table 5–4 for details on scoring.
Blood pressure (BP)	The systolic blood pressure is the pressure that the heart pumps blood, while the diastolic blood pressure is the pressure that the heart relaxes and refills with blood. Normal blood pressure is lower than 120 (systolic) over 80 (diastolic) millimeters of mercury (mmHg).
Centrum semiovale	Mass of axons superior to the lateral ventricles/corpus callosum. Inferiorly these fibers are continuous with the corona radiata.
Diffuse myopathy	A disease affecting the muscle fibers (primary defect, as opposed to neuropathy, in which the primary defect is in the nerves) and resulting in muscular weakness.
Dysarthria/clumsy hand	A rare syndrome characterized by dysarthria and clumsiness in one hand. Its cause is a lacunar stroke in the pons.
Dysarthria	Motor speech disorder involving muscular weakness, dyscoordination, and alteration of muscle tone. It includes slow movement of the muscles used for speech production, including the lips, tongue, vocal folds, and/or muscles of respiration.
Dyskinesia	Abnormal involuntary movement. The patient does not have the ability to inhibit this movement.
Dysphagia	Difficulty with one of the stages of swallowing.
Electroencephalogram (EEG)	Neurophysiological test that shows electrical activity in the brain.
Electromyography (EMG)	Laboratory technique to record the electrical activity (electric potential) of skeletal muscles.
Fainting episodes	Temporary loss of consciousness due to the lack of oxygen in the brain.
Frenchay Dysarthria Assessment (FDA)	A standardized test to assess nonspeech and speech movements of lips, jaw, tongue, phonation, intelligibility, etc. (see Table 5–4 for details concerning scoring of the FDA).
Gabapentin (active ingredient), Neurontin (brand name) 300 mg	An anti-epileptic medication used to treat neuropathic pain and seizures.
Hydroxychloroquine (active ingredient), Plaquenil (brand name) 200 mg	As an antirheumatoid drug, it is a medication used to treat autoimmune diseases such as lupus erythematosus and rheumatoid arthritis, as well as malaria.
Inderal	See propranolol.
Inflammatory	Swelling, heat, pain, and redness in the specific part of the body that is infected.
Isolated dysarthria	Condition in which dysarthria is the only sign.
Lyrica	See pregabalin.
Neurontin	See gabapentin.
od	Medical shorthand for "every day."
Orthostatic hypotension	Orthostatic hypotension refers to a marked reduction in blood pressure when a patient moves from sitting to standing posture (a decrease of 20 mmHg [systolic pressure] or 10 mmHg [diastolic pressure] between the two positions.
Oxcarbazepine (active ingredient), Trileptal (brand name)	An anti-epileptic drug.
Paroxysmal dyskinesia	This includes involuntary movements that occur at certain times.

continues

TABLE 5–6.	*continued*
Pinprick sensation	Sensation of pinprick on the skin, mediated by the spinothalamic pathway.
Plaquenil	See hydroxychloroquine.
Postural tremor	A type of tremor that occurs during voluntary contraction of the muscles and more specifically when the body part is held against gravity.
Pregabalin (active ingredient), Lyrica (brand name) 75 mg	Medication used to treat epilepsy, neuropathic pain, and generalized anxiety disorder.
Propranolol (active ingredient), Inderal (brand name)	Medication used to treat hypertension.
Sensorimotor stroke	This involves a lesion in the thalamus, posterior internal capsule, and lateral pons with symptoms such as hemiparesis/hemiplegia and a contralateral sensory impairment.
Systemic lupus erythematosus (SLE)	An autoimmune disease that may affect the skin, joints, brain, etc.
T2 lesion	Lesion shown in the MRI that is considered to be active. It shows a degree of edema in the normal appearance of the axons (white matter).
tds	3 times a day.
Trileptal	See oxcarbazepine.

radiata with a diameter of almost 1 cm. No change from the results of the last MRI was found. Normal imaging was found for the ventricular system and the subarachnoid space.

Four Years, 2 Months Following Intake

The patient was diagnosed with a probable **systemic lupus erythematosus (SLE)** but has not received treatment yet. She stated that over the past months, when she sits or lies down, she has dizziness and tends to faint. When she moves around, she feels better. She also complained of muscle pains.

On examination, there was postural tremor of the right limbs with limited movements of the joints due to pain. **BP:** 110/70 mmHg. She was on Lyrica 75 mg **od**. The patient was scheduled for reexamination in two months.

Seven Years, 1 Month Following Intake

The patient presented with a past history of involuntary movements in the right upper limbs and had started **Plaquenil 200 mg** on alternate days. There has been some improvement of the pains in the small joints but not in the shoulder joints. The patient also described a burning sensation in the right gastrocnemius muscle. The pain, tiredness, and involuntary movements of the right upper limb continue, and I was wondering whether this consists of paroxysmal **dyskinesia**. The patient also told me that she has some difficulties in the movement of the tongue, and indeed I noticed some difficulty in turning the tongue to the right side. Since there were some mild swallowing difficulties for a short period, I requested an evaluation by the speech language pathologist. Also, an **EMG** study was conducted and revealed normal findings. There was no electrophysiological evidence suggestive of **diffuse myopathy** in this patient. A follow-up was scheduled in four months.

Medical Diagnosis

Systemic lupus erythematosus (SLE)

Speech Examination: Six Years, 10 Months Following Intake

The patient was alert, and when asked about familiar topics, she was eager to answer the questions. Her speech during dialogue was characterized perceptually by slow rate and slow tongue alternate movements.

The *Frenchay Dysarthria Assessment* (**FDA**) was administered to the patient (see Table 5–4 for details of Frenchay scoring). The results correlated with the neurologist's impression for slower tongue movement. There was found moderate to severe difficulty, with scores of **"c"** or **"d"** in the domains of the tongue. More specifically:

- Reflexes (swallow): Normal
- Respiration in speech: Normal
- Lip seal: Normal
- Lips alternate: Normal
- Lips in speech: Normal
- Laryngeal component time: Normal
- Laryngeal component pitch: Normal
- Laryngeal component volume: Normal
- Tongue component (protrusion): Patient was able to protrude/retract tongue to lip (5 times in 7 seconds) (c). The movement was irregular or accompanied by facial grimace.
- Tongue component elevation: Gross movement of the tongue when the patient tried to elevate it (5 times) (d).
- Tongue component lateral: Labored lateral tongue movement (5 times) produced in 7 seconds (c).
- Tongue component: Diadochokinetic rate of the bisyllable /kala/ (10 times) with tongue changes in position, and imprecise consonants/distorted vowels were present (d). Time to complete was 11 seconds.
- Intelligibility: During the production of 10 cards with written words the patient was intelligible for all words (normal finding).

Speech-Language Diagnosis: Dysarthria

In this case, differential diagnosis reveals several potential etiologies. The tongue symptomatology mimics a rare lacunar stroke syndrome, specifically the lacunar syndrome of "**isolated dysarthria**." If this is the case, the corticolingual tract function should be impaired. However, in this case no sensory functions should be affected. The location of the infarct could involve the posterior limb of the internal capsule, basis pontis, and corona radiata producing marked hemiparesis or hemiplegia affecting the face, arm, or leg of the contralateral side and **dysarthria**, **dysphagia**, and transient sensory symptomatology. Other lacunar states that could affect this patient could be **dysarthria/clumsy hand** syndrome, involving the basis pontis, the anterior limb or genu of the internal capsule, corona radiata, basal ganglia, and cerebral peduncle and producing dysarthria and clumsiness (weakness) of the hand, which often are most prominent when the patient is writing. Finally, the symptoms could arise from a mixed **sensorimotor stroke**, with an infarct location in the thalamus and adjacent posterior internal capsule and lateral pons and producing hemiparesis or hemiplegia with contralateral sensory impairment. A variant of these lacunar stroke syndromes could easily produce the current patient's symptomatology.

Questions Concerning This Case

1. The MRI revealed a 1-cm lesion in the corona radiata. Would this involve sensory or motor fibers, or potentially both? Given the symptoms provided by the patient, can you hypothesize which fibers were involved?
2. The SLP provided several potential sites of lesion, based on the findings. Which one of these best matched the symptoms of the patient?

Case provided by Dr. Kostas Konstantopoulos, European University Cyprus.

CHAPTER 5
STUDY QUESTIONS

1. The primary nuclei of the basal ganglia include the _____ _____, _____ _____ and _____.

2. Please identify the structures and landmarks indicated on the figure.

   a. _____ _____

   b. _____

   c. _____ of caudate

   d. _____ limb of internal capsule

   e. _____ tract

   f. _____ _____ (nucleus of basal ganglia)

   g. _____ tract

   h. _____

   i. _____ geniculate body

   j. _____ (nucleus of thalamus)

   k. _____ geniculate body

   l. _____ ventricle

3. The head/body/tail (circle one) of caudate protrudes into the anterior horn of the lateral ventricle.

4. The _____ is responsible for synchronizing the various areas of the cerebral cortex.

5. The term _____ refers to a movement disorder resulting in excessive, uncontrollable movement. The disorder typically arises from damage to the basal ganglia.

6. GABA/dopamine (circle one) is an inhibitory neurotransmitter.

7. The striate body/globus pallidus (circle one) serves as the input for the basal ganglia.

8. The direct/indirect (circle one) pathway is involved in maintenance of background function, such as muscle tone or antagonist muscle control.

9. The _____ is important for placing memory into long-term storage.

10. The diencephalon consists of the _____, _____, _____, and _____.

11. The _____ is the final relay for nearly all sensory information directed toward the cerebral cortex.

12. All sensory information except _____ passes through the thalamus.

13. The _____ (nucleus of the thalamus) is related to language function, and a lesion to this nucleus can cause subcortical aphasia.

14. The _____ _____ body is a visual relay of the thalamus.

15. The _____ _____ body is an auditory relay of the thalamus.

16. The _____ _____ of the thalamus are components of the reticular activating system, which is responsible for arousing the cerebral cortex.

17. Damage to the _____ nucleus can cause ballism, a hyperkinesia.

18. The _____ is considered to be the organizational structure of the limbic system.

REFERENCES

Amaral, D., & Lavenex, P. (2007). Hippocampal anatomy. In P. Andersen, R. Morris, D. Amaral, T. Bliss, & J. O'Keefe (Eds.), *The hippocampus book* (pp. 37–114). New York, NY: Oxford University Press.

Andersen, P., Morris, R., Amaral, D., Bliss, T., & O'Keefe, J. (2007). The hippocampal formation. In P. Anderson, R. Morris, D. Amaral, T. Bliss, & J. O'Keefe (Eds.), *The hippocampus book* (pp. 3–6). New York, NY: Oxford University Press.

Baehr, M., & Frotscher, M. (2012). *Duus' topical diagnosis in neurology: Anatomy, physiology, signs, symptoms* (5th ed.). New York, NY: Thieme.

Bamiou, D. E., Musiek, F. E., & Luxon, L. M. (2003). The insula (Island of Reil) and its role in auditory processing: Literature review. *Brain Research Reviews, 42*(2), 143–154.

Carpenter, M. B. (1978). *Core text of neuroanatomy.* Baltimore, MD: Williams & Wilkins.

Corkin, S. (2013). *Permanent present tense.* New York, NY: Basic Books.

Crick, F. C., & Koch, C. (2005). What is the function of the claustrum? *Philosophical Transactions of the Royal Society of London B: Biological Sciences, 360*(1458), 1271–1279.

DeLong, M. R., & Wichmann, T. (2007). Circuits and circuit disorders of the basal ganglia. *Archives of Neurology, 64*(1), 20–24.

Ettlinger, G., & Wilson, W. A. (1990). Cross-modal performance: Behavioural processes, phylogenetic considerations and neural mechanisms. *Behavioural Brain Research, 40*(3), 169–192.

Horn, J. P., & Swanson, L. W. (2012). The autonomic motor system and the hypothalamus. In E. R. Kandel, J. H. Schwartz, T. M. Jessell, S. A. Siegelbaum, & A. J. Hudspeth (Eds.), *Principles of neural science* (5th ed., pp. 1956–1078). New York, NY: McGraw Hill.

Kreitzer, A. C., & Malenka, R. C. (2008). Striatal plasticity and basal ganglia circuit function. *Neuron, 60*(4), 543–554.

Netter, F. H. (1983). *The CIBA collection of medical illustrations. Vol. 1. Nervous system. Part I. Anatomy and physiology.* West Caldwell, NJ: CIBA Pharmaceutical.

Noback, C. R., Demarest, R. J., & Strominger, N. L. (1991). *The nervous system: Introduction and review.* Philadelphia, PA: Williams & Wilkins.

Redgrave, P., Rodriguez, M., Smith, Y., Rodriguez-Oroz, M. C., Lehericy, S., Bergman, H., . . . Obeso, J. A. (2010). Goal-directed and habitual control in the basal ganglia: Implications for Parkinson's disease. *Nature Reviews Neuroscience, 11*(11), 760–772.

Seikel, J. A., Drumright, D. G., & King, D. W. (2016). *Anatomy & physiology for speech, language and hearing* (5th ed.). Clifton Park, NY: Cengage Learning.

Seikel, J. A., King, D. W., & Drumright, D. G. (1997). *Anatomy & physiology for speech, language and hearing* (3rd ed.). San Diego, CA: Singular.

Tsao, D. Y., Freiwald, W. A., Tootell, R. B., & Livingstone, M. S. (2006). A cortical region consisting entirely of face-selective cells. *Science, 311*(5761), 670-674.

Wichmann, T., & DeLong, M. R. (2013). The basal ganglia. In E. R. Kandel, J. H. Schwartz, T. M. Jessell, S. A. Siegelbaum, & A. J. Hudspeth (Eds.), *Principles of neural science* (5th ed., pp. 982–998). New York, NY: McGraw-Hill.

Yin, B., Terhune, D. B., Smythies, J., & Meck, W. H. (2016). Claustrum, consciousness, and time perception. *Current Opinion in Behavioral Sciences, 8,* 258–267.

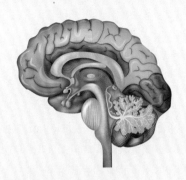

6 ANATOMY OF THE BRAINSTEM

Learning Outcomes for Chapter 6

• Visually identify the 3 levels of the brainstem, including medulla, pons, and midbrain.

• Visually identify landmarks of the superficial medulla.

• Discuss the prominent deep landmarks and functional significance of the medulla, including the reticular formation, decussation of the pyramids, fasciculi cuneatus and gracilis, nucleus solitarius, hypoglossal and dorsal vagal nuclei, inferior olivary nucleus, and nucleus ambiguus.

• Discuss the prominent deep landmarks and functional significance of the pons, including posterior tegmentum, basilar portion, pontine nuclei, medial longitudinal fasciculus, vestibular nuclei, trapezoid body, and the superior olivary complex.

• Discuss the prominent deep landmarks and functional significance of the midbrain, including the tectum, tegmentum, crus

INTRODUCTION

The brainstem is physically and functionally an intermediary between the cerebral cortex above and the spinal cord below. From the perspective of the spinal cord, the brainstem houses significantly more complex responses to environmental stimuli in the form of elegant reflexes and hard-wired motor plans. From the view of the cerebral cortex, the brainstem is an intermediate step toward complex processing of multiple stimuli, as well as a means of executing complex acts that arise from the cortex. From our viewpoint as speech-language pathologists and audiologists, the brainstem is a vitally important structure.

The brainstem can be broken into three large components: the **medulla oblongata**, the **pons**, and the **midbrain**. **Cranial nerve nuclei** found within the brainstem provide a means of interacting with the environment and a gateway to higher cortical function (Carpenter, 1991; Crossman, 2008; Noback, Demarest, & Strominger, 1991). Take a look at the views in Figure 6–1 as we discuss the surface anatomy of the brainstem. Following that discussion, we will examine its internal architecture.

SUPERFICIAL BRAINSTEM LANDMARKS

The surface of the brainstem has a number of landmarks that will help orient us to the structures within the brainstem. The brainstem serves as a significant integration center for sensory and motor function, so understanding the parts is very useful to seeing the whole. We'll begin with the medulla oblongata, the component of the brainstem closest to the spinal cord, and move up to the pons and midbrain. Realize that these components represent artificial and arbitrary divisions, based upon physical appearance. That having been said, there are certainly some significant functional differences among the three levels.

Superficial Medulla Oblongata

The superficial **medulla oblongata** (also simply known as the "medulla") is the inferior-most of the substructures of the brainstem. As you look at it, it appears to be an enlargement of the spinal cord below. The medulla is approximately 2.5 cm long (Nolte, 2002). You may want to take a look at Figure 6–1A to orient yourself to this small but mighty structure.

The superficial medulla has several landmarks that will help navigate the discussion of this structure. The **anterior median fissure** (Figure 6–1A) is an extension of the same landmark of the spinal cord, although in the medulla it is blurred at the decussation of the pyramids. The **pyramidal decussation** is an cerebri, inferior colliculus, superior cerebellar peduncle, superior colliculus, inferior colliculus, red nucleus, Edinger–Westphal nucleus, and substantia nigra.

• Identify the components of the VIII vestibulocochlear nerve and discuss the function of the auditory pathway nuclei.

• Explain the significance of the components of the cochlear nucleus, including the anteroventral, dorsal, and posteroventral cochlear nucleus.

• Discuss the role of the octopus cells, globular cells, and bushy cells in signal processing in the cochlear nucleus.

• Discuss the role of the superior olivary complex in signal processing, particularly differentiating the role of the lateral and medial superior olive.

• Discuss the relationship between the inferior colliculus and superior olivary complex, as well as the function of the inferior colliculus in auditory processing.

• Describe the relationship between the medial geniculate body, the pulvinar, and the lateral geniculate body in terms of information processing.

• Discuss the difference between the function of the core, belt, and parabelt in the auditory cortex.

• Describe the differential pathway of the vestibular and auditory branches of the VIII vestibulocochlear nerve after entering the brainstem.

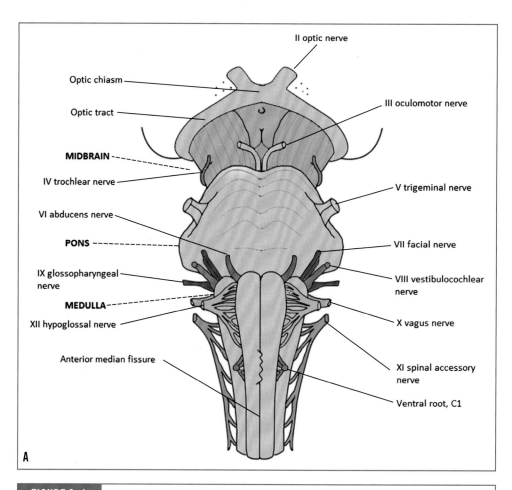

FIGURE 6–1. Views of brainstem. **A.** Anterior brainstem showing cranial nerves. *continues*

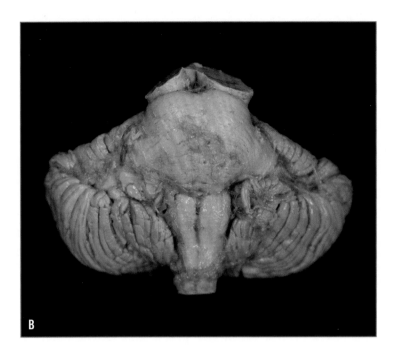

B

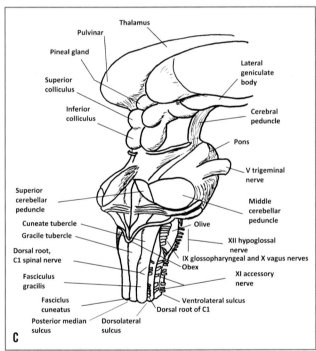

C

Thalamus
Pulvinar
Pineal gland
Superior colliculus
Inferior colliculus
Lateral geniculate body
Cerebral peduncle
Pons
V trigeminal nerve
Middle cerebellar peduncle
Superior cerebellar peduncle
Cuneate tubercle
Gracile tubercle
Olive
Dorsal root, C1 spinal nerve
XII hypoglossal nerve
IX glossopharyngeal and X vagus nerves
Obex
Fasciculus gracilis
XI accessory nerve
Fasciclus cuneatus
Ventrolateral sulcus
Posterior median sulcus
Dorsolateral sulcus
Dorsal root of C1

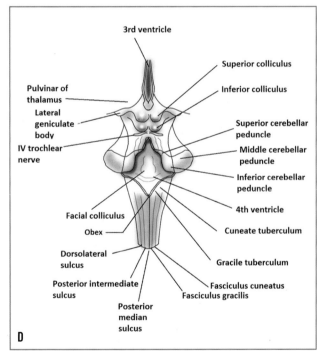

D

3rd ventricle
Superior colliculus
Inferior colliculus
Pulvinar of thalamus
Lateral geniculate body
IV trochlear nerve
Superior cerebellar peduncle
Middle cerebellar peduncle
Inferior cerebellar peduncle
4th ventricle
Facial colliculus
Obex
Cuneate tuberculum
Dorsolateral sulcus
Gracile tuberculum
Posterior intermediate sulcus
Fasciculus cuneatus
Fasciculus gracilis
Posterior median sulcus

FIGURE 6–1. *continued* **B.** Photograph of anterior brainstem. **C.** Lateral brainstem. *Source:* After view of Netter (1983). **D.** Posterior brainstem. *continues*

---

internal phenomenon wherein most of the descending motor fibers of the corticospinal tract from one hemisphere decussate (crossover) to continue descending on the opposite side. This blurring of the anterior median fissure is an outer manifestation of this very important phenomenon that we will see repeatedly as we talk about pathways of the brain. This pyramidal decussation occurs at the lower medulla.

If you now look at Figure 6–1C for the side view of the medulla, you will see the ventrolateral sulcus and dorsolateral sulcus. The **ventrolateral sulcus** is the location from which

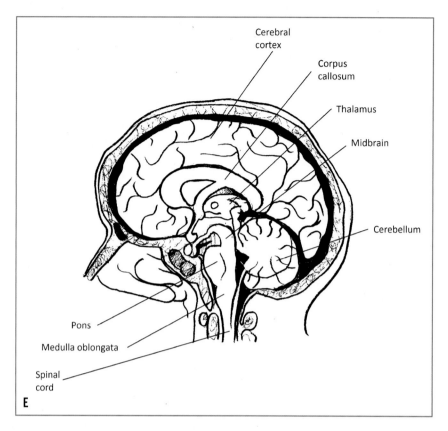

Cerebral cortex

Corpus callosum

Thalamus

Midbrain

Cerebellum

Pons

Medulla oblongata

Spinal cord

E

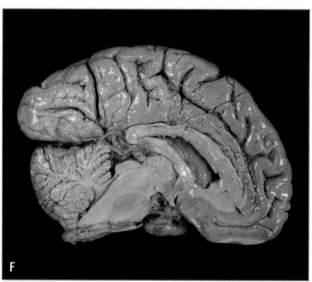

F

FIGURE 6–1.   *continued* **E.** Sagittal section through brain showing relation of brainstem to cerebral structures. **F.** Photograph of sagittal sections through brain.

the **XII hypoglossal nerve** exits the medulla (this nerve innervates the muscles of the tongue). The **ventrolateral sulcus** is the point at which the **XI accessory, X vagus,** and **IX glossopharyngeal nerves** exit. Between the ventrolateral and dorsolateral sulci is the olive, the prominence associated with the **inferior olivary nuclear complex.** This will be familiar to you in the context of learning the auditory

pathway, since the inferior olive is an important nucleus associated with localizing sound in space (Bear, Connors, & Paradiso, 1996).

If you look at Figure 6–1D, you can see the posterior landmarks. In this view, the cerebellum has been removed to reveal the fourth ventricle immediately posterior to the medulla. As discussed earlier, CSF is produced within the ventricles, and the fourth ventricle is the last of the series of ventricles through which CSF circulates.

The inferiormost point on the posterior medulla is the **obex**, which marks the beginning of a region known as the **calamus scriptorius**, which is the inferior 1/3 of the 4th ventricle. Lateral to the obex is the **clava** or **gracilis tubercle**, a bulge reflecting the **nucleus gracilis** within. The **cuneate turbercle** can be seen lateral to the clava: this marks the terminal point of the fasciculus cuneatus (to be discussed).

The vagal trigone and hypoglossal trigones are found within the calamus scriptorius. The vagal trigone is a bulge that marks the dorsal vagal nucleus of the X vagus nerve, and the **hypoglossal trigone** is caused by the XII hypoglossal nucleus.

Superficial Pons

Superior to the medulla is the pons. Pons is Latin for "bridge," and its function is to provide a bridge among the medulla, midbrain, and cerebellum. The anterior bulge of the pons overlies the fibers that serve as the communication links among these structures. Four cranial nerve nuclei reside at the level of the pons, and the middle cerebellar peduncle is found here as well. The cerebellar peduncles are pathways between the cerebellum and other brain regions.

The prominent bulge in Figure 6–1A represents the transverse fibers that provide communication between the cerebellum and the pons known as the **pontocerebellar tract**. At the anterior midline, you can see the **basal sulcus**, which marks the course of the basilar artery of the cerebrovascular supply (to be discussed). On the inferior superficial pons, the VI abducens nerve exits from the **inferior pontine sulcus** (not shown).

Figure 6–1B shows the lateral surface of the pons. The **middle cerebellar peduncle (brachia pontis)** is the intermediate communicating attachment of the pons to the cerebellum. Important for audiologists, the juncture of the cerebellum and the pons marks the **cerebellopontine angle**, a point at which tumors may develop that affect both vestibular and auditory function. The VII facial and VIII vestibulocochlear nerves arise from this point, so tumors at this location may cause sensorineural hearing loss, vestibular dysfunction, and facial paralysis. The V trigeminal nerve exits the pons at the middle cerebellar peduncle, and it is responsible for facial sensation and the activation of the muscles of mastication.

In Figure 6–1C, you can see the posterior pons. In this figure, the cerebellum has been removed, showing that the fourth ventricle is between the pons and the cerebellum. The upper limit of the ventricle is the upper margin of the pons. The **superior cerebellar peduncles (brachia conjunctiva)** of the midbrain makes up the upper lateral surface of the fourth ventricle, and the **superior** and **inferior medullary veli** and cerebellum are the superior border. The paired **facial colliculi** represent the location of the nucleus of the VI abducens nerve.

Superficial Midbrain

The midbrain is the third and most superior structure of the brainstem. Look again at Figure 6–1A. The largest component of the anterior midbrain is the paired **crus cerebri**. These are extremely important structures that connect the cerebrum with the rest of the CNS and PNS, by means of the **cerebral peduncles**. While the peduncles appear large in this picture, realize that they are really quite small (for comparison, the medulla is about the size of your pinky finger in diameter). A lesion to the midbrain could have profound effects on the function of the entire body, because nearly all motor and sensory fibers pass through this crus (Chusid, 1985).

The posterior midbrain (Figure 6–1C) is called the **tectum**. There are four important landmarks on the tectum, known as the **corpora quadrigemina** (literally, "four bodies"). The corpora quadrigemina consists of the **superior** and **inferior colliculi**, which are important nuclei of the visual and auditory system, respectively. The IV trochlear nerve emerges near the inferior colliculus and courses around the crus cerebri.

The superficial landmarks of the brainstem provide a means of navigating and discussing the structures you see. Now let's look at the inner structures of the brainstem.

DEEP STRUCTURES OF THE BRAINSTEM

The organization of the brainstem is primarily in the vertical dimension, being made up of columnar nuclei and tracts that serve the periphery, spinal cord, cerebral, cerebellar, and subcortical structures. Figure 6–2 may help you navigate the internal brainstem.

Deep Structures of the Medulla Oblongata

The **central canal** is the upper extension of the spinal canal, and it expands in the medulla to become the fourth ventricle. **Cerebrospinal fluid** (CSF) passes through this canal. Around the canal is the **central gray matter**, which expands to the **reticular formation**. The reticular formation actually extends through medulla, pons, and midbrain. It is a vitally important set of nuclei that forms the "oldest" part of the brainstem and reflects an early evolutionary effort at complex processing. The importance of the reticular formation cannot be overstated: it contains nuclei associated with respiration and the maintenance of blood pressure and works with the intralaminar nuclei of the thalamus to keep the cerebral cortex awake. Damage to the reticular formation may leave a person in a persistent vegetative state, absent of conscious thought. Refer to Tables 6–1 and 6–2.

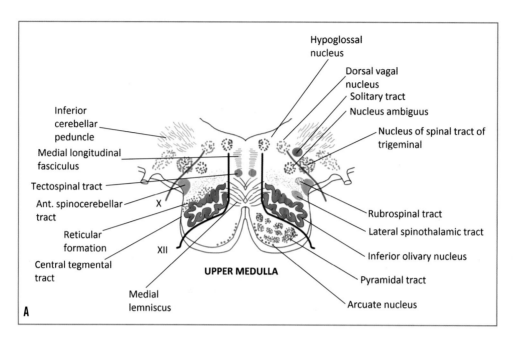

Hypoglossal nucleus

Dorsal vagal nucleus

Solitary tract

Nucleus ambiguus

Nucleus of spinal tract of trigeminal

Inferior cerebellar peduncle

Medial longitudinal fasciculus

Tectospinal tract

Ant. spinocerebellar tract

Reticular formation

Central tegmental tract

X

XII

Rubrospinal tract

Lateral spinothalamic tract

Inferior olivary nucleus

Pyramidal tract

Arcuate nucleus

Medial lemniscus

UPPER MEDULLA

A

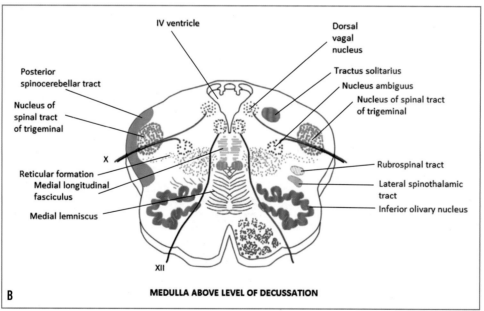

IV ventricle

Dorsal vagal nucleus

Tractus solitarius

Nucleus ambiguus

Nucleus of spinal tract of trigeminal

Posterior spinocerebellar tract

Nucleus of spinal tract of trigeminal

Reticular formation

Medial longitudinal fasciculus

Medial lemniscus

X

XII

Rubrospinal tract

Lateral spinothalamic tract

Inferior olivary nucleus

MEDULLA ABOVE LEVEL OF DECUSSATION

B

FIGURE 6–2. Cross-sections of medulla oblongata at four levels. **A.** Upper medulla, immediately inferior to pons. **B.** Medulla, above level of decussation. *continues*

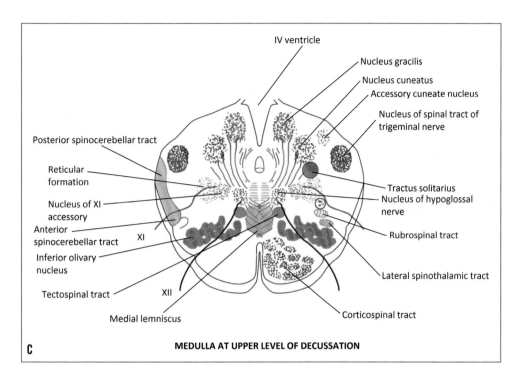

C

MEDULLA AT UPPER LEVEL OF DECUSSATION

Labels (clockwise from top):
IV ventricle
Nucleus gracilis
Nucleus cuneatus
Accessory cuneate nucleus
Nucleus of spinal tract of trigeminal nerve
Tractus solitarius
Nucleus of hypoglossal nerve
Rubrospinal tract
Lateral spinothalamic tract
Corticospinal tract
Medial lemniscus
XII
Tectospinal tract
Inferior olivary nucleus
Anterior spinocerebellar tract
XI
Nucleus of XI accessory
Reticular formation
Posterior spinocerebellar tract

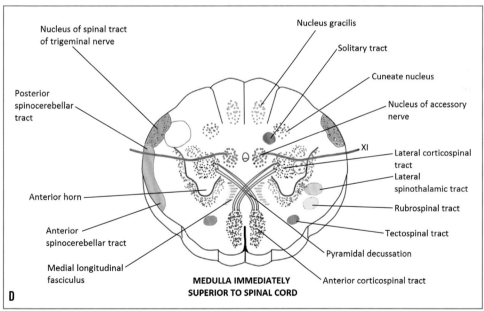

D

MEDULLA IMMEDIATELY SUPERIOR TO SPINAL CORD

Labels:
Nucleus of spinal tract of trigeminal nerve
Nucleus gracilis
Solitary tract
Cuneate nucleus
Nucleus of accessory nerve
XI
Lateral corticospinal tract
Lateral spinothalamic tract
Rubrospinal tract
Tectospinal tract
Pyramidal decussation
Anterior corticospinal tract
Medial longitudinal fasciculus
Anterior spinocerebellar tract
Anterior horn
Posterior spinocerebellar tract

FIGURE 6–2. *continued* **C.** Medulla at upper level of decussation. **D.** Lower medulla, immediately above spinal cord. *Source:* Republished with permission of Georg Thieme Verlag, from Baehr, M., and Frotscher, M. (2012). *Duus' Topical Diagnosis in Neurology: Anatomy, Physiology, Signs, Symptoms*, 5th ed. Stuttgart, Germany: Thieme; permission conveyed through Copyright Clearance Center, Inc.

TABLE 6–1.	Nuclei of the Medulla	
Level	Nucleus	Function
Medulla oblongata	Cuneate nucleus	Fine touch and proprioception, upper body
	Gracile nucleus	Kinesthetic and light touch information from lower body
	Inferior olivary nucleus (cerebellum)	Mediates information from cerebrum to cerebellum via inferior cerebellar peduncle
	Hypoglossal nucleus (XII)	Motor innervation of tongue muscles
	Nucleus ambiguus (IX, X, XI)	Motor nucleus for velum, pharynx, larynx muscles in conjunction with dorsal motor nucleus of X; significant nucleus for swallowing function
	Spinal nucleus of trigeminal (V)	Mediates touch, pain and temperature sense from face; projects to ventral posteromedial nucleus of thalamus
	Dorsal motor nucleus of vagus (X)	Parasympathetic function for gastrointestinal tract, lungs, and abdomen
	Vestibular nuclei (VIII) (medial, lateral, inferior, superior nuclei)	Project to cerebellum, oculomotor nerve, tectum; serve as input for position and movement of body in space
	Nucleus solitarius (VII, IX, X)	Taste from VII and IX; mediate gag reflex; mediate cough, gag, carotid sinus, aortic baroreceptor and chemoreceptor reflexes (blood oxygen); output to hypothalamus and other centers
	Superior and inferior salivatory (VII)	Motor innervation of sublingual, parotid, and submandibular glands; lacrimal glands; mucous membranes of oral and nasal cavity
	Lateral reticular nucleus	Nucleus of reticular activating system

Brainstem Strokes

Since the brainstem is the center for control of breathing, heartbeat, blood pressure, and swallowing, a stroke affecting it produces a range of symptoms such as dizziness, difficulty in breathing, **dysphagia**, **incoordination**, **diplopia**, and nausea. "**Locked-in syndrome**" is considered a severe state in brainstem stroke, in which the patient is paralyzed and mute even though he/she understands sensory stimuli (Baehr & Frotscher, 2012).

A stroke within the middle midbrain is the most common of the midbrain strokes. Individuals with this stroke exhibit **vertical gaze paresis**, **pure hemiparesis**, as well as **ataxia of arms and legs**. Individuals with upper or lower midbrain infarct showed no consistent clinical findings (Bogousslavsky, Maeder, Regli, & Meuli, 1994).

The medulla is particularly vulnerable to stroke. A bilateral medial medullary infarction results in **tetraparesis** (paresis involving all four limbs), bilateral loss of deep sensation, dysphagia, **dysphonia**, and **anarthria** (Kumral, Afsar, Kirbas, Balkir, & Ozdemirkiran, 2002). Dysphagia is also prominent in unilateral medullary infarction rostrally (Kwom, Lee, & Kim, 2005). Pure **lateral medullary infarction** also results in dysphagia, facial paresis, and dysarthria (Duffy, 2013; Kim, 2003). Finally, dysphagia is also prominent and frequent in a pontine infarction, when the location of the infarct is in the upper part of the pons and in the anterolateral vascular territory (Lapa, Luger, Pfeilschifter, Henke, Wagner, & Foerth, 2017).

TABLE 6–2.	Tracts Found Within the Medulla	
Level	Tract	Function
Medulla oblongata	Inferior cerebellar peduncle	Afferent input to cerebellum, carrying posterior spinocerebellar tract (proprioception, trunk and lower limbs), cuneocerebellar tract (proprioception, upper limbs and neck), trigeminocerebellar tract (proprioception from muscles of face), olivocerebellar tract (input from cortex and spinal cord, to climbing fibers), vestibulocerebellar tract (vestibular information)
	Posterior spinocerebellar tract	Proprioception, trunk and lower limbs to cerebellum via inferior cerebellar peduncle
	Anterior spinocerebellar tract	Proprioceptive information to cerebellum via superior cerebellar peduncle
	Spinal lemniscus (spinothalamic tract)	Touch, pain, thermal to ventral posteromedial nucleus of thalamus
	Medial longitudinal fasciculus	Arises from vestibular nuclei; important for generation of vestibulo-ocular reflex; tract within brainstem connecting III, IV, VI cranial nerves for ocular movement; interacts with VIII vestibular nerve for head-eye movement coordination; descends to olivary complex as tectospinal and medial vestibulospinal tracts
	Trigeminothalamic tract (spinal tract of V trigeminal)	From sensory nucleus of V trigeminal to thalamus (ventral posteromedial nucleus)
	Medial lemniscus	Axons of nucleus gracilis and nucleus cuneatus
	Fasciculus gracilis	Conveys somatic (touch, vibration, pain) sensation from limbs to nucleus gracilis
	Fasciculus cuneatus	Conveys somatic (touch, pressure, vibration, pain) and proprioception from cervical to upper thorax regions to nucleus cuneatus
	Pyramidal decussation	Point at which corticospinal tract fibers cross midline. ~75% decussate to form the lateral corticospinal tract, while ~25% remain ipsilateral to form anterior corticospinal tract
	Lateral corticospinal tract	Motor efferent from cerebral cortex to spinal nerve nuclei
	Anterior corticospinal tract	Motor efferent from cerebral cortex to spinal nerve nuclei
	Decussation of lemnisci	Point at which fibers of cuneate and gracile fasciculi decussate prior to reaching nuclei
	Lateral spinothalamic tract	Conveys somatic (pain, touch, thermal) information to thalamus
	Spinotectal tract	Conveys sensory information from spinal cord to inferior and superior colliculi
	Rubrospinal tract	Carries information from red nucleus to tectum and then spinal cord; facilitates upper body flexion
	Tectospinal tract	Part of extrapyramidal system; conveys visual orienting information from superior colliculus to ocular muscles
	Tractus solitarius	Descending fibers of VII facial, IX glossopharyngeal, X vagus through medulla

In Figure 6–2D, you can see the **decussation of the pyramids**, which are the fibers of the corticospinal tracts as they cross from one side to the other. The corticospinal tract is the communication pathway between the cerebrum and skeletal muscle. The pyramidal decussation explains why a left cortical lesion may result in right side paralysis of the body, since commands to activate the right side of the body arise from the left hemisphere. At the decussation, the fibers separate into **lateral** and **anterior corticospinal tracts**. The lateral corticospinal tract is the decussated corticospinal tract, while the smaller anterior tract is made up of uncrossed nerve fibers. The anterior corticospinal tract is a redundant feature that helps maintain your survival should you have unilateral damage to the tract.

The **fasciculus gracilis** and **fasciculus cuneatus** are very important landmarks. (The term "fasciculus" refers to a group of fibers banded together, but you can simply think of it as a fiber tract.) The nuclei of these tracts are in the posterior medulla (see Figure 6–2C), and the tracts themselves mediate kinesthetic sense, muscle stretch, and proprioceptive sense from the lower and upper body. Sensations pass from the upper body, arrive at the **accessory cuneate nucleus**, and are relayed to the cerebellum by means of the **cuneocerebellar tract**. The cuneocerebellar tract passes through the inferior cerebellar peduncle. Also in the posterior portion of the medulla are the trigeminal nerve nucleus and the spinal tract of the trigeminal.

Take a look at the upper medulla. At this point, the corticospinal tract has not yet divided into anterior and lateral corticospinal tracts. Also notice that the central canal has expanded to become the fourth ventricle. The **nucleus solitarius**, an important nucleus of the X vagus nerve, is found lateral to the **hypoglossal** and **dorsal vagal nuclei**. The **hypoglossal nucleus** serves the XII hypoglossal nerve, while the IX glossopharyngeal, X vagus, and XI accessory nerves arise from the **nucleus ambiguus**, dorsal vagal nucleus, and solitary tract nucleus, respectively. These three nerves (IX, X, and XI) tend to function together, and we will discuss them in detail shortly.

Effect of Lesions at the Midbrain Level

The brainstem is quite compact and yet is home to nearly all motor and sensory pathways that either arise from the cortex or reach consciousness. Because of this compactness, small lesions can have a very significant effect.

Lesions of the cerebral peduncle, often arising from hemorrhage, embolus, or tumor, can cause **contralateral spastic paresis** due to the presence of both pyramidal and extrapyramidal tracts within the peduncles. **Weber syndrome** is a condition that arises from occlusion of the posterior cerebral artery or choroidal artery and results in a large constellation of problems, including **hemiataxia** (ataxic signs in half of the body), **intention tremor**, **dysdiadochokinesis** (loss of coordination of alternating movements), and **ataxic dysarthria** (Baehr & Frotscher, 2012). The red nucleus resides within the midbrain, and a lesion to this nucleus will result in contralateral hyperkinesia because of its interaction with the basal ganglia via the extrapyramidal system. Similarly, a lesion of the substantia nigra can result in contralateral **parkinsonism** signs, including **pill-rolling tremor**, **muscular rigidity**, and reduced **range of motion** in the affected side. Because the III oculomotor nucleus and fibers are within the midbrain, midbrain lesion can cause ipsilateral **oculomotor paresis** or paralysis as well as fixed and dilated pupils.

Now look for the **inferior olivary nucleus** (see Figures 6–2B and C). This is in the anterolateral aspect of the medulla and looks a little like an intestine doubled over on itself. Some of the fibers arising from this complex decussate and enter the cerebellum by means of the inferior cerebellar peduncle. Axons from the **principal inferior olivary nucleus** decussate at the **median raphe** to ascend to the cerebellum and comprise the bulk of the inferior cerebellar peduncle. Lateral to the inferior cerebellar peduncle, you will find the trigeminal spinal tract and its nucleus. The anterior boundary of the reticular formation within the medulla is the **nucleus ambiguus**.

In the posterior aspect of the upper medulla and lower pons is a critically important set of nuclei, the **medial** and **inferior vestibular nuclei**. Recall from your audiology course that these nuclei are involved with knowing and maintaining one's position in space (vestibular sense). These nuclei receive input from the vestibular portion of the VIII vestibulocochlear. Also identify the **lateral spinothalamic tracts**: these tracts carry pain and touch information from the spine to the thalamus.

If you reflect for a moment on the functions we have described as we discussed the medulla, you can recognize the critical nature of this part of the brainstem and the devastating effect a small lesion would have on body function. The list of affected functions is long: balance, motor function for the larynx, respiration, cardiac function, tongue movement, control of muscles of mastication, all motor function in the periphery (via the corticospinal tract), and all sensations that reach the cerebrum or cerebellum.

Deep Structures of the Pons

The pons is divided into two parts, the **posterior tegmentum** and the **anterior basilar portion**. First, let's discuss the **basilar portion**. At the level of the lower pons (Figure 6–3),

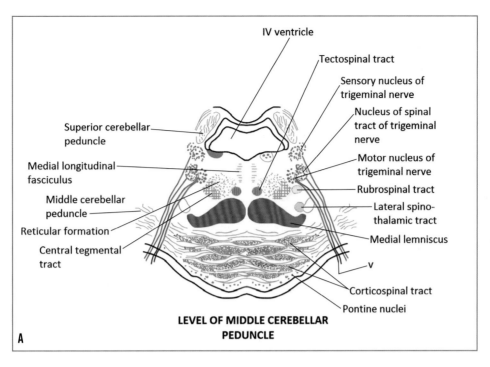

LEVEL OF MIDDLE CEREBELLAR PEDUNCLE

A

Labels in part A:
- IV ventricle
- Tectospinal tract
- Sensory nucleus of trigeminal nerve
- Nucleus of spinal tract of trigeminal nerve
- Motor nucleus of trigeminal nerve
- Rubrospinal tract
- Lateral spino-thalamic tract
- Medial lemniscus
- v
- Corticospinal tract
- Pontine nuclei
- Superior cerebellar peduncle
- Medial longitudinal fasciculus
- Middle cerebellar peduncle
- Reticular formation
- Central tegmental tract

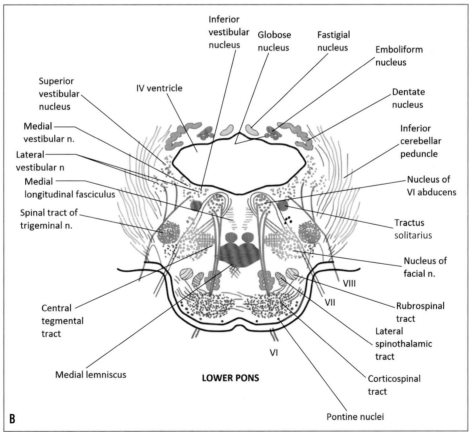

LOWER PONS

B

Labels in part B:
- Inferior vestibular nucleus
- Globose nucleus
- Fastigial nucleus
- Emboliform nucleus
- Dentate nucleus
- Inferior cerebellar peduncle
- Nucleus of VI abducens
- Tractus solitarius
- Nucleus of facial n.
- Rubrospinal tract
- Lateral spinothalamic tract
- Corticospinal tract
- Pontine nuclei
- Superior vestibular nucleus
- IV ventricle
- Medial vestibular n.
- Lateral vestibular n
- Medial longitudinal fasciculus
- Spinal tract of trigeminal n.
- Central tegmental tract
- Medial lemniscus
- VIII
- VII
- VI

FIGURE 6–3. Transverse sections through the midbrain and pons. **A.** Section through pons at level of middle cerebellar peduncle. **B.** Lower pons, immediately above medulla oblongata. *Source:* Republished with permission of Georg Thieme Verlag, from Baehr, M., and Frotscher, M. (2012). *Duus' Topical Diagnosis in Neurology: Anatomy, Physiology, Signs, Symptoms*, 5th ed. Stuttgart, Germany: Thieme; permission conveyed through Copyright Clearance Center, Inc.

the corticospinal tract is coalescing as it enters the medulla. In the upper pons (Figure 6–3A), you'll see that these tracts are not as organized and are harder to identify. You can see the **pontine nuclei** (see Figures 6–3A and B), which receive information from the cerebrum and spinal cord and project that information to the cerebellum via the pontocerebellar tract of the middle cerebellar peduncle. The **medial lemniscus** can be found here as well (see Figure 6–3B). The **lemniscal pathway** is a set of ascending fibers that convey somatic sense to the brain. Refer to Tables 6–3 and 6–4.

Effects of Lesion at the Level of the Pons

The pons is one of the most vulnerable regions of the brainstem due to the high number of functions related to it. Besides the fact that the motor tracts from the cerebrum and sensory pathways from the body pass through the pons, the pons also is home to many cranial nerve nuclei and pathways to and from the cerebellum. We will only touch on a few of the problems that can arise from a lesion affecting the pons.

The pontine tegmentum makes up the posterior aspect of the pons. The motor nucleus of the V trigeminal nerve resides in the tegmentum, and a lesion to this nerve can result in ipsilateral paralysis of the muscles of mastication as well as the tensor veli palatine and the tensor tympani muscles. Lesion to the sensory nucleus of the trigeminal will result in **impaired discriminatory sensation** of the ipsilateral face, while damage to the lateral spinothalamic tract will result in reduced sensation to pain and thermal stimulation on the contralateral side. The lateral lemniscus passes through the midbrain, and damage to it can cause loss of hearing, while damage to the medial

TABLE 6–3. Nuclei of the Pons

Level	Nucleus	Function
Pons	Principal motor nucleus of trigeminal nerve (V)	Motor innervation of muscles of mastication, tensor tympani, and tensor veli palatini
	Principal (pontine) sensory nucleus of trigeminal nerve (V)	Sensory innervation for face and scalp
	Mesencephalic nucleus of trigeminal nerve (V)	Proprioception of muscles of mastication
	Abducens nucleus (VI)	Motor innervation of lateral rectus muscle; rotates eye outward
	Facial nucleus (VII)	Motor innervation of muscles of facial expression; sensory taste information from anterior 2/3 of tongue
	Nucleus of trochlear nerve (IV)	Motor innervation to superior oblique eye muscle to depress eye
	Cochlear nuclei (anteroventral, dorsal, posteroventral)	First relay in brainstem auditory pathway
	Vestibular nuclei	Balance and orientation in space
	Superior olivary complex (medial superior olive, lateral superior olive), medial nucleus of trapezoid body	Auditory localization of sound in space
	Periolivary nuclei (dorsomedial, dorsal, lateral, medial periolivary nuclei, and nucleus of trapezoid body)	Auditory sources for olivocochlear bundle (efferent auditory system)

lemniscus can cause loss of position sense and ataxia. Because the corticobulbar tract passes through the tegmentum, a lesion involving this tract can affect all motor cranial nerves, all of which are involved in speech production. Damage to the central tegmental tract can result in palatopharyngeal myoclonus, a rhythmic oscillation of the velum. In contrast, damage to the tectospinal tract can result in loss of the blink reflex.

Lesion to the **basis pontis** (anterior pons) can cause ipsilateral flaccid paralysis of the muscles of mastication as well as loss of sensation of the face, due to damage to the fibers of the V trigeminal. Because the middle cerebellar peduncle arises from the basis pontis, lesions can cause ipsilateral hemiataxia, which is presence of ataxic signs on the same side as the lesion. Lesions affecting the corticospinal tract will result in contralateral spastic paresis, and lesion to the pontine nuclei serving the cerebellum will result in ipsilateral ataxia.

The caudal pons is particularly vulnerable because of the large number of functions residing in its small space. Lesions to the medial longitudinal fasciculus can result in **nystagmus** (oscillatory movements of the eyeball) as well as **gaze paralysis**, while lesions to the nucleus of the VI abducens nerve will result in abductor paralysis of the eyeball. If the vestibular nuclei are damaged, the patient will demonstrate nystagmus and rotary vertigo (sensation of rotatory movement). Involvement of the nucleus of the facial nerve or its pathway can result in flaccid facial paralysis on the side of the lesion. A lesion affecting the tegmental tract can result in **palatopharyngeal myoclonus**. Lesions affecting the lateral lemniscus will result in hearing loss.

TABLE 6–4.	Tracts Found in the Pons	
Level	Tract	Function
Pons	Superior cerebellar peduncle	Output of cerebellum; efferent fibers of cerebellothalamic tract; project to thalamus and red nucleus
	Anterior (ventral) spinocerebellar tract	Proprioceptive information to cerebellum via superior cerebellar peduncle
	Posterior (dorsal) spinocerebellar tract	Proprioception (muscle spindle and Golgi tendon organ [GTO]) from lower limbs and trunk to cerebellum via inferior cerebellar peduncle
	Medial longitudinal fasciculus	Arises from vestibular nuclei; important for generation of vestibulo-ocular reflex; tract within brainstem connecting III, IV, VI cranial nerves for ocular movement; interacts with VIII vestibular nerve for head-eye movement coordination; descends to olivary complex as tectospinal and medial vestibulospinal tracts
	Tectospinal tract	Part of extrapyramidal system; connects midbrain tectum with spinal cord; reflex posture of head relative to visual and auditory stimuli
	Lateral lemniscus	Auditory tract between cochlear nucleus and inferior colliculus
	Middle cerebellar peduncle	Carries somatic sensory information to cerebellum
	Pontocerebellar fibers	Fibers from pons to cerebellum via middle cerebellar peduncle; input to pons is cerebral cortex
	Corticopontine fibers	Fibers from cortex; carry motor plan to cerebellum via pontocerebellar tract
	Corticospinal tract	Motor efferent from cerebral cortex to spinal nerve nuclei
	Corticobulbar tract	Motor efferent from cerebral cortex to brainstem cranial nerve nuclei

When we talk about the spinal cord, we discuss the **medial longitudinal fasciculus** (MLF). It is responsible for maintaining flexor tone. You can see most of the ascending fibers of the MLF ascending the pons as they arise from the vestibular nuclei and project to muscles of the eye for the regulation of eye movement with relation to head position in space. You can see the relationship between the **vestibular nuclei** and the MLF (lower pons), which underlies the relationship between the vestibular system and ocular tracking: without the vital information from the vestibular system, the eyes would interpret every movement as external to the body. The vestibular system notifies the visual system of head movement so the ocular muscles can adjust for these changes.

You might also notice that the vestibular nuclei project into the lower pons as well. The inferior vestibular nucleus is within the medulla, and the lateral, medial, and superior vestibular nuclei are found in the pons. You can also see the **trapezoid body**, which is a mass of small nuclei and fibers seen at this level. The trapezoid body is a relay within the auditory pathway. Lateral to the trapezoid body is the **superior olivary complex**, which contains nuclei that are critical for localization of sound in space.

In the posterior pons, you'll find the **posterior tegmentum**, which is an upper extension of the reticular formation we discussed in the section on the medulla. The tegmentum is home to the nuclei for many cranial nerves, including the V trigeminal (see Figure 6–3A), VI abducens, and VII facial (see Figure 6–3B). In the ventral pons, you will see fibers of the corticospinal, corticobulbar, and corticopontine tracts. The motor nucleus of the VII facial nerve is found near the **superior olive**. Axons from the facial nucleus course around the nucleus of the VI abducens nerve at the **internal genu** and then exit the brainstem. The **superior cerebellar peduncle** arising from the midbrain forms the lateral margin of the fourth ventricle, and the **anterior medullary velum** is the roof of the ventricle. You can see this peduncle dorsal to the nuclei of the trigeminal nerve.

Deep Structures of the Midbrain

Take a look at Figure 6–4 for our discussion of the midbrain. The midbrain is deceptively small considering its importance in communication between the brainstem and cerebrum. We divide the midbrain into three areas: the posterior **tectum** (a.k.a. the *quadrigeminal plate*), the medial **tegmentum** (a continuation of the pontine tegmentum), and the **crus cerebri**.

The tectum is made up mostly of the **inferior colliculus**, an important auditory relay related to localization of sound in space as well as integration of body sense with auditory sense. This nucleus receives input from the lateral lemniscus, and those fibers encapsulate it. You can see the decussation of the **superior cerebellar peduncle** here (tegmental decussation). The critically important **crus cerebri** enter the brainstem at the midbrain. The crus cerebri are the efferent and afferent pathways between the cerebrum and the rest of the nervous system. Within the crus cerebri are the corticobulbar and corticospinal tracts, as well as the **frontopontine** fibers, which terminate in the pons. The **substantia nigra** is found between the crus cerebri and tegmentum. This is a dark brown mass of cells that are critical for control of movement and muscle tone. The substantia nigra manufactures dopamine, which is a neurotransmitter used in control of movement. Destruction of these nuclei results in **Parkinson's disease**. Refer to Tables 6–5 and 6–6.

The **cerebral aqueduct** connects the fourth ventricle with the third ventricle. Around the aqueduct is a mass of cells known as the periaqueductal or central gray. Within this region, you can find the nucleus of the IV trochlear nerve. The **superior colliculus** is located in the tectum of the superior midbrain. The superior colliculus integrates information from the cerebrum, optic tract, inferior colliculus, and spinal cord for the purpose of tracking visual stimuli through head movement. The relationship between the **inferior colliculus** (audition) and superior colliculus (vision) provides the means for visually localizing the source of a sound in space.

Find the **red nucleus** within the tegmentum. This nucleus is a critical component of the rubrospinal tract. Information from the cerebellum and cerebrum arises at the red nucleus, which controls background movement related to flexion. The **Edinger–Westphal** nucleus can be found near the red nucleus, and it is responsible for accommodation to light by the iris. Look also at the III oculomotor nucleus and the medial geniculate body. The III oculomotor nerve is largely responsible for eye movement. **The medial geniculate body** is a nucleus of the thalamus, making up the final nucleus of the subcortical auditory pathway.

In summary, the brainstem consists of the medulla, pons, and midbrain and mediates higher-level body function.

- The medulla contains the pyramidal decussation, an important location wherein the motor commands from one cerebral hemisphere cross to serve the opposite side of the body. The IX glossopharyneal, X vagus, XI accessory, and XII hypoglossal cranial nerves arise at the level of the medulla, as does the inferior cerebellar peduncle. At the decussation of the pyramids, the descending corticospinal tract has condensed from the less-structured form at higher levels to a well-organized tract. In the rostral medulla, the expansion to accommodate the fourth ventricle is apparent, marking a clear divergence from the minute central canal of the spinal cord and lower medulla.
- The pons contains the middle cerebellar peduncle, as well as four cranial nerve nuclei, the V, VI, VII, and VIII nerves.
- The midbrain contains the cerebral peduncles and gives rise to the III and IV cranial nerves. The superior cerebellar peduncle arises from the midbrain.
- The reticular formation is a set of nuclei essential for life function.

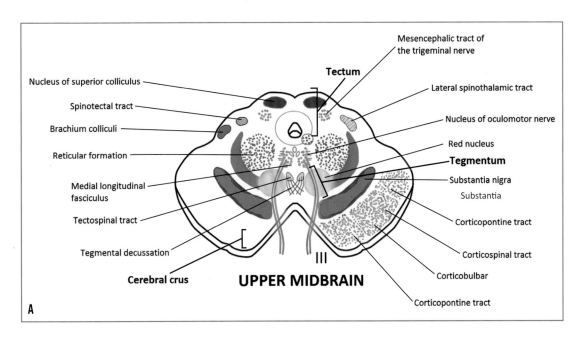

A

UPPER MIDBRAIN

Nucleus of superior colliculus
Spinotectal tract
Brachium colliculi
Reticular formation
Medial longitudinal fasciculus
Tectospinal tract
Tegmental decussation
Cerebral crus

Tectum
Mesencephalic tract of the trigeminal nerve
Lateral spinothalamic tract
Nucleus of oculomotor nerve
Red nucleus
Tegmentum
Substantia nigra
Substantia
Corticopontine tract
Corticospinal tract
Corticobulbar
Corticopontine tract

III

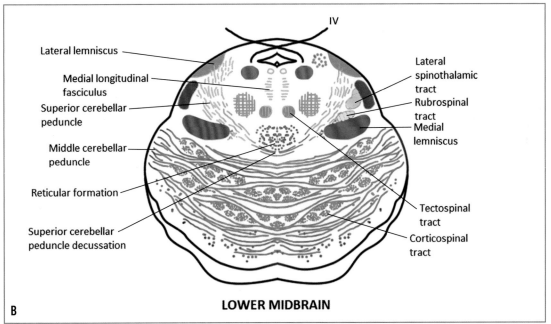

B

LOWER MIDBRAIN

IV

Lateral lemniscus
Medial longitudinal fasciculus
Superior cerebellar peduncle
Middle cerebellar peduncle
Reticular formation
Superior cerebellar peduncle decussation

Lateral spinothalamic tract
Rubrospinal tract
Medial lemniscus
Tectospinal tract
Corticospinal tract

FIGURE 6–4. Transverse section through the midbrain. **A.** Upper midbrain. **B.** Lower midbrain. *Source:* Republished with permission of Georg Thieme Verlag, from Baehr, M., and Frotscher, M. (2012). *Duus' Topical Diagnosis in Neurology: Anatomy, Physiology, Signs, Symptoms*, 5th ed. Stuttgart, Germany: Thieme; permission conveyed through Copyright Clearance Center, Inc.

TABLE 6–5.	Nuclei Found in the Midbrain	
Level	Nucleus	Function
Midbrain	Medial geniculate body (nucleus of thalamus but apparent at this level)	Auditory relay
	Substantia nigra	Supplies dopamine to basal ganglia
	Superior colliculus	Visual relay (localization of visual stimuli)
	Inferior colliculus	Auditory relay (localization of sound in space)
	Red nucleus	Motor coordination; component of extrapyramidal pathway
	Oculomotor nucleus (III)	Motor innervation medial rectus, superior rectus, inferior rectus, inferior oblique, and levator palpebrae superioris muscles of eye
	Edinger–Westphal nucleus (III)	Sphincter muscle of iris

TABLE 6–6.	Tracts Found at the Level of the Midbrain	
Level	Tract	Function
Midbrain	Corticospinal tract	Motor efferent from cerebral cortex to spinal nerve nuclei
	Corticobulbar tract	Motor efferent from cerebral cortex to brainstem cranial nerve nuclei
	Temporopontine fibers	Fibers arising from temporal lobe and terminating in pontine nuclei
	Frontopontine fibers	Fibers arising from frontal lobe, passing through cerebral peduncle and terminating in pons
	Medial longitudinal fasciculus	Arises from vestibular nuclei; important for generation of vestibulo-ocular reflex; tract within brainstem connecting III, IV, VI cranial nerves for ocular movement; interacts with VIII vestibular nerve for head-eye movement coordination; descends to olivary complex as tectospinal and medial vestibulospinal tracts
	Medial, spinal lemniscus	Information from nuclei gracilis and cuneatus of medulla to thalamus
	Spinothalamic tract (anterolateral and ventrolateral)	Touch, pain, thermal to ventral posteromedial nucleus of thalamus
	Trigeminal lemniscus	Pain, tactile, thermal sense of face to ventroposteromedial nucleus of thalamus

AUDITORY PATHWAY

While we will discuss afferent and efferent pathways that involve the brainstem in Chapter 9, there is a very specific pathway that we need to discuss in the context of the brainstem. The central auditory pathway transits the entire brainstem on its way to the cerebral cortex, so it deserves special attention now.

There are two components to the **vestibulocochlear nerve**: **cochlear** and **vestibular**. Both of these afferent pathways arise from sensors deep within the inner ear. Cochlear afferents arise from the hair cells of the basilar membrane: bipolar cells of the VIII vestibulocochlear nerve synapse with outer and inner hair cells, and the dendrites pass into the bony space in the inner ear known as the modiolus. Cell bodies in the modiolus are collectively known as the **spiral ganglion**. The second set of afferents, the vestibular nerve, arises from the motion and position sensors of the vestibular mechanism. These fibers exit the vestibule of the inner ear and combine with the auditory nerve as it exits the temporal bone. The auditory nerve enters the brainstem at the level of the juncture of the pons and medulla, entering the first waystation of the central auditory pathway, the **cochlear nucleus**. We'll discuss the auditory pathway in terms of the nuclei in the pathway.

Cochlear Nucleus

The central auditory pathway begins with the cochlear nucleus (CN) (Figure 6–5). It is important to note that the tonotopic array of information arising as a result of the basilar cochlear processing is retained throughout the auditory pathway, including the cerebral cortex (Hackett, Preuss, & Kaas, 2001; Morel, Garraghty, & Kaas, 1993; Lauter, Herscovitch, Formby, & Raichle, 1985). The VIII vestibulocochlear nerve divides into three components, serving the three major subdivisions of the CN: the **dorsal cochlear nucleus** (DCN), the **anteroventral cochlear nucleus** (AVCN), and the **posteroventral cochlear nucleus** (PVCN). All three of these areas receive full tonotopic representation, such that the cochlea is fully represented in each subdivision of the CN.

The DCN and PVCN are both considered to be part of the sound identification stream of the auditory pathway, while the AVCN is a major contributor to the sound localization stream. To fulfill the role of signal identification, the PVCN and DCN perform the first level of auditory processing that occurs in the auditory pathway. In contrast, the AVCN performs little or no processing, instead transmitting a faithful neural copy of the auditory signal to the primary signal localization center of the auditory pathway, the olivary complex. The DCN and PVCN both perform feature analysis of the auditory signal, such that the CN detects a broad range of features present in the acoustic signal. This information is then passed to the **medial nucleus of the trapezoid body**, **inferior colliculus**, and **lateral lemniscus**. The outflow of the DCN passes as the dorsal stria (also known as the **stria of Monaco**), while that of the PVCN is the intermediate stria (also known as the **stria of Held**). The AVCN output is by means of the ventral stria.

The AVCN, DCN, and PVCN are endowed with a rich and diverse set of neuron types with a variety of sensitivities (Pickles, 2012). For example, large spherical cells in the AVCN are highly sensitive to timing of the acoustic signal, and the output of these cells is routed to the medial superior olive. Small spherical cells are sensitive to minute differences in intensity, and the output is sent to the lateral superior olive. Neurons known as **octopus cells** also have high timing precision, but they are found predominantly in the PVCN and may project to other nuclei. Neurons known as **bushy cells** (Figure 6–6) extract and sharpen temporal and spectral information, sending the information to the superior olivary complex, as do stellate cells. Stellate cells also send information to the **periolivary region** (the region around the superior olivary complex) for the purpose of affecting some inhibitory control of the auditory output by means of the olivocochlear pathway (to be discussed). **Octopus cells** sense onset and offset of the acoustic signal, and fire synchronously to steady-state firing. **Globular cells** sharpen high frequency information. Notably, many cells are known predominantly for their responses, rather than morphology. Onset-sensitive neurons respond to the onset of a signal, just as offset-sensitive neurons respond to their termination. There are neurons that fire with up-sweep and down-sweep of the frequency of a signal, presumably responding to transitions in speech. Some neurons respond to continuous, unchanging acoustics, while others are sensitive to intensity variations. The feature detectors of the CN very likely evolved well before the advent of speech in humans, so we probably simply capitalized on them as we, as a species, developed oral communication.

Superior Olivary Complex

The **superior olivary complex** (SOC) consists of three major nuclei and a group of satellite nuclei. The primary nuclei of the SOC are the **lateral superior olive** (LSO) and **the medial superior olive** (MSO), as well as the **medial nucleus of the trapezoid body** (MNTB). The LSO receives sound intensity information from both ears, compares the signal, and determines the location in horizontal space from which the signal arose. The MSO, in contrast, uses frequency information to compare the arrival time of the signal to the two ears, again to locate the sound source in horizontal space. The LSO uses high frequency information for binaural intensity comparison, while the MSO uses low frequency information for the arrival time comparisons between the two ears. This, of course, is the reason that the AVCN must provide an unmodified copy of the auditory signal: output from the

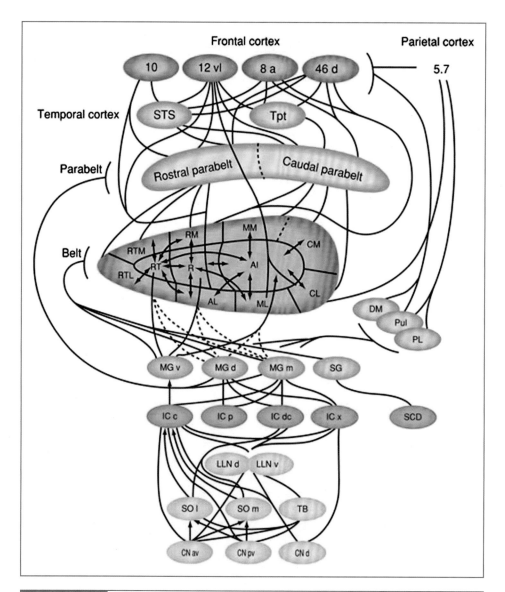

FIGURE 6–5. Auditory pathway. *Source:* From Seikel/Drumright/King. *Anatomy & Physiology for Speech, Language, and Hearing,* 5th ed. (with Anatesse Software Printed Access Card). © 2016 Delmar Learning, a part of Cengage, Inc. Reproduced by permission. www.cengage.com/permissions

two cochleae must be precisely compared, and to do this requires that the original signals be represented flawlessly. A group of six satellite nuclei reside superficial to the LSO and MSO (Figure 6–7). These nuclei receive input not only from the AVCN, but also from cortical efferents, and provide the output for the olivocochlear bundle (OCB). The **olivocochlear bundle** is the efferent component of the auditory pathway, responsible for attenuating the signal coming from the cochlea in order to maximize the signal-to-noise ratio for discrimination purposes.

Inferior Colliculus

The **inferior colliculus** (IC) is sometimes referred to as the auditory reflex center. It is also involved in localization of sound in space and interacts with the **superior colliculus** (a nucleus of the visual pathway) to support visual localization of a sound source. The IC has output to the XI accessory nerve, which provides the mechanism for turning the head toward a sound source via the sternocleidomastoid muscle. The IC receives its input from all three of the outputs of the CN.

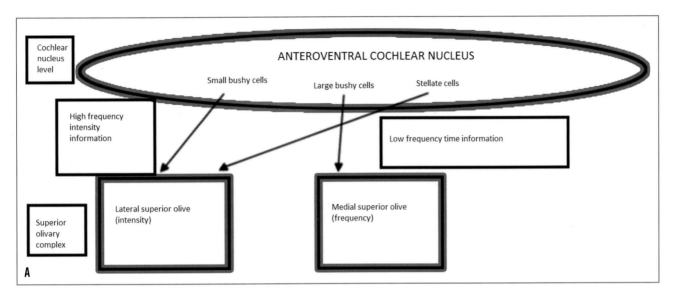

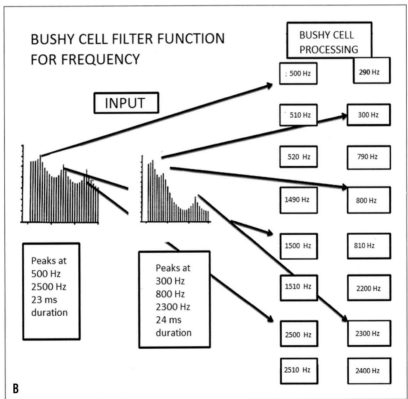

FIGURE 6–6. Example hypothesized analysis function of bushy cells from the cochlear nucleus. **A.** Projection of bushy cell outputs to the superior olivary complex. Note that the small bushy cells send output to the LSO, providing sharpened intensity information for localization of sound in space, while the large bushy cells provide sharpened temporal information to the MSO of the superior olivary complex. The stellate cells also contribute to the intensity processing. **B.** Note the mechanism for spectral analysis of speech by bushy cells. Bushy cells have very sharp spectral and temporal analysis capacity, so they can identify spectral peaks of vowels as well as the duration of the spectral information. On the left, spectral slice of the vowel peaks at 500 Hz, 1500 Hz, and 2500 Hz are identified, by the spectral and temporal characteristics, and this information is ultimately transmitted to the cortex for rapid extraction of vowel identity.

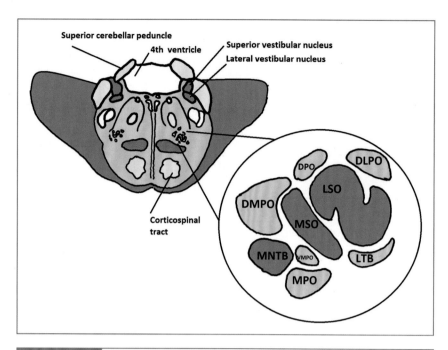

FIGURE 6–7. Nuclei of the olivary complex in the context of the pons. Note LSO = lateral superior olive; MSO = medial superior olive; MNTB = medial nucleus of trapezoid body; DLPO = dorsolateral periolivary nucleus; DMPO = dorsomedial periolivary nucleus; DPO = dorsal periolivary nucleus; LTB = lateral nucleus of trapezoid body; MPO = medial pre-olivary nucleus; VMPO = ventromedial periolivary nucleus. *Source:* From view and data of Pickles (1988).

Lateral Lemniscus

The **lateral lemniscus** (LL) consists of the striae of Held and Monaco, as well as the trapezoid body. It receives input from the CN and SOC. The **dorsal nucleus of the lateral lemniscus** (DNLL) receives bilateral input from the LL and is involved in binaural hearing. The **ventral nucleus of the lateral lemniscus** (VNLL) only receives input from the contralateral ear.

Medial Geniculate Body

The **medial geniculate body** (MGB) is the last stop before the cerebral cortex: all auditory fibers terminate on this nucleus. The MGB consists of ventral, dorsal, and medial divisions (Figure 6–8). The ventral portion receives input from the IC, SC, and the regions surrounding the thalamus and projects to the primary auditory cortex (core, BA 41). The dorsal portion projects to the auditory association areas (BA 42) and other regions of the temporal lobe (likely the belt region) (see Figure 6–8).

AUDITORY RECEPTION AT TEMPORAL LOBE

At this point, we come full circle in our discussion. If you once again look at Figure 6–5, you can see all of the players in the auditory pathway. Turn your attention to the medial geniculate body of Figure 6–8 and the **belt, parabelt,** and temporal cortex of Figures 6–9A and B for this part of the discussion. As you can see, the belt surrounds the **core,** which is A1, R, and RT (referring to the classical **Heschl's gyrus,** rostral, and rostro-temporal portions, respectively). The three regions of the core receive identical input, in that they receive all frequency components of the auditory pathway. Interestingly, the tonotopic arrangement of A1 and R are reversed, as indicated in Figure 6–9A. Note that the belt region of Figures 6–5 and 6–9 includes a number of subregions, all of which have different analysis functions. Some regions are critical for species-specific call identification (part of the auditory "what" stream), while others are responsible for localization (the auditory "where" stream). As Figure 6–5 shows, the

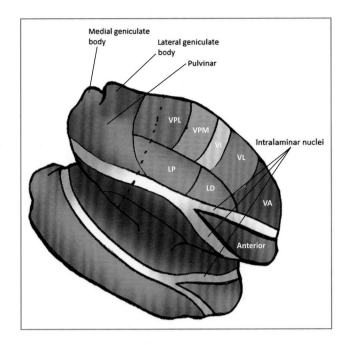

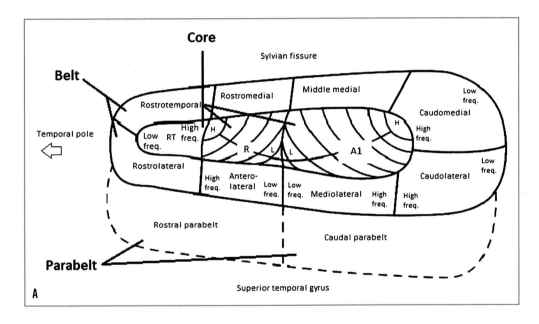

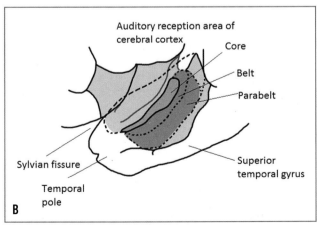

FIGURE 6–8. Medial geniculate body within context of thalamus. Note that the medial geniculate body is in close proximity to the pulvinar (involved in language processing) and the lateral geniculate body (a visual relay) and receives its input from the acoustic pathway. VPL = ventral posterolateral nucleus; VPM = ventral posteromedial nucleus; VI = ventral intermedial nucleus; VL = ventral lateral nucleus; VA = ventral anterior nucleus; LD = lateral dorsal nucleus; LP = lateral posterior nucleus. *Source:* After view of Seikel, Drumright, and King (2016).

FIGURE 6–9. Auditory cortex. **A.** Schematic showing relationships of core (auditory reception area, BA41), belt (auditory association area, typically considered to consist of eight different regions), and parabelt. *Source:* Modified from Kaas and Hackett (2000). **B.** Physical relationship of Heschl's gyrus region on temporal lobe to the schematic. *Source:* Modified from Seikel, Drumright, and King (2016).

outputs of the belt and parabelt regions project to the temporal (superior temporal sulcus, temporal pole), parietal (BA 5 and 7 from MGB), and frontal (BA 10, 12, 8, and 46) lobes for processing.

Efferent Pathways

The efferent pathways are also known as the centrifugal pathways. They are the means by which the nervous system modifies the output of the cochlea at the source (Guinan, 1996, 2010; Zheng, Henderson, McFadden, & Hu, 1997). The efferent pathways are largely responsible for our ability to separate signal from noise. There are two basic systems that perform this task. The **rostral system** involves efferents from the core of the auditory reception portion of the cerebral cortex (Figure 6–10) that communicate with the SOC, IC, and MGB. It is assumed that the cortex is involved in identifying important areas of the auditory signal. This information is used to attenuate information output at the cochlea level that is deemed to be less important. The **caudal system** (Figure 6–11) arises from the region of the MSO, coursing contralaterally to synapse with outer and inner hair cells. At the inner hair cell (IHC) level, the VIII nerve output of the non-signal IHC is attenuated. At the outer hair cell (OHC) level, it is presumed that the OHC amplifier action in non-signal regions is reduced as a result of the activation. **The lateral olivocochlear bundle** arises from the region of the

LSO, with fibers coursing ipsilaterally to terminate in the CN and hair cells, serving the same function as the caudal system (Figure 6–12).

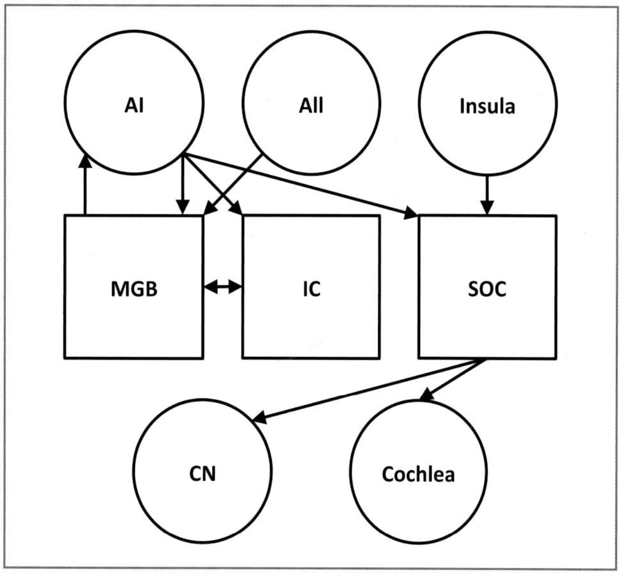

Vestibular Pathway

The **vestibular pathway** arises from the ampullae, utricle, and saccule of the vestibular mechanism. Each semicircular canal of the vestibular mechanism has an ampulla that is responsible for converting movement of the endolymph

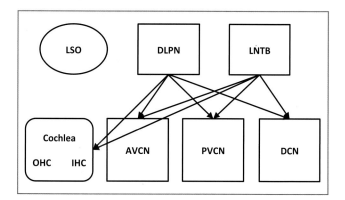

FIGURE 6–11. The caudal efferent system arises from the region of the MSO and courses contralaterally to synapse with outer and inner hair cells. The caudal system acts on the inner hair cells (IHC) to attenuate the output of the non-signal information coded by the outer hair cells (OHC). It is presumed that the OHC amplifier action in non-signal regions is reduced as a result of the activation.

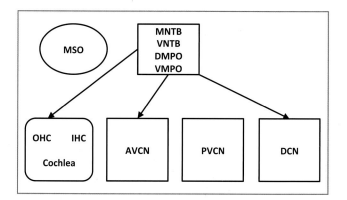

FIGURE 6–12. The lateral olivocochlear bundle emerges from the periolivary region surrounding the LSO. Fibers course ipsilaterally, terminating at the CN and hair cells. In this manner, amplifier activity of the cochlea is reduced in non-signal areas, thereby improving signal in noise performance.

FIGURE 6–10. Rostral auditory efferent system. Efferents from the core terminate in the superior olivary complex, inferior colliculus, and medial geniculate body. This information is used to attenuate information output at the cochlea level that is deemed to be less important.

in the canals into electrochemical signals. The **utricle** and **saccule** are responsible for converting acceleration-related information. The output of these mechanisms gives rise to the vestibular portion of the **VIII vestibulocochlear nerve**. The superior and inferior vestibular branches converge at the **vestibular ganglion** of the **internal acoustic meatus** and join with the auditory component and exit the temporal bone. The VIII vestibulocochlear nerve enters the brainstem at the juncture of the pons and medulla, where the auditory and vestibular components diverge. The vestibular component proceeds to innervate the superior, lateral, medial, and inferior vestibular nuclei of the pons and medulla, which give rise to the vestibulocerebellar pathway discussed in Chapter 8, as well as the vestibulospinal tract (Chapter 9).

Acoustic Reflex

The acoustic reflex is a final pathway we should consider in our discussion of auditory function. The **acoustic reflex**, also sometimes referred to as the **stapedial reflex**, is considered a protective response to loud auditory stimuli (Moller, 2003). Output of the cochlea by means of the VIII vestibulocochlear nerve arrives at the ventral cochlear nucleus, which in turn synapses with the VII facial nerve nucleus and the contralateral MSO via the trapezoid body. The stapedius muscle is innervated by the VII facial nerve, and its activation by means of the reflex circuit results in stiffening of the ossicular chain and reduction in signal amplitude reaching the cochlea.

In summary, the cochlear and vestibular nerves make up the afferent vestibulocochlear nerve.

- The spiral ganglion is the nucleus of the auditory nerve, receiving input from the hair cells. Afferents for the vestibular nerve arise from the motion and position sensed by the vestibular mechanism. The cochlear and vestibular components combine as the nerve exits the temporal bone and enter the brainstem at the level of the juncture of the pons and medulla.
- The cochlear nucleus is the first stop in the auditory pathway. The dorsal cochlear nucleus and posteroventral cochlear nucleus perform complex feature analysis on the acoustic signal, while the anteroventral cochlear nucleus sends an unmodified copy of the signal to the olivary complex for use in localization of sound in space.
- The superior olivary complex consists of the lateral superior olive, the medial superior olive, and the medial nucleus of the trapezoid body, as well as satellite nuclei. The lateral superior olive localizes sound in space using sound intensity information, while the medial superior olive localizes sound using interaural phase difference.
- The inferior colliculus is also involved in localization of sound in space and interacts with the superior colliculus (a nucleus of the visual pathway) to support visual localization of a sound source.

- The lateral lemniscus receives input from the cochlear nucleus and superior olivary complex and is involved in binaural hearing.
- The medial geniculate body is a nucleus of the thalamus and is the last nucleus in the auditory pathway before arriving at the cortex.
- The temporal lobe of the cerebral cortex is the site of auditory reception. The core of the auditory reception area is classically referred to as Heschl's gyrus, while the belt is the site of higher-level processing. The belt performs complex feature extraction, with results going to the parabelt and other cortical regions.
- The efferent pathways are also known as the centrifugal pathways and are responsible for our ability to separate signal from noise. The rostral system arises from the cortex and communicates with the superior olive, inferior colliculus, and medial geniculate body. It attenuates the less relevant output of the cochlea. The caudal system arises from the region of the medial superior olive and acts on the inner and outer hair cells to attenuate output. The lateral olivocochlear bundle arises from the region of the lateral superior olive, also acting on the hair cell output.
- The vestibular pathway arises from the ampullae, utricle, and saccule of the vestibular mechanism. The superior and inferior vestibular branches join with the auditory component of the vestibulocochlear nerve.
- The acoustic reflex is considered a protective response to loud auditory stimuli. Output of the VIII vestibulocochlear nerve is passed to the ventral cochlear nucleus, the VII facial nerve nucleus, and the contralateral medial superior olive, activating the stapedius muscle.

CHAPTER SUMMARY

The brainstem consists of the medulla oblongata, pons, and midbrain. It mediates higher-level body function. The medulla contains the pyramidal decussation, and the IX glossopharyneal, X vagus, XI accessory, and XII hypoglossal cranial nerves arise from this level. The decussation of the pyramids marks the point where efferent information arising from one cerebral hemisphere via the pyramidal tract crosses to innervate the opposite side of the body. The inferior cerebellar peduncle is found at the level of the medulla. The pons contains the middle cerebellar peduncle, as well as four cranial nerve nuclei, the V, VI, VII, and VIII nerves. The midbrain contains the superior cerebellar peduncle and the cerebral peduncles and gives rise to the III and IV cranial nerves. The reticular formation is a set of nuclei essential for life function.

The cochlear and vestibular nerves make up the afferent vestibulocochlear nerve. Afferents for the cochlear nerve arise from the cochlea, while vestibular nerve input arises from the vestibular mechanism. The cochlear and vestibular components combine to form the vestibulocochlear nerve.

The cochlear nucleus consists of the dorsal, ventral, and posteroventral-cochlear nuclei. The dorsal cochlear nucleus and the posteroventral cochlear nucleus perform complex feature analysis on the acoustic signal. The anteroventral cochlear nucleus sends an unmodified copy of the signal to the olivary complex for localization in space. In the superior olivary complex, the lateral superior olive localizes sound in space using interaural intensity cues, while the medial superior olive uses phase differences to identify location of sound in space. The inferior colliculus is also involved in localization of sound in space, and the lateral lemniscus is involved in binaural hearing. The medial geniculate body is a nucleus of the thalamus and is the last nucleus in the auditory pathway before arriving at the cortex. The temporal lobe of the cerebral cortex is the site of auditory reception. The core is the primary reception area, the belt performs

feature extraction, and the parabelt performs high-level processing.

The efferent or centrifugal pathways are responsible for separating signal from noise. The rostral system arises from the cortex and works with the superior olive, inferior colliculus, and medial geniculate body to attenuate output of the cochlea that is less important. The caudal system arises from the region of the medial superior olive and acts on the inner and outer hair cells to attenuate output. The lateral olivocochlear bundle arises from the region of the lateral superior olive, also acting on the hair cell output.

The vestibular pathway arises from the ampullae, utricle, and saccule of the vestibular mechanism. The superior and inferior vestibular branches join with the auditory component of the vestibulocochlear nerve. The acoustic reflex is considered to be a protective mechanism for hearing. Output of the VIII vestibulocochlear nerve is passed to the ventral cochlear nucleus, the VII facial nerve nucleus, and the contralateral medial superior olive, activating the stapedius muscle.

CASE STUDY 6–1

Physician's Notes on Initial Physical Examination and History

This is a 50-year-old male who around three years ago noticed weakness of the right hand without significant sensory symptoms following by dyspnea. A short while later, a spinal cord MRI showed **cervical compression**, and the patient underwent surgery (see Table 6–7 for terminology. Note that we are presenting the data of this case in chronological order to show the emerging speech and language signs and symptoms as the condition progresses). After the surgical procedure, the patient was treated with **cortisone** but exhibited difficulty weaning from the ventilator. Two years following the procedure, the patient exhibited neurological symptomatology, including weakness in the left arm, difficulty in walking, speech difficulties, neck weakness, and **dysphagia**. The **EMG** showed active denervation affecting all four limbs.

Three Years, 3 Months Following Intake

There were obvious tongue fasciculations and atrophy, as well as upper limb fasciculations. Even though the tone was normal there was weakness of the upper limbs (proximal > distal) affecting the right side more than the left (see Table 6–8 for details of muscle testing). An EMG in the hospital showed clear active denervation-reinnervation changes in upper and lower limb muscles.

There was clear evidence of **lower motor neuron** degeneration affecting the bulbar and cervical segments.

No **UMN** signs were noted. It was recommended that the patient continue **SSRI** medication for both mood and **pseudobulbar affect**. The patient was referred for speech and language therapy, occupational therapy, physiotherapy, and consultation with the dietitian to avoid possible weight loss. I explained to the patient and the relatives that continued weight loss or episodes of choking should prompt serious consideration of PEG insertion. I prescribed continued **riluzole** 50 mg 2×/day with follow-up of liver function and blood count every month, continued physical activity, and monthly weighing and consultation with dietitian to avoid weight loss. Finally, I prescribed monthly consultation with the pulmonologist after receiving results of respiratory function tests.

Three Years, 9 Months Following Intake

The patient was seen for follow-up for his disease condition. His condition remains unchanged. He is now using the **BiPAP** throughout the night and for a couple of hours in the afternoon when he is at rest. He continues receiving Rilutek 50 mg 2×/day and **amitriptyline** 20 mg daily for saliva control. He is being followed by the pneumonologist and is planned to have a **gastrostomy** tube placement at the end of the month. On examination, he exhibits **dysarthria** and **dysphonia** and severe weakness of the right more than left arm with **muscle atrophy**. The legs are strong and he walks without difficulty. He is clinically stable and will be reevaluated after the **PEG** tube insertion.

TABLE 6–7.	**Terminology for Case Study 6–1**

"c" or "d" scores	Scoring on the *Frenchay Dysarthria Assessment* (FDA). See Table 6–9 for details on Frenchay scoring.
2×/day	Two times a day.
Amitriptyline (active ingredient), Elavil (brand name) 20 mg	Used to treat depression. In neurology, it is also used for the reduction of saliva to avoid choking, a sign of dysphagia.
Amyotrophic lateral sclerosis (ALS) (motor neuron disease)	A disease in which there is degeneration of motor neurons. The signs include lack of voluntary movement for walking, talking, swallowing, etc. The affected muscles present atrophy and fasciculations, as well as alternating high and low muscle tone, dependent upon the site of lesion activity. The survival rate is 3–5 years from the beginning of symptomatology.
Bilevel positive airway pressure (BiPAP)	The BiPAP (also known as CPAP, continuous positive airway pressure) is a machine used for therapy for sleep apnea. BiPAP provides pressurized air through a mask to the patient's airway, preventing apnea.
Cervical compression	In this condition there are symptoms such as neck pain, stiffness, etc. Its cause may be a compression of the spinal cord and/or nerves (myelopathy, radiculopathy).
Cortisone (active ingredient), Cortone acetate (brand name)	A medication that treats inflammation. Cortisone is used to treat a wide variety of conditions (by suppressing inflammation), such as multiple sclerosis, lupus erythematosus, etc.
Cortone acetate	See cortisone.
Dysarthria	Motor speech disorder involving muscular weakness, dyscoordination, and alteration of muscle tone. It includes slow movement of the muscles used for speech production, including the lips, tongue, vocal folds, and/or muscles of respiration.
Dysphagia	Difficulty with one of the stages of swallowing.
Dysphonia	Voice that sounds hoarse, breathy, etc.
EMG	Results of a laboratory technique to record the electrical activity (electric potential) of skeletal muscles.
Fasciculation	Small involuntary muscle contraction.
Frenchay Dysarthria Assessment (FDA)	A standardized test to assess nonspeech and speech movements of lips, jaw, tongue, phonation, intelligibility, etc. (see Table 6–9 for details concerning scoring of the FDA).
Gastrostomy (PEG)	A surgical operation that results in an external opening into the stomach for nutrition and feeding.
Lower motor neuron	Motor nerve cells that are located in the anterior gray columns of the spinal cord or the cranial nerve nuclei in the brainstem.
Muscle atrophy	Reduction in muscle mass starting from muscle weakness and leading to total atrophy.
PEG (percutaneous endoscopic gastronomy) tube	See gastrostomy.
Pseudobulbar affect (emotional incontinence)	Neurological sign characterized by involuntary crying or laughing.
Riluzole (active ingredient), Rilutek (brand name) 50 mg	Used to protect the nerve cells and is prescribed in amyotrophic lateral sclerosis.

continues

TABLE 6–7.	*continued*
Selective serotonin reuptake inhibitors (SSRIs)	A group of medications used to treat depression (antidepressants).
Upper motor neuron (UMN) sign	Upper motor neuron lesions are located in the neural pathway superior to the anterior horn cells in the spinal cord or the motor nuclei of the cranial nerves in the brainstem and through the cerebral cortex. This sign involves muscle weakness in the limbs and/or tongue, slowness of movement, and spasticity (continuous contraction of a muscle that causes stiffness).

TABLE 6–8.   Examining Muscle Strength

When examining a patient, identifying specific areas of muscular weakness helps to localize the site of lesion. Strength testing is completed for each muscle group, making sure that you test one side and then the next for each group, so you can compare strength for the two sides. Here is a muscle strength rating scale.

0/5	No contraction of muscle
1/5	Indication of muscle flicker, but no movement noted
2/5	Movement occurs, but not against gravity when tested in the horizontal plane
3/5	Movement occurs against, but not when there is resistance provided by the the examiner
4/5	Movement occurs against some resistance provided by the examiner
5/5	Normal strength

Medical Diagnosis

Overall impression of progressive ALS (motor neuron disease, LMN predominant)

Speech Examination (Flaccid Dysarthria)

The *Frenchay Dysarthria Assessment* was administered to the patient (see Table 6–9 for details of Frenchay scoring). The results correlated with the neurologist's impression for primarily flaccid involvement rather than spastic involvement in this patient. There was found moderate to severe difficulty, **"c" or "d"** scores, in most of the domains assessed. More specifically:

- Reflexes (cough): Patient chokes 1–2 times per day and is having difficulty clearing phlegm from throat (c).
- Reflexes (swallow): Patient exhibited slow eating of a cookie and choked once during drinking of water via a cup (c).

TABLE 6–9.   Frenchay Scoring Details

The *Frenchay Dysarthria Assessment* (FDA) utilizes a rating scale for all testing.

a score	Normal for age
b score	Mild abnormality noticeable to skilled observer
c score	Obvious abnormality but the patient can perform task/movements with reasonable approximation
d score	Some production of task but poor in quality, unable to sustain, inaccurate, or extremely labored
e score	Unable to undertake task/movement/sound

- Respiration at rest: Patient exhibited marked interruptions of inhalation/exhalation and shallow breathing (c).
- Respiration in speech: Speech was very shallow (only 3–4 words per exhalation produced) (d).
- Palate fluids: When asked whether food or drink comes through nose, the patient reported moderate problems with occurrence of several times a week (c).
- Palate maintenance: Inability to elevate palate for all sounds when instructed to say "ah-ah-ah" five times (c).
- Palate in speech: Moderate hypernasality when patient asked to say "may pay" and "nay bay" (c).
- Laryngeal time: Sustained phonation for /a/ in 5 seconds (c).
- Laryngeal volume: Limited change in volume when the patient counted from 1 to 5 and great difficulty in the control of voice volume (d).
- Laryngeal in speech: Patient exhibited difficulty in producing clear phonation and adjusting volume to environment (c).
- Tongue at rest: Apparent fasciculations in the tongue (c).
- Tongue protrusion: Patient was able to protrude/retract tongue to lip only (5 times in 8 seconds) (d).
- Tongue elevation: Gross movement of the tongue when the patient tried to elevate it (5 times) (d).

- Tongue lateral: Labored lateral tongue movement (5 times) produced in 8 seconds (c).
- Tongue component: Diadochokinetic rate of the word /kala/ (10 times) with tongue changes in position, and imprecise consonants/distorted vowels were present (d).
- Tongue during speech: Articulation was grossly distorted (d).
- Intelligibility: During the production of 10 cards with written words, the patient was intelligible for only 5 words (d).

Speech-Language Diagnosis

Mixed spastic-flaccid dysarthria

Questions Concerning This Case

1. **Amyotrophic lateral sclerosis** results in both upper and lower motor neuron degeneration. How is this related to the dysarthria components, which are both spastic and flaccid?
2. Fasciculations can occur in lower motor degeneration. What part of the neuron must be damaged for there to be fasciculations?

Case provided by Dr. Kostas Konstantopoulos, European University Cyprus.

CHAPTER 6
STUDY QUESTIONS

1. The superiormost structure of the brainstem is the _____.

2. The inferiormost structure of the brainstem is the _____ _____.

3. On the figure please identify the structures indicated.

   a. _____

   b. _____

   c. _____ _____

   d. _____ _____ fissure

   e. _____ decussation

4. The _____ ventricle is immediately posterior to the pons and medulla.

5. The prominent bulge on the anterior pons consists of fibers of the _____ tract.

6. The groove on the anterior pons into which the basilar artery will rest is termed the _____ sulcus.

7. The _____ cerebellar peduncle arises at the level of the pons.

8. The _____ cerebellar peduncle arises at the level of the medulla.

9. The _____ angle is the point on the posterior aspect of the brainstem that marks the juncture of pons and cerebellum.

10. The _____ peduncles are fibers passing from and to the cerebral cortex, and which enter the brainstem at the level of the midbrain.

11. The _____ formation is a component of the reticular activating system, which is involved in arousing the cerebral cortex.

12. At the _____ of the _____ the corticospinal tract divides into anterior and lateral corticospinal tracts.

13. The IX glossopharyneal, X vagus, XI accessory, and XII hypoglossal cranial nerves arise at the level of the _____.

14. The _____ nerve mediates the sense of audition.

15. The nucleus of the VIII vestibulocochlear nerve is the _____ ganglion.

16. The first brainstem nucleus of the auditory pathway is the _____ nucleus.

17. In the cochlear nucleus, the _____ _____ _____ (subdivision) sends a direct copy of the auditory signal to the olivary complex.

18. The _____ _____ _____ (subdivision of cochlear nucleus) is involved in localization of sound in space.

19. The first level of auditory processing occurs at the _____ _____ _____ and _____ _____ _____ (levels of the cochlear nucleus).

20. The _____ _____ _____ (nucleus of the olivary complex) is responsible for processing differences in signal intensity between left and right ears.

21. The _____ _____ _____ (nucleus of the olivary complex) is responsible for processing differences in signal timing between the two ears.

22. The _____ bundle is an efferent auditory pathway that attenuates the signal coming out of the cochlea.

23. The _____ _____ body is an auditory relay of the thalamus.

24. True or False: The tonotopic array of the cochlea is preserved at the level of the cortex.

25. True or False: The belt region of the auditory cortex consists of regions that perform analysis of the acoustic signal.

26. The _____ auditory pathways are also known as the centrifugal pathways and are responsible for our ability to separate signal from noise.

REFERENCES

Baehr, M., & Frotscher, M. (2012). *Duus' topical diagnosis in neurology: Anatomy, physiology, signs, symptoms* (5th ed.). New York, NY: Thieme.

Bear, M. F., Connors, B. W., & Paradiso, M. A. (1996). *Neuroscience: Exploring the brain*. Baltimore. MD: Williams & Wilkins.

Bogousslavsky, J., Maeder, P., Regli, F., & Meuli, R. (1994). Pure midbrain infarction. Clinical syndromes, MRI, and etiologic patterns. *Neurology, 44*(11), 2032–2040.

Carpenter, M. B. (1991). *Core text of neuroanatomy* (4th ed.). Baltimore, MD: Williams & Wilkins.

Chusid, J. G. (1985). *Correlative neuroanatomy and functional neurology* (17th ed.). Los Altos, CA: Lange Medical.

Crossman, A. R. (2008). Overview of the nervous system. In S. Standring (Ed.), *Gray's anatomy: The anatomical and clinical basis of practice* (40th ed., pp. 225–236). London, UK: Churchill Livingstone.

Duffy, J. R. (2013). *Motor speech disorders—e-book: Substrates, differential diagnosis, and management*. Elsevier Health Sciences.

Guinan, Jr, J. J. (1996). Physiology of olivocochlear efferents. In *The cochlea* (pp. 435–502). New York, NY: Springer.

Guinan, Jr, J. J. (2010). Cochlear efferent innervation and function. *Current Opinion in Otolaryngology & Head and Neck Surgery, 18*(5), 447.

Hackett, T. A., Preuss, T. M., & Kaas, J. H. (2001). Architectonic identification of the core region in auditory cortex of macaques, chimpanzees, and humans. *Journal of Comparative Neurology, 441*(3), 197–222.

Kaas, J. H., & Hackett, T. A. (2000). Subdivisions of auditory cortex and processing streams in primates. *Proceedings of the National Academy of Sciences, 97*(22), 11793–11799.

Kim, J. S. (2003). Pure lateral medullary infarction: Clinical-radiological correlation of 130 acure, consecutive patients. *Brain, 126*(8), 1864–1872.

Kumral, E., Afsar, N., Kirbas, D., Balkir, K., & Ozdemirkiran, T.

(2002). Spectrum of medial medullary infarction: Clinical and magnetic resonance imaging findings. *Journal of Neurology, 249*(1), 85–93.

Kwom, M., Lee, J. H., & Kim, J. S. (2005). Dysphagia in unilateral medullary infarction: Lateral vs medial lesions. *Neurology, 65*(5), 714–718.

Lapa, S., Luger, S., Pfeilschifter, W., Henke, C., Wagner, M., & Foerth, C. (2017). Predictors of dysphagia in acute pontine infarction. *Stroke, 48*(5), 1397–1399.

Lauter, J. L., Herscovitch, P., Formby, C., & Raichle, M. E. (1985). Tonotopic organization in human auditory cortex revealed by positron emission tomography. *Hearing Research, 20*(3), 199–205.

Moller, A. R. (2003). *Sensory systems: Anatomy and physiology*. New York, NY: Academic Press.

Morel, A., Garraghty, P. E., & Kaas, J. H. (1993). Tonotopic organization, architectonic fields, and connections of auditory cortex in macaque monkeys. *Journal of Comparative Neurology, 335*(3), 437–459.

Netter, F. H. (1983). *The CIBA collection of medical illustrations. Vol. 1. Nervous system. Part I. Anatomy and physiology*. West Caldwell, NJ: CIBA Pharmaceutical.

Noback, C. R., Demarest, R. J., & Strominger, N. L. (1991). *The nervous system: Introduction and review*. Philadelphia, PA: Williams & Wilkins.

Nolte, J. (2002). *The human brain* (5th ed.). St. Louis, MO: Mosby Year Book.

Pickles, J. O. (2012). *An introduction to the physiology of hearing* (4th ed.). Leiden, The Netherlands: Brill.

Seikel, J. A., Drumright, D. G., & King, D. W. (2016). *Anatomy & physiology for speech, language, and hearing* (5th ed.). Clifton Park, NY: Cengage Learning.

Zheng, X. Y., Henderson, D., McFadden, S. L., & Hu, B. H. (1997). The role of the cochlear efferent system in acquired resistance to noise-induced hearing loss. *Hearing Research, 104*(1), 191–203.

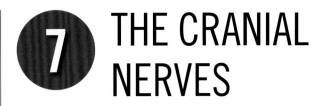

THE CRANIAL NERVES

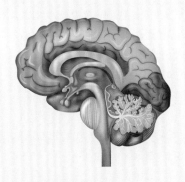

Learning Outcomes for Chapter 7

- Identify each cranial nerve by name, number, and general function.

- Identify the individual cranial nerve as being sensory, motor, or mixed in nature.

- Discuss the major differentiation among the classifications of cranial nerves as being general versus special, efferent versus afferent, somatic versus visceral, and special.

- Discuss the I olfactory nerve in terms of the functional significance of olfaction, physical location of the sensors, olfactory bulb and tract, and relationship between olfaction and the limbic system.

- Discuss the II optic nerve in terms of visual field (nasal and temporal components), decussation of the optic nerve, projection of field onto optic tract, nucleus of the thalamus related to the visual system, projection onto the cerebral cortex of visual information.

INTRODUCTION

To the speech-language pathologist or audiologist, knowledge of cranial nerves is bedrock to the assessment and treatment of neurogenic disorders. Figure 7–1 summarizes the function of the cranial nerves.

CRANIAL NERVE CLASSIFICATION

Cranial nerves can be classified broadly as sensory, motor, or mixed nerves. **Sensory nerves** only mediate sensation (e.g., II optic), **while motor nerves** only mediate movement (e.g., VI abducens). Most cranial nerves are of the **mixed** variety, activating muscle and mediating sensation (Gilman, Newman, Manter, & Gatz, 1996).

Cranial nerves also can be classified based upon the type of tissue they innervate, or variously, their source during neural development. In this case, we would talk about **somatic nerves** (nerves that serve skeletal muscles) and **visceral nerves** (nerves that serve the viscera and autonomic function).

Finally, we can categorize cranial nerves based upon their general or special function. **General nerves** are those that mediate body function from most areas of the body, such as the sense of touch. **Special nerves** are those that mediate sensation from only a single sensor, such as taste sensors (gustation). We need this variety of descriptors because individual cranial nerves can serve many of these functions, and we need to be able to differentiate them.

We have found that one of the best ways to learn cranial nerves is to refer to them by name and number, although you will hear people refer to either name or number separately. When you say "fifth trigeminal," you will always link those two together, thereby building the relationship between name and number. We also hold the convention of using Roman numerals (I, II, III), although some authors use Arabic numerals instead (e.g., cranial 1, cranial 2, cranial 3).

Cranial nerve numbers relate to their location in the brainstem. Cranial nerves I through IV are the highest, being found at the level of the midbrain (although I olfactory is not really <u>within</u> the midbrain). Cranial nerves V through VIII are found at the level of the pons, and IX through XII are found at the medulla level. Earlier, when we discussed the spinal reflex arc, we introduced the notion that the dorsal root ganglion was afferent in nature with its nucleus outside of the spinal cord, while the anterior motor component was found within the spinal cord itself. We find a similar pattern in the brainstem: the motor nuclei are found within the brainstem, while many sensory ganglia are found outside of the brainstem, including the I olfactory, II optic, V trigeminal, VIII vestibulocochlear, and XI accessory nerves. There are also aggregating centers of neurons that collect and integrate sensory information within the brainstem (Table 7–1).

- Define the terms of visual pathology, including hemianopsia, bitemporal, binasal, and homonymous.

- State the cranial nerves involved in movement of the eye and the location within the brain of the nuclei controlling them.

- Discuss the branches of the V trigeminal, their functions, and territory served.

- Identify the location of the motor and sensory nuclei for the V trigeminal nerve.

- Discuss the somatic and visceral functions of the VII facial nerve in both sensory and motor domains.

- Discuss the effect of cortical versus brainstem UMN lesion on muscles of the face.

- Discuss the auditory pathway, including auditory nuclei and their functions, and efferent pathway.

- Discuss the difference in function between the outer and inner hair cells.

- Discuss the role of the IX glossopharyngeal nerve in terms of visceral motor, somatic motor, and sensory activation.

- Discuss the branches of the X vagus nerve involved in speech production and swallowing, identifying specific branches for vocal fold function, changes of fundamental frequency, control of the cricopharyngeus muscle, sense of taste for pharynx, larynx, and trachea.

- Discuss the role of the XI accessory nerve as it relates to the IX glossopharyngeal and X vagus nerves.

- Discuss the contribution of the XII hypoglossal nerve to speech and swallowing function.

General Somatic Afferent (GSA) Nerves

General somatic afferent nerves convey information to the brain about the state of the body, pressure or movement across the skin, temperature, pain, length of muscles, and movement and position of joints. GSA information may reach consciousness, but is generally retained in the background and below the level of conscious awareness. The position of your joints, the temperature of your body, and the multiple pressures on your body at any instant are not critical to your conscious activity unless they become relevant as dangers or are interesting for some other reason. The difference here is that GSA information can be conscious—I'm aware of being cold or of a fly on my arm, but only if I bring it to my conscious attention as a matter of choice and mental priorities.

Special Somatic Afferent (SSA) Nerves

Special somatic afferent (SSA) nerves serve body sensations that are truly special. These senses are mediated by very specialized sensors. These SSA sensors include vision and our favorite, hearing and balance. SSA sensors are localized rather than global (I don't hear with my knees, although

grasshoppers do) and they are highly specialized to the specific stimulus they process.

General Visceral Afferent (GVA) Nerves

General visceral afferent (GVA) nerves mediate information from the body's viscera, such as the digestive tract. Unlike GSA, GVA information does not typically reach consciousness. The exception to this, of course, is nature's early warning system, pain. For example, gas pain in the intestines arises from the expansion of the intestinal wall, and this information reaches consciousness so you are alert to the fact that an abnormal and potentially dangerous condition exists. Information about the breakdown of your breakfast in the intestines, in contrast, doesn't need to be consciously processed: your body knows what to do about breakfast without your having to intervene.

Special Visceral Afferent (SVA) Nerves

Special visceral afferent (SVA) nerves also involve specialized and localized sensors, but these are sensing specialized (taste or smell) information. The sense of smell (olfaction) and taste (gustation) arise from chemical reactions in sensors of the nasal mucosa and oral cavity, respectively.

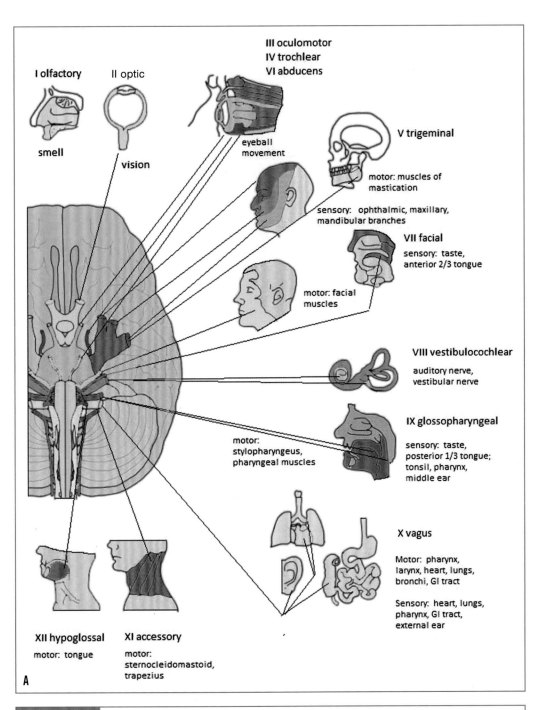

I olfactory
smell

II optic
vision

III oculomotor
IV trochlear
VI abducens
eyeball
movement

V trigeminal

motor: muscles of
mastication

sensory: ophthalmic, maxillary,
mandibular branches

VII facial
sensory: taste,
anterior 2/3 tongue

motor: facial
muscles

VIII vestibulocochlear
auditory nerve,
vestibular nerve

IX glossopharyngeal
sensory: taste,
posterior 1/3 tongue;
tonsil, pharynx,
middle ear

motor:
stylopharyngeus,
pharyngeal muscles

X vagus

Motor: pharynx,
larynx, heart, lungs,
bronchi, GI tract

Sensory: heart, lungs,
pharynx, GI tract,
external ear

XII hypoglossal
motor: tongue

XI accessory
motor:
sternocleidomastoid,
trapezius

A

FIGURE 7–1.   Cranial nerves. **A.** Graphic illustration of primary cranial nerve functions. *continues*

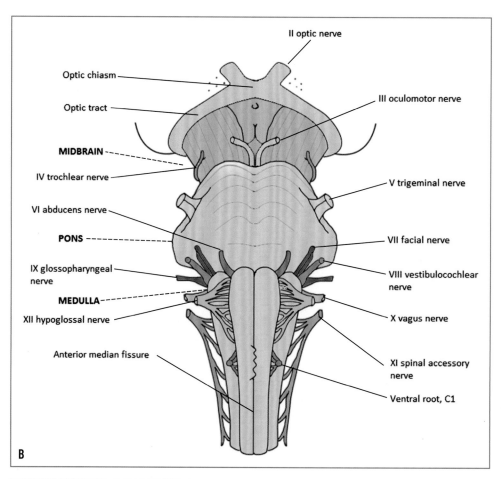

B

FIGURE 7–1. *continued* **B.** Location on brainstem of cranial nerves. *Source:* After view of Carpenter (1991).

TABLE 7–1.	Classification System for Cranial Nerves		
	Classification	Function	Specific cranial nerves in class
Afferent fibers	General somatic afferent (GSA)	These fibers convey information about pain, temperature, and touch and proprioception information from skin, muscle, tendons, and joints.	V trigeminal VII facial IX glossopharyngeal X vagus
	General visceral afferent (GVA)	These fibers convey information from hollow organs and glands (viscera) in head, neck, and thorax, as well as abdomen and thorax.	IX glossopharyngeal X vagus
	Special somatic afferent (SSA)	This special sense conveys information about hearing and vestibular sensation (VIII vestibulocochlear nerve), as well as vision (II optic nerve).	VIII vestibulocochlear nerve II optic nerve
	Special visceral afferent (SVA)	This special sense category carries information the special sensors of taste (gustation; VII facial, IX glossopharyngeal, and X vagus) and smell (olfaction; I olfactory).	VII facial nerve IX glossopharyngeal nerve X vagus I olfactory
Efferent fibers	General somatic efferent (GSE)	This class of nerves innervates skeletal muscle, specifically the tongue and ocular muscles.	III oculomotor IV trochlear VI abducens XII hypoglossal
	General visceral efferent (GVE)	These fibers innervate cardiac muscle and smooth muscle, as well as glandular secretion.	III oculomotor VII facial IX glossopharyngeal X vagus
	Special visceral efferent (SVE)	These fibers innervate skeletal muscle from the branchial arches, specifically including mandibular, facial, pharyngeal and laryngeal muscles.	V trigeminal VII facial IX glossopharyngeal X vagus XI accessory

Source: Based on data of Gilman, Newman, Manter, & Gatz (1996); Stominger, Demarest, & Laemle (2012); Seikel, Drumright, & King (2016).

General Visceral Efferent (GVE) Nerves

General visceral efferent (GVE) nerves are those that activate autonomic muscles and glands. These are not considered to be under voluntary control (i.e., we can't readily control glandular secretions, although you <u>can</u> avoid crying through conscious, cortical control, and tearing is definitely a GVE function).

General Somatic Efferent (GSE) Nerves

General somatic efferent (GSE) nerves are those that activate skeletal muscle. GSE nerves are critically important to speech production and are under voluntary control. Special visceral efferent (SVE) also innervate skeletal muscles, but specifically skeletal muscles of branchial arch origination.

These include the larynx, pharynx, velum, facial muscles, and the muscles of mastication. As you can see, GSE and SVE are both very important in our fields!

SPECIFIC CRANIAL NERVES

I Olfactory Nerve (SVA)

The **I olfactory nerve** is something of an anomaly, because it doesn't actually enter the brainstem. Olfaction is a phylogenetically old system and predates the brainstem in evolution (Buck & Barmann, 2013). Olfaction is deeply involved in emotional responses, particularly those mediated by the amygdala (Zald & Pardo, 1997). The sense of smell is sensitive to degenerative condition as well, resulting in loss of appetite in individuals with Alzheimer's disease (Mesholam, Moberg, Mahr, & Doty, 1998).

Olfactory sensors of this special visceral afferent nerve are embedded in the nasal mucosa. The olfactory nerve is primarily housed within the brain case, with its dendrites protruding into the nasal cavity through the perforated cribriform plate of the ethmoid bone. (The perforation of this bone makes it vulnerable to fracturing, and trauma to the face can cause cerebrospinal fluid rhinorrhea, or leakage of CSF into the nasal cavity. This is a dangerous condition since this can allow bacteria to circumvent the blood-brain barrier.)

There is a related nerve that we won't discuss here, but is called the vomeronasal nerve, sometimes referred to as cranial nerve 0 (zero). The vomeronasal nerve is variable in humans and mediates a sensation similar to smell, the sense of pheromones. For more on this, see Fields (2007), Fuller and Burger (1990), and Whitlock (2004).

Damage to the I Olfactory Nerve

The I olfactory nerve is particularly susceptible to facial trauma, such as that inflicted in motor vehicle accidents. Blunt force trauma to the midface region can readily sever the olfactory nerve at its vulnerable entry point through the nasal mucosa, through the cribriform plate, and into the brain case. Trauma can result in **cerebrospinal fluid rhinorrhea**, or leakage of cerebrospinal fluid from the nose, and the trauma site can allow bacteria to enter the brain space, allowing meningeal infection. Loss of the sense of smell (**anosmia**) is a common result of trauma.

Olfactory bulbs within the cranial vault are the nuclei of the olfactory nerve, with dendrites passing through the cribriform plate to receive the input (Figure 7–2). Output of the olfactory bulb is through the olfactory tract, which divides into lateral and medial components. The medial portion enters the septal area, synapses with nuclei of the septal region and decussates to the contralateral limbic system via the anterior commissure of the corpus callosum. The lateral portion projects to the amygdala, prepyriform region, and ultimately to the parhippocampal gyrus by means of an anterior projection. The parahippocampal gyrus (BA 28) provides the cortical association connection of the olfactory system (Baehr & Frotscher, 2012). Notice that the olfactory sensation is delivered directly to the cortex without passing first through the thalamus. Rather, the information is relayed to the mediodorsal nucleus of the thalamus from the olfactory cortex, and is subsequently routed to the ipsilateral insula and ipsilateral orbitofrontal cortex.

Realize the strong relationship between olfaction and emotion. "Good" smells evoke positive emotions, while "bad" smells evoke revulsion. These primary reactions can be damped by cortical control, but they really are bedrock responses. Table 7–2 might help summarize this information for you.

II Optic Nerve (SSA)

The **II optic nerve** provides the neurologist with a useful diagnostic tool and helps those of us in speech-language pathology and audiology recognize the effects of cerebrovascular accident as well. This special somatic afferent nerve is specifically related to the process of vision, rather than eye movement, which is mediated by other nerves. Retinal cells of the eye are activated by light, and output from rod and cone cells is relayed to bipolar cells and subsequently interneurons. From there, bipolar cells within the **lateral geniculate body** (LGB) transmit the information as the optic nerve. The nerve continues to the optic chiasm (the point of decussation of information), after which the pathway is referred to as the optic tract.

Lesions of the II Optic Nerve and Tract

The II optic nerve and tract provide the neurologist with information about the site of lesion, based upon the clinical evaluation. Examination of Figure 7–3A will be useful for this discussion. A lesion of point A on this figure produces complete blindness in one eye because of transection of the optic nerve. Point B represents a lesion at the optic chiasm. The **chiasm** is the point of decussation of the optic nerve. This decussation is special, in that all the information from the left visual field crosses over to the right optic tract, and the information from the right visual field crosses to the left optic tract. This is an important point.

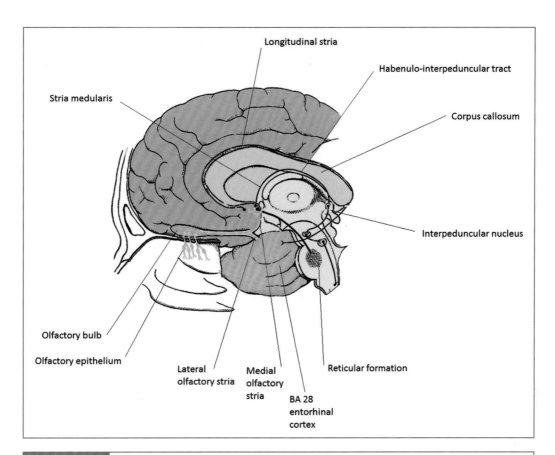

Longitudinal stria

Habenulo-interpeduncular tract

Stria medularis

Corpus callosum

Interpeduncular nucleus

Olfactory bulb

Olfactory epithelium

Lateral olfactory stria

Medial olfactory stria

BA 28 entorhinal cortex

Reticular formation

FIGURE 7–2. Olfactory bulb, nerve, and tract. Note that the olfactory tract divides into two major components, the medial and lateral olfactory stria. The lateral branches terminate in ipsilateral prepyriform cortex (also known as the primary olfactory cortex), the amygdala, and parahippocampal gyrus (BA 28). The medial branch enters the anterior commissure of the corpus callosum, with fibers terminating in the corresponding areas on the side contralateral to stimulation. *Source:* Republished with permission of Georg Thieme Verlag, from Baehr, M. and Frotscher, M. (2012). *Duus' Topical Diagnosis in Neurology: Anatomy, Physiology, Signs, Symptoms*, 5th ed. Stuttgart, Germany: Thieme; permission conveyed through Copyright Clearance Center, Inc.

TABLE 7–2. Summary of Cranial Nerve Function

Cranial nerve	Function	Classification	Primary nucleus
I olfactory	Sense of smell	SVA	Mitral cells, olfactory bulb
II optic	Vision	SSA	Retinal ganglion cells
III oculomotor	Innervation of all extrinsic ocular muscles except superior oblique and lateral rectus	GSE	Oculomotor nucleus, midbrain
	Light accommodation reflexes of iris	GVE	Edinger–Westphal nucleus, midbrain
IV trochlear	Superior oblique eye muscles	GSE	Trochlear nucleus, pons
V trigeminal	Exteroceptive sensation, including pain, tactile, and thermal sense from face and forehead, mucous membrane of mouth, upper teeth, gums, temporomandibular joint, stretch receptors of mastication	GSA	Sensory nucleus of trigeminal, pons

continues

TABLE 7–2.   *continued*

Cranial nerve	Function	Classification	Primary nucleus
V trigeminal *continued*	Motor innervation to muscles of mastication (temporalis, masseter, medial and lateral pterygoid), tensor veli palatini, and tensor tympani	SVE	Motor nucleus of trigeminal, pons
VI abducens	Motor innervation of lateral rectus ocular muscle	GSE	Abducens nucleus, pons
VII facial	Motor innervation of facial muscles	SVE	Motor nucleus of VII, pons
	Taste, anterior 2/3 of tongue	SVA	Solitary nucleus, medulla
	Tactile sense of external auditory meatus and epithelium of pinna	GSA	Trigeminal nuclei, pons
	Lacrimal glands for tearing; sublingual and submandibular glands for saliva; mucous membrane of nose and mouth	GVE	Superior salivatory and lacrimal nuclei, pons
VIII vestibulocochlear	Auditory sensation	SSA	Spiral ganglion of auditory branch
	Vestibular sensation	SSA	Vestibular ganglion of vestibular branch
IX glossopharyngeal	Somatic sense (pain, tactile, and thermal) from posterior 1/3 of tongue, pharynx (mediation of gag reflex), tonsils, mastoid cells	GVA	Solitary nucleus, medulla
	Taste in posterior 1/3 of tongue	SVA	Inferior salivatory nucleus, pons
	Somatic sense (pain, thermal, tactile), auditory tube, faucial pillars, nasopharynx, uvula, middle ear	GSA	Trigeminal nuclei, pons
	Motor innervation, stylopharyngeus, and superior pharyngeal constrictor	SVE	Inferior salivatory nucleus, pons
	Motor innervation of parotid gland	GVE	Inferior salivatory nucleus, pons
X vagus	Cutaneous sensation, external auditory meatus	GSA	Trigeminal nuclei, pons
	Sensory information from pharynx, larynx, trachea, esophagus, viscera of thorax, abdomen	GVA	Solitary nucleus, medulla
	Taste sensors of epiglottis, laryngeal aditus, valleculae	SVA	Solitary nucleus, medulla
	Motor innervation of parasympathetic ganglia, thorax, and abdomen	GVE	Dorsal motor nucleus of vagus, medulla
	Striated muscle of larynx and pharynx	SVE	Nucleus ambiguus, medulla
XI accessory	Anastomoses with X vagus to form recurrent laryngeal nerve; motor innervation of laryngeal muscles (except cricothyroid), and cricopharyngeus	SVE, cranial component	Nucleus ambiguus, medulla
	Motor innervation, sternocleidomastoid and trapezius	SVE, spinal component	Anterior horn, C1–C5 spinal cord
XII hypoglossal	Motor innervation of muscles of the tongue	GSE	Nucleus of hypoglossal nerve, medulla

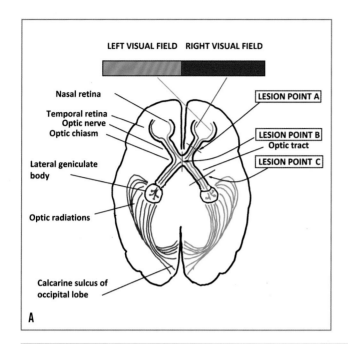

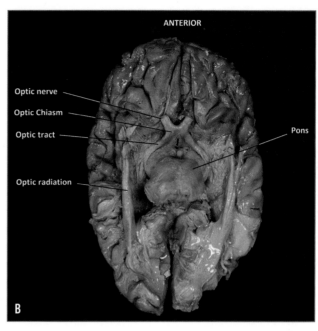

FIGURE 7–3. **A.** Optic nerve and effect of lesion of lesions on visual field. *Source:* Modified from Seikel, Drumright, and King (2016). **B.** Photograph of optic radiation.

Because of the lens of the eye, all information is reversed left-for-right and up-for-down. To understand this discussion, we refer to the areas related to the visual field as temporal or nasal: temporal refers to the side of the field nearest the temporal bone, while nasal refers to the side of the field nearest the nose (there are also temporal and nasal portions of the eye, but we'll refer to these as lateral and medial to avoid confusion). The information in the left visual field is projected to the right-eye lateral aspect and the left-eye medial aspect of the retina. Each eye receives both left and right visual fields, but the left visual field information from the right eye will not decussate, as you can see on the figure. In this manner, each eye gets both fields of vision, but the left hemisphere gets only right visual field, and the right hemisphere gets only left visual field. For example, a lesion caused by pressure from a tumor at the optic chiasm results in loss of information that would have decussated. This means that the right eye will lose the right temporal visual field, and the left eye loses the left temporal visual field, a condition known as **heteronymous** (different fields) **hemianopsia** (blindness of half of the visual field). A cut to point C on the optic tract would result in **homonymous hemianopsia**, specifically loss of the right visual field (projected to the left cortex).

From the LGB, visual information can take three pathways. Most of the information passes from the LGB to the calcarine sulcus via the optic radiation. The calcarine sulcus (BA 17) of the occipital lobe is the site of primary visual input, and information following this route is involved in form analysis and spatial discrimination. Information that is needed for immediate motor responses passes to the pulvinar of the thalamus and then to the cerebrum. That information required for vision-related reflexes (e.g., pupillary dilation) will terminate in the superior colliculus of the brainstem. The **superior colliculus** (visual relay) interacts with the inferior colliculus (auditory relay) to aid in localization of sound sources. Information from the thalamus and superior colliculus will ultimately be routed to the calcarine cortex as well (Meister & Tessier-Lavigne, 2013).

When the optic nerve or tract is damaged, specific changes occur to a person's vision. When physicians talk about visual changes occurring from lesions, they will always refer to changes in the *visual field*. Let's examine Figure 7–3 to get a notion of how the visual field reflects the underlying neuroanatomy. Take a look at the left eye. Because of lenses in the eyes, the image received by the retina is turned upside down and right-for-left. We talk about **temporal** and **nasal portions** of the visual field: the nasal portion is that which is near the nose, while the temporal portion is the lateral aspect of the visual field, near the temporal area. If you look at the left visual field and the object being viewed, you'll see that the temporal portion of the image (visual field) projects to the medial portion of the retina. The nasal portion of the image (visual field) projects to the lateral portion of the retina. This turns out to be important. Follow the path of the optic nerve from the medial portion of the retina and see that it crosses from left to right at the optic chiasm. We have seen this decussation before in the nervous system, so it isn't surprising. Now look at the information arising from the lateral aspect of the retina: it remains ipsilateral. This configuration (medial retina information decussating and lateral retina information remaining ipsilateral) results in the entire right visual field projecting to the left hemisphere, and entire left visual field projecting to the right hemisphere.

When you talk about a visual field cut, you need to identify how much cut there is and where the cut is found. **Hemianopsia** (or "hemianopia") refers to loss of half of the visual field (left or right visual field), which describes how much cut there is. If the visual field cut results in loss of both temporal fields of vision, it is termed **bitemporal hemianopsia**. This occurs from a lesion to the optic chiasm, since that would eliminate all information decussating. Sometimes a lesion at the chiasm can affect only the ipsilateral fibers of each side, resulting in **binasal hemianopsia** (loss of the nasal portion of the visual fields). Both bitemporal and binasal hemianopsia are referred to as **heteronymous hemianopsia**. Heteronymous refers to "different origin," and in this case, it means that the visual field cut is different in each eye. You can have **homonymous hemianopsia** by damaging fibers of one side of the optic tract. In this case, you could lose the entire left visual field or entire right visual field.

Returning to Figure 7–3, we are now in a position to describe cuts at different locations. A lesion at point A would result in **monocular blindness** because it completely bisects the optic nerve before decussation at the optic chiasm. A cut at point B (affecting the contralateral fibers) results in bitemporal heteronymous hemianopsia, as we discussed above. A cut at point C would result in a complete left visual field cut.

Eye Movement: III Oculomotor Nerve (GSE, GVE), IV Trochlear Nerve (GSE), VI Abducens Nerve (GSE)

We have combined our discussion of these three nerves because they serve movement of the eye. Although we'll treat this as movement of one eye, realize that we have two eyes that must work together: this will require some cortical activity for conjugate eye movement.

The **III oculomotor** nerve is responsible for a great deal of the movement of the eyeball, as well as light accom-

modation and focus by the eye. This nerve consists of two components: GSE and GVE. The general somatic efferent component serves most of the extrinsic muscles of the eye, including the superior levator palpebrae; superior, medial, and inferior rectus muscles; and the inferior oblique muscle (Figure 7–4A). The nuclei for the III oculomotor nerve are found within the midbrain, about the level of the superior colliculus. Axons arise from the nuclei and course through the red nucleus of the midbrain and medial to the cerebral peduncles. The fibers exit the brainstem at that level, dividing into superior and inferior branches. The superior rectus muscle rotates the eye up and out, while activation of the inferior rectus muscle rotates the eye down and out. The medial rectus muscle rotates the eye medially, and the inferior oblique muscles rotate the eyes up and in. Movement of both eyes together will require a complex process of contraction and inhibition to attain the goal.

The III oculomotor has a second, very important function, and that is to govern the amount of light that reaches the retina and to alter focus. The general visceral efferent component is mediated by the **Edinger–Westphal nucleus** (also known as the accessory oculomotor nucleus), which allows the iris of the eye to constrict and focus in response to light and distance from the visual target. The nuclei can be found just anterior to the cerebral aqueduct in the midbrain, and fibers emerge from the brainstem medial to the cerebral peduncles. The fibers pass into the orbit by means of the superior orbital fissure of the skull.

The **IV trochlear** is a general somatic efferent nerve that arises from the trochlear nucleus of the midbrain region. Its sole responsibility is to innervate the superior oblique muscle of the eye, turning the eye down and slightly out.

The **VI abducens nerve** (also known as the abducent) is responsible for abduction of the eyeball. General somatic efferent innervation of the lateral rectus muscle rotates the eye laterally. The nerve arises from the abducens nucleus within the pons and emerges from the brainstem at the juncture of the pons and medulla. The VI abducens enters the eye socket through the superior orbital fissure.

Lesions to the nerves of oculomotor function provide important diagnostic information to physicians. The III oculomotor nerve can be compressed by tumors or **aneurysms** (ballooning of arteries), and damaged by hemorrhage. If the lesion is ipsilateral, one will see problems with adduction of the eye, elevation of the eyelid, pupil constriction, and focus. Because the forces of the lateral rectus are unopposed, the affected eye will rotate out (termed **divergent strabismus**) and the drooping eyelid will be termed **ptosis**. **Mydriasis** is the term for abnormal dilation of the pupil.

Lesion affecting the IV trochlear nerve affects the superior oblique muscle, which rotates the eye down, and lesion will eliminate this ability. Because the VI abducens controls the lateral rectus, a lesion of this nerve will re-

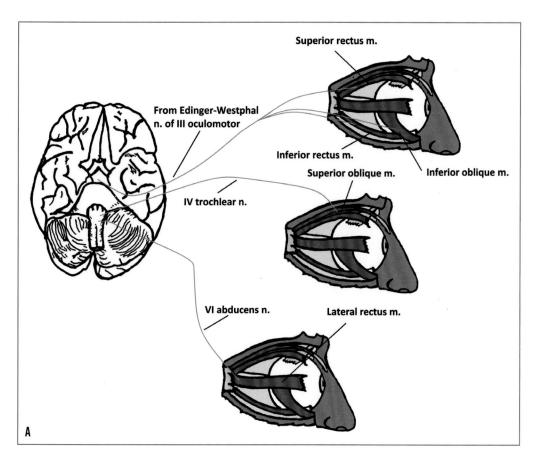

Superior rectus m.

From Edinger-Westphal
n. of III oculomotor

Inferior rectus m.

Superior oblique m.

Inferior oblique m.

IV trochlear n.

VI abducens n.

Lateral rectus m.

A

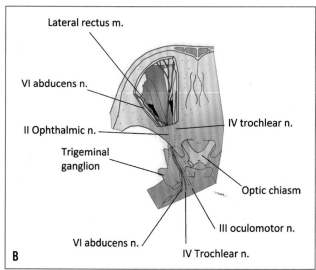

Lateral rectus m.

VI abducens n.

II Ophthalmic n.

Trigeminal
ganglion

IV trochlear n.

Optic chiasm

VI abducens n.

III oculomotor n.

IV Trochlear n.

B

FIGURE 7–4. **A.** Muscle innervation for ocular movement, entailing III oculomotor, IV trochlear, and VI abducens nerves and muscles of ocular movement. **B.** Innervation pattern for muscles of the eye. *Source:* Modified from Seikel, Drumright, and King (2016).

sult in loss of ability to move the eye laterally. Forces of other muscles will pull the eye medially, termed internal strabismus.

The III oculomotor nerve is controlled cortically by BA 8, which projects to the superior colliculus and ultimately the nucleus for the III oculomotor nerve, as well as the IV trochlear and VI abducens nerves. **Conjugate movement** (moving the eyes together to look at the same side) and **convergence** (rotating both eyes medially to focus on close objects) are governed by cortical activity, and lesions that affect the superior frontal lobe can affect these two ocular functions.

V Trigeminal Nerve (GSA, SVE)

The **V trigeminal nerve** is a player in both speech-language pathology and audiology. It has two very important functions in the speech realm: motor activation of the muscles of mastication and mediation of somatic sense for the face. In the hearing realm, this nerve innervates the tensor tympani, one of the muscles responsible for the acoustic reflex. Let's examine this important nerve.

Lesions of the V Trigeminal Nerve

The V trigeminal nerve innervates the entire face and oral cavity by means of its three branches. **Trigeminal neuralgia** (also known as *tic douloureux*) is a significant sensory deficit, often resulting in extreme burning or shocking sensation of the face or cheek area. The attacks can be sudden and brief or long-lasting, and the pain can be quite intense. The condition may be caused by a blood vessel compressing the trigeminal nerve or a disease process such as multiple sclerosis, or it may arise from trauma or surgery.

Motor problems of the trigeminal nerve arise from lesions affecting the mandibular branch. This branch innervates the muscles of mastication, so the dominant sign of lesion to this nerve is unilateral flaccid paralysis (bilateral paralysis is rare), which results in deviation of the mandible toward the strong side upon elevation.

As you can see in Figure 7–5, the trigeminal nerve lives up to its name: "tri" refers to the three roots of the nerve, and "gemina" refers to *birth* or *origin*. The trigeminal nerve has three branches that arise from the brainstem and has several important functions. The V trigeminal nerve arises from the **sensory nucleus** and **motor trigeminal nucleus** in the pons. There is an enlargement of the nerve after it exits the brainstem, and that enlargement is known as the **trigeminal gan-**

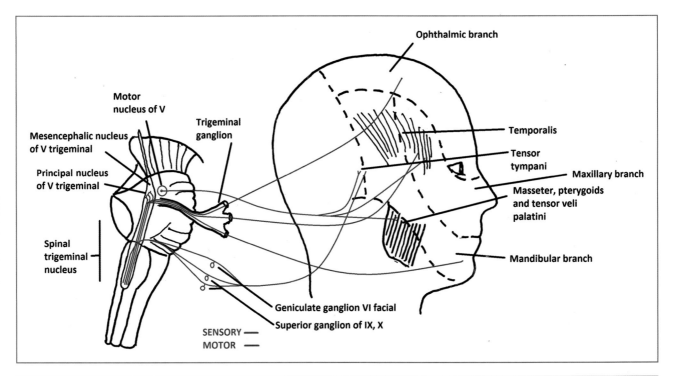

FIGURE 7–5. Origins and area served by the trigeminal nerve. Note that the ophthalmic nerve mediates somatic sense from the upper face, including pain, touch, and pressure sense for the skin above the level of the eyelids, the forehead, scalp, iris, cornea, upper eyelid, conjunctiva, and nasal mucous membrane. The maxillary nerve conveys somatic sensation from the areas of the lower eyelid, maxilla, upper teeth and lip, mucosal lining of the nasal and buccal cavities, maxillary sinuses, and nasopharynx. The mandibular nerve is both sensory and motor. The sensory component conveys somatic information from the mandible, including the skin, lower teeth, gums, and lip, as well as some of the mucosal lining of the buccal cavity. It conveys tactile sense from the external auditory meatus, auricle, and temporomandibular joint, and the region of the temporal bone, as well as kinesthetic and proprioceptive sense from muscles of mastication. The motor component innervates the muscles of mastication, the mylohyoid, anterior digastricus, tensor veli palatine, and tensor tympani of the middle ear.

glion. From there the nerve divides into three components: the ophthalmic, maxillary, and mandibular nerves.

The **ophthalmic** is a general somatic afferent nerve, serving the upper face. It conveys general sensory information such as pain, touch, and pressure from the forehead, scalp, iris, cornea, upper eyelid, conjunctiva, and nasal mucous membrane. It's important to note that although it conveys sensation from the iris and cornea, this is somatic sense rather than vision. When something touches your eye, that sensation is conveyed by the ophthalmic nerve.

The **maxillary nerve** is also only sensory, again being a general somatic afferent nerve. Somatic information from lower eyelid, maxilla, upper teeth and lip, mucosal lining of the nasal and buccal cavities, maxillary sinuses, and nasopharynx are transmitted via this nerve to the brainstem.

The **mandibular nerve** is both motor and sensory in nature. It exits the skull by means of the foramen ovale of the sphenoid bone. The general somatic afferent component conveys information from the mandible (skin, lower teeth, gums, and lower lip); the skin and some of the mucosal lining of the buccal cavity; tactile sense from the external auditory meatus and auricle; temporomandibular joint; and the region of the temporal bone. It also conveys the kinesthetic and proprioceptive information from the muscles of mastication. The lingual branch of the mandibular nerve conveys somatic sense from the anterior mucous membrane of the tongue and the floor of the mouth.

The mandibular nerve also provides motor innervation to the muscles of mastication. This special visceral efferent component innervates the muscles of mastication, including temporalis, masseter, and lateral and medial pterygoids. It also innervates the tensor veli palatini of the velum and the tensor tympani of the middle ear, as well as the mylohyoid and anterior digastricus muscles. The nerve arises from the trigeminal nucleus within the pons (Carpenter, 1991).

Damage to the V trigeminal nerve can have a significant impact upon speech production and mastication. If the lesion is of the upper motor neuron (UMN) system, you may see a strong **jaw jerk reflex** arising from the muscle spindles of the masseter and temporalis. Lower motor neuron lesion (LMN) will result in muscle weakness of the affected muscles, which will cause the mandible to deviate toward the strong side if the lesion is unilateral. If the sensory component of the V trigeminal is affected, one can lose sensation for the anterior two-thirds of the tongue (note that taste is mediated by a different nerve), as well as loss of the **corneal blink reflex**. Loss of tactile or pain sense for any of the facial areas served by the nerve may be seen, but the patient may also experience the extreme pain of **trigeminal neuralgia**.

VII Facial Nerve (SVE, SVA, GVE)

The **VII facial nerve** innervates all of the muscles of the face, some of the salivary glands, and tear glands (see Figure 7–6). It also is an important mediator of the sense of taste. The special visceral afferent component of the VII facial nerve terminates in the geniculate ganglion, located in the facial canal of the temporal bone. You will remember that we discussed this nucleus when we examined the pons in the last chapter. The muscles of the face have an interesting innervation pattern that has surprising results when upper motor neuron lesions occur. Notice that the upper half of the face (from the eyes up) has bilateral innervation arising from the cortex. This means that each side is innervated by both right and left hemispheres, so that if there is a unilateral cortical lesion or unilateral lesion to the UMN pathway, both sides of the muscles of the forehead will function normally. The lower face, in contrast, has the classic contralateral innervation pattern that we've come to expect, which means that unilateral cortical or UMN lesion can result in contralateral weakness. Realize that if the lower motor neuron is affected, you <u>can</u> see unilateral forehead muscle weakness.

Lesions of the VII Facial Nerve

The VII facial nerve has two significant responsibilities: movement of facial muscles and sense of taste for the anterior two-thirds of the tongue. This nerve has a rather unique innervation pattern, in that the lower face is contralaterally innervated and the upper face is bilaterally innervated. Essentially, both sides of the upper face receive activation from both cerebral hemispheres, so that upper motor neuron control of movement above the level of the eyes is redundant and resistant to neurological problems. In contrast, a lesion to the right hemisphere can cause muscular weakness on the left lower face (from the eyes down), so that a stroke that affects muscle activity will often cause weak facial musculature on the side contralateral to the lesion.

Lower motor neuron lesion will cause ipsilateral paralysis or paresis, and may involve drooping and non-responsive musculature. During the oral mechanism examination, the clinician will notice that attempts to smile will result in the affected side being drawn toward the non-affected side, and **facies** (facial presentation) will be asymmetrical. On speaking, the cheek may tend to puff out for plosives due to loss of muscle tone, and the patient may experience buccal pocketing of food while eating, since the buccal musculature may no longer assist in keeping food on the molars.

Bell's palsy is another condition of interest. Bell's palsy appears to arise from inflammation of the VII facial nerve, often from viral origin. In this case, the inflammation causes compression of the nerve as it leaves the skull. Bell's palsy will result in facial paralysis on the side of the lesion, but will often remit after a few months.

Trauma is a common cause of VII facial nerve damage. Trauma to the facial nerve, such as that found in motor vehicle accidents, will result in a flaccid paralysis, with loss of function occurring on the side of the lesion.

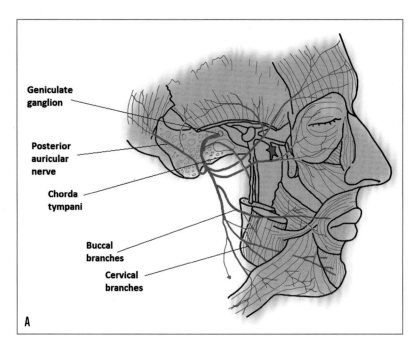

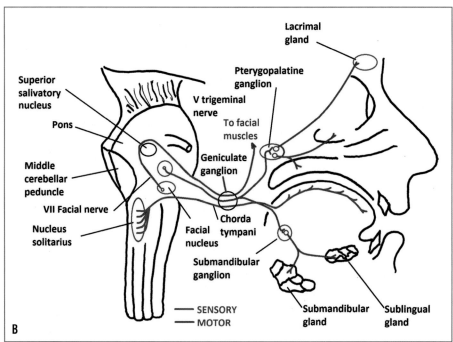

The facial nerve arises from the pons and exits at the cerebellopontine angle (juncture of the cerebellum and pons) via the internal auditory meatus and facial canal of the temporal bone. The **geniculate ganglion** of the VII facial nerve serves the sensory component of the VII facial nerve. A small branch from that nerve, the **chorda tympani**, enters the middle ear space and passes between the tympanic membrane and the malleus. This component mediates the sense of taste for the anterior tongue. It will ultimately join the lingual nerve of the V trigeminal, which mediates somatic sense for the tongue. The facial nerve emerges from the skull at the stylomastoid foramen of the temporal bone and branches into the cervicofacial and temporofacial divisions. The temporofacial division further divides into the zygomatic and temporal branches, while the cervicofacial division branches into the lingual, buccal, and marginal mandibular nerves. In this manner, all muscles of the face are innervated by the VII facial nerve.

The other motor component of the VII facial nerve is the general visceral efferent component. This component originates at the nucleus intermedius with input from the superior salivatory nucleus of the pons, innervating the glandular tissue of the **submandibular glands** and sublingual glands, as well as the **lacrimal glands** for tearing and intranasal glands for mucus secretion within the nose. The **superior salivatory nucleus** has input from the olfactory system, so that the aroma of supper cooking can trigger the secretion of saliva.

One more very important function is served by the special visceral afferent component of the VII facial nerve. **Gustation** (the sense of taste) for the anterior two-thirds of the tongue is mediated by this component of the VII facial nerve via the chorda tympani, as was discussed earlier. Information about taste passes through the geniculate ganglion to the solitary tract nucleus, and ultimately arises at the thalamus on its way to the insula of the cerebral cortex. The insula, as noted earlier, is considered the gustatory cortex.

Lesions of the VII facial nerve can certainly affect speech, particularly bilabial sounds. If the lesion is of the cranial nerve (lower motor neuron), a person may have facial paralysis on the affected side with reduced ability to wrinkle the chin or elevate the lips for smiling on one side. The individual may drool due to loss of labial continence. A condition known as **Bell's palsy** (palsy is an older word for paralysis) can occur as a result of compression of the facial nerve due to inflammation, and damage to the VII facial secondary to motor vehicle accidents is common, particularly in accidents involving fractures of the temporal bone. Loss of the sense of taste is also a frequent event in temporal bone trauma.

VIII Vestibulocochlear Nerve (SSA)

This is one of the most critical cranial nerves to our field. The **VIII vestibulocochlear** is a special somatic afferent nerve that conveys information about both sound and balance to the central nervous system. In the previous chapter we talked about the auditory pathway, so now we'll talk about the VIII vesitbulocochlear nerve itself. There is an unclassified efferent component to the auditory system, but since it arises from within the brainstem pathway rather than as a cranial nerve nucleus, we don't consider it a component of the VIII vestibulocochlear nerve (Guinan, 2010). This nerve has two branches: the acoustic branch and the vestibular branch.

Lesions of the VIII Vestibulocochlear Nerve

Lesions of the VIII vestibulocochlear nerve are quite significant for both the speech-language pathologist and audiologist. Clearly, we use hearing for development of our phoneme repertoire, and oral language is the primary means of communication for hearing individuals. The vestibular mechanism is critical for balance, but it can also play a significant role in cognitive performance.

Damage to the auditory pathway can occur secondary to cerebrovascular accident if the brainstem or temporal lobe is involved. If you examine Figure 6–5 of the auditory pathway, you can see that **audition** (the process of hearing) is not restricted to the temporal lobe, but rather involves parietal and frontal lobe locations as well. Indeed, there is occipital input to the temporal lobe so that sound and vision are integrated to aid in identification of a sound source. Damage to diverse cortical centers can result in a person having intact auditory thresholds for sound and speech but having deficiencies in making sense of those sounds. This disorder, termed **(central) auditory processing disorder**, arises from a variety of issues, including neural asynchrony and poor connectivity, and its complete elaboration remains a goal for the profession. For a foundational discussion on the topic, see Musiek and Chermak (2013).

A common cause of damage to the VIII nerve is an auto accident. The "T-bone" motor vehicle accident, where a person's car is hit from the side, can result in a fracture of the temporal bone and damage to the nerve. For a review of traumatic brain injury, see Mackay, Chapman, and Morgan (1997).

Disruption of the auditory pathway can also occur at the source: the hair cells. Damage to these sensors can arise from a number or causes, including noise exposure, exposure to **ototoxins** (toxins that target hair cell function), or even the immune system. Indeed, immune system dysfunction can result in **sudden sensorineural hearing loss** (SSNH), with profound loss of hearing occurring within minutes. In this case, a course of prednisone must be initiated within 24 hours of onset if there is to be any hope of return to normal function. The mechanism for SSNH is not entirely understood. (Parenthetically, one of the authors of this text [J.A.S.] had a sudden, severe loss of hearing during a faculty meeting. Beginning an immediate course of prednisone began the reversal process within eight hours, with a return to baseline level within a day. The disorder was ultimately diagnosed as immune system mediated, and to this day J.A.S. never leaves home without prednisone!)

Brainstem tumors can compress the VIII nerve, resulting in hearing dysfunction. A **cerebellopontine angle tumor** affects the juncture of the cerebellum and pons, the point where the V, VII, and VIII nerves enter the brainstem. As the tumor grows, the functions mediated by these nerves will decline ipsilateral to the tumor. A tumor within the brainstem itself can also compress the nerve or nuclei of the vestibular mechanism causing balance dysfunction. Tumors at the site of the internal auditory meatus, where the VIII nerve exits the temporal lobe, can cause both auditory and vestibular dysfunction.

Vestibular dysfunction can result in **vertigo**, which is the perception of movement in space in the absence of physical movement. Vertigo can result in feelings of nausea and disorientation and can be very debilitating. It can also result in cognitive problems, perhaps as a result of the inevitable distraction of a constant physiological mismatch between internal perception of movement and visual reality (Mast & Ellis, 2015; McNaughton, Knierim, & Wilson, 1995; Smith, Zheng, Horii, & Darlington, 2005).

Acoustic Branch

Acoustic information arrives at the cochlea, where it is transduced into information that can be transmitted to the central nervous system. The transduction process involves three major steps. First, acoustic information is translated into mechanical information at the middle ear. Then this information is translated into wave information within the fluid of the cochlea. Finally, wave information is translated into a neural code by the hair cells of the cochlea and is conveyed to the VIII vestibulocochlear nerve. For our purposes here, we will only discuss hair cell function and VIII nerve activation.

There are two types of hair cells: inner and outer (Figure 7–7). **Inner hair cells** are predominantly responsible for conveying place and timing information concerning the point of maximum perturbation by the traveling wave (Hudspeth, 2013, 2014). **Outer hair cells** are responsible for amplifying the sound arriving at the cochlea by means of active response to the incoming auditory signal. This amplification serves to sharpen the basilar membrane response, improving auditory discrimination (the ability to discriminate changes in the auditory signal) while increasing the signal strength that will activate the VIII vestibulocochlear nerve.

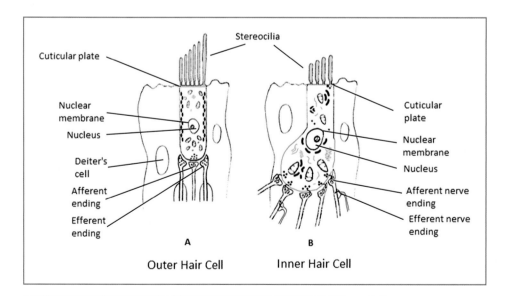

FIGURE 7–7. Hair cells of the human auditory system. Note the presence of cilia connected by tip links. **A.** Outer hair cells. Note that the dendrite of the VIII vestibulocochlear nerve makes synapse directly with the base of the hair cell, as do efferent axons of the olivocochlear bundle. **B.** Inner hair cells. Note that there are many more afferent dendrites than on outer hair cells and that efferent fibers terminate on the afferent fibers.

Both inner and outer hair cells are endowed with **cilia** on the distal surface. Deflection of the cilia by the traveling wave of the cochlea causes depolarization of the hair cell, with subsequent activation of the VIII nerve. There are **tip links** that connect the cilia so that they move as a linked unit: movement of the cilia opens ion channels, allowing K+ to enter the hair cell. Potassium depolarizes the hair cell in the same manner as depolarization of a neuron, initiating a response in the VIII nerve fiber (Pickles, 2012).

The responses of the two types of hair cells are categorically different. The inner hair cell, with rich innervation by the VIII vestibulocochlear nerve, responds much as a neuron does, in that it depolarizes and activates the nerve. The outer hair cell responds to depolarization by shortening. The effect of the change in outer hair cell length is to pulse the basilar membrane in precise response to the traveling wave. This pulsing amplifies the effect of the traveling wave and thus the signal itself. The outer hair cells are thus poorly represented at the VIII vestibulocochlear nerve, with the bulk of the nerve being made up of fibers that arise from the inner hair cells (Spoendlin, 1984). Information from the inner hair cells is used to identify frequency, intensity, and duration of the components of the acoustic signal (Figure 7–8).

From the scala media of the cochlea, the nerve fibers pass through the **habenula perforata** of the osseous spiral lamina (medial wall), to coalesce within the **modiolus** of the cochlea as the **spiral ganglion**. The spiral ganglion of the VIII vestibulocochlear nerve is the collection of cell bodies

of that nerve. Axons arising from the neurons of the ganglion combine with the axons from the vestibular branch and exit the temporal bone via the internal auditory meatus and enter the brainstem at the level of the upper medulla (see Figures 7–1 and 7–9). The acoustic branch divides into three branches, serving three areas of the cochlear nucleus: **dorsal cochlear nucleus**, **anteroventral cochlear nucleus**, and **posteroventral cochlear nucleus** (see Figure 6–5).

Vestibular Branch

The vestibular branch of the VIII vestibulocochlear nerve is responsible for conveying information concerning the position of the body in space, as well as its movement through space. Unlike the cochlea, whose cell bodies lie within the modiolus of the cochlea, the cell bodies of the vestibular branch reside within the internal auditory meatus of the temporal bone. Sensors of the vestibular mechanism share overall design with hair cells of the cochlea, in that they are mechanoreceptors endowed with cilia that are deflected by motion of fluid. Hair cells of the vestibular mechanism rely on inertial forces acting on the fluid coursing through the vestibular apparatus to move the cilia, and the forces are enhanced by presence of a gelatinous **cupola** overlying the cilia and superior aspect of the hair cell. Thus, similar functional cells and their ciliary appendages serve markedly different purposes, with cochlear hair cells sensing minute perturbations in wave

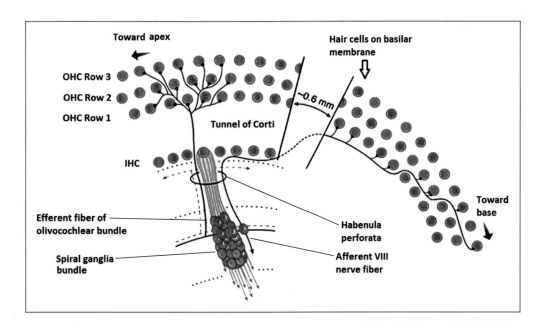

FIGURE 7–8. Innervation pattern of outer and inner hair cells. Note that outer hair cells are only nominally represented in the VIII vestibulocochlear nerve, whereas inner hair cells are richly represented. *Source:* From Seikel/King/Drumright. *Anatomy and Physiology for Speech, Language, and Hearing*, 3rd ed. © 2005 Delmar Learning, a part of Cengage, Inc. Reproduced by permission. www.cengage.com/permissions

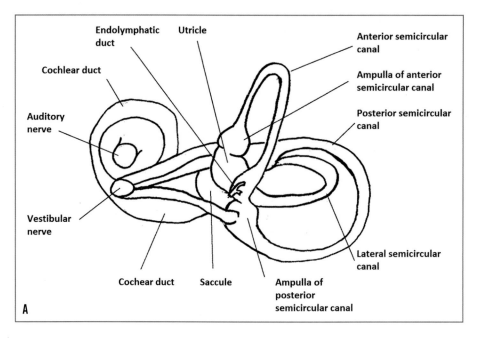

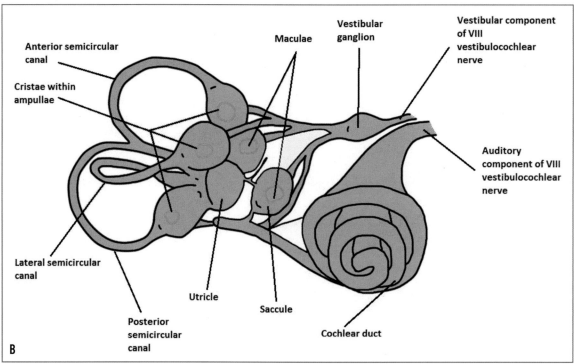

FIGURE 7–9. Acoustic and vestibular branches of VIII vestibulocochlear nerve. **A.** Cochlea and vestibular mechanism viewed from lateral aspect. **B.** Vestibulocochlear nerve and its sources, as viewed from medial aspect.

dynamics relative to sound, and vestibular hair cells sensing larger movement of fluid as a unit (Goldberg, Walker, & Hudspeth, 2013).

Axons of the vestibular ganglion enter the brainstem at the level of the lower pons, subsequently branching to syn- apse with the **superior**, **medial**, **lateral**, and **inferior vestibular nuclei** in the lower pons and upper medulla. Some fibers also project directly to the flocculonodular lobe of the cerebellum. Output of vestibular nuclei is sent to the spinal cord, cerebellum, thalamus, and cerebral cortex.

Damage to the VIII vestibulocochlear nerve can result in either hearing loss or vestibular dysfunction or both. The auditory component of the nerve is arrayed such that the fibers serving higher frequencies are on the outside of the nerve, while the inner fibers represent lower-frequency areas of the cochlea. Compression of the nerve through tumor will first be seen in the high frequencies of one ear, since bilateral tumors would be rare. Tumors are frequently located at the juncture of the cerebellum and pons (**cerebellopontine angle**) as well as within the internal auditory meatus. Physical trauma to the temporal bone housing the nerve is a frequent occurrence in motor vehicle accidents involving lateral impact, and both hearing loss and vestibular disturbance can occur in these instances. Indeed, vestibular disturbance following trauma is a typical event due to the disturbance of the vestibular mechanism and its components. **Nystagmus** and **vertigo** may be found with vestibular trauma.

Efferent Component

There is an **efferent component** associated with the VIII vestibulocochlear nerve, although it is not a component of the nerve itself. The **olivocochlear bundle**, arising from the superior olivary complex of the brainstem, is a feedback system whose fibers enter the cochlea and synapse with outer and inner hair cells. Activation of this bundle will result in damping the output of hair cells, and it is widely thought that the function is to improve the signal-to-noise ratio for hearing. We discussed this in detail in Chapter 6.

IX Glossopharyngeal Nerve (GSA, GVA, SVA, GVE, SVE)

The **IX glossopharyngeal nerve** has both sensory and motor components as well as a special visceral afferent component related to taste. It is an important nerve for swallowing function (Figure 7–10) (Barlow & Estep, 2006). Much of the activity of the IX glossopharyngeal nerve is accomplished in coordination with the X vagus and XI accessory nerves, and some authors refer to this combination as the vagal system (Baehr & Frotscher, 2012). The motor component of the IX glossopharyngeal nerve arises from the **nucleus ambiguus** and **inferior salivatory nuclei** (nucleus solitarius) of the medulla. (You will remember that we ran across the inferior

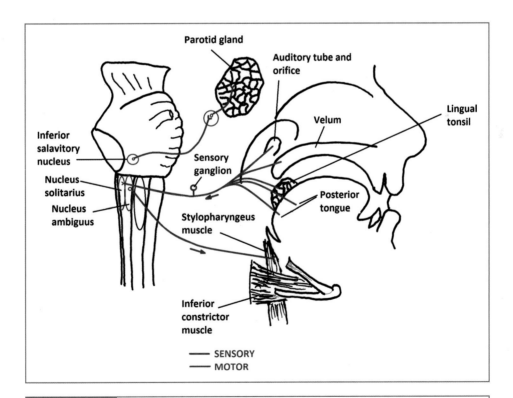

FIGURE 7–10. IX glossopharyngeal origins and actions. Note that the SVE component serves the pharyngeal constrictors and stylopharyngeus, while the SVA component mediates the sense of taste for the posterior tongue. The GVA component (not shown) innervates the parotid gland. The GVA component mediates tactile, pain, and temperature sensation, which is critical for activation of the swallowing response via the nucleus of the reticular formation.

salivatory nucleus in our discussion of the VII facial nerve and activation of the submandibular and sublingual glands. We will now see parallel activation in the parotid gland.) The somatic sensory component terminates in the **solitary tract nucleus** and **spinal tract nucleus of the V trigeminal nerve**. The sensory component emerges from the medulla in the ventrolateral aspect, exiting the skull through the jugular foramen of the temporal bone. It courses past the styloid process, lateral to the stylopharyngeus muscle to innervate the tongue base. The nerve nuclei include the superior and inferior (petrosal) ganglia.

Taste for the posterior one-third of the tongue is mediated by the special visceral afferent component of the IX glossopharyngeal nerve. Taste receptors on the posterior tongue and part of the velum send taste information to the solitary tract nucleus. Arterial pressure information, sensed within the carotid sinus, is also delivered to the solitary tract nucleus. The general sense component (general somatic afferent) conveys information about touch, pain, and pressure to the posterior tongue, fauces, upper pharynx, and auditory tube to the inferior ganglion of the medulla. Somatic information is conveyed from the posterior auricle and external auditory meatus to the nucleus of the spinal trigeminal nerve by means of the superior branch of the IX glossopharyngeal.

The IX glossopharyngeal also has efferent components. The special visceral efferent component activates the stylopharyngeus and superior constrictor muscles via the nucleus ambiguus. **Parotid glands** are activated by means of the general visceral efferent component, arising from the inferior salivatory nucleus.

Lesions of the IX glossopharyngeal nerve can have widespread consequences. If you examine Figure 7–10, you can see that the glossopharyngeal nerve is intrinsic to the swallow function, with afferents providing input to the reticular nucleus swallowing center. If the afferents are compromised, the pharyngeal swallow response will also be compromised, with potentially delayed or absent swallow trigger and absence of the protective gag response. Further, the sense of taste for the posterior one-third of the tongue may be compromised. This aspect of taste focuses on the more bitter tastes, but perhaps more importantly, taste sensation at the posterior tongue stimulates the parotid gland to release a serous saliva that is critical to effective swallowing. Notice the relationship between the IX glossopharyngeal and the X vagus (to be discussed next). The X vagus is responsible for protection of the airway through adduction of the vocal folds and other actions. In swallowing, these actions are linked through glossopharyngeal function. Finally, the muscular contribution of the IX glossopharyngeal nerve to swallowing includes the peristaltic contraction of the pharyngeal constrictors and elevation of the pharynx via the stylopharyngeus.

X Vagus Nerve (GSA, GVA, SVA, GVE, SVE)

The **X vagus** is a complex nerve that has a great deal of significance for speech and swallowing. The X vagus arises at the level of the medulla oblongata and exits from the skull at the jugular foramen with the IX glossopharyngeal and XI accessory nerves (Figure 7–11). In the brainstem, the motor component of the vagus arises from the dorsal motor nucleus of the vagus (vagal nucleus) and the nucleus ambiguus. The vagal nucleus mediates the general visceral efferent parasympathetic responses of the body based on sensory information conveyed by the inferior vagal ganglion: this includes motor innervation of intestines, pancreas, stomach, esophagus, trachea, bronchial smooth muscle and mucosal glands, kidneys, liver, and the heart. The nucleus ambiguus is particularly important to our discipline because it is responsible for innervation of the muscles of the larynx (*special visceral efferent*).

Lesions of the X Vagus Nerve

The X vagus is quite extensive in range and function. Damage to the vagus can take many forms, from trauma to degenerative disease, and the cause of some lesions remains unknown. We have particular interest in the recurrent and superior laryngeal nerves, which are branches of the vagus. The recurrent laryngeal nerve may be injured during thyroid surgery or as a result of trauma from a collision or aneurysm of the aorta. Viral infection can cause temporary or permanent injury to the nerve. Unilateral lesion to the recurrent laryngeal nerve will result in ipsilateral vocal fold paralysis, as well as potential deficiency related to the cricopharyngeus muscle, responsible for control of the upper esophageal sphincter. Lesion to the superior laryngeal nerve will result in reduction in the ability to adjust the fundamental frequency, potential cricopharyngeal deficit (Uludag, Aygun, & Isgor, 2016), and loss of sensation in the upper larynx.

Bilateral damage to the pharyngeal branch of the vagus can result in dysphagia, loss of the gag reflex (because of its facilitative relationship with the IX glossopharyngeal), or hypernasality. Unilateral damage may result in deviation of the velum toward the unaffected side upon elevation. Both lesions may result in nasal regurgitation.

Pain, touch, and temperature sense are mediated by the general somatic afferent component of the X vagus. Regions served by this function include the skin overlying the posterior auricle, the tympanic membrane, and the external auditory meatus. This somatic information is relayed to the

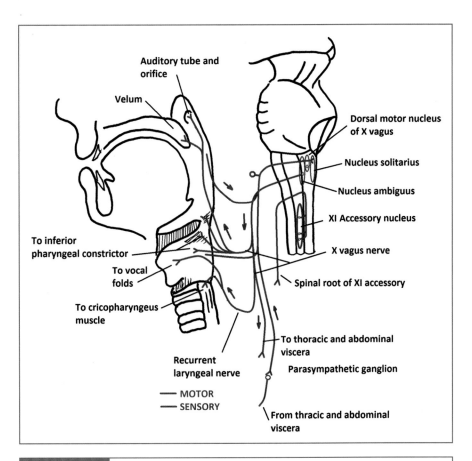

Auditory tube and orifice

Velum

Dorsal motor nucleus of X vagus

Nucleus solitarius

Nucleus ambiguus

XI Accessory nucleus

To inferior pharyngeal constrictor

To vocal folds

X vagus nerve

To cricopharyngeus muscle

Spinal root of XI accessory

Recurrent laryngeal nerve

To thoracic and abdominal viscera

Parasympathetic ganglion

—— MOTOR
—— SENSORY

From thracic and abdominal viscera

FIGURE 7–11. X vagus and XI accessory nerves. Notice that the X vagus is responsible for activation of the muscles of the larynx, including those responsible for protection of the airway. The X vagus also has responsibility for elevation of the velum and sensation within the airway. It is responsible for tonic contraction of the cricopharyngeus (and thus for maintaining separation between the esophagus and pharynx) via the recurrent laryngeal nerve. Also notice that the X vagus has significant visceral responsibility. The XI accessory nerve is responsible for motor innervation of the sternocleidomastoid and trapezius muscles and works in conjunction with the X vagus for innervation of the pharyngeal muscles.

spinal nucleus of the V trigeminal. The general visceral afferent component of the X vagus mediates the sense of pain from the lower pharynx, the larynx, viscera of the thorax and abdomen, and bronchi of the lungs. This component also mediates the sense of nausea and hunger. This information is received by the nucleus solitarius and dorsal vagal nucleus. This GVA component also monitors heartbeat, blood pressure, respiration, and digestion.

Four branches of the vagus perform these functions. The pharyngeal, recurrent laryngeal, and superior laryngeal branches arise from the inferior ganglion, while the auricular branch arises from the superior ganglion. The **recurrent laryngeal nerve** (RLN) is particularly important for speech-language pathologists. The right RLN courses behind the subclavian artery, ascending to the larynx between the trachea and esophagus. The left RLN courses under the aortic arch before ascending to the trachea and esophagus. The RLN enters the larynx between the cricoid and thyroid cartilages to provide general visceral afferent innervation to the mucosa of the vocal folds. The special visceral efferent component innervates all but one of the intrinsic muscles of the larynx, including the thyrovocalis, thyromuscularis, oblique and transverse arytenoid muscles, lateral cricoarytenoid, and posterior cricoarytenoid muscles. The RLN innervates the inferior constrictor and the lowest component of that muscle, the cricopharyngeus muscle, providing tonic contraction of that muscle to isolate the esophagus from the pharynx until swallowing occurs. The auricular branch is responsible for conveying sensory information from the tympanic membrane and external auditory meatus.

The special visceral afferent component of the **pharyngeal branch** mediates the sense of taste from the epiglottis, valleculae, larynx, and trachea to the inferior ganglion of the X vagus (Gilman & Winans, 1992), as well as the general visceral afferent sense of touch, pain, and pressure for those regions. It is likely that the taste receptors found within the intestines are also mediated by this component of the X vagus. The pharyngeal branch also combines with the IX glossopharyngeal to provide special visceral efferent innervation to the superior and middle pharyngeal constrictors (pharyngeal peristalsis), as well as to the palatoglossus (elevation of posterior tongue or velar depression), palatopharyngeus (velar depression), salpingopharyngeus (constriction of auditory tube), levator veli palatine, and musculus uvulae muscles (elevation of velum). The **superior laryngeal nerve** mediates general visceral afferent sensation for the region above the vocal folds via the internal branch of the superior laryngeal nerve. The external branch of this nerve is responsible for activating the cricothyroid muscle for changing the vocal fundamental frequency.

The X vagus has many responsibilities, and lesions to this nerve can have far-reaching consequences. (One of our biology colleagues, Dr. Curt Anderson, says, tongue in cheek, that when someone asks you a question about a nerve, most of the time you'll be correct if you answer "vagus!") Lesion affecting the pharyngeal branch can result in loss of airway protection in swallowing, velar paralysis or paresis, inappropriate patency of the upper esophageal sphincter or, alternatively, inability to relax the sphincter. The recurrent laryngeal nerve is responsible for vocal fold adduction and abduction, so a lesion to this nerve would have a profound impact on the ability to product phonation for speech. The superior laryngeal nerve is responsible for changing the vocal fundamental frequency, so a lesion to this branch would result in monopitch phonation. To put it another way, incapacitation of the X vagus could result in hypernasality, aphonia, life-threatening dysphagia, nasal regurgitation, gastroesophageal reflux and aspiration, and a host of disorders that reside within these dysfunctions.

XI Accessory Nerve (SVE)

The **XI accessory nerve** lives up to its name: its primary responsibility is to work with the IX glossopharyngeal and X vagus nerves to perform their functions. The XI accessory nerve has spinal and cranial components and is responsible for direct innervation of the sternocleidomastoid and trapezius muscles via its special visceral efferent component (see Figure 7–11). It also works with the X vagus to innervate muscles of the pharynx, larynx, and velum (except the tensor veli palatini, which is innervated by the V trigeminal, and the cricothyroid muscle of the larynx).

Motor activation is by means of two sets of nuclei and two branches. The cranial root of the XI accessory nerve arises from the nucleus ambiguus of the medulla, exiting the cranial vault through the jugular foramen. The **cranial component** serves the X vagus functions of the recurrent laryngeal nerve. The **spinal component** of the XI accessory arises from the first five spinal segments and exits the central nervous system with the cranial component. The spinal root innervates the sternocleidomastoid and trapezius muscles.

The primary dysfunction arising from a lesion to the XI accessory is paralysis of the trapezius or sternocleidomastoid. A lesion affecting one side of the sternocleidomastoid muscle will result in the individual not being able to turn his or her head toward the side of the lesion. Trapezius paralysis results in reduced ability to elevate one's arm, as well as causing a drooping shoulder on the side of the lesion.

XII Hypoglossal Nerve (GSE)

The **XII hypoglossal** is a general somatic efferent nerve whose function is to activate muscles of the tongue (Figure 7–12). Needless to say, this is a critical muscle for speech function but also is important for swallowing. In the medulla, the hypoglossal nucleus gives rise to this nerve, which exits the skull through the hypoglossal foramen. It innervates all intrinsic muscles of the tongue and all extrinsic tongue muscles as well, with the exception of the palatoglossus, which is technically a muscle of the velum.

Lesions of the XII Hypoglossal Nerve

The XII hypoglossal nerve is responsible for activating all muscles of the tongue. The tongue is the most important and widely used articulator for speech, so damage to this nerve will have deep and profound impact on speech intelligibility. Unilateral lower motor neuron lesion will cause the tongue to protrude toward the side of the lesion, with the injured side being low in muscle tone. Atrophy will ensue, and fasciculations may be present due to damage to the cell body. Upper motor neuron lesion may result in hypertonia and impaired movement, resulting in a spastic component.

Lesion to the XII hypoglossal nerve will result in muscular weakness of tongue muscles. If the lesion is of the cranial nerve itself, the paralysis will be ipsilateral relative to the lesion. This means a left cranial XII lesion will paralyze the left tongue muscles. The classic test for ipsilateral weakness is to protrude the tongue. Protrusion of a non-paralyzed tongue is accomplished through bilateral contraction of several muscles and results in a non-deviated tongue. When one side of the tongue is paralyzed, the other, non-paralyzed side over-

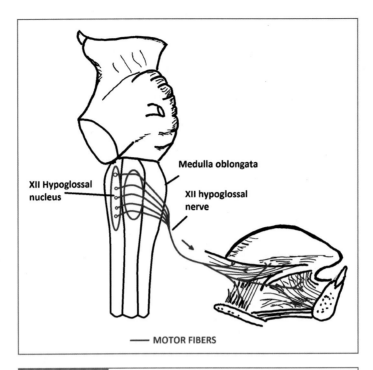

FIGURE 7–12. Origins of XII hypoglossal nerve. Note that the hypoglossal nerve innervates all muscles of the tongue.

XII Hypoglossal nucleus

Medulla oblongata

XII hypoglossal nerve

—— MOTOR FIBERS

whelms it, causing the tongue to deviate toward the weak side (or toward the lesion). If the lesion is an upper motor neuron lesion (such as in the corticobulbar tract), the deficit will be seen on the side opposite the lesion because of decussation of the tract. The differentiating characteristics will include atrophy and perhaps tongue fasciculations for lower motor neuron lesion, and hypertonicity and even spasticity for the upper motor neuron lesion. In all cases, the tongue protrudes toward the side of the paralyzed muscles.

CHAPTER SUMMARY

Cranial nerves are a bedrock concept for speech-language pathology and audiology.

- Cranial nerves may be classified as either sensory, motor, or mixed sensory-motor. They are also categorized relative to function: general or specialized and as visceral or somatic.
- The I olfactory nerve mediates smell, and the II optic nerve communicates visual information.
- The III oculomotor, IV trochlear, and VI abducens nerves are motor nerves that provide eye movement.
- The V trigeminal nerve innervates muscles of mastication, as well as the tensor veli palatini and tensor tympani. It mediates sensation from the face, mouth, teeth, mucosal lining, and tongue.
- The VII facial nerve is responsible for activation of muscles of the face. The sensory component serves taste of the anterior two-thirds of the tongue.
- The VIII vestibulocochlear nerve mediates auditory and vestibular sensation.
- The IX glossopharyngeal nerve mediates the sense of taste in the posterior tongue, as well as somatic sense from the tongue, fauces, pharynx, and auditory tube. Motor function of the IX glossopharyngeal includes the stylopharyngeus and superior pharyngeal constrictor.
- The X vagus nerve serves many autonomic and somatic motor functions. Somatic sensation of pain, touch, and temperature from the region of the eardrum is mediated by the vagus, as well as pain sense from pharynx, larynx, esophagus, and other areas. The recurrent laryngeal nerve (RLN) and superior laryngeal nerve (SLN) activate the intrinsic laryngeal muscles. The pharyngeal branch of the X vagus combines with the IX glossopharyngeal nerve to innervate muscles of the pharynx, with the RLN innervating the cricopharyngeus muscle associated with swallowing.
- The XI accessory nerve innervates the sternocleidomastoid and trapezius muscles and collaborates with the vagus in the activation of palatal, laryngeal, and pharyngeal muscles.
- The XII hypoglossal nerve innervates the muscles of the tongue with the exception of the palatoglossus.

CASE STUDY 7–1

Physician's Notes on Initial Physical Examination and History

This is a 22-year-old male who was referred for neurological assessment regarding dysar-thria. The patient completed high school and was referred from the army. He has 3 siblings, all alive and well. His family has a negative history of epilepsy (see Table 7–3 for terminology. Note that we are presenting the data of this case in chronological order to show the emerging speech

TABLE 7–3.	Terminology for Case Study 7–1
"e" score	Scoring on the *Frenchay Dysarthria Assessment* (FDA). See Table 7–4 for details on scoring the Frenchay.
1-0-2	Medical shorthand for 1 tablet in the morning, none in midday, and 2 tablets in the evening.
Babinski sign	This refers to the plantar reflex that is elicited when the sole of the foot is stimulated with a blunt instrument. This sign involves an extension of the hallux.
Benzhexol	See trihephenidyl hydrochloride.
Brain volume or weight	Brain volume refers to the volume of either the gray or white matter, or both. Brain volume decreases with atrophy.
Encephalitis	Inflammation of the brain due to viral infection. Its symptomatology mimics influenza (fever and/or headache) with confused thinking.
Epilepsy	This neurological disorder includes a disruption in the activities of the neurons. Its symptomatology involves seizures, unusual sensations, and typically loss of consciousness.
Frenchay Dysarthria Assessment (FDA)	A standardized test to assess nonspeech and speech movements of lips, jaw, tongue, phonation, intelligibility, etc. (see Table 7–4 for details concerning scoring of the FDA).
Gliosis	Damage to the central nervous system may create gliosis or proliferation of glial cells (astrocytes, microglia, etc.).
Levetiracetam (active ingredient), Keppra (brand name) 500 mg	Used to treat seizures in epilepsy.
Nocte	Every night.
Olanzepine (active ingredient), Zyprexa (brand name) 2.5 mg	Used to treat schizophrenia and bipolar disorders.
Phenobarbitone (active ingredient)	Used to treat seizures in epilepsy by reducing brain activity.
Phenytoin (active ingredient), Dilantin (brand name)	Used to treat seizures in epilepsy by reducing brain activity.
tid	3 times a day.
Tonic clonic seizure	One type of seizure involving stiffening in the muscles (tonic) and rhythmical jerking (clonic).
Trihephenidyl hydrochloride (active ingredient), Benzhexol (brand name) 2 mg	Used for the treatment of Parkinson's disease.
Valproic acid (active ingredient), Depakene (brand name) 500 mg	Used to treat various types of seizure disorders and manic depression.

and language signs and symptoms as the condition progresses.). The patient was admitted to the hospital at the age of 8½ months for treatment of encephalitis. The disease left the patient with dysarthria, decreased tongue movements, reduced mental function, dysphagia especially in liquids, and learning difficulties. During admission, the patient exhibited seizures and was treated with a combination of **phenytoin** and **phenobarbitone** for a few years. Thereafter, the medications were discontinued. At the age of 16, the patient started having complex partial seizures with occasional secondary generalization to **tonic-clonic seizures**. At that point, he was given **valproic acid**, to which levetiracetam was added later on. The EEG captured focal and generalized epileptiform discharges. An MRI scan of the brain five years previously showed high involvement of the cortex (to a lesser extent the subcortical white matter) surrounding the Sylvian fissure and along the central sulcus bilaterally. There was also a concomitant loss of cortical **brain volume** of the insular cortex bilaterally. The basal ganglia, brainstem, cerebellum, ventricular system, and basal cisterns all appeared to be normal. The impression for this patient is **gliosis** with loss of volume involving the perisylvian fissure and insula bilaterally.

Current Physical Examination and Medications

The patient's vital signs were normal. He exhibited frequent head tremor and adventitious movements in his upper and lower extremities. Speech was not possible because his tongue was immobile. Reflexes were increased throughout, and he had bilateral **Babinski** responses. Medications at examination were valproic acid 500 mg **tid**, **levetiracetam** 500 mg **1-0-2**, **olanzepine** 2.5 mg **nocte**, and **Benzhexol** 2 mg in the morning.

Medical Diagnosis

Encephalitis-induced **epilepsy** and moderate dysfunction especially affecting speech areas

Three Months Following Intake: Speech Examination

The patient was alert to time and place. During the assessment, no speech was produced by the patient except grunting.

The *Frenchay Dysarthria Assessment* was given to the patient (see Table 7–4 for details of Frenchay scoring). The patient demonstrated severe difficulty resulting in "e" **scores** in most of the domains assessed regarding tongue movement. More specifically:

TABLE 7–4.	Frenchay Scoring Details

The *Frenchay Dysarthria Assessment* (FDA) utilizes a rating scale for all testing.

a score	Normal for age
b score	Mild abnormality noticeable to skilled observer
c score	Obvious abnormality but the patient can perform task/movements with reasonable approximation
d score	Some production of task but poor in quality, unable to sustain, inaccurate, or extremely labored
e score	Unable to undertake task/movement/sound

- Reflexes (swallow): Patient able to swallow ice cream or purees, but no choking was observed ("d" score).
- Tongue component (protrusion): Patient was unable to protrude/retract tongue to lip ("e" score).
- Tongue component elevation: No movement of the tongue when the patient tried to elevate it (e).
- Tongue component lateral: No lateral tongue movement produced (e).
- Tongue component: Diadochokinetic rate of the word /kala/ was not attained by the patient at all (e).
- Tongue during speech: No tongue movement during speech (e).

Speech-Language Diagnosis

Flaccid dysarthria or severe apraxia of speech. The results correlated with the neurologist's impression of primarily flaccid dysarthria. A differential diagnosis for this patient may be severe apraxia of speech, but further testing is needed to rule out the planning component.

Questions Concerning This Case

1. This patient contracted encephalitis in infancy. What is the mechanism of encephalitis, and what are the potential sites of lesion for the disease condition?
2. Do the areas of the brain identified in the MRI explain the flaccid dysarthria? Do they explain presence of apraxia of speech?

Case provided by Dr. Kostas Konstantopoulos, European University Cyprus.

CASE STUDY 7–2

Physician's Notes on Initial Physical Examination and History

This 62-year-old male was seen by the audiology clinic in January 2010 for sudden hearing loss. His history was remarkable for having worked in construction during his youth, at which time he was involved with demolition using a jackhammer in highly reverberant environments (concrete grain elevators). Despite this ongoing construction noise exposure, his audiogram from 2002 (at 53 years of age) showed essentially normal hearing for his age, with no threshold exceeding 25 dB HL (Figure 7–13; note that we are presenting the data of this case in chronological order to show the emerging speech

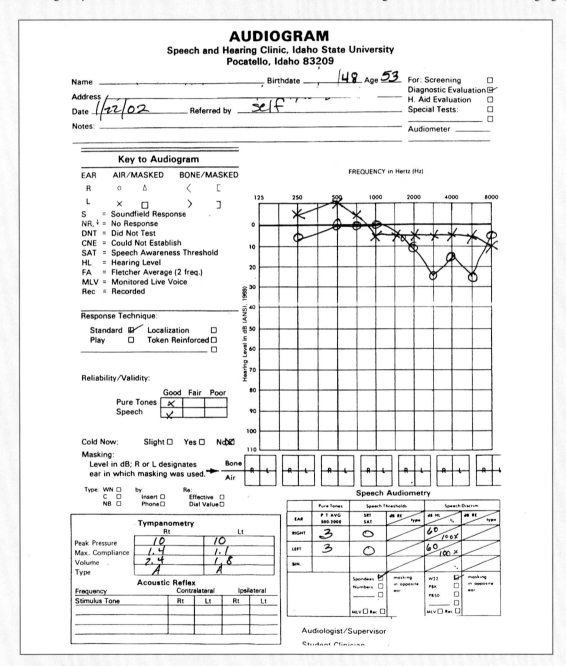

FIGURE 7–13. Premorbid audiogram showing normal thresholds at age 53 despite extreme noise exposure in youth.

and language signs and symptoms as the condition progresses). Notably, he had exercised excellent hearing care, including always wearing hearing protection in noisy environments, beginning in his mid 30s. His thresholds in September 2009 (Figure 7–14) revealed that his loss had increased to 40 dB HL in the right ear at 4 kHz, and less significant high-frequency loss in the left ear. At the time of the consultation the patient was a faculty member in speech and hearing at a state university.

The patient reported that on January 29, 2010 he was sitting in a faculty meeting when he had a sudden and severe hearing loss (Figure 7–15), with right ear loss of 70 dB HL at 4 kHz, and five frequencies in the right ear exceeding 40 dB HL. The left ear configuration was similar, but with approximately 10 dB less loss. The patient reported that, at the time, speech and music were severely distorted, sounding like a sound system that was overdriven and peak-clipped. The patient immediately called his otolaryngologist and acquired a prescription for a cor-

ticosteroid (prednisone), taken orally. Within 10 hours his hearing began to improve, returning to its previous levels within a day. The otolaryngologist diagnosed the patient as having sudden sensorineural hearing loss (SSHL).

This scenario repeated on April 2 of the same year (Figure 7–16), again with right ear thresholds reaching 70 dB HL. Again prednisone was prescribed, with the resulting declination of threshold maximum to 50 dB HL in the left ear at 4 kHz. The patient was fitted with binaural open hearing aids and adapted successfully to their use. He experienced bouts of hearing loss at a rate of approximately three times per year, always treated with prednisone to good result.

Otolaryngological Consultation and Assessment

The patient was referred to the University of Utah medical school otolaryngological clinic and was seen in February 2011 by a specialist in Meniere's disease. Assessment included pure-tone and speech testing, as well as consultation

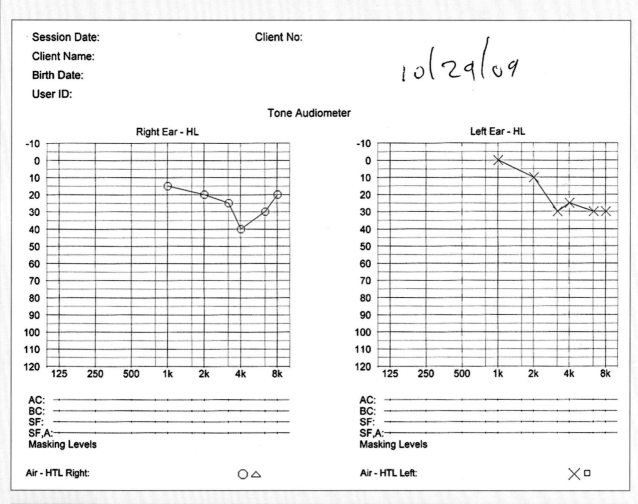

FIGURE 7–14. Increased hearing loss at age 61, showing right-ear 4 kHz notch indicative of noise-induced hearing loss. Note that this is prior to the acute stage of sudden sensorineural hearing loss.

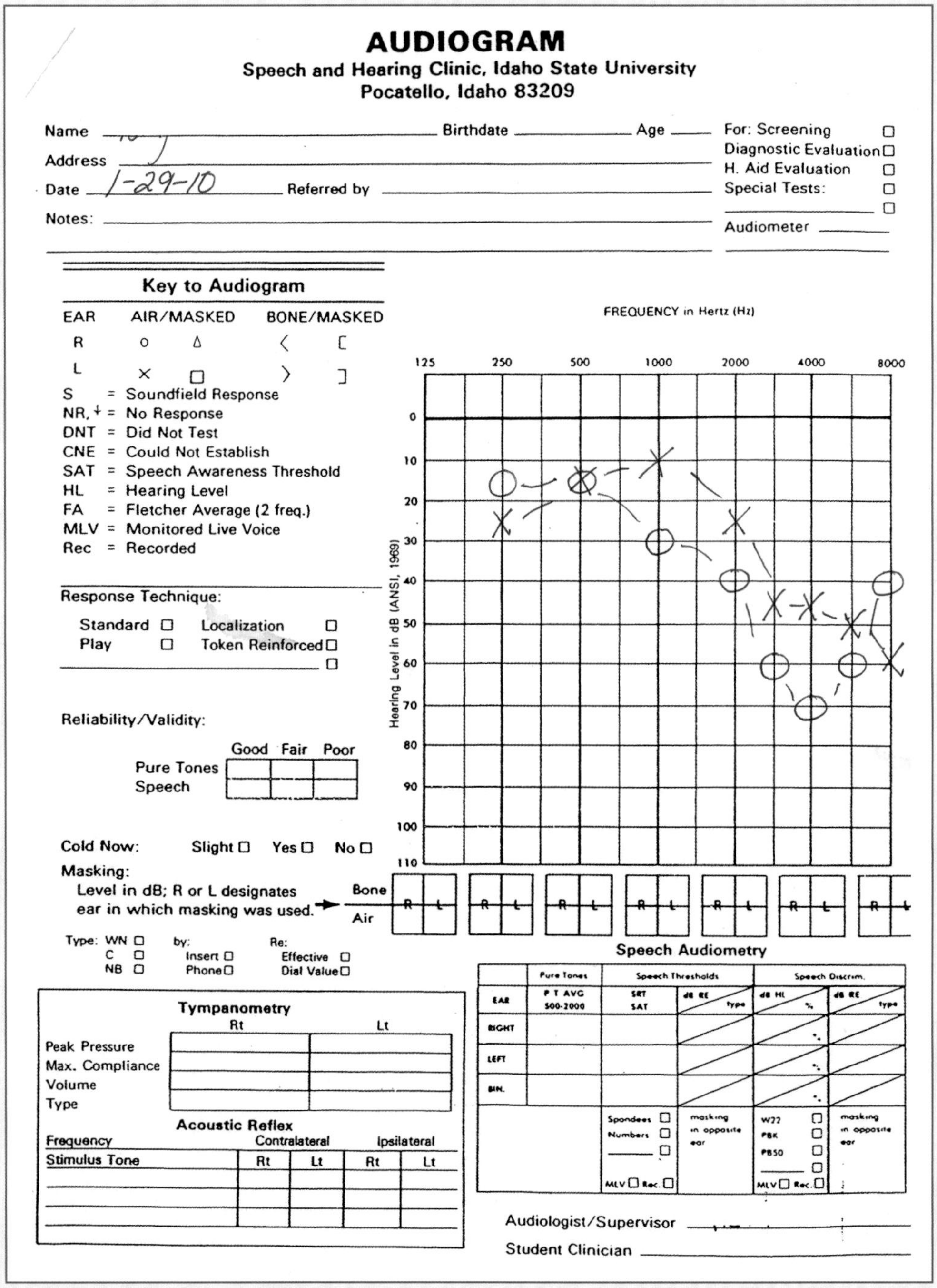

FIGURE 7–15. Acute stage of first attack of sudden sensorineural hearing loss. Note that the right ear 4 kHz loss is now 75 dB HL, and the left ear has increased hearing loss as well.

concerning the patient's history. A tentative diagnosis of immune-mediated hearing loss was made, and the patient was placed on a chemotherapy medication that has the effect of damping immune function. The effects of the medication were sufficiently noxious that the patient discontinued its use.

At one point approximately two years after terminating the medication the patient received inoculation for the influenza virus and shingles on the same day. Subsequently he had a return of hearing loss that was treated with prednisone. Unlike previous events, once the course of prednisone was terminated the hearing declined again and a second

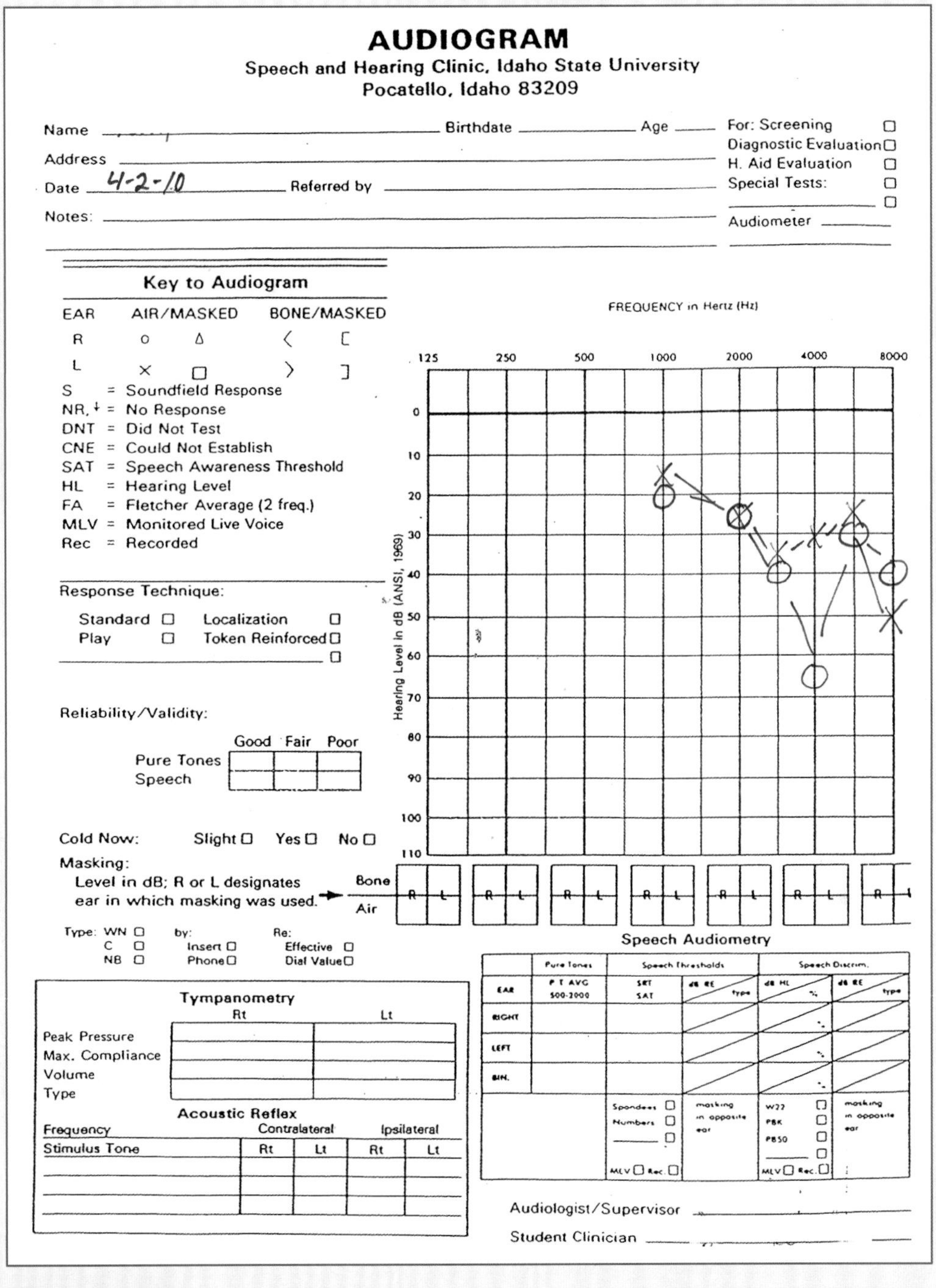

AUDIOGRAM
Speech and Hearing Clinic, Idaho State University
Pocatello, Idaho 83209

Name _____ Birthdate _____ Age ____
Address _____
Date **4-2-10** _____ Referred by _____
Notes: _____

For: Screening ☐
Diagnostic Evaluation ☐
H. Aid Evaluation ☐
Special Tests: ☐
☐
Audiometer _____

Key to Audiogram

EAR	AIR/MASKED	BONE/MASKED
R	o Δ	< [
L	× ☐	>]

S = Soundfield Response
NR,↓ = No Response
DNT = Did Not Test
CNE = Could Not Establish
SAT = Speech Awareness Threshold
HL = Hearing Level
FA = Fletcher Average (2 freq.)
MLV = Monitored Live Voice
Rec = Recorded

Response Technique:

Standard ☐   Localization ☐
Play ☐   Token Reinforced ☐
_____ ☐

Reliability/Validity:

	Good	Fair	Poor
Pure Tones			
Speech			

Cold Now: Slight ☐ Yes ☐ No ☐

Masking:
Level in dB; R or L designates
ear in which masking was used.

Type: WN ☐   by: Re:
C ☐   Insert ☐   Effective ☐
NB ☐   Phone ☐   Dial Value ☐

Tympanometry

	Rt	Lt
Peak Pressure		
Max. Compliance		
Volume		
Type		

Acoustic Reflex

	Contralateral		Ipsilateral	
Stimulus Tone	Rt	Lt	Rt	Lt

FREQUENCY in Hertz (Hz)

Speech Audiometry

Audiologist/Supervisor _____
Student Clinician _____

FIGURE 7–16. Acute stage of second SSHL attack.

course was initiated, with successful outcome. It was hypothesized that the vaccinations had activated his immune response, thereby causing reactivation of the hair cell damage.

Current Status

The patient was fitted for new hearing aids in March 2017. His audiogram showed a 60 dB loss at 4 kHz in both ears, with similar but lesser losses in the frequencies above 4 kHz (Figure 7–17).

Discussion

Immune-mediated sudden hearing loss is reasonably uncommon, and in this manifestation was considered to be a variant of Meniere's disease. The confirmation arising

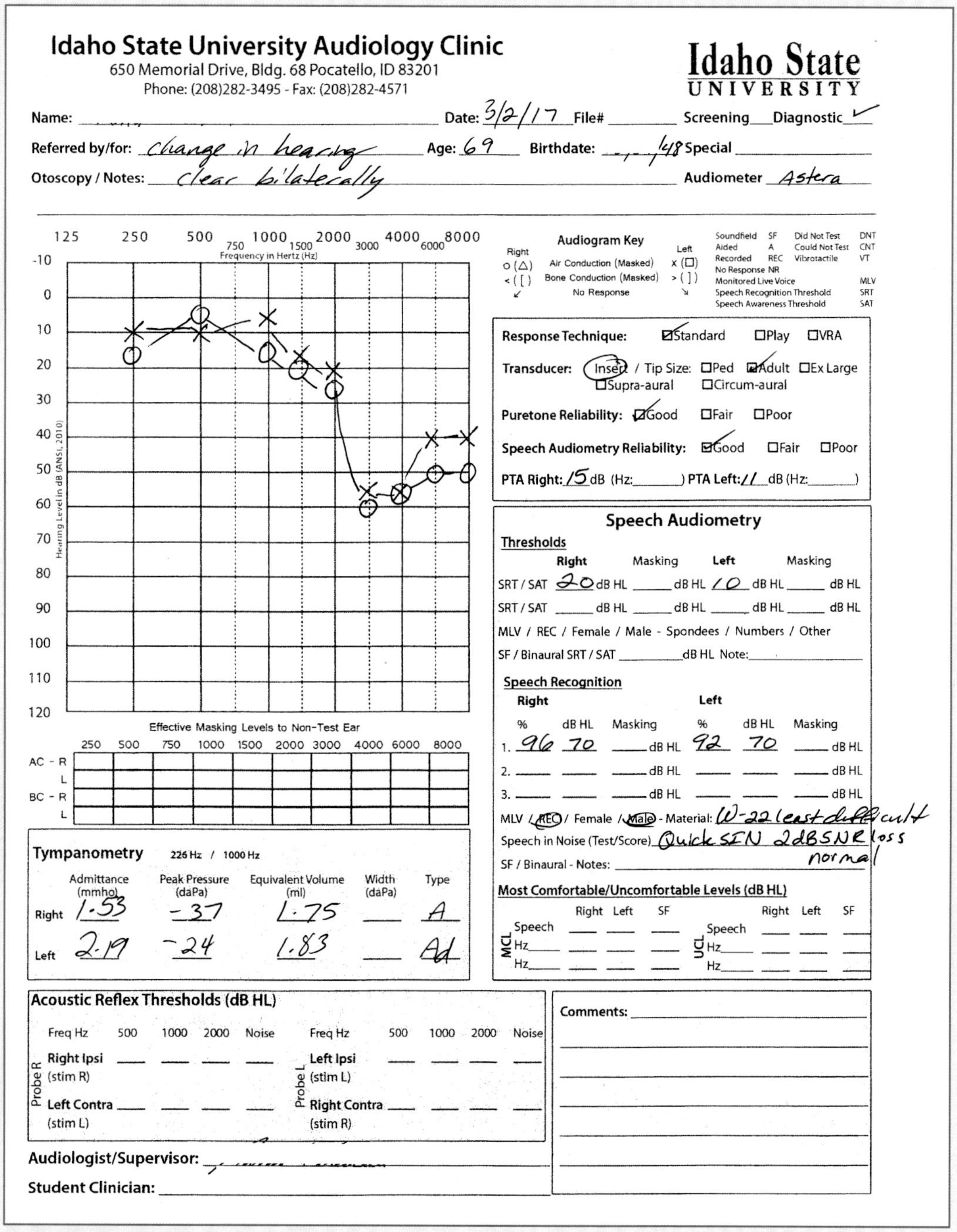

FIGURE 7–17. Stable hearing at hearing aid fitting, age 69. Note that the right ear 4 kHz loss has stabilized at 60 dB HL.

from the vaccination response gives strong support to the diagnosis. It is hypothesized that the early noise exposure made the hair cells more vulnerable to immune attack, since the 4 kHz region is a classical sign of noise-induced hearing loss.

Questions Concerning This Case

1. The double inoculation seemed to trigger a significant hearing loss that required a second dose of prednisone to reduce the effects. How could vaccination trigger a hyperfunctional immune response?

2. This individual had a history of noise exposure that should have left him with the classic "Carhart notch" at 4 kHz much earlier in life than it occurred. How is it that he managed so many years without showing signs of noise exposure, only to have them emerge as a result of his autoimmune disease? Recall that he had begun using hearing protection in his third decade of life and had continued this practice.

From the cases of the Idaho State University Hearing Clinic.

STUDY QUESTIONS FOR CHAPTER 7

1. Cranial nerves that mediate both sensation and motor function are termed _____ _____.

2. Cranial nerves that innervate skeletal muscle are termed somatic/visceral (circle one) nerves.

3. The sense of pressure on the skin would be considered a special/general (circle one) sensation.

4. Please match term and descriptor

   a. general somatic afferent

   b. special somatic afferent

   c. special somatic afferent

   d. general visceral afferent

   e. special visceral afferent

   f. general visceral efferent

   g. general somatic efferent

   _____ This class of nerves mediate special senses of taste and olfaction through chemoreceptors.

   _____ This class of nerve mediates sensation from special sensors, including vision and hearing.

   _____ This class of nerve mediates information from the viscera of the body, such as the digestive tract.

   _____ This class of nerves activate autonomic muscles and glands that are not under voluntary control.

   _____ This class of nerve conveys information to the brain about the state of the body, pressure or movement across the skin, temperature, pain, length of muscles, and movement and position of joints.

   _____ This class of nerves activate skeletal muscle.

5. True or False: Hemianopsia refers to loss of half of the visual field.

6. True or False: Bitemporal hemianopsia occurs from a lesion to the calcarine sulcus.

7. _____ This term means drooping of the eyelid.

8. Please identify number and name of the nerve being described.

a. I have a toothache in my upper lateral incisor. This nerve and branch mediate the sense of pain from that tooth.

_____ _____; _____ branch

b. This nerve (number and name) mediates the sense of smell.

_____ _____

c. Sensors for this nerve (number and name) are embedded in the nasal mucosal lining.

_____ _____

d. This nerve (number and name) does not synapse in the thalamus.

_____ _____

e. This nerve (number and name) mediates the sense of vision.

_____ _____

f. This nerve (number and name) is the only cranial nerve that does not enter the brainstem.

_____ _____

g. Output of this nerve (number and name) ultimately arrives at the calcarine sulcus of the occipital lobe.

_____ _____

h. Light accommodation occurs as a result of this cranial nerve (number and name).

_____ _____

i. Muscles innervated by this nerve (number and name) turn the eyeball down and out.

_____ _____

j. Muscles innervated by this nerve (number and name) abduct the eyeball.

_____ _____

k. I feel a fly walking above my eye. This nerve and branch mediate the perception.

_____ _____; _____ branch

l. The lateral geniculate body is a thalamic nucleus that is served by this nerve (number and name).

_____ _____

m. I have an itch on my chin. This nerve and branch mediate the sense to my brain.

_____ _____; _____ branch

n. I chew my food. This nerve and branch activate the muscles of mastication.

_____ _____; _____ branch

o. I taste my food with the front of my tongue. This nerve (number and name) mediates the sense of taste for that part of my tongue.

____ _____

p. I move my lips. This nerve (number and name) mediates the motor function of the facial muscles.

____ _____

q. I hear my name called. This nerve and branch mediate the sense of hearing.

____ _____; _____ branch

r. I am dizzy because I have labyrinthitis. This nerve and branch mediate the sense of balance.

____ _____; _____ branch

s. I taste something on the back of my tongue. This nerve (number and name) mediates the sense of taste for the posterior tongue.

____ _____

t. My parotid glands fire. This nerve (number and name) mediates activation of the posterior salivary glands.

____ _____

u. My sublingual glands fire. This nerve (number and name) activates the anterior salivary glands.

____ _____

v. My vocal folds adduct when I cough. I can thank this nerve and branch for adducting my vocal folds.

____ _____; _____ _____ nerve

w. My fundamental frequency changes when I sing. I can thank this nerve and branch for control of fundamental frequency.

____ _____; _____ _____ nerve

x. Bell's palsy arises from damage to this nerve (number and name).

____ _____

y. This nerve and branch mediate the sense of taste of the epiglottis.

____ _____; _____ branch

z. This nerve (number and name) is responsible for innervating the sternocleidomastoid, although it also works with the IX glossopharyngeal and X vagus.

____ _____

aa. This nerve (number and name) innervates the muscles of the tongue.

____ _____

9. The outer/inner (circle one) hair cells are responsible for the amplifier function of the cochlea.

10. The outer/inner (circle one) hair cells are responsible for frequency resolution in the cochlea.

11. Afferent fibers from the outer/inner (circle one) hair cells are sparsely represented in the VIII vestibulocochlear nerve.

REFERENCES

Baehr, M., & Frotscher, M. (2012). *Duus' topical diagnosis in neurology: Anatomy, physiology, signs, symptoms* (5th ed.). New York, NY: Thieme.

Barlow, S. M., & Estep, M. (2006). Central pattern generation and the motor infrastructure for suck, respiration, and speech. *Journal of Communication Disorders, 39*(5), 366–380.

Buck, L. B., & Bargmann, C. I. (2013). Smell and taste: The chemical senses. In E. R. Kandel, J. H. Schwartz, T. M. Jessell, S. A. Siegelbaum, & A. J. Hudspeth (Eds.), *Principles of neural science* (5th ed., pp. 712–743). New York, NY: McGraw-Hill.

Carpenter, M. B. (1991). *Core text of neuroanatomy* (4th ed.). Baltimore, MD: Williams & Wilkins.

Fields, R. D. (2007). Sex and the secret nerve. *Scientific American Mind, 18*, 20–27.

Fuller, G. N., & Burger, P. C. (1990). Nervus terminalis (cranial nerve zero) in the adult human. *Clinical Neuropathology, 9*(6), 279–283.

Gilman, S., Newman, S. W., Manter, J. T., & Gatz, A. J. (1996). *Manter and Gatz's essentials of clinical neuroanatomy and neurophysiology*. Philadelphia, PA: F. A. Davis.

Goldberg, M. E., Walker, M. F., & Hudspeth, A. J. (2013). The vestibular system. In E. R. Kandel, J. H. Schwartz, T. M. Jessell, S. A. Siegelbaum, & A. J. Hudspeth (Eds.), *Principles of neural science* (3rd ed., pp. 917–934). Norwalk, CT: Appleton & Lange.

Guinan Jr., J. J. (2010). Cochlear efferent innervation and function. *Current Opinion in Otolaryngology & Head and Neck Surgery, 18*(5), 447.

Hudspeth, A. J. (2013). The inner ear. In E. R. Kandel, J. H. Schwartz, T. M. Jessell, S. A. Siegelbaum, & A. J. Hudspeth (Eds.), *Principles of neural science* (3rd ed., pp. 654–681). Norwalk, CT: Appleton & Lange.

Hudspeth, A. J. (2014). Integrating the active process of hair cells with cochlear function. *Nature Reviews. Neuroscience, 15*(9), 600.

Mackay, L. E., Chapman, P. E., & Morgan, A. S. (1997). *Maximizing brain injury recovery*. Gaithersburg, MD: Aspen.

Mast, F. W., & Ellis, A. W. (2015). Internal models, vestibular cognition, and mental imagery: Conceptual considerations. *Multisensory Research, 28*(5–6), 443–460.

McNaughton, B. L., Knierim, J. J., & Wilson, M. A. (1995). Vector encoding and the vestibular foundations of spatial cognition: Neurophysiological and computational mechanisms. In M. S. Gazzaniga (Ed.), *The cognitive neurosciences* (pp. 585–595). Cambridge, MA: MIT Press.

Meister, M., & Tessier-Lavigne, M. (2013). Low-level visual processing: the retina. In E. R. Kandel, J. H. Schwartz, T. M. Jessell, S. A. Siegelbaum, & A. J. Hudspeth (Eds.), *Principles of neural science* (3rd ed., pp. 577–601). Norwalk, CT: Appleton & Lange.

Mesholam, R. I., Moberg, P. J., Mahr, R. N., & Doty, R. L. (1998). Olfaction in neurodegenerative disease: A meta-analysis of olfactory functioning in Alzheimer's and Parkinson's diseases. *Archives of Neurology, 55*(1), 84–90.

Musiek, F. E., & Chermak, G. D. (Eds.) (2013). *Handbook of central auditory processing disorder, Nolume I: Auditory neuroscience and diagnosis*. San Diego, CA: Plural.

Pickles, J. O. (2012). *An introduction to physiology of hearing* (4th ed.). Bingley, UK: Emerald Group.

Seikel, J. A., Drumright, D. G., & King, D. W. (2016). *Anatomy & physiology for speech, language, and hearing* (5th ed.). Clifton Park, NY: Cengage Learning.

Smith, P. F., Zheng, Y., Horii, A., & Darlington, C. L. (2005). Does vestibular damage cause cognitive dysfunction in humans? *Journal of Vestibular Research, 15*(1), 1–9.

Spoendlin, H. H. (1984). Primary neurons and synapses. In I. Friedmann & J. Ballantyne, *Ultrastructural atlas of the inner ear* (pp. 133–164). London, UK: Butterworth.

Strominger, N. L., Demarest, R. J., & Laemle, L. B. (2012). *Noback's human nervous system: Structure and function*. New York, NY: Springer Science & Business Media.

Uludag, M., Aygun, N., & Isgor, A. (2017). Innervation of the human cricopharyngeal muscle by the recurrent laryngeal nerve and external branch of the superior laryngeal nerve. *Langenbeck's Archives of Surgery, 402*(4), 683–690.

Whitlock, K. E. (2004). Development of the nervus terminalis: Origin and migration. *Microscopic Research Techniques, 65*(1–2), 2–12.

Zald, D. H., & Pardo, J. V. (1997). Emotion, olfaction, and the human amygdala: Amygdala activation during aversive olfactory stimulation. *Proceedings of the National Academy of Sciences, 94*(8), 4119–4124.

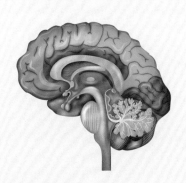

8 CEREBELLAR ANATOMY AND PHYSIOLOGY

INTRODUCTION

Above all, we are sensate beings. You can envision the cerebral cortex as the structure responsible for integrating sensory information and making cognitive and linguistic sense of it. In the same fashion, you can envision the cerebellum as the mechanism by which we make physical sense of our world, in a very real way. The cerebellum integrates all of the disparate sensations of the body into a non-cognitive, non-linguistic whole for the purpose of knowing our physical universe and for acting through that physical universe on our environment.

The cerebellum makes up the largest component of the central nervous system, being made up of 69 billion neurons (compared with the 18 billion neurons of the cerebral cortex) (Azevedo et al., 2009; Herculano-Houzel, 2009). Despite this extreme neural density, the cerebellum has exquisitely organized cellular structure, which supports its vital function. The cerebellum is responsible for coordinating the motor plan arising from the cerebral cortex with an extraordinary variety and density of body sensory information. In addition to coordination, the cerebellum has a role in memory, cognitive function, and motor skill learning (Akshoomoff & Courchesne, 1992; Raymond, Lisberger, & Mauk, 1996). It interacts with the limbic system, cortical association areas, and the reticular activating system of the brainstem and thalamus.

STRUCTURE OF THE CEREBELLUM

The cerebellum is located at the base of the skull, posterior to the brainstem and ventral to the occipital lobe, and rests in the posterior cranial fossa. If you look at the picture of the central nervous system in sagittal section (Figure 8–1), you will see that the cerebellum is inferior to the cerebral cortex and posterior to the brainstem. The fourth ventricle resides between the brainstem and the cerebellum. The cerebellum is unique in the study in the human brain, in that it receives inputs from multiple areas of the nervous system and sends outputs primarily to three regions: the premotor cortex, the motor cortex, and the brainstem. The cerebellum accomplishes its work through structural division into distinct regions to coordinate balance, accuracy, and movement. While the cerebellum does not affect the strength of muscle contraction, it has a very powerful influence on the coordination of the muscular activity in space and time (Lisberger & Thach, 2013).

Three major fiber bundles hold the cerebellum to the brainstem: the inferior, middle, and superior cerebellar peduncles (Figure 8–2B). You will want to

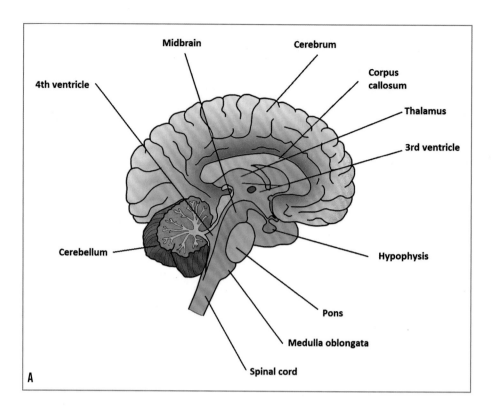

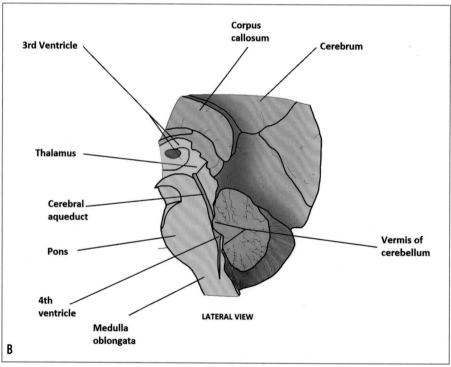

FIGURE 8–1. Cerebellum of the central nervous system. **A.** As seen in sagittal view, posterior to brainstem and inferior to cerebral cortex. **B.** As seen in detail. Note from the sagittal view that the fourth ventricle separates the cerebellum from the brainstem at the level of the pons. *Source: From Seikel/Drumright/King. Anatomy & Physiology for Speech, Language, and Hearing, 5th ed. (with Anatesse Software Printed Access Card). © 2016 Delmar Learning, a part of Cengage, Inc. Reproduced by permission. http://www.cengage.com/permissions*

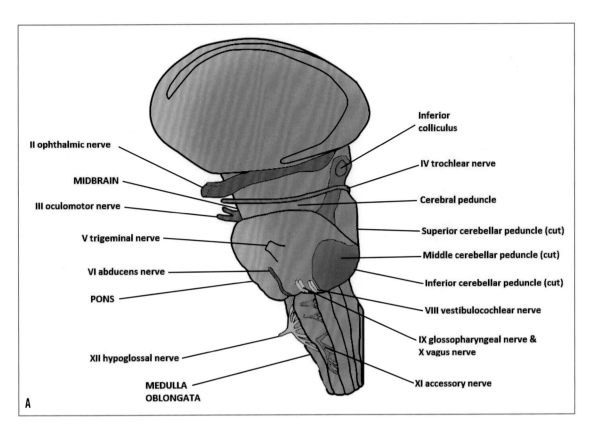

II ophthalmic nerve

MIDBRAIN

III oculomotor nerve

V trigeminal nerve

VI abducens nerve

PONS

XII hypoglossal nerve

MEDULLA OBLONGATA

Inferior colliculus

IV trochlear nerve

Cerebral peduncle

Superior cerebellar peduncle (cut)

Middle cerebellar peduncle (cut)

Inferior cerebellar peduncle (cut)

VIII vestibulocochlear nerve

IX glossopharyngeal nerve & X vagus nerve

XI accessory nerve

A

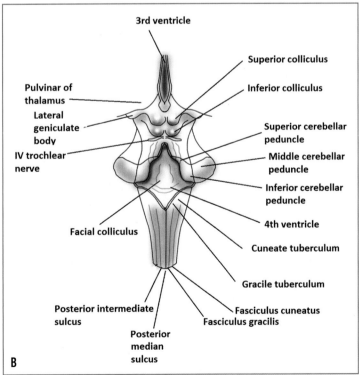

3rd ventricle

Pulvinar of thalamus

Lateral geniculate body

IV trochlear nerve

Facial colliculus

Posterior intermediate sulcus

Posterior median sulcus

Superior colliculus

Inferior colliculus

Superior cerebellar peduncle

Middle cerebellar peduncle

Inferior cerebellar peduncle

4th ventricle

Cuneate tuberculum

Gracile tuberculum

Fasciculus cuneatus

Fasciculus gracilis

B

FIGURE 8–2. Lateral and posterior views of brainstem showing superior, middle, and inferior peduncles. **A.** Lateral view. **B.** Posterior view. Note that with cerebellum removed in the posterior view, the fourth ventricle is revealed. *continues*

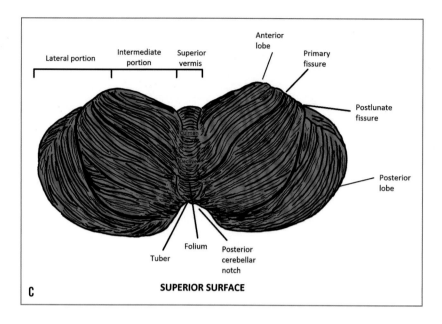

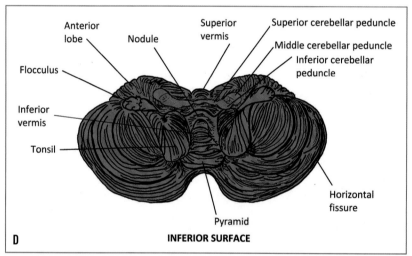

FIGURE 8–2. *continued* **C.** Superior view of cerebellum. **D.** Inferior view of cerebellum, removed from brainstem. On the superior view, note the significant landmarks of vermis, anterior lobe, primary fissure, and posterior lobe. On the anterior view, note the cerebellar tonsil, pyramid, and the important flocculonodular lobe, made up of flocculus and nodulus. *continues*

remember that there are also *cerebral* peduncles that serve as communication conduits for the cerebrum, and these two sets of peduncles can be confused. The **inferior cerebellar peduncle** enters the brainstem at the level of the medulla, while the **middle cerebellar peduncle** makes up the significant bulge that you see on the pons. The **superior cerebellar peduncle** enters the brainstem at the level of the midbrain. These peduncles contain tracts (to be discussed) that bring

sensory information to the cerebellum and that mediate the output of the cerebellum.

You can see from Figures 8–1 and 8–2 that there are some important landmarks that will help us navigate this structure.

In the posterior aspect, you can see the **primary fissure** (see Figure 8–21). The cerebellum is divided into two hemispheres. Each hemisphere is divided into an **anterior** and

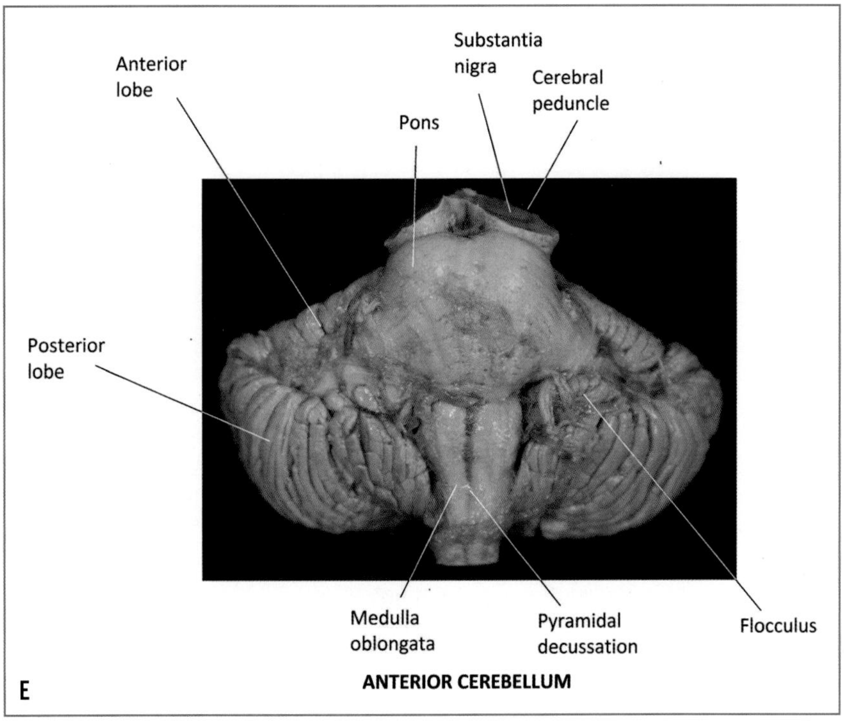
Substantia
nigra
Cerebral
peduncle
Anterior
lobe
Pons
Posterior
lobe
Medulla
oblongata
Pyramidal
decussation
Flocculus
E
ANTERIOR CEREBELLUM

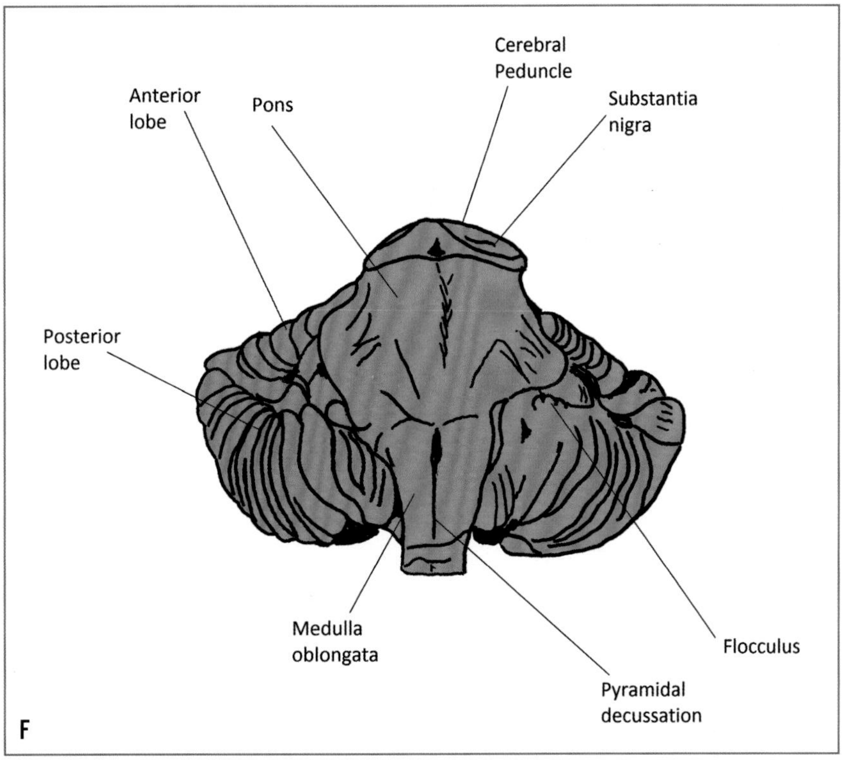
Cerebral
Peduncle
Anterior
lobe
Pons
Substantia
nigra
Posterior
lobe
Medulla
oblongata
Flocculus
Pyramidal
decussation
F

FIGURE 8–2. *continued* Photograph (**E**) and drawing (**F**) of anterior cerebellum *continues*

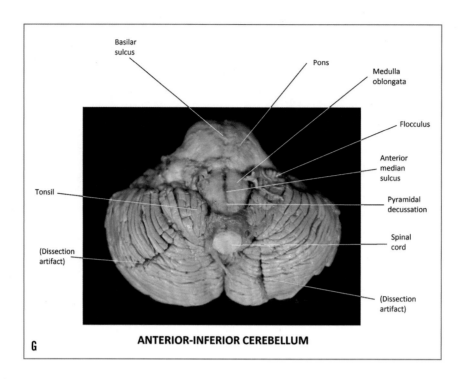

ANTERIOR-INFERIOR CEREBELLUM

G

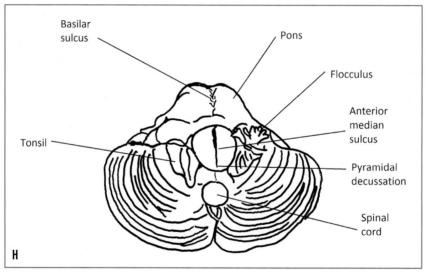

H

FIGURE 8–2.   *continued* Photograph (**G**) and drawing (**H**) of anterior-inferior surface of cerebellum. *continues*

posterior lobe (also known as **superior** and **inferior lobes**), as well as a pair of structures that combine to form a third lobe, the **flocculonodular lobe**.

To see the flocculonodular lobe, you have to remove the cerebellum from the brainstem so you can peer at its anterior surface. The flocculonodular lobe is made up of left and right **flocculi**, with a medially located **nodule** or **nodulus**.

(The term "flocculus" means "tuft of wool," and apparently someone thought that the flocculi of the cerebellum looked like a tuft of wool sticking out from the anterior surface!) The flocculonodular lobe turns out to be a very important lobe for our professions because it mediates information from the vestibular portion of the inner ear. Also in this anterior view, you can see the superior, middle, and inferior peduncles

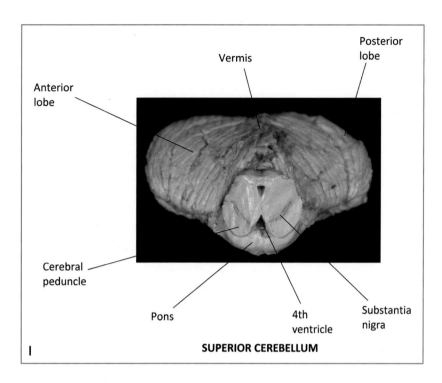

SUPERIOR CEREBELLUM

I

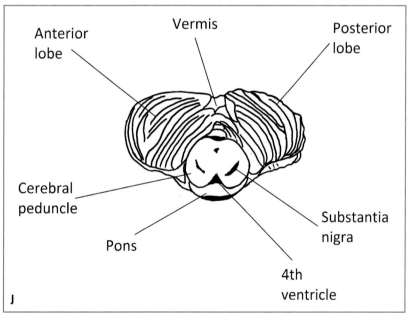

J

FIGURE 8–2. *continued* Photograph (**I**) and drawing (**J**) of superior cerebellum. *continues*

that provide communication with the brainstem. You can also see the **vermis** of the cerebellum. The word "vermis" means "worm," a term describing what the middle portion of the cerebellum looked like. The vermis wraps around the cerebellum so that it is visible from both posterior and inferior views.

These lobes are further separated into lobules and are convoluted by folds or **folia**. Lobules I through V are within

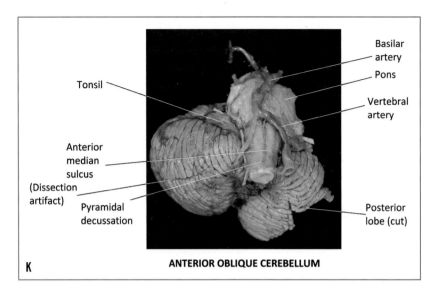

ANTERIOR OBLIQUE CEREBELLUM

K

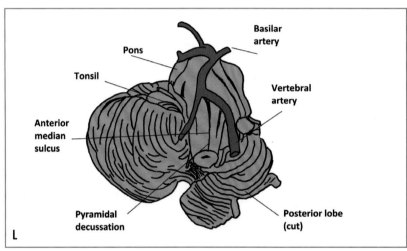

L

FIGURE 8–2. *continued* Photograph (**K**) and drawing (**L**) of anterior-oblique cerebellum.

the anterior lobe, while the posterior lobe includes lobules VI–IX. The flocculonodular lobe includes lobule X.

Besides these anatomical divisions, you can also divide the cerebellum into functional regions: vestibulocerebellum, spinocerebellum, and pontocerebellum (Figure 8–3).

The **vestibulocerebellum** (also known as the archicerebellum because of its age in development of the brain) is critically important for the function of balance. The vestibulocerebellum is made up of the flocculus and nodulus (**flocculonodular lobe**), and projections from the vestibular mechanism arise in this area. The **spinocerebellum** (also known as the **paleocerebellum**: "paleo" means old or ancient) is made up of the anterior lobe and the portion of the posterior lobe that relates to the legs, whose sensory information is conveyed through the spinal cord. The **neocerebel-**

lum (pontocerebellum) derives its original name from the fact that it attaches to the brainstem at the pons. The neocerebellum is the phylogenetically newer component of the cerebellum, and it has a very important relationship with the cerebral cortex. The **neocerebellum** includes the **anterior** lobes and the intermediate vermis.

A cross-section of the cerebellum bears a resemblance to the cerebral cortex. The outer layer (the *cerebellar* cortex) is composed of a very dense set of neurons (to be discussed), with the core of the cerebellum being made up of white matter. Similar to the cerebrum with its subcortical nuclei, at the base of the cerebellum is a set of nuclei that are part of the input and output circuits of the cerebellum.

In summary, the gross structure of the cerebellum consists of two hemispheres and three lobes.

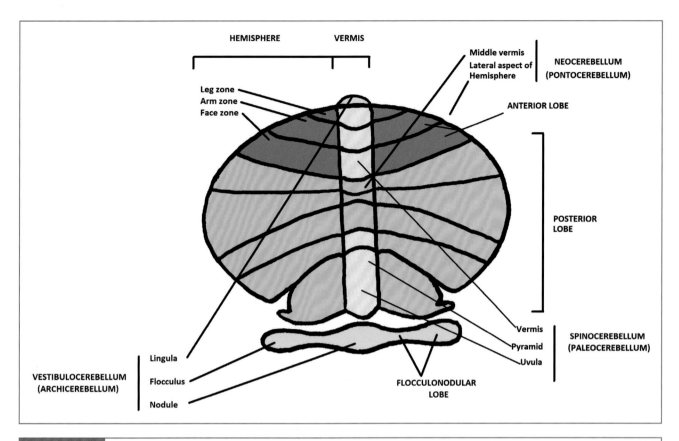

FIGURE 8–3.   Schematic of cerebellum revealing the relationship of components. This view is created by unfolding the cerebellum. Note the proximity of the anterior and posterior lobes to the vermis and flocculonodular lobe. Also, note the important notation relating spatiotopic organization of the cerebellum (leg, arm, and face zone). Finally, recognize the zones indicated by the vestibulocerebellum (flocculonodular lobe), spinocerebellum (vertebral column and cerebrum), and neocerebellum (serving the cerebral cortex).

- The cerebellum is posterior to the brainstem, inferior to the cerebrum, and ventral to the occipital lobe. The fourth ventricle resides between the brainstem and the cerebellum.
- The cerebellum receives inputs from multiple areas of the nervous system and sends output to the premotor and motor cortex and to the brainstem.
- The inferior cerebellar peduncle enters the brainstem at the level of the medulla, the middle cerebellar peduncle enters at the pons, and the superior peduncle enters at the midbrain. These peduncles contain sensory and motor tracts serving the cerebellum.
- The primary fissure divides the cerebellum into two hemispheres, with each hemisphere divided into anterior and posterior lobes. A third lobe is the flocculonodular lobe, which mediates vestibular information. The vermis of the cerebellum wraps around the cerebellum so that it is visible from both posterior and inferior views.
- The vestibulocerebellum (the archicerebellum) is important for balance. It consists of the flocculus and nodulus (flocculonodular lobe). The spinocerebellum (paleocere-

bellum) consists of the anterior lobe and the portion of the posterior lobe related to legs. The pontocerebellum (neocerebellum) interacts primarily with the cerebral cortex. It includes the posterior lobes and the intermediate vermis.

Ataxia

The term **ataxia** refers to a condition involving impaired coordination of motor function, typically including difficulties with regulation of force, timing, and rate of activation. The site of lesion for ataxia is the cerebellum, its pathways, and/or its nuclei. Within this umbrella term, there is a range of symptomatology that shows the complexity and multi-functionality of the cerebellum and that also reflects disruption of specific loops that involve the cerebellum, cerebral cortex, brainstem, and thalamus. While the dominant sign of ataxia is motor dyscoordination, the symptoms can also include cognitive and affective components.

The signs of cerebellar ataxia are diverse, and not all signs are present in all individuals with the condition. Dyscoordination of movement (also known as **asynergia**) is loss of the ability to coordinate movements within systems (e.g., coordinating walking by integrating the leg and trunk muscles with vestibular input) or among systems (e.g., difficulty integrating the motor function of the larynx with that of the respiratory system in speech). A person with ataxia may also exhibit **dysmetria**, which is difficulty predicting distance, and which results in target overshoot and undershoot, as well as range of motion. Individuals with ataxia will also demonstrate **dysdiadochokinesis**, which is difficulty with rapid alternating movements (such as turning the hand from supine to prone position or repeating the syllables "puh-tuh" rapidly). Cerebellar lesions can also result in an **intention tremor**, which is tremor that is seen during a motor act. Intention tremor is particularly strong at termination of the motor act. An example of tremor at termination would be seen in the act of reaching for a glass of water: as your hand reaches the glass, agonist and antagonist muscles work precisely together to guide the final stages of grasping the glass, and this attempt at fine interaction between muscle groups results in a large tremor at termination. Gait of a person with ataxia may be wide-based, and a person with ataxia may have a tendency to fall. A person with ataxia may demonstrate **hypotonia** (low muscle tone), slurred speech (**ataxic dysarthria**), and abnormal eye movements (**nystagmus**).

Disruptions due to lesions in the cortico-ponto-cerebellar loop and cerebello-thalamo-cortical loop are responsible for the major cerebellar signs (Bodranghien et al., 2016). Overt movement activates sensorimotor cortices of the brain together with cerebellar lobules IV–V and VIII contralaterally, while more cognitively demanding tasks activate prefrontal and parietal cortices of the brain together with cerebellar lobules VI and VII. There is evidence that finger-tapping activates the right lobules (IV–V, VII), verb generation activates the right lobules (VI, Crus I, VIIB, VIIIA), and working memory tasks activate bilateral regions of lobules (VI–VII) (Stoodley, Valera, & Schmahmann, 2012). Ataxic dysarthria appears to result from bilateral lesions in the superior areas of the cerebellum, and the right cerebellar hemisphere is implicated in the planning and processing of speech (Spencer & Slocomb, 2007). Focal lesions of the cerebellum that produce ataxic dysarthria may involve the lateral hemispheres and posteromedial or paravermal regions (Duffy, 2013). Similarly, damage to the rostral paravermal region of the anterior lobe was correlated with in articulatory dysfunction of the tongue and orofacial musculature (Urban, Marx, Hunsche, Gawehn, Vucurevic, Wicht, Massinger, Stoeter, & Hopf, 2003).

CELLULAR STRUCTURE OF THE CEREBELLUM

There are three major layers of the cerebellum: the outer molecular layer, the intermediate layer, and the deep granular layer (Figure 8–4). The **outer layer** is made up of **Golgi cells**, **basket cells**, and **stellate cells**. The **intermediate layer** is also referred to as the **Purkinje** layer because of the presence of Purkinje cells (you will recall that we ran across these cells in the cerebrum as well). Purkinje cells are large cells with a prominent dendritic tree and marked single axonal root. In the cerebellum they are arrayed in highly regular rows, much like trees in an orchard. There are 15 million Purkinje cells in the human cerebellum, and their axons project to the cerebellar nuclei. When a Purkinje cell is activated, it inhibits the nucleus with which it synapses. Golgi cells within the outer layer have their dendrites in the outer layer, while their axons project through the Purkinje layer to terminate in the granular layer, which houses granule cells and mossy fibers. Basket cells and stellate cells of the outer molecular layer communicate with the dendrites of Purkinje cells.

The cellular level of the cerebellum is a complex set of excitations and inhibitions, faintly reminiscent of the circuitry of the basal ganglia. The players in this activity include the Purkinje cells, which provide the sole output for the cerebellum, climbing fibers (arising from the olivary nuclei of the pons), mossy fibers (also arising from the olivary nucleus), Golgi cells, stellate cells, and parallel fibers. Parallel fibers run through the dendritic trees of Purkinje cells, effectively linking many cells.

Afferent input to the cerebellum comes from all regions of the body and takes many forms. Much input comes directly from the ipsilateral vestibular nuclei and the ipsilateral spinal cord. Very important input is from the cerebral cortex via the contralateral pontine nuclei and the **olivary nuclei** of the medulla. The olivary nuclei receive input from the spinal cord, the cerebral cortex, the red nucleus, and the optic tract, and the olive gives rise to climbing fibers. Climbing fibers ascend through the granular layer to make strongly excitatory synapse with the dendrites of the Purkinje cells. Mossy fibers, on the other hand, make up the majority of the afferent inputs, but have a lesser effect on the Purkinje cells. Mossy fibers arise from the same sources (spinal cord, cerebral cortex, olivary complex, vestibular nuclei), but don't synapse directly with Purkinje cells. Instead, mossy fibers synapse with Golgi cells and granule cells. Golgi cell output inhibits the granule cell, which in turn inhibits the Purkinje cells. When granule cells are excited, they cause excitation in the Purkinje cells. The role of the Purkinje cell is to either cause excitation or inhibition of the final output nuclei of the cerebellum (to be discussed). *If the Purkinje cell related to a specific input is excited, it will inhibit the output related to that input. If the Purkinje cell is inhibited relative to a specific input, the nuclei will have an excitatory response in relation to*

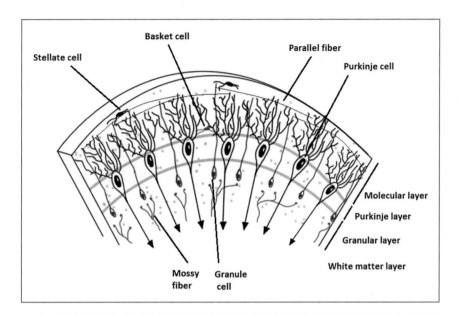

FIGURE 8–4.   Cellular representation within the cerebellar cortex. Note that the outer molecular layer is largely populated by the stellate cells, basket cells, Golgi cells (not shown), and dendrites of Purkinje cells. The intermediate Purkinje layer consists predominantly of Purkinje cells. The inner granular layer is made up of granule cells and mossy fibers.

a specific input. In this way, Purkinje activity in response to a stimulus (e.g., joint position information) damps the output of the cerebellar nuclei relative to that stimulus. If there is no sensory input, the Purkinje will allow activation of the cerebellar nuclei. Granule fibers project into the outer layer, with their axons, called parallel fibers, running parallel to the array of Purkinje cells and making synapse with the dendrites of many Purkinje cells, much like a power line or telephone wire running through the branches of a tree. In this manner, the granule cells excite Purkinje cells and thus inhibit cerebellar output.

The cerebellum doesn't initiate movement, but rather is responsible for error-checking. Essentially, the cerebellum is a computer. Just as the computer in an automobile takes information about the air pressure, temperature of the air and engine, and humidity and calculates precisely the best fuel mix to optimize gasoline mileage, the cerebellum takes the body's information about joint position, muscle tone and contraction, pressure on the skin, and so on, and calculates the amount of force that will be required to complete a given targeted task.

There are zones of sensation and response in the motor system, referred to as **multizonal microcomplexes** (MZMC), which monitor different sensory/motor subunits for errors. The cerebellum is functionally divided into sagittal zones of approximately 1 to 2 mm in width, and Purkinje cells within a zone are innervated by climbing fibers arising from a specific neuron in the olivary nuclei. The output of those specific

Purkinje cells is sent to specific, mapped regions of the cerebellar nuclei. In this manner, the climbing fibers precisely organize the Purkinje cells and their output based on the spatiotopic maps of the olivary nuclei, making the function of the climbing fibers critical to the error-correction function itself (Apps & Garwicz, 2005). Mossy fibers provide a more diverse input to the cerebellum, since mossy fibers cross microzones to innervate multiple Purkinje cells. It appears that mossy fibers are responsible for the plasticity seen in the cerebellum, supporting modification of output based on motor skill learning. The climbing fiber terminates the action of the Purkinje when a specific microcomplex reports successful completion, and the Purkinje will actively stimulate output of the cerebellar nuclei as long as that condition has not been met. The mossy fibers interact with the climbing fibers through the parallel fibers, and it appears that this interaction allows not only motor learning but storage of motor plans (Apps & Garwicz, 2005).

The cellular architecture of the cerebellum is so highly organized that some authors have referred to it as "crystalline" (Apps & Garwicz, 2005). This exquisite structure underlines the notion that there is typically a reason that a structure evolved. The climbing fibers and granule cells are clear examples of that. The climbing fibers communicate directly with Purkinje cells, strongly exciting them. Granule cells project into the outer layer and then project into a "T" formation whose arms extend to interact with over 1,000 Purkinje cells within the arborization of the dendrite. This input inhibits a field of Purkinje cells from firing, while the specific climbing fiber excites the specific Purkinje cell <u>to</u> fire.

To summarize, there are three major layers of the cerebellum.

- The outer molecular layer is made up of Golgi cells, basket cells, and stellate cells. The intermediate (Purkinje) layer is dominated by Purkinje cells, with a prominent dendritic tree and marked single axonal root. When a Purkinje cell is activated, it inhibits the nucleus with which it synapses. Axons of Golgi cells project through the Purkinje layer to terminate in the granular layer that houses granule cells and mossy fibers. Basket cells and stellate cells of the outer molecular layer communicate with the dendrites of Purkinje cells.
- Much afferent input to the cerebellum comes from the ipsilateral vestibular nuclei and the ipsilateral spinal cord. The cerebral cortex sends information through the contralateral pontine nuclei and to olivary nuclei of the medulla, which also receive input from the spinal cord, the red nucleus, and the optic tract.
- Climbing fibers ascend and synapse with Purkinje cells. Mossy fibers synapse with Golgi cells and granule cells. Golgi cell output inhibits the granule cell, which in turn inhibits the Purkinje cells. When granule cells are excited, they will cause excitation in the Purkinje cells. When the Purkinje cell is excited, it will inhibit the output related to a given input.
- The cerebellum is responsible for error-checking. The cerebellum integrates the body's information about joint position, etc. and calculates the amount of force that will be required to complete a given targeted task.
- There are zones of sensation and response in the motor system, referred to as multizonal microcomplexes (MZMC), which monitor different sensory/motor subunits for errors. Climbing fibers precisely organize Purkinje cells and their output based on the spatiotopic maps of the olivary nuclei. Mossy fibers are responsible for the plasticity seen in the cerebellum, supporting modification of output based on motor skill learning.

Ataxic Cerebral Palsy

A child with perinatal involvement of the cerebellum and its pathways will demonstrate the same difficulties with gait, dysmetria, and dyscoordination that you see with adults. This disorder in children is termed ataxic cerebral palsy. Two separate and very large issues play into the disorder in children. First, the disorder is not immediately diagnosed at birth. The signs of ataxia aren't present until between 18 and 24 months of age, when muscle groups and systems become coordinated. The second large dif-

ference between ataxic cerebral palsy and acquired ataxia is that the disorder is part of the background of motor development for the child, as opposed to a new condition to which someone must adapt. Because of this, therapy for a child with ataxic cerebral palsy should begin as soon as diagnosis is made.

Treatment for a child with ataxic cerebral palsy may include speech-language therapy, occupational therapy (OT), and physical therapy (PT). Because this is an issue with the act of coordinated motor execution, therapy will focus on practicing the motor act across all of these domains (speech, OT, and PT). The child may have experienced feeding problems as an infant, and will likely have difficulties with bolus manipulation and swallowing as a child, and this will be an important focus of therapy as well. As a speech-language pathologist, you will have the job of helping this child learn the skilled patterns of speech and swallowing necessary for life.

NUCLEI OF THE CEREBELLUM

The cerebellum has four pairs of nuclei: the fastigial, dentate, emboliform, and globose (or blobular) nuclei. All of these nuclei receive their input from the Purkinje cells (Figure 8–5) and project exclusively to the ventrolateral and ventromedial nuclei of the thalamus. The ventromedial and ventrolateral nuclei are the "motor nuclei" of the thalamus, projecting in turn to both motor planning and motor execution regions of the cerebral cortex.

All nuclei project to either the ventromedial nucleus or ventrolateral nucleus (Paek et al., 2015). These nuclei project to areas of the cerebrum associated with motor planning and execution areas. Specifically these are areas for executive function (BA 46 and 9), areas associated with planning complex movement (supplemental motor area [SMA], pre-SMA, and the premotor region BA 6) (Morel, Liu, Wannier, Jeanmonod, & Rouiller, 2005), and the areas associated with motor execution (BA 4 and BA 7b of the intraparietal sulcus) (Voogd, 2003). You will recall that BA 4 is the precentral gyrus (a.k.a., motor strip), while BA 7b of the parietal lobe is part of the intraparietal sulcus region associated with the dorsal visual stream motor integration region that is responsible for reaching and grasping. Thus, the nuclei associated with leg (intermediate zone) and arm/face (lateral zone) project to regions associated with planning and executing fine motor acts. In addition to direct cortical control, the **fastigial nucleus**, which receives its input from the vermis, projects to the vestibular nuclei of the brainstem, the reticular formation of the pons and medulla, and the inferior olivary complex. The **emboliform** and **globose nuclei** provide input

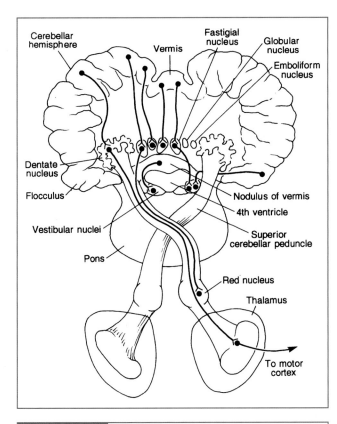

reticular formation of the brainstem (via the **uncinate fasciculus**). The vermis sends its input to the fastigial nucleus, and from there the efferent information is sent via the inferior cerebellar peduncle to reticular nuclei (**reticulospinal tract**) and vestibular nuclei (**vestibulospinal tract**) in the brainstem. Thus, output of the vestibular nuclei projects to the fastigial nucleus and then is sent back to the vestibular nuclei and the reticular formation in the brainstem, forming a "functional loop," providing maintenance of balance.

Globose and Emboliform Nuclei

Cerebral cortex efferents serve the vermis (**spinocerebellum**), which in turn serves the globose and emboliform nuclei. The efferents from these nuclei terminate in the red nucleus, the source of the rubrospinal tract involved in maintenance of muscle tone and background movement. Dorsal and ventral spinocerebellar tracts convey information from muscle, joint, and cutaneous receptors to the vermis and paravermis, and subsequently to the globose and emboliform nuclei. Efferent information from the globose and emboliform nuclei is sent through the rubrospinal tract to the lower motor neurons, controlling muscle tone and posture.

Dentate Nucleus

This is the largest of the cerebellar nuclei. The cerebral cortex motor command is transmitted to the pontine nuclei to the cerebrocerebellum. Efferent stimulation from the Purkinje cells of that region terminate on the dentate nucleus, which, in turn, project through the superior cerebellar peduncle to the contralateral red nucleus and ventral lateral nucleus of the thalamus. The thalamic nucleus projects back to the motor strip (BA 4 and 6), supplemental motor area (SMA), and premotor cortices to provide feedback and correction of the motor plan. Some authors suggest there are four closed cerebro-cerebellar loops that connect cerebellar regions with regions in the frontal cortex associated with the processing of motor and cognitive tasks (Krienen & Buckner, 2009). This element of the cerebellum provides precision in planning (premotor BA 6), mental rehearsal (SMA), and fine control of movement (BA 4 and 6), particularly of more complicated motor actions (BA 6), by directing the efferent information to the corticospinal and corticobulbar pathways.

To summarize, the cerebellum has four pairs of nuclei.

- All of these nuclei receive their input from the Purkinje cells and project exclusively to the ventrolateral and ventromedial nuclei of the thalamus.
- The dentate nuclei ultimately project to both motor planning and motor execution regions of the cerebral cortex. Output of the dentate nuclei project to either the ventromedial or ventrolateral nucleus, which project to motor planning areas of the cerebrum.

FIGURE 8–5. Schematic of output of cerebellar nuclei. Nuclei within the deep white matter of the cerebellum include the globose, emboliform, fastigial, and dentate nuclei. Note that nuclei receive their input from the Purkinje cells of the cerebellar cortex. All nuclei project output to either the ventrolateral or ventromedial nucleus of the thalamus. Output from these nuclei then project to areas associated with body sensation (BA 7, part of the motor planning area for reaching, and a component of the dorsal visual stream), motor planning (BA 4, 6 and supplementary motor area), or motor execution (BA 4). *Source:* From Seikel/King/Drumright, *Anatomy and Physiology for Speech, Language, and Hearing*, 3E. © 2005 Delmar Learning, a part of Cengage, Inc. Reproduced by permission. http://www.cengage.com/permissions

to the red nucleus (source of the rubrospinal tract), supporting muscle tone to the legs (Voogd, 2003; Voogd, 2011; Voogd & Glickstein, 1998). Here are brief summaries of each nucleus.

Fastigial Nucleus

This nucleus receives its input from the vestibular mechanism via the vestibulocerebellum, and it sends its output as feedback either to the ipsilateral vestibular nuclei (via the **fastigiobulbar tract**) or the contralateral vestibular nuclei and

- The fastigial nucleus receives its input from the vermis and projects to the vestibular nuclei of the brainstem, the reticular formation of the pons and medulla, and the inferior olivary complex.
- The emboliform and globose nuclei provide input to the red nucleus (source of the rubrospinal tract), supporting muscle tone to the legs. They receive input from the vestibular mechanism and are important for balance function. These nuclei also provide input to the red nucleus for maintenance of muscle tone and background movement.
- The dentate nuclei are the largest of the cerebellar nuclei. The motor command from the cerebrum is transmitted to the pontine nuclei and then to the cerebrocerebellum. Output of the dentate nuclei provides feedback and correction of the motor plan of the cerebrum.

TRACTS SERVING THE CEREBELLUM

Because the cerebellum has the responsibility for integrating somatic sense with motor function, it must receive detailed information concerning all of the body senses that could play into movement (Figure 8–6). There are many afferent and efferent pathways, consisting of tracts that provide information about body sense, as well as those that supply output of the cerebellum to the cerebrum. Figure 8–7 may help in this discussion, as well as examination of Table 8–1.

Input to the Cerebellum

The cerebellum consists of three functional zones: the leg zone, the arm zone, and the face zone (Voogd, 2003, 2011). These zones are reminiscent of the topographical maps we've discussed in the cerebral cortex (e.g., the tonotopic map of the primary auditory cortex; the somatosensory maps of the postcentral gyrus and the insular cortex; the motor strip homunculus; the map of the intraparietal sulcus). In contrast to these maps, however, the zonal map is coarser, in that the resolution seen in the other maps has not been as clearly elucidated. Another interesting aspect is that the cerebellar maps are patchy, with areas of non-activity interspersed with clear spatial map to body region. This lack of clarity in the maps most likely reflects our lack of knowledge concerning cerebellar anatomy and physiology as opposed to its actual function. (For a thorough and fascinating review of the discovery of the cerebellar map, see Voogd, 2011.) The presence of these representational zones will aid our discussion of the tracts.

In addition to these zonal features, the cerebellum is divided anatomically into regions based on area served. Vestibular input is received by the vestibulocerebellum, which consists of the flocculonodular lobe, also known as the archicerebellum). Input from the trunk and abdominal regions is directed to the vermis, uvula, and the pyramids, known as

the paleocerebellum. The neocerebellum includes the middle portion of the vermis (lobule VI) and the cerebellar hemispheres. The region of the neocerebellum receiving input from the spinal cord is termed the spinocerebellum, while the region of the neocerebellum receiving input from the cerebral cortex is referred to as the pontocerebellum because these cortical fibers terminate in the pontine nuclei before entering the cerebellum.

The pathways that serve these regions of the cerebellum receive input from diverse sensors throughout the body. Here we'll briefly describe them.

Vestibulocerebellar Pathways

The vestibular pathways transmit information generated in the vestibular mechanism of the inner ear. Afferent information passes through the vestibular branch of the VIII vestibulocochlear nerve to the vestibular nuclei of the pons and to the flocculonodular lobe of the cerebellum via the inferior cerebellar peduncles. This vestibular input provides information about the precise location of the head in space, as well as its acceleration.

Dorsal Spinocerebellar Tract

The dorsal spinocerebellar tract transmits information concerning temperature, proprioception (muscle spindle), and touch that arises in the lower body and legs. This information is conveyed to the ipsilateral cerebellum, with afferents arising from the nucleus dorsalis (Clarke's column) in the spinal cord and projecting to both the anterior and posterior lobes of the cerebellum.

Cuneocerebellar Tract

This tract mediates the sense of temperature, proprioception (muscle spindle stretch), and tactile sensation from the arms and upper trunk. Information originates in the external cuneate nucleus of the cervical region and enters the cerebellum through the inferior cerebellar peduncle.

Ventral Spinocerebellar Tract

This tract sends information about proprioception (Golgi tendon organs [GTOs]) and pain sense arising in the legs and lower trunk to the ipsilateral cerebellar cortex. The fibers of this pathway decussate in the spinal cord, ascend, and enter through the superior cerebellar peduncle. They then decussate again to project to the cerebellar cortex.

Rostral Spinocerebellar Tract

This tract arises from the cervical spinal cord, providing proprioception (GTO) and pain sense from the upper trunk and

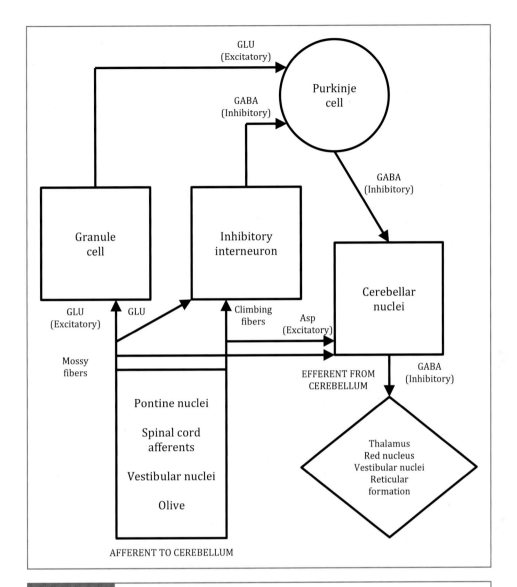

FIGURE 8–6.   Cellular actions in the cerebellum. Note that the inputs to the cerebellum are the pontine nuclei, spinal cord, vestibular nuclei, and olivary nuclei. Mossy fibers and climbing fibers are excitatory to granule cells, which in turn excite Purkinje cells. Excitation of Purkinje cells causes inhibition of the cerebellar nuclei, eliminating or reducing the output of those nuclei relative to that specific input information. Both mossy and granule fibers can have an inhibitory effect if they activate inhibitory interneurons, in which case the output of the cerebellum will be excitatory to the cerebellar nuclei. Note: GLU = glutamate; ASP = Aspartate aminotransferase; GABA = Gamma aminobutyric acid. *Source:* Based on model of Baehr and Froscher (2012).

arms. It also undergoes a double decussation, similar to the ventral spinocerebellar pathway.

Pontocerebellar Tract

Fibers of the pontocerebellar tract are vital to smooth and accurate motor function. Projection from the parietal, occipital, temporal, and frontal lobes of the cerebral cortex synapse on the pontine nuclei, and efferents from these nuclei project via pontocerebellar fibers to mossy fibers of the opposite cerebellar cortex via the middle cerebellar peduncle. Mossy fibers synapse with granule cells, which in turn synapse with Purkinje cell dendrites. The Purkinje cell output to the dentate nucleus is routed back to the cerebellar cortex and, importantly, to the motor cortex of the cerebrum via the superior cerebellar peduncle and thalamus. This mechanism

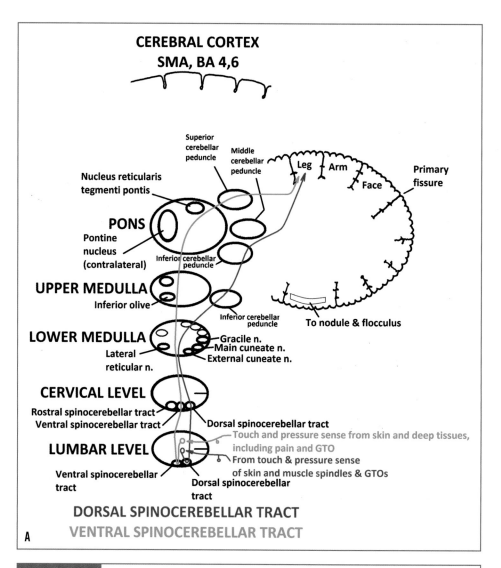

FIGURE 8–7. Schematic of afferent pathways of the cerebellum. **A.** The dorsal spinocerebellar tract mediates somatic information from the skin (touch and pressure) and muscle (muscle spindle and GTO) through the inferior cerebellar peduncle, terminating in the cerebellar cortex. The ventral spinocerebellar tract conveys pain and GTO information from skin and deep tissues, through the superior cerebellar peduncle and terminating in the cerebellar cortex. *continues*

allows the motor command for voluntary movement that arises in the cerebral cortex to be modified by the cerebellum to meet the immediate conditions of the body in space. By sending the output back to the cerebellum, the new plan can be compared with cerebral cortex output to ensure that the corrected plan was followed.

Olivocerebellar Tract

Fibers from this tract arise from the inferior olivary and medial accessory olivary nuclei of the medulla. They decus-

sate and project to the contralateral cerebellum, terminating as climbing fibers. Input to the olive includes visual information, motor plan information from the cerebral cortex, afferent information from the spinal cord, and output of the red nucleus.

Cerebellar Peduncles

One final cerebellar topic concerns specific pathways of the peduncles. In a way, the cerebellar peduncles are the interchanges of a vast network of highways.

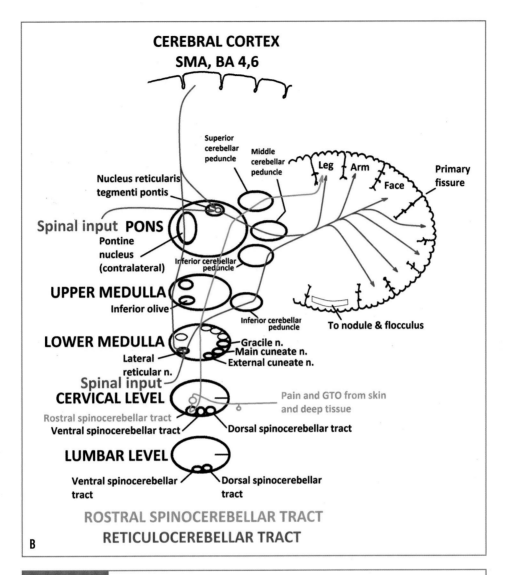

FIGURE 8–7. *continued* **B.** The rostral spinocerebellar tract conveys information from skin and deep tissues concerning touch, pressure, and GTO, passing through the inferior peduncle and terminating in the cerebellar cortex. The reticulocerebellar tract conveys cortical input concerning the motor plan. This information descends through the anterior pons, synapsing with pontine nuclei before descending to the lateral reticular nucleus of the lower medulla. It combines with spinal cord afferents and ascends through the inferior peduncle to terminate on the cerebellum. *continues*

Superior Cerebellar Peduncle

The **superior cerebellar peduncle** (also known as the *brachium conjunctivum*) arises from the anterior cerebellar hemisphere, coursing through the lateral wall of the fourth ventricle. Most pathways within the superior cerebellar peduncle are efferent in nature and decussate at the level of the inferior colliculi. Dentatorubral and dentatothalamic fibers arise from the dentate nucleus and synapse in the opposite red nucleus and thalamus. The ventral spinocerebel-

lar tract ascends within this peduncle, and fibers from the fastigial nucleus descend in conjunction with this peduncle as they course to the lateral vestibular nucleus. This feedback loop provides a mechanism for adjusting the motor plan even as it is being executed.

Middle Cerebellar Peduncle

The **middle cerebral peduncle** (a.k.a., *brachium pontis*) consists of the afferent fibers of the pontocerebellar tract that

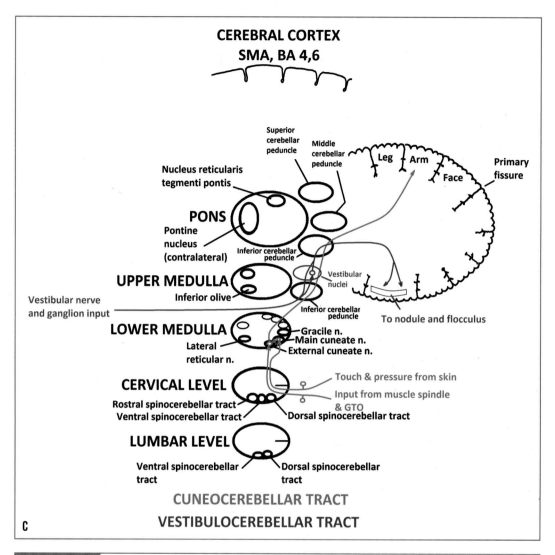

CEREBRAL CORTEX
SMA, BA 4,6

FIGURE 8–7. *continued* **C.** The vestibulocerebellar mediates information concerning the position of body in space through the inferior cerebellar peduncles, terminating at the flocculonodular lobe. The cuneocerebellar tract carries touch and pressure information from the skin, passing through the inferior cerebellar peduncle and terminating in the cerebellar cortex.

project from the contralateral pontine nuclei. These fibers are a continuation of the input from the cerebral cortex, with most of the input arising from the frontal lobe of the cerebrum.

Inferior Cerebellar Peduncle

The **inferior cerebellar peduncle** (a.k.a., restiform body) provides the conduit for the spinocerebellar tracts, and contains the largest diversity of pathways of the three peduncles.

To summarize, input to the cerebellum takes many forms.

- The vestibulocochlear nerve afferents arising from the vestibular nuclei converge on the flocculonodular lobe of the cerebellum within the vestibulocerebellum.
- The olivocerebellar tract arises from the inferior olive of the brainstem and projects to the cerebrocerebellum. The accessory olive provides input to the vestibulocerebellum and spinocerebellum. Both inferior and accessory olivary nuclei process sensory information from the limbs.
- The posterior spinocerebellar tract arises from the thoracic nucleus of Clarke's column within the gray matter of the spinal cord, conveying muscle spindle information from

TABLE 8–1.	Some Pathways Providing Input to the Cerebellum	
Category	**Pathway**	**Function**
Afferent from cortex concerning motor plan	Corticopontine tract	Information about the motor plan to the pontine nuclei and inferior olive
	Olivocerebellar tract and pontocerebellar tract	Delivers information from the corticopontine tract efferent to the cerebellum: this provides the motor plan from BA 4 and 6 (motor and premotor)
Information about where the body is in space	Vestibulocerebellar tract	Balance from vestibular system
	Reticulocerebellar tract	Muscle tension (Golgi tendon organ [GTO]) from spinal cord (joins with cortical output)
	Cuneocerebellar tract	This mediates upper limb stretch sensors (muscle spindle)
	Dorsal and rostral spinocerebellar tract	Muscle spindles (stretch) and GTO (tension)
	Ventral (anterior) spinocerebellar tract	Skin, deep tissue (pain and GTO)
Output from the cerebellum to the cortex	Dentothalamic and dentorubral tracts	Efferent from the cerebellum to the cerebral cortex

the lower limbs to the vermis region of the anterior and posterior lobes of the cerebellum.

- The fastigiobulbar tract provides feedback to the vestibular nuclei from the vestibulocerebellum.
- The cerebelloreticular tract carries information from the fastigial nuclei to the reticular formation of the brainstem.
- The cerebello-olivary tract carries information from the dentate nucleus to the olivary complex.

CEREBELLUM AND MOTOR CONTROL

You can't help but marvel at the exquisitely "clean lines" of the cerebellum: it is like a fine timepiece, in more ways than one! The cerebellum is endowed with very graceful architecture that undergirds its abilities, and its ultimate role is to regulate the rate, range, and force of motor function through integration of body sense with the motor plan.

It is important to realize that the cerebellum doesn't initiate motor function. Its role is to monitor body states, through information supplied to it by the millions of sensors throughout the body, and to use that information to inform the motor control process. Second, it is not solely involved in

motor function. There is growing evidence that the cerebellum is involved in cognitive function, emotional control, and language function (Baillieux, De Smet, Paquier, De Deyn, & Mariën, 2008; Rapoport, van Reekum, & Mayberg, 2000; Schmahmann & Caplan, 2006). The cerebellum is also deeply involved in motor learning, and perhaps some other types of learning, but damage to the cerebellum does not result in an inability to learn.

The cerebellum is the means by which we achieve fine motor control, and anything that degrades the cerebellum will affect our ability to execute motor actions efficiently and effectively. We can look at cerebellar control function from the view of the anatomical divisions described earlier. One of our phylogenetically earliest needs was to navigate in space, so the input from the vestibular system to the flocculonodular lobe (archicerebellum) is obviously critical to smooth and organized fine motor control. Damage to the archicerebellum will result in trunk ataxia, staggering, and generally reduced response to motion (as in reduced vestibular responses or motion sickness).

The anterior lobe is phylogenetically newer and is involved in integration of sensory information associated with antigravity muscles. You may recall that the muscle stretch reflexes are responsible for maintaining muscle state against continuous forces such as gravity, and damage to the paleocerebellum can result in excessive stretch reflexes of support musculature.

The newest of these structures is the posterior (inferior) lobe (neocerebellum), which is involved in termination of movements, particularly of the hands. Because the hands are so involved in fine motor activity, damage to this lobe will cause **dysmetria**, which is the inability to control target acquisition due to overshoot and undershoot, as well as a tremor associated with termination of movement. Damage to this lobe can also result in low muscle tone (**hypotonia**) and gait problems. The cognitive deficit we alluded to earlier can arise from damage to the neocerebellum, and there can be loss of emotion control with damage to the vermis (Akshoomoff & Courchesne, 1992). Durisko and Fiez (2010) found that the motor component of simple, monosyllable speech retrieval and working memory involve the superior-medial cerebellum more than other areas, while the superior-lateral and inferior cerebellar regions are engaged in working memory not involving speech. When the speech is more complex (e.g., production of three-syllable words), lobule VI and crus I/II in the superior cerebellum and lobule VIII in the inferior cerebellum are involved (Bohland & Guenther, 2006). Bilateral activation is essential to these tasks.

One overarching theory of cerebellar function in cognition holds that the cerebellum seems to work as an internal timing system for providing temporal knowledge in cognitive tasks (Keren-Happuch, Chen, Ho, & Desmond, 2014; Koch, Oliveri, Torriero, Salerno, Gerfo, & Caltagirone, 2007). The cerebellum has specific multiple roles in emotion identification, executive function (decision making), music (rhythmic synchronization tasks), and working memory (Keren-Happuch et al., 2014; Stoodley, Valera, & Schmahmann, 2012). For language function, multiple areas of the cerebellum are activated during both expressive <u>and</u> receptive language tasks such as verb generation and reading, covert word repetition, and semantic discrimination (Keren-Happuch et al., 2014; Stoodley et al., 2012). Again, reflect on the fact that our prior views of the cerebellum were purely motor in nature, and the significant revision to this concept is that non-vocalized expression and the act of perception both activate the cerebellum.

In speech, the cerebellum is responsible for sequencing and adapting the motor sequence for overlearned syllables in order to produce words and sentences (Ackermann, 2008). Damage due to an ischemic stroke in the right anterior vermal and paravermal regions (supplied by the superior cerebellar artery) will produce speech characteristics of ataxic dysarthia (see a relevant case study at the end of the chapter).

In summary, the cerebellum is a critical system of motor control for the cerebrum.

- The cerebellum regulates the rate, range, and force of motor function through integration of body sense with the motor plan. The cerebellum doesn't initiate motor function, rather it monitors body states and uses that information to inform the motor control process. The cerebellum is involved in motor learning, and perhaps some other types of learning, but damage to the cerebellum does not result in an inability to learn.

- The cerebellum is the means by which we achieve fine motor control. The flocculonodular lobe is critical to smooth and organized fine motor control. The anterior lobe is involved in integration of sensory information associated with anti-gravity muscles. The posterior lobe is involved in termination of movements, particularly of the hands.

CHAPTER SUMMARY

The cerebellum is a critically important structure that supplies a means of integrating body sense with motor function.

The cerebellum receives inputs from multiple areas of the brain and sends outputs primarily to three regions: the premotor cortex, the cortex, and the brainstem.

The cerebellum is divided into both anatomical and functional regions. Anatomically, the inferior cerebellar peduncle enters the brainstem at the level of the medulla, the middle cerebellar peduncle enters at the pons, and the superior peduncle enters the brainstem at the midbrain. Tracts in these peduncles provide communication with the rest of the body. There are two cerebellar hemispheres divided by the primary fissure. Each hemisphere has anterior, posterior, and flocculonodular lobes. The flocculonodular lobe consists of the left and right flocculi and the nodulus. The vermis is the middle portion of the cerebellum.

Functional divisions of the cerebellum include the vestibulocerebellum, spinocerebellum, and pontocerebellum. The vestibulocerebellum is important for the function of balance, while the spinocerebellum relates to leg function. The neocerebellum is involved in monitoring the motor command arising from the cerebral cortex for the purpose of integrating the command with sensory information arriving at the cerebellum.

The cellular structure of the cerebellar cortex is highly organized, based on cortical layers. The outer molecular layer consists of Golgi cells, basket cells, and stellate cells, while the intermediate layer contains Purkinje cells, which inhibit the deep nuclei of the cerebellum and receive input from outer layer Golgi cells, basket cells, and stellate cells. Golgi cells within the outer layer have their dendrites in the outer layer, while their axons project through the Purkinje layer to terminate in the inner granular layer, which houses granule cells and mossy fibers. Afferent input to the cerebellum comes from all regions of the body and includes input from vestibular nuclei, the spinal cord, the cerebral cortex via the contralateral pontine nuclei, and the olivary nuclei of the medulla, muscle spindle, and Golgi tendon organ output, and other proprioceptive sensors.

The cerebellum doesn't initiate movement but is responsible for error-checking. Multizonal microcomplexes (MZMC) monitor different sensory/motor subunits for errors. The cerebellum Purkinje cells within a zone are innervated by climbing fibers arising from a specific neuron in the olivary nuclei, and the Purkinje output is sent to specific cerebellar nuclei.

Nuclei of the cerebellum within the central white matter include the fastigial, dentate, emboliform, and globose nuclei. All receive input from the Purkinje cells and project exclusively to the ventrolateral and ventromedial nuclei of the thalamus. The dentate nuclei ultimately project to both motor planning and motor execution regions of the cerebral cortex. The fastigial nucleus projects to vestibular nuclei, the reticular formation, and the inferior olivary complex. The efferents from the globose and emboliform nuclei terminate in the red nucleus, controlling muscle tone and background movement.

Tracts serving the cerebellum include the vestibulocerebellar pathways, providing information from the vestibular mechanism; the dorsal spinocerebellar tract, with input concerning temperature, proprioception (muscle spindle), and touch from the lower body and legs; the cuneocerebellar tract, which mediates temperature, proprioception (muscle spindle stretch), and tactile sensation from the arms and upper trunk; the ventral spinocerebellar tract, which sends information about proprioception (GTOs) and pain sense arising in the legs and lower trunk; the rostral spinocerebellar tract, which provides proprioception (GTO) and pain sense from the upper trunk and arms; the pontocerebellar tract, providing information from the cerebral cortex via the pontine nuclei; and the olivocerebellar tract, providing visual input, motor plan information, afferent information from the spinal cord, and output of the red nucleus.

There are three cerebellar peduncles. Most pathways within the superior cerebellar peduncle are efferent in nature and decussate within the pons at the level of the inferior colliculi. The middle cerebral peduncle consists of the afferent fibers of the pontocerebellar tract that project from the contralateral pontine nuclei. The inferior cerebellar peduncle provides the conduit for the spinocerebellar tracts and contains the largest diversity of pathways of the three peduncles.

The cerebellum doesn't initiate motor function and is not involved directly in cognitive function, although damage can result in some cognitive deficit and it is involved in some forms of learning. The cerebellum is the means by which we achieve fine motor control, and lesions that degrade the cerebellum affect our ability to execute motor actions efficiently and effectively. Lesions to the anterior lobe can result in excessive stretch reflexes of support musculature. Damage to the neocerebellum can cause dysmetria (the inability to control range of movement), tremor associated with termination of movement, low muscle tone, and gait problems.

CASE STUDY 8–1

Physician's Notes on Initial Physical Examination and History

This is a 26-year-old female who started suffering from **EBV infection** two years previously (see Table 8–2 for terminology. Note that we are presenting the data of this case in chronological order to show the emerging speech and language signs and symptoms as the condition progresses.). Earlier this year, the patient began complaining of **blurred vision**, then **hypoesthesia** in both legs and perhaps on the right side of the body. The symptoms subsided without treatment. Seven years previously, she suffered a sudden left eye visual loss and was diagnosed with **optic neuritis**. She was treated with **steroids (1000 Solu-Medrol i.v.)** and Medrol, with partial response. One month later, she had an episode of loss of speech (dysarthria/anarthria) and difficulty in swallowing (dysphagia). She was examined and admitted to the hospital. **Lumbar puncture** showed **oligoclonal bands** in the cerebrospinal fluid (CSF) using CSF electrophoresis, and the MRI of the head revealed several **hyperintense lesions in the T2** of round shape and moderate size, including within the corpus callosum.

Subsequently, **Rebif 22 mg three times a week** was started as a treatment, but she suffered significant side effects and complained of dizziness and vomiting. Then, Rebif at 40% of the dose was followed and her **symptoms** greatly improved. Due to the clinical history of optic neuritis, long lesion in the spinal cord and **neuromyelitis** were suspected, and treatment with **plasmapheresis, IVIG,** and **methotrexate** was initiated with partial response. Her condition continued to deteriorate and lately, following treatment with IVIG, she stopped walking at all.

Results of the Neurological Examination

Initially, the blurring in the left eye had improved but it now has worsened. There was no **diplopia** or **nystagmus** or

TABLE 8–2. Terminology for Case Study 8–1

"b-c" score	Scoring on the *Frenchay Dysarthria Assessment* (FDA) indicating "obvious abnormality but the patient can perform task/movements with reasonable approximation." See Table 8–4 for details of the Frenchay scoring.
1-2/5 promixal paresis	See Table 8–3 for details of muscle testing.
4/5 in quadriceps	See Table 8–3 for details of muscle testing.
Blurred vision	Lack of sharpness of vision and a subsequent inability to see fine detail.
Diplopia	Double vision. A single object is seen as two images.
Dysmetria	Discoordination of movement or inability to judge distance. The result is that the hand, arm, or leg undershoots or overshoots an intended position. It is considered to be the result of ataxia and is caused by impairment in the cerebellum.
Epstein–Barr virus (EBV) infection	Infection of the human virus EBV. EBV causes mononucleosis. The symptoms of mononucleosis include fatigue, fever, lack of appetite, sore throat, swollen glands in the neck, and weakness in the muscles.
Expanded Disability Status Scale (EDSS)	This scale measures movement ability. It ranges from 0 to 10, with 0 considered to be normal and 10 being no movement. Lower numbers in EDSS indicate less severe disability. The score of 7 in this patient indicates severe disability affecting daily activities. The patient needs assistance in walking.
Fingolimod	Medication specialized in decreasing the number of episodes of worsening in multiple sclerosis by preventing the immune system from attacking the nerve cells.
Hypoesthesia	Also called numbness, it is considered to be a reduced sense of touch.
Hyperintense lesions in the T2	Lesions shown in the MRI that are considered to be active. They show a degree of edema in the normal appearance of the axons (white matter).
Immunoglobulin infusions (IVIG)	Therapy that is based on proteins (antibodies) used by the immune system to neutralize bacteria and viruses.
Interferon	A protein that is made and released by cells in response to the presence of viruses, bacteria, parasites, and tumor cells. A virus-infected cell will release interferons, causing nearby cells to heighten their antiviral defenses.
Intravenous methylprednisolone	A corticosteroid hormone used to treat immune system disorders by decreasing the response of the immune system and thus reducing symptoms such as swelling, pain, and allergic-type reactions.
Left arm weakness 4/5	See Table 8–3 for muscle function scoring.
Lumbar puncture	Medical procedure used to collect cerebrospinal fluid (CSF) via a needle that is inserted into the spinal canal. CSF analysis aids the diagnosis of neurological diseases.
Medrol	A steroidal medication that reduces inflammation and is used to treat exacerbations in multiple sclerosis.

TABLE 8–2. *continued*	
Methotrexate	A chemotherapy agent that suppresses the immune system and is used to treat cancer, autoimmune diseases, etc.
Multiple sclerosis (MS)	An autoimmune neurological disease that affects 400,000 people in the US. The disease causes damage to the brain and spinal cord. Its signs and symptoms may include problems with movement, muscle control, balance, vision, or speech. In MS, the body's immune system attacks the covering of axons of neurons (myelin). The axons are responsible for conveying electrical signals to the following neuron or muscle.
Natalizumab	A protein (monoclonal antibody) that, as a medication, is used to treat multiple sclerosis by preventing the immune system from attacking the brain and spinal cord. It aids in decreasing the number of attacks.
Neuromyelitis or neuromyelitis optica	A disease that affects the eyes, occurring when the immune system attacks healthy cells in the central nervous system.
Nystagmus	Involuntary saccadic movement of the eye.
Oligoclonal bands	Bands of proteins (immunoglobulins) seen when analyzing the blood serum or CSF.
One-and-a-half syndrome	Weakness in eye movement affecting both eyes but with different degrees. For example, one eye may not be able to move while the other eye can move in only one lateral direction (inward or outward).
Optic neuritis	Demyelination of the optic nerve caused by inflammation. It may lead to complete or partial loss of vision in one or both eyes.
Plasmapheresis	A type of therapy that removes, treats, and returns (exchanges) blood plasma (liquid part of the blood including certain proteins that may attack the immune system) from blood circulation. It is used in multiple sclerosis to manage severe attacks by eliminating the harmful effect of these proteins and improving the symptomatology of the disease.
Rebif 22 mg three times a week subcutaneous (sc)	A beta-1a interferon (see above) that, as a protein, is used to decrease the frequency of relapses and delay the occurrence of physical disability in multiple sclerosis.
Right leg plegia 0/5	See Table 8–3 for muscle function scoring.
Signs	Characteristics of a disease apparent upon objective clinical observation.
Symptoms	Characteristics of a disease experienced as perceptions by the patient.
Spastic paraparesis	Muscular weakness and spasticity (stiffness) in the legs.
Spastic tetraparesis	Muscle weakness that affects all four limbs (both arms and legs) and is characterized by spasticity. Synonymous with quadriplegia.
Steroids (1000 Solu-Medrol intravenous, i.v.)	A corticosteroid that helps to suppress the immune system and decrease inflammation.

other cranial nerve disability. She still demonstrated some mild **dysmetria** in her left arm, as well as **left arm weakness 4/5** and right leg **plegia 0/5** and **4/5 in quadriceps** with full drop foot (see Table 8–3 for definitions of muscle testing). In the left leg she demonstrated **1-2/5 promixal paresis**. Hypoesthesia was found in right leg and left arm. The patient could not stand or walk. **EDSS**: 7.0. Earlier MRI showed large lesions in white matter of brain hemispheres and brainstem. New MRI results showed reduction in some lesions but also appearance of new ones without gadolinium enhancement.

Eight Years Following Intake

This patient had been followed at the neurology clinic for eight years and was just taken into care in fall of this year. Following physical examination she was treated with interferon for one year, and she had regular immunoglobulin infusions of 0.4 mg/kg per month during that time. This gain did not prevent any relapses, and the next year treatment with **natalizumab** was begun. While on natalizumab she did not have further relapses for at least seven months, but unfortunately she developed severe side effects, including severe chest pain and low backache. This treatment was discontinued in the following year, and she had a major relapse five months later, with optic neuritis as well as **spastic tetraparesis**. There was no response to **intravenous methylprednisolone** and she was therefore transferred for

plasmapheresis, which improved her vision, but she was left with severe **spastic paraparesis**.

In the last 10 days she had a brainstem relapse with **one-and-a-half syndrome** and mild bilateral cerebellar signs for a five-day course of i.v. Solu-Medrol. She is due to start **fingolimod**.

Medical Diagnosis

Multiple sclerosis

Speech Examination

The *Frenchay Dysarthria Assessment* was administered. The results showed moderate difficulty, with a **"c" score**, revealing a mixed type dysarthria (spastic-ataxic in nature), with a predominance of the spastic components (see Table 8–4 for details of Frenchay scoring). More specifically:

- Laryngeal component: Sustained phonation for /a/ in 6 seconds (spastic component).
- Laryngeal component: Changes in volume when the patient counts from 1 to 5 with a noticeably uneven progression (ataxic component).
- Tongue component: Slow movement (5 times) protrusion/retraction of the tongue (7 seconds) (spastic component).
- Tongue component: Incomplete in movement (5 times) elevation of the tongue (spastic component).
- Tongue component: Incomplete lateral tongue movement (5 times) produced in 8 seconds (spastic component).
- Tongue component: Diadochokinetic rate of the word /kala/ (10 times) with one sound to be well articulated

TABLE 8–3.	Examining Muscle Strength

When examining a patient, identifying specific areas of muscular weakness helps to localize the site of lesion. Strength testing is completed for each muscle group, making sure that you test one side and then the next for each group, so you can compare strength for the two sides. Here is a muscle strength rating scale.	
0/5	No contraction of muscle
1/5	Indication of muscle flicker, but no movement noted
2/5	Movement occurs, but not against gravity when tested in the horizontal plane
3/5	Movement occurs against, but not when there is resistance provided by the the examiner
4/5	Movement occurs against some resistance provided by the examiner
5/5	Normal strength

TABLE 8–4.	Frenchay Scoring Details

The *Frenchay Dysarthria Assessment* (FDA) utilizes a rating scale for all testing.	
a score	Normal for age
b score	Mild abnormality noticeable to skilled observer
c score	Obvious abnormality but the patient can perform task/movements with reasonable approximation
d score	Some production of task but poor in quality, unable to sustain, inaccurate, or extremely labored
e score	Unable to undertake task/movement/sound

and further deterioration as the numbers increased (9 seconds) (spastic component).

- Respiration during speech (counting from 1 to 20) was characterized by fading of the voice as numbers increased. The patient took four breaths to complete the count (spastic component).
- Moderate hypernasality was found when the patient was asked to say "may pay" "nay bay," making the plosive sounds to sound like the nasal sounds (spastic component).
- During dialogue, the patient's voice was characterized by breathiness and voice production that required extra effort and attention by the patient. The patient demonstrated pitch variation while attempting to control her voice quality (spastic component).
- The tongue movements in conversational speech were characterized by slow alternating movements and labored speech, as well as omissions of the sounds /t/, /k/, and /s/ (spastic component).

Medical Diagnosis

Relapsing-remitting multiple sclerosis

Speech-Language Diagnosis

Mixed spastic-ataxic dysarthria

Questions Concerning This Case

1. This is considered relapsing-remitting multiple sclerosis. Can you identify the periods of relapse and remission in this case? What is the time course of the progression of this disease?
2. What were the early signs of this disease (as opposed to early symptoms)?
3. What is the neuropathological basis of multiple sclerosis, and which part of the cell is affected?
4. Why is there mixed dysarthria in multiple sclerosis?

Case provided by Dr. Kostas Konstantopoulos, European University Cyprus.

CASE STUDY 8–2

Physician's Notes on Initial Physical Examination and History

This is a 64-year-old female who described having **burning paresthesias** in the feet and impairment of balance for the last five or six years. (See Table 8–5 for terminology. Note that we are presenting the data of this case in chronological order to show the emerging speech and language signs and symptoms as the condition progresses.) She also experienced a tendency to fall forward and to the side. She has fallen several times while on the stairs and now is afraid to climb stairs. She feels that her symptoms are worse when she closes her eyes. She denies any weakness or mental impairment. Her past medical history and family history are unremarkable. Her medications included Vastarel, administered symptomatically. She was a heavy smoker and used to drink socially. Recent evaluation included an MRI of the brain a few years ago that showed beginning vermian atrophy without any focal lesions in the brain. She also had an encephalogram that was unremarkable. The blood studies including B12 vitamin were normal. Thyroid function and routine biochemistry as well as hematological studies were normal. Finally, **brainstem evoked potentials** two years previously were also normal. During current examination, her mental status was found to be normal. She demonstrated a scan-

ning dysarthric speech. Eye movements were not impaired and her vision was intact. There were no other cranial nerve deficits. On motor examination, muscle bulk and tone were normal (see Table 8–3 for definitions of muscle testing). Reflexes were brisk in the lower extremities but plantar responses were flexor bilaterally. She exhibited mild **dysmetria** in both arms. In the lower extremities there was discoordination. Her gait was broad based and she demonstrated impairment of balance, especially when turning. Her performance deteriorated slightly when her eyes were closed. She had impaired vibration and pinprick sensation in a stocking glove distribution.

Medical Diagnosis

Cerebellar ataxia, perhaps a variant of Friedreich's ataxia. The patient has a clinical picture of slowly progressive midline cerebellar ataxia as well as length-dependent polyneuropathy, most likely axonal in nature. We planned to complete her workup for vitamin E levels as well as inflammatory markers and repeat B12 level. She needed to have a nerve conduction study to document the exact nature of the neuropathy. The MRI analysis two years previously showed clear atrophy of the midline cerebellum, which is in keeping with her clinical presentation.

TABLE 8–5.   **Terminology for Case Study 8–2**

"b-c" score	Scoring on the *Frenchay Dysarthria Assessment* (FDA). See Table 8–4 for scoring information concerning for the FDA.
Alendronate substance (active ingredient), Fosamax (brand name)	Medication used to treat osteoporosis by slowing bone loss and reducing the possibility of fractures.
Appendicular ataxia	Disorder characterized by irregular movements that affect the extremities. It is caused by damage to the cerebellar hemispheres and its pathways.
Aprataxin	A DNA binding protein.
Aspiration	Pathological admission of food or liquid into the airway below the level of the vocal folds.
Ataxia	A motor disorder arising from discoordination of the motor act, and frequently including low muscle tone. Ataxia is most frequently seen in cerebellar damage.
Ataxic broad-based gait	This gait is described as abnormal, unsteady, staggering, and uncoordinated.
Ataxic dysarthria (cerebellar dysarthria)	A motor speech disorder that is characterized by abnormalities in all subsystems for speech (respiration, phonation, resonation, articulation, and prosody), but it is more prominent in articulation and prosody. In this disorder the movement for speech is slow and inaccurate due to the incoordination that is caused by cerebellar damage.
Barium swallow	An x-ray swallow exam of the oral cavity, pharynx, and esophagus.
Biochemistry	Biochemical analysis is a set of methods that analyze the substances of organisms and their chemical reactions.
Brainstem evoked potentials	These are electrical potentials that are recorded through electrodes that are placed on the scalp as a response of the nervous system following a presentation of a stimulus, typically visual or auditory.
Burning paresthesia	A paresthesia causing a burning, painless sensation in the hands, arms, legs, or feet.
Cerebellar dysarthria	See ataxic dysarthria.
CT (computerized tomography) scan	Series of x-ray images used to show images of the brain and the body. The CT scan is used to diagnose many diseases or injuries.
DAB classification	Classification system for dysarthria, referring to the pioneering work of Darley, Aronson, and Brown at Mayo Clinic. For further information, see Darley, Aronson, & Brown (1969).
Dexa bone scan	A technique that is used to measure bone mineral density through an advanced x-ray technology.
Dysarthria	Motor speech disorder involving muscular weakness, dyscoordination, and alteration of muscle tone. It includes slow movement of the muscles used for speech production, including the lips, tongue, vocal folds, and/or muscles of respiration.

TABLE 8–5. *continued*

Dysmetria	Incoordination of movement or inability to judge distance. The result is that the hand, arm, or leg undershoots or overshoots an intended position. It is considered to be the result of ataxia and is caused by impairment in the cerebellum.
Dysphonia	Voice that is hoarse, breathy, etc.
Echocardiogram	An ultrasound test that is used to create a 2-dimensional or 3-dimensional image of the heart through sonography.
Episode of passing out (fainting)	Sudden temporary loss of consciousness caused by the lack of oxygen in the brain.
Excess and equal stress	A perceptual feature in the DAB classification in which there is excessive stress (increased vocal intensity and/or fundamental frequency) on unstressed syllables.
Finger-to-nose test	A neurological test in which the patient touches the tip of his/her nose with his/her index finger as quickly as possible.
Frenchay Dysarthria Assessment **(FDA)**	A standardized test to assess nonspeech and speech movements of lips, jaw, tongue, phonation, intelligibility, etc. (see Table 8–4 for details concerning scoring of the FDA).
Friedreich's ataxia	An autosomal neurological inherited disease that affects the normal function of the nervous system. Its symptomatology involves incoordination of movement, heart disease, and diabetes.

One Year Following Intake

The patient was seen for a follow-up for cerebellar ataxia of late onset most likely of genetic etiology. She has vermian atrophy in the MRI, and all other investigations have been unrevealing. She also had negative screening for all available SCA genes. She is clinically unchanged. On examination, there was **cerebellar dysarthria**, hypometric and saccadic eye movements, **ataxic broad-based gait**, and impairment of balance. There was no significant **appendicular ataxia**. There was no muscle weakness, and no extrapyramidal features. We planned to proceed with further genetic testing, including examination for Friedreich's ataxia, as she may have an atypical form; we considered checking some more recent genes, including **aprataxin** and senataxin.

Two Years Following Intake

The patient was seen for a follow-up for cerebellar ataxia of unclear etiology. Since her last visit, she reported worsening in her condition, with frequent falls on the ground.

Her thyroid function test results were within normal limits. On examination, she demonstrated **dysphonia** and a **scanning speech** as well as saccadic eye movements. Her gait was ataxic and broad based and there was impairment of balance. There was no muscular weakness, although there was mild intention tremor. We emphasized the need for regular physiotherapy. We planned to initiate **alendronate** once weekly and calcium daily.

Three Years Following Intake

The patient was seen for a follow-up for cerebellar ataxia with midline dysfunction. She reported deterioration of her symptoms with difficulty in preserving her balance, frequent falls on the ground, and difficulty in swallowing, although her weight has been stable since her last visit. On examination, she demonstrated dysarthria and an ataxic broad-based gait. She was unable to preserve her balance. She also demonstrated dysmetria on the **finger-to-nose test**, and there is decreased vibration sensation in the lower limbs.

She was referred to the speech-language therapist and will be seen again in four months with up-to-date blood tests.

Four Years, 3 Months Following Intake

The patient was seen for a follow-up for cerebellar ataxia. Her condition was unchanged since her last visit, although she described an **episode of passing out** at night when she got up to **void**. She described loss of consciousness without any other symptoms. She was taken to the emergency room and blood studies were normal, but no other investigations were done. A recent **barium swallow** study revealed that she has some **aspiration** of liquids, and thickening of liquids was recommended. In addition, she was found to have an enlarged stomach that was also displaced down to the pelvis. On examination, she had unchanged midline cerebellar **ataxia** mostly with gait ataxia, cerebellar dysarthria, and saccadic eye movements. I suggested that she continue vitamins. She needed to have a **Dexa bone scan** to reassess the osteoporosis issue because she had not been taking the alendronate regularly. I also gave her a referral for cardiological evaluation with a Holter monitor and **echocardiogram** to rule out any cardiac cause of the problem, and she was referred to a gastroenterologist for the findings of the barium swallow.

Five Years, 3 Months Following Intake

The patient was seen today for a follow-up for cerebellar ataxia. Her neurological condition was generally stable with gait unsteadiness, limb ataxia, and slurred speech. Furthermore, the patient complained about occasional swallowing problems. The blood analysis from earlier this year was satisfactory. The patient was to continue with multivitamins and she will repeat the blood analysis. An appointment in the dysphagia clinic was also arranged, and she was scheduled to have clinical evaluation again in six months.

Speech-Language Assessment

The patient was administered a modified barium swallow study in a standing position and viewed in a lateral and antero-posterior plane. She was administered various consistencies of liquids (thin and thick 5 cc and 10 cc) and pureed solid consistencies mixed with barium suspension. The oral phase was functional. In the pharyngeal phase there was aspiration of trace thin liquid prior to the swallow, secondary to poor oral control and premature spillage to the pharynx. The cough reflex was suppressed and did not aid in airway protection. No aspiration was noted for other consistencies. There was mild pharyngeal residue in the valleculae, with higher-viscosity consistencies. Esophageal clearance was unobstructed, and the esophageal peristaltic wave was within functional limits. However, the clinician noted a severely dilated stomach. The impression was of mild pharyngeal phase dysphagia characterized by silent aspiration of thin liquids. It was recommended that she modify her diet to change from thin liquids to thickened liquids or nectar.

The *Frenchay Dysarthria Assessment* (FDA) was given to the patient (see Table 8–4 for details of Frenchay scoring). The results showed moderate difficulty, **"b-c"** score, with signs of ataxic **dysarthria**. The **DAB classification** shows a cluster of speech characteristics typical of the perceptual impression of scanning speech. This cluster involves **excess and equal stress**, prolonged phonemes, prolonged intervals, and slow rate. More specifically:

- Reflexes cough: Patient has occasional difficulty with choking, or food sometimes entering the airway (b).
- Reflexes swallow: Patient observed drinking 1/2 cup of water and eating a cookie and eating was markedly slow (c).
- Respiration in speech: When asked to count from 1 to 20 as quickly as possible, there were occasional breaks in fluency due to poor respiratory control. An extra breath was required for the patient to complete the task (b).
- Lips alternate: Labored movement when the patient was asked to repeat "oo ee" 10 times. One movement was within normal limits, while other movements were severely distorted (c).
- Laryngeal time: Sustained phonation for /a/ with clear voice only for 7 seconds (c). Note, however, that the patient is a heavy smoker.
- Laryngeal pitch: Minor difficulty with pitch breaks when the patient was asked to sing a scale (b).
- Laryngeal in speech (intonation): Voice during speech was mostly effective—there was occasional inappropriate use of volume and pitch noticeable to the examiner (b).
- Tongue protrusion: Irregular movement accompanied by facial grimace (5 times in 7 seconds) (c).
- Tongue elevation: Incomplete gross movement of the tongue (c).
- Tongue lateral: Slow labored or incomplete tongue movement (5 times in 7 seconds) (c).
- Tongue alternate: Diadochokinetic rate of the word /kala/ (10 times) with one sound well articulated and the other poorly presented (10 seconds to complete the task) (c).
- Tongue in speech: Correct articulation points on the whole, but slow alternating movements made speech labored. There were found several omissions of consonants (c).

Speech-Language Diagnosis

Ataxic dysarthria

Questions Concerning This Case

1. Imaging revealed "vermian atrophy." What part of the anatomy is being referred to?

2. What are the characteristics of scanning speech, and how does it relate to the dysfunction of the cerebellum?

Case provided by Dr. Kostas Konstantopoulos, European University Cyprus.

CASE STUDY 8–3

Physician's Notes on Initial Physical Examination and History

This is a 45-year-old female who in the last six years noticed an unsteady gait that has gradually become worse. In addition, she presented with difficulty holding heavy objects, and her handwriting was particularly affected and disorganized. On direct questioning, she also admitted some change in her speech. There was also occasional urinary incontinence but no other **bladder disturbance** (see Table 8–6 for terminology. Note that we are presenting the data of this case in chronological order to show the emerging speech and language signs and symptoms as the condition progresses). Finally, she reported numbness early in the morning affecting both hands, and says that she is more unsteady in the dark.

Family History

There are four siblings in the family. She has a younger brother aged 42 who has a similar disorder and has been severely involved since his late 20s. He now walks very unsteadily and has to lean on the walls to do so. There are also two other healthy siblings, a 48-year-old brother and a 50-year-old sister, neither of whom have the presenting condition. The parents apparently did not have the disorder, although her mother died at a young age.

During the examination, the cranial nerves were normal, but she exhibited mild scanning speech and no nystagmus. In the arms there was no **atrophy**. There was mild **finger-to-nose** ataxia but no weakness or any sensory loss. In the lower limbs there was no atrophy. **Hip flexion was 4+/5** (see Table 8–3 for definitions of muscle testing). The rest of the examination was normal. The patient had **down-going plantar** responses. She also had **heel-to-shin unsteadiness** and exhibited an **ataxic gait.**

She presented mainly with a late-onset **cerebellar syndrome.** She was scheduled to have evoked response studies

as well as a battery of blood tests. In my clinical view, the patient presented with a genetic cerebellar syndrome even though I was unsure about the specific etiology.

One Year, 5 Months Following Intake

I reviewed this adult female with late-onset cerebellar ataxia. It appears that she is **homozygous** for the disorder, which might explain the possibility that her mother also had a similar disorder, although we are not certain. Blood was drawn from the patient today to confirm the **mutation**.

Medical Diagnosis

Friedreich's ataxia

Two Years, 1 Month Following Intake

I examined today this 47-year-old right-handed female with a diagnosis of late-onset Friedreich's ataxia. On neurological examination, she presented with mild to moderate speech disturbances (cerebellar speech) without nystagmus. The examination of the upper and lower limbs revealed generalized **areflexia**, **truncal ataxia,** and mild to moderate disturbance in finger-to-nose examination bilaterally. The patient was unable to complete the **heel-to-toe examination,** and she was unable to walk in a straight line. My impression was that her health condition had been stable over the last year. She continued with the same dose of medication (vitamin E, four tablets per day).

Sixteen Years, 9 Months Following Intake

I was glad to see this patient with long-standing Friedreich's ataxia. The patient was able to walk indoors with the help of a **Zimmer frame** and was still able to prepare her food at home, dress herself, and do her ironing. Her speech

TABLE 8–6.	Terminology for Case Study 8–3
"c" or "d" scores	Scoring on the *Frenchay Dysarthria Assessment* (FDA). See Table 8–4 for details concerning the Frenchay scoring.
Alendronate (active ingredient), Fosamax (brand name) 70 mg	Medication used to treat osteoporosis (bone loss).
Areflexic	This denotes the absence of reflexes.
Ataxic gait	Gait described as abnormal unsteady, staggering, and uncoordinated.
Atrophy	Decrease (wasting) in a size of an organ, especially muscles.
Biochemical examination (biochemistry)	Methods that analyze the substances of organisms and their chemical reactions.
Bladder disturbance or dysfunction	Neurological condition in which there is urinary incontinence in a patient (sometimes described as urgency, changes in frequency, etc.). It is caused by neurologic damage.
Cerebellar syndrome (disorder)	This can be caused by cerebellar damage due to hereditary ataxias or congenital conditions, and it involves impaired muscle coordination (ataxia).
Deferiprone (active ingredient), Ferriprox (brand name)	Medication used for the treatment of thalassemia major (inherited blood disease). This medication is a compound of iron.
Down-going plantars	Considered a normal response of plantar reflex in infants, stimulated by rubbing a blunt object on the sole of the foot with moderate force (see plantar response). It should not be present in adults.
Finger-to-nose ataxia	Incoordination (ataxia) in a neurological test in which the patient touches the tip of his/her nose with his/her index finger as quickly as possible.
Frenchay Dysarthria Assessment (FDA)	A standardized test to assess nonspeech and speech movements of lips, jaw, tongue, phonation, intelligibility, etc. (see Table 8–4 for details concerning scoring of the FDA).
Friedreich's ataxia	An autosomal neurological inherited disease that affects the normal function of the nervous system. Its symptomatology involves incoordination of movement, heart disease, and diabetes.
Heel-to-shin unsteadiness	A neurological test in which the patient is in the supine position and needs to place the heel on the opposite knee and slide it up and down as quickly as possible.
Heel-to-toe examination	A neurological test in which the patient walks heel-to-toe to demonstrate coordination and vestibular stability.
Hip flexion was 4+/5	See Table 8–3 for discussion of muscle testing.
Homozygous	This happens when an individual has two of the same alleles (forms of a gene), as opposed to heterozygous, where an individual has one each of two different alleles.
Lovastatin (active ingredient), Mevacor (brand name) 20 mg	A medication used to lower "bad" (low-density lipoprotein [LDL]) cholesterol and fats.

TABLE 8–6.	*continued*
Mevacor	See lovastatin.
Mutation	A change in the structure of a gene. It becomes a variant form that is transmitted through generations.
Nystagmus	Involuntary saccadic movement of the eye.
Pramipexole (active ingredient), Mirapexin (brand name) 0.18 mg	A medication (dopamine agonist) used to treat Parkinson's disease by mimicking the action of dopamine.
Restless leg syndrome	A disease with symptoms such as abnormal sensations in the legs and an urge to move them.
Scanning speech (scanning dysarthric speech)	Characteristic speech of cerebellar damage in which the words are pronounced as separate, equally stressed syllables.
Truncal ataxia	Inability or difficulty making coordinated voluntary movements, affecting the limbs, trunk, pharynx, larynx, etc.
Zimmer frame	Metal frame with four legs that the patient uses to aid in walking.

remained unchanged and perhaps slightly improved. Her voice seemed to be louder to me compared with the pre-**deferiprone** period. The patient did not complain about choking. Her major complaint was **restless leg syndrome**. She cannot sleep at night because she needs to get up and walk before returning to sleep. This happens every two hours. She is taking 300 mg of deferiprone a week and her hematologic and **biochemical examinations** seem to be unaffected by this medication.

Nineteen Years, 2 Months Following Intake

This patient with Friedreich's ataxia was seen today for a follow-up appointment. Regarding her ataxia, she seemed to be stable, wheelchair-bound, and unable to walk without assistance. She denied difficulty with her swallowing but I referred her to the dysphagia clinic because previously she had admitted choking with liquids. She is currently on **alendronate** 70 mg once weekly, **lovastatin** 20 mg daily, and **pramipexole** 0.18 mg 1/2 tablet daily.

Speech Examination

The *Frenchay Dysarthria Assessment* was administered to the patient (see Table 8–4 for details of Frenchay scoring). The results correlated with the neurologist's impression for primarily ataxic involvement in this patient. There was moderate to severe difficulty, with **"c" or "d"** scores in most of the domains assessed. More specifically:

- Reflexes (cough): Patient chokes 1–2 times per day on water (c).
- Reflexes (swallow): Patient exhibited slow eating of a cookie and choked once during drinking of water via a cup (c).
- Laryngeal time: Strained-strangled voice quality and sustained phonation for /a/ in 5 seconds (c).
- Laryngeal pitch: Patient able to represent four distinct pitch changes with uneven progression while singing a scale (at least six notes) (c).
- Laryngeal volume: Limited change in volume when the patient counted from 1 to 5 and great difficulty in control of the volume (d).
- Laryngeal in speech: Patient's voice requires effort and attention, deteriorates, and can be unpredictable. There are difficulties with modulation, clarity of phonation, and pitch variation, but the patient is able to control these on occasion (c).
- Tongue protrusion: Patient was able to protrude/retract tongue to lip with an irregular movement accompanied by noticeable tremor (5 times in 6 seconds) (c).
- Tongue elevation: Labored movement of the tongue when the patient tried to elevate it (5 times) (c).
- Tongue lateral: Labored lateral tongue movement (5 times) produced in 7 seconds (c).

- Tongue alternate: Diadochokinetic rate of the word /kala/ (10 times) with one sound to be well articulated but the other poorly presented. Task takes 10 seconds to complete (c).
- Tongue during speech: There was grossly distorted articulation (d).

Speech-Language Diagnosis

Ataxic dysarthria

Questions Concerning This Case

1. The physician diagnosed **Friedreich's ataxia**, which involves cerebellar degeneration. The physician reported the perception of **scanning speech**. Knowing what you do about cerebellar function, why is scanning speech a sign of ataxia?
2. What is the neuropathological basis of Friedreich's ataxia?

Case provided by Dr. Kostas Konstantopoulos, European University Cyprus.

CHAPTER 8
STUDY QUESTIONS

1. _____ This cerebellar peduncle enters the brainstem at the level of the medulla.

2. _____ This cerebellar peduncle enters the brainstem at the level of the pons.

3. The _____ lobe receives input concerning vestibular function.

4. The cerebellum is posterior/anterior (circle one) to the brainstem.

5. The _____ ventricle is immediately anterior to the cerebellum.

6. True or False: The cerebellum receives inputs from multiple areas of the nervous system and sends output to the premotor and motor cortex and to the brainstem.

7. True or False: The vestibulocerebellum (the archicerebellum) is important for balance.

8. The outer cell layer of the cerebellum is termed the _____ layer.

9. The intermediate layer of the cerebellum is referred to as the _____ layer.

10. True or False: When a Purkinje cell is activated, it excites the nucleus with which it synapses.

11. Afferent input to the cerebellum concerning balance function arises from the _____ mechanism.

12. The cerebral cortex sends information to the cerebellum through the contralateral _____ nuclei.

13. True or False: The cerebellum is responsible for error-checking by integrating somatic information about joint position, etc. with the motor plan.

14. The _____ nuclei project to the premotor and motor regions of the cerebral cortex.

15. The _____ nucleus outputs project to the vestibular nuclei of the brainstem, the reticular formation of the pons and medulla, and the inferior olivary complex.

16. The _____ and _____ nuclei provide input to the red nucleus in support of muscle tone to the legs.

17. These nuclei are important for maintaining muscle tone. _____ _____

18. The _____ nucleus projects its output to the cerebral cortex, modifying the motor plan, supporting fine motor function.

19. The _____ nucleus receives its input from the vermis and projects to the vestibular nuclei of the brainstem, the reticular formation of the pons and medulla, and the inferior olivary complex.

20. True or False: Vestibular input is received by the archicerebellum.

21. True or False: The dorsal spinocerebellar tract transmits information concerning temperature, proprioception (muscle spindle), and touch that arises in the lower body and legs.

22. The _____ _____ tract sends information about proprioception (GTOs) and pain sense arising in the legs and lower trunk to the ipsilateral cerebellar cortex.

23. The _____ _____ tract arises from the cervical spinal cord, providing proprioception (GTO) and pain sense from the upper trunk and arms to the cerebellar cortex.

24. The _____ tract projects from the parietal, occipital, temporal, and frontal lobes of the cerebral cortex to synapse on the pontine nuclei. Efferents from these nuclei project to the cerebellar cortex via the middle cerebellar peduncle.

25. The _____ tract arises from the inferior olivary and medial accessory olivary nuclei of the medulla. The tract projects to the climbing fibers of the cerebellum. The important function of this tract is to integrate visual and motor plan information from the cortex with afferent information from the spinal cord.

26. The _____ tract arises from the inferior olive of the brainstem and projects to the cerebrocerellum.

27. The posterior _____ tract arises from the thoracic nucleus of Clarke's column within the gray matter of the spinal cord, conveying muscle spindle information from the lower limbs to the vermis region of the anterior and posterior lobes of the cerebellum.

28. True or False: The cerebellum regulates the rate, range, and force of motor function through integration of body sense with the motor plan.

29. True or False: Fine motor control is possible without the cerebellum.

REFERENCES

Ackermann, H. (2008). Cerebellar contributions to speech production and speech perception: Psycholinguistic and neurobiological perspectives. *Trends in Neuroscience, 31*(6), 265–272.

Akshoomoff, N. A., & Courchesne, E. (1992). A new role for the cerebellum in cognitive operations. *Behavioral Neuroscience, 106*(5), 731–738.

Apps, R., & Garwicz, M. (2005). Anatomical and physiological foundations of cerebellar information processing. *Nature Reviews Neuroscience, 6*(4), 297–311.

Armstrong, D. M., Eccles, J. C., Harvey, R. J., & Matthews, P. B. C. (1968). Responses in the dorsal accessory olive of the cat to stimulation of hind limb afferents. *The Journal of Physiology, 194*(1), 125–145.

Azevedo, F. A., Carvalho, L. R., Grinberg, L. T., Farfel, J. M., Ferretti, R. E., Leite, R. E., . . . & Herculano-Houzel, S. (2009). Equal numbers of neuronal and nonneuronal cells make the human brain an isometrically scaled-up primate brain. *Journal of Comparative Neurology, 513*(5), 532–541.

Baehr, M., & Frotscher, M. (2012). *Duus' topical diagnosis in neurology*. New York, NY: Thieme.

Baillieux, H., De Smet, H. J., Paquier, P. F., De Deyn, P. P., & Mariën, P. (2008). Cerebellar neurocognition: Insights into the bottom of the brain. *Clinical Neurology and Neurosurgery, 110*(8), 763–773.

Bodranghien, F., Bastian, A., Casali, C., Hallett, M., Louis, E. D., Manto, M., . . . van Dum, K. (2016). Consensus paper: Revisiting the symptoms and signs of cerebellar syndrome. *Cerebellum, 15*(3), 369–391.

Bohland, J. W., & Guenther, F. H. (2006). An fMRI investigation of syllable sequence production. *NeuroImage, 32*, 821–841.

Carpenter, M. B. (1996). *Core text of neuroanatomy* (4th ed.). Baltimore, MD: Williams & Wilkins.

Darley, F. L., Aronson, A. E., & Brown, J. R. (1969). Clusters of deviant speech dimensions in the dysarthrias. *Journal of Speech and Hearing Research, 12*(3), 462–496.

Duffy, J. R. (2013). *Motor speech disorders-E-book: Substrates, differential diagnosis, and management*. St. Louis, MO: Elsevier Health Sciences.

Durisko, C., & Fiez, J. A. (2010). Functional activation in the cerebellum during memory and simple tasks. *Cortex, 46*, 896–906.

Gellman, R., Gibson, A. R., & Houk, J. C. (1985). Inferior olivary neurons in the awake cat: detection of contact and passive body displacement. *Journal of Neurophysiology, 54*(1), 40–60.

Herculano-Houzel, S. (2009). The human brain in numbers: A linearly scaled-up primate brain. *Frontiers in Human Neuroscience, 3*, 31.

Keren-Happuch, E., Chen, S. H. A., Ho, M. H. R., & Desmond, J. E. (2014). A meta-analysis of cerebellar contributions to higher cognition from PET and fMRI studies. *Human Brain Mapping, 35*(2), 593–615.

Koch, G., Oliveri, M., Torriero, S., Salerno, S., Gerfo, E. L., & Caltagirone, C. (2007). Repetitive TMS of cerebellum interferes with millisecond time processing. *Experimental Brain Research, 179*(2), 291–299.

Lisberger, S. G., & Thach, W. T. (2013). The cerebellum. In E. R. Kandel, J. H. Schwartz, T. M. Jessell, S. A. Siegelbaum, & A. J. Hudspeth (Eds.), *Principles of neural science* (5th ed., pp. 960–981). New York, NY: McGraw-Hill.

Morel, A., Liu, J., Wannier, T., Jeanmonod, D., & Rouiller, E. M. (2005). Divergence and convergence of thalamocortical projections to premotor and supplementary motor cortex: A multiple tracing study in the macaque monkey. *European Journal of Neuroscience, 21*(4), 1007–1029.

Paek, S. B., Min, H. K., Kim, I., Knight, E. J., Baek, J. J., Bieber, A. J., . . . Chang, S. Y. (2015). Frequency-dependent functional neuromodulatory effects on the motor network by ventral lateral thalamic deep brain stimulation in swine. *NeuroImage, 105*, 181–188.

Raymond, J. L., Lisberger, S. G., & Mauk, M. D. (1996). The cerebellum: A neuronal learning machine. *Science, 272*, 1126–1131.

Rapoport, M., van Reekum, R., & Mayberg, H. (2000). The role of the cerebellum in cognition and behavior: A selective review. *Journal of Neuropsychiatry and Clinical Neurosciences, 12*(2), 193–198.

Schmahmann, J. D., & Caplan, D. (2006). Cognition, emotion and the cerebellum. *Brain, 129*(2), 290–292.

Seikel, J. A., Drumright, D. G., & King, D. W. (2016). *Anatomy & physiology for speech, language, and hearing* (5th ed.). Clifton Park, NY: Cengage Learning.

Spencer, K. A., & Slocomb, D. L. (2007). The neural basis of ataxic dysarthria. *Cerebellum, 6*(1), 58–65.

Stoodley, C. J., Valera, E. M., & Schmahmann, J. D. (2012). Functional topography of the cerebellum for motor and cognitive tasks: An fMRI study. *NeuroImage, 59*(2), 1560–1570.

Urban, P., Marx, J., Hunsche, S., Gawehn, J., Vucurevic, G., Wicht, S., Massinger, C., . . . Hopf, H. C. (2003). Cerebellar speech representation: lesion topography in dysarthria as derived from cerebellar ischemia and functional magnetic resonance imaging. *Archives of Neurology, 60*(7), 965–972.

Voogd, J. (2003). The human cerebellum. *Journal of Chemical Neuroanatomy, 26*(4), 243–252.

Voogd, J. (2011). Cerebellar zones: A personal history. *The Cerebellum, 10*(3), 334–350.

Voogd, J., & Glickstein, M. (1998). The anatomy of the cerebellum. *Trends in Cognitive Sciences, 2*(9), 307–313.

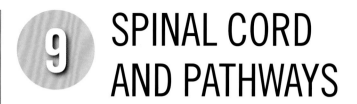

9 SPINAL CORD AND PATHWAYS

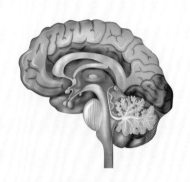

Learning Outcomes for Chapter 9

• Differentiate vertical and transverse anatomy of the spinal cord, the roles of white and gray matter within the spinal cord, and the configuration of the spinal meninges.

• Discuss the concept of dermatomes and myotomes with relation to spinal nerves in general.

• Define dorsal root ganglion, funiculus, and fasciculus, filum terminale, cauda equine, relationship between the central canal and the ventricles of the cerebral cortex.

• Identify the ascending pathways of the posterior, anterior and lateral funiculi and the information those pathways convey.

• Explain the course of the corticospinal tract from cerebrum to internal capsule, brainstem, spinal cord, ending with activation of a muscle.

INTRODUCTION

The spinal cord consists of a set of central nervous system pathways that allow communication to and from the periphery. All movement of skeletal structures is mediated by means of the pathways of the spinal cord, and all somatic sensation from the periphery is sent to the CNS by this means as well.

The spinal cord must be viewed from both longitudinal and cross-sectional orientations in order to make sense of its components and function. Longitudinally, the spinal cord is made up of **tracts** consisting of many neuron fibers that arise from either upper CNS structures (efferent pathways) or from peripheral sensors (afferent pathways). The vertical or longitudinal structure can be likened to a series of strands of a rope, where the rope is the entire spinal cord and the strands are the various tracts.

The spinal cord is also divided structurally by the vertebrae, providing a segmental view of the spinal cord. This segmental view isn't arbitrary: the spinal cord segments mark the points of exit for the spinal nerves that serve specific parts of the torso, arms, and legs, with some significant functional implications. We'll talk about both longitudinal and segmental views as we discuss this "superhighway of the CNS."

All of these tracts must pass through the brainstem, and some brainstem pathways do not continue through the spinal cord. Realize how important the spinal cord and brainstem pathways are. We are sensate creatures, and our cerebrum is designed to take the sensation it receives, make some sort of sense of it, and act on that sensation. This total function <u>requires</u> the existence of pathways that convey sensory information from the periphery, as well as the mechanism for sending motor commands to the periphery. Without afferent (sensory) and efferent (motor) pathways, our cerebral cortex would be out of a job! It would have, literally, nothing to do. As a thought experiment, imagine being born with no sensory input to the brain and no way to act through muscular contraction. This new brain that had never had any sensory input would have no history, no memory to work with, and no information to process. It is frankly unimaginable. You might want to take a look at Table 9–1 to see how much work your spinal cord does!

Spinal Cord Injury

In the United States, spinal cord injury affects approximately 11,000 people annually, with nearly 230,000 living with spinal cord injury at the present time (Crewe & Krause, 2009). The average age of injury is 31½ years, meaning that many of those receiving these life-altering injuries will live more than half of their lives following

- Explain the course of the corticobulbar tract from cerebrum to internal capsule and then to the
- brainstem level, including decussation and activation of cranial nerves.
- Discuss the role of the extrapyramidal system, and identify the tracts that make up this system.

the trauma. Almost 50% of spinal cord injuries are from motor vehicle accidents (MVAs). While loss of mobility is a significant and striking issue for those with spinal cord injury, there are many other conditions that arise from the injury, including loss of bladder control, loss of arm and hand strength, and affected sexual function.

Injury at the cervical level will result in loss of upper and lower body function, a condition known as **tetraplegia**. Injury at the thoracic level will spare the arms but will result in **paraplegia** (affecting both lower limbs). Loss of bowel and bladder function following spinal cord injury is typical, although therapy can aid in regaining control for many individuals. Damage above the T6 level can place the patient at risk for **autonomic hyperreflexia**, in which the body responds to a noxious stimulus with a dangerous spike in blood pressure, placing the patient at acute risk for stroke. **Spasticity** of muscles below the level of the

spinal cord injury is typical, as are **contractures** (Crewe & Krause, 2009).

Pediatric spinal cord injury makes up approximately 5% of all spinal cord injuries (Proctor, 2002). Epidemiology reveals that the most common spinal injury in children under 2 years of age is to the cervical spinal cord, typically from MVAs and falling. Because neck pain is emblematic of spinal cord injury, the ability of a small child to report focal injury is limited, making diagnosis difficult. Neonatal spinal cord injuries are relatively rare, and typically involve the cervical vertebrae. These injuries can occur when physical manipulation of the neonate during birth is required, damaging the spinal cord. Child abuse is another contributor to the injuries received by young children. Odontoid fracture (fracturing of the odontoid process of C2 due to rotatory force) can occur, but congenital odontoid malformation is a more common cause of C2 damage (Proctor, 2002).

VERTICAL ANATOMY OF THE SPINAL CORD

From the vertical perspective, the spinal cord is a mass of longitudinal columns running along the length of the cord. In reality, it is actually a set of columns, but these columns have different sites of origination and termination. The columns consist of the nervous system components we have discussed earlier. If you look at a cross-section through the spinal cord (Figure 9–1), you can see the **gray matter**, which is composed of cell bodies of the neurons. The **white matter** in this figure is apparent around the gray matter. That white matter you see actually represents the various tracts of the spinal cord. As with the rest of the central nervous system, the spinal cord is wrapped in meningeal linings.

The superior aspect of the spinal cord is at the foramen magnum of the skull. The medulla oblongata of the brainstem is an upward extension of the spinal cord, both physically and in terms of function. The spinal cord has aggregates of neuron cell bodies that serve motor function, and there are cell bodies in ganglia lying outside of the spinal column that provide input for afferent information. This structure is parallel to that found in the brainstem. The spinal cord has numerous basic reflexive functions, similar to those found in the brainstem. The critical difference between the function of the spinal cord and brainstem is one of complexity. The basic spinal reflex arc that we discussed in Chapter 3

is expanded into a set of exquisite reflexes and groups of reflexes (known as **central pattern generators**, or CPGs). As we'll discuss in Chapter 11, CPGs are composed of individual reflexive responses that are organized into coordinated and often sequential units responsible for execution of complex reflexive responses such as swallowing. The spinal cord really does reflect the basic unit of the nervous system, with the structures above it being more complex versions of the basic functions seen at this level.

The spinal cord is about 46 cm long and between 1 and 1.5 cm in diameter. It is housed within the protective vertebral canal of the vertebral column, which is a set of vertebrae categorized by location within the column as well as by anatomical difference (Figure 9–2A and Table 9–1). Vertebrae are designated by letter and number reflecting that structure: C1 through C7 represent the seven vertebrae of the cervical spinal column, T1 through T12 correspond to the thoracic vertebrae, L1 through L5 reflect the lumbar region, and the sacrum (S) is a fused unit. The cervical vertebrae begin with the atlas (C1), which supports the skull and marks the superior end of the spinal cord, and the axis (C2), which is immediately below the atlas. These vertebrae have unique features that set them apart from all other vertebrae. The other five cervical vertebrae have similar structure but are unique in the vertebral column for having a passageway for vascular supply to the brain (the transverse foramina), to be discussed.

TABLE 9–1.		Segments of Spinal Cord and Muscles Served
Segment	Function	Muscles innervated
C3–C4	Respiration	Diaphragm, via cervical plexus
C2–C7	Head and neck stability and respiration	Sternocleidomastoid (with XI spinal accessory)
		Scalenus anterior, medius, posterior (C3–C8)
		Serratus anterior (C5–C7)
		Subclavius (C5–C6)
		Levator scapulae (C1–C4)
		Trapezius (XI accessory, C2–C5)
C1–T1	Arm and hand function	Pectoralis major
		Pectoralis minor
		Levator scapulae (C1–C4)
		Rhomboideus major and minor (C5)
		Deltoids and biceps (C5–C6)
		Extensor carpi radialis pronator teres (wrist: C6–C7)
		Triceps (C7–C8)
		Flexor digitorum superficialis (finger flexion: C8–T1)
		Opponens pollicis inerossei (finger spread, close: C8–T1)
C7–T12	Respiration and thorax stability	Levator costarum brevis, longis (C7–T11)
		Serratus posterior superior (T1–T5)
		Serratus posterior superior inferior (T9–T12)
		External and internal intercostals (T1–T11)
		Subcostals (T1–T12)
C1–L5	Respiration and trunk stability	Transversus abdominis (T7–T12)
		Internal oblique abdominis (T7–T12)
		External oblique abdominis (T7–T12)
		Rectus abdominis (T7–T12)
		Quadratus lumborum (T12–L4)
		Serratus posterior superior (T1–T5)
		Iliocostalis lumborum (thoracis, cervicis (lower cervical, all thoracic, lumbar nerves)
		Longissimus thoracis, cervicis, capitis (lower cervical, all thoracic, lumbar nerves)
		Spinalis thoracis, cervicis, capitis (lower cervical, all thoracic, lumbar nerves)
L1, L2, L3	Hip flexion	Iliopsoas adductors
L3, L4	Knee extension	Quadriceps
L4, l5, S1	Hip adduction, foot dorsiflexion	Gluteus medius
		Tibialis anterior
L5, S1, S2	Hip extensor, foot plantar flexion	Gluteus maximus
		Gastrocneumius
S2, S3, S4	Bowel function Bladder control	Anal sphincter
		Urethral sphincter

Source: Based on data of Seikel, Drumright, & King (2016) and Stolov & Clowers (1981).

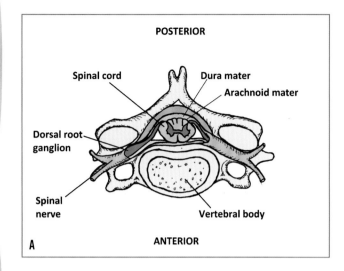

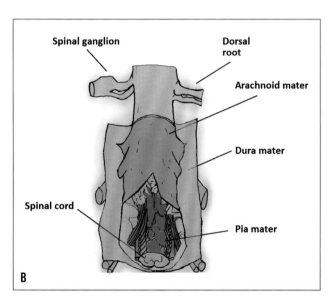

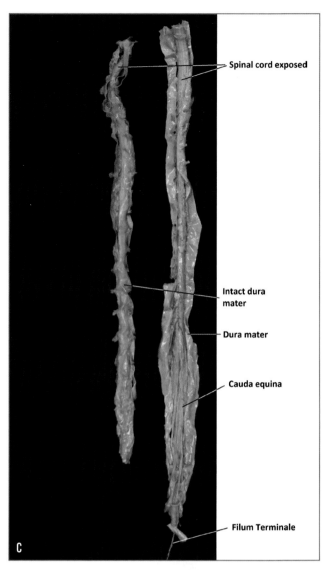

FIGURE 9–1. Meningeal linings of the spinal cord. **A.** Transverse section of spinal cord showing meningeal linings. **B.** Dorsal view of spinal cord revealing meningeal linings. *Source:* After view of Carpenter (1978). **C.** Photograph of spinal cord with intact dissected (*right*) and intact (*left*) meningeal linings.

The spinal cord is contained within **spinal meningeal linings** and suspended by **denticulate ligaments**. The denticulate ligaments arise from the pia mater and attach the spinal cord to the vertebral column. At the lower end of the spinal cord is a cone-shaped projection known as the **conus medullaris**. A fibrous projection from the conus medullaris called the **filum terminale** ("end filament") joins with the **dural tube** and then becomes the **coccygeal ligament**. The coccygeal ligament is attached to the posterior coccyx.

Now focus your attention on the spinal nerves of Figure 9–2B. There are 31 pairs of spinal nerves, correspond-

ing to the vertebral segments. The spinal nerves are related to each vertebra: the first spinal nerve (C1) arises from the spinal cord on the superior surface of the atlas (C1 vertebra), while spinal nerve C2 arises from below C1. Thus, there are 8 pairs of cervical spinal nerves instead of 7 (corresponding to seven cervical vertebrae). The subsequent nerve origins make logical sense with reference to the vertebrae: there are 12 pairs of thoracic nerves, 5 pairs of lumbar and sacral nerves, and 1 pair of coccygeal nerves. The spinal nerve notation follows the notation we talked about for vertebrae, with the first thoracic spinal nerve being T1, and so forth.

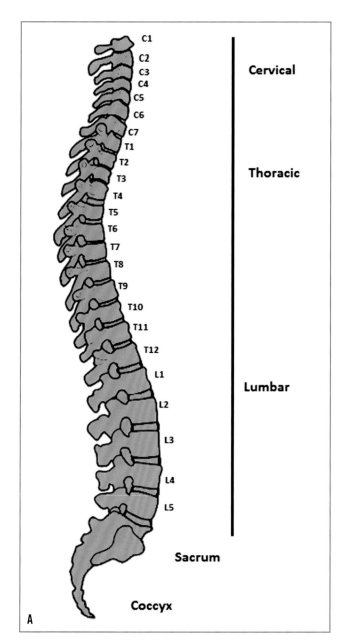

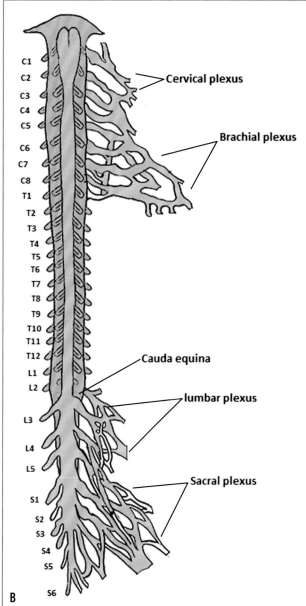

FIGURE 9–2. Vertebral column and spinal cord. **A.** Vertebral column, showing cervical, thoracic, lumbar, sacral, and coccygeal portions. Note notation relative to segments, such that the third cervical vertebra is labeled C3. *Source:* After view of Seikel, Drumright, and King (2016). **B.** Spinal cord. Note that spinal nerves are numbered similar to vertebral segments, such that C3 is shorthand for the third spinal nerve. Note that spinal nerve C1 emerges above the vertebral segment C1, so that all numbered nerves correspond with the vertebral segment above the nerve. *Source:* After view of Seikel, Drumright, and King (2016). *continues.*

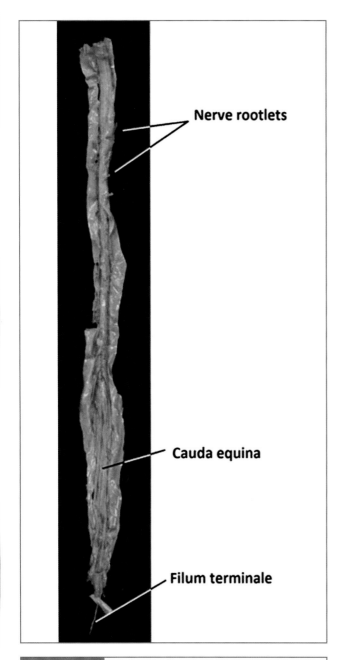

Nerve rootlets

Cauda equina

Filum terminale

FIGURE 9–2. *continued* **C.** Photograph of spinal cord showing spinal nerve roots.

During prenatal development, the spinal cord fits perfectly within the canal, but as the body develops, the canal becomes larger than the spinal cord. The result of this is that the spinal cord is shorter than the vertebral column, leaving a space in the lower aspect that has only nerves passing through it to serve the lumbar and coccygeal regions. Because of this, when a child is born, the conus medullaris is found in the L3 vertebral level, but by adulthood you will find it at the L1 level. At the inferior aspect of the spinal cord you can see the cauda equina ("horse's tail"), ending in the filum terminale ("end filament"). The reason lumbar punctures to sample cerebrospinal fluid are given here is that the risk of injury to the spinal cord is greatly reduced.

Electrical Stimulation for Spinal Cord Injury

Electrical stimulation (e-stim) following spinal cord injury can provide many benefits to the patient. Because mobility is an issue following injury, treatment of pressure ulcers is critical. Electrical stimulation has been shown to be an effective treatment for these ulcers. Electrical stimulation can also aid in bladder control (Liu, Moody, Traynor, Dyson, & Gall, 2014) and in reducing muscle atrophy (Baldi, Jackson, Moraille, & Mysiw, 1998).

Computer-controlled electrical stimulation is being used to provide movement and control for individuals with spinal cord injury (Ragnarsson, 2008). Functional electrical stimulation (FES) refers to use of computer-aided electrical stimulation to improve or stimulate complex function. The goal of FES is to stimulate motor patterns, such as standing, stepping, reaching, etc. As Ragnarsson notes, FES not only provides movement, but also increases independence and helps to maintain muscle tone and bulk.

Spinal nerves can have both afferent and efferent components. Spinal nerves serve specific body regions, known as "**dermatomes**." If you look at Figure 9–3, you can see how the sensory dermatomes are arrayed, reflecting the function served by each nerve. This is important information for the neurologist because it allows her or him to identify areas of nerve damage based upon a person's ability to feel stimulation at a body region. In reality, there is overlap in the dermatomes, which provides a degree of redundancy. The motor representation is not as clearly represented because muscles span various distances that cross dermatome regions, and activation of these muscles often uses networks of nerves, known as plexuses.

TRANSVERSE ANATOMY OF THE SPINAL CORD

Now let's think about the transverse anatomy of the spinal cord. Remember that we likened the spinal cord to a series of cords bundled together. Each of these cords would have

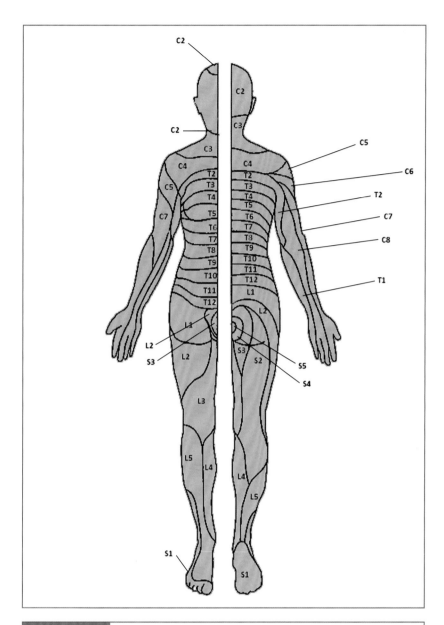

FIGURE 9–3. Dermatome map of the sensory component of spinal and cranial nerves. Recognize that the dermatomes actually have overlap, so that two nerves will serve some of each dermatome.

a cross-sectional aspect, and that is what you can see in Figure 9–4.

As you can see, there is a central gray area, surrounded by white. The gray area represents cell bodies of neurons, while the white is composed of myelinated fibers of the neurons. The gray matter is further divided into the posterior gray column (also known as the posterior horn) and anterior gray column. The **posterior gray** includes cell bodies of interneurons that connect, among other things, the efferent input to the motor fibers that serve muscle.

These myelinated fibers make up the tracts of the spinal cord that allow communication between the brain and the periphery. On the same figure, you can see the **central canal**, which is continuous with the fourth ventricle of the brain. Ultimately, we'll talk about the white matter in terms of **funiculi** and **fasciculi**, which are bands of fibers that make up tracts.

The dorsal root fibers are sensory in nature. Sensory information from the periphery, such as muscle tension or muscle stretch, enters the dorsal root ganglion, which lies

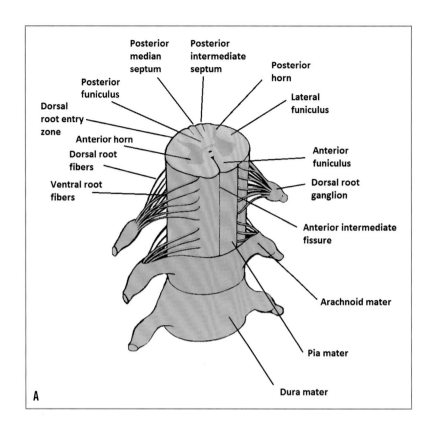

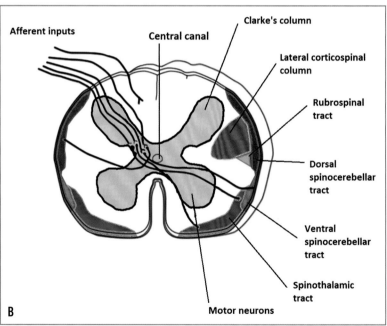

outside of the spinal cord (see Figure 9–4A). The ventral root consists of fibers that are exiting the spinal cord as spinal nerves and which are destined to activate muscle. Realize that there are no "ventral root ganglia" here, because a ganglion is an aggregate of cell bodies with a functional purpose, and the cell bodies for the motor nerves are within the ventral gray of the spinal cord. We saw this same design with several of the cranial nerves of the brainstem, where we found the motor cranial nerve nuclei within the brainstem, but some of the afferent nuclei (such as the trigeminal ganglion) outside of the brainstem. The brainstem is, of course, more complex, and you'll see nuclei <u>within</u> the brainstem, such as the nucleus solitarius, that accumulate sensory information. The spinal nerves divide into separate rami or divisions: the dorsal rami serve the muscles of the posterior body, while the ventral rami serve the anterior body. Some of the fibers of the ventral rami serve the autonomic nervous system, which resides as a parallel system outside of the spinal cord.

We've talked many times about synapses, but there are specialized synapses for motor function. Efferent neurons communicate with muscle through motor endplates. You will recall the basic reflexive unit, the reflex arc (Chapter 3). It's worth remembering that the most basic response to the environment that the body has resides at the segment level: the spinal reflex arc is our very first level of defense.

In summary,

- The spinal cord is suspended by denticulate ligaments that arise from the pia mater and attach the spinal cord to the vertebral column.
- The conus medullaris is the lower section of the spinal cord, with the final projection called the filum terminale. The filum terminale joins with the dural tube of the spinal cord and becomes the coccygeal ligament, which attaches to the coccyx.
- There are 31 pairs of spinal nerves related to each vertebra. The spinal cord is shorter than the vertebral column, leaving a space in the lower aspect.
- Spinal nerves can have both afferent and efferent components. Afferent spinal nerves serve specific body regions, known as dermatomes.
- The transverse anatomy of the spinal cord includes a central gray area surrounded by white matter. The gray area is composed of neuron cell bodies and the white, myelinated fibers of the neurons.
- The gray matter is divided into posterior and anterior gray columns. The myelinated fibers make up the tracts of the spinal cord for communication to and from the higher CNS structures. The central canal is continuous with the fourth ventricle of the brain.
- Dorsal root fibers are sensory in nature, and sensory information from the periphery enters the dorsal root ganglion that lies outside of the spinal cord. The ventral root con-

sists of fibers that are exiting the spinal cord as spinal nerves and that will activate muscle.

PATHWAYS OF THE SPINAL CORD

Clearly, if information from the periphery (touch, kinesthetic sense, pain, etc.) is to be received, processed, and acted upon by the upper levels of the CNS, there must be a means of getting that information there. This is where the afferent and efferent pathways come in. At the most basic level, afferent pathways of the spinal cord convey information from peripheral sensors to the central nervous system, where it can be processed. In contrast, efferent pathways convey impulses from the CNS that allow some sort of action by muscles or glands. In between these two conduits lies the actual processing of the afferent signal and a "decision" about how to (or whether to) act on it. This decision making may be conscious ("I just felt a tickle on my leg and I'm going to scratch it") or unconscious, such as slight postural adjustment associated with terrain changes while walking. In all cases, however, information has to be received in order to be processed and acted upon. Refer to Tables 9–2 and 9–3.

The pathways of the spinal cord are longitudinal in nature, but are best seen in transverse slices of the spinal cord. Generally, the spinal cord gets larger as it ascends because more pathways are added.

Take a look at Figure 9–5. This is a transverse section that shows the major pathways of the spinal cord. The spinal cord is grossly divided into **dorsal**, **lateral**, and **ventral funiculi** made up of white matter (a *funiculus* is a large column). These funiculi are further divided into **fasciculi**. We mentioned the cervical and lumbar enlargements earlier: there will be more gray matter in areas that serve more muscle (segments C3 to T2 and T9 to T12). Tracts of white matter are widest in the cervical region because all descending and ascending fibers must pass through those segments. Sensory pathways are in the posterior (dorsal) portion of the spinal cord, and motor pathways tend toward the anterior (ventral) aspect. Let's look at the pathways.

In summary,

- Afferent and efferent pathways are responsible for communicating between the periphery and the higher levels of the CNS.
- Afferent pathways of the spinal cord convey information from peripheral sensors to the central nervous system, where it can be processed.
- Efferent pathways convey impulses from the CNS that allow some sort of action by muscles or glands.
- The pathways of the spinal cord are longitudinal in nature and the spinal cord gets larger as it ascends because more pathways are added.

TABLE 9–2.	Motor Pathways of the Spinal Cord and Brainstem			
Tract	Origination	Pathway	Termination	Function
Corticospinal tract (pyramidal tract)	Precentral gyrus of cerebral cortex, BA 4 and 6	Pyramidal tract: Descends as anterior and lateral corticospinal tract after medulla decussation	Spinal nerve nuclei	Motor innervation of skeletal muscle of neck, trunk, and extremities
Corticobulbar tract (corticonuclear)	Dorsolateral precentral gyrus of cerebral cortex and frontal eye field for cranials III, IV, VI (BA 4, 6, and 8)	Pyramidal tract: Brainstem corticobulbar tract	Brainstem cranial nerve nuclei	Motor innervation of cranial nerves
Corticotectal tract	Occipital and inferior parietal cortex and superior colliculus, interstitial nucleus of Cajal, nucleus of Darkschewitsch	Medial longitudinal fasciculus	III, IV, VI cranials	Eye movement for visual orientation and acquisition
Tectospinal tract	Occipital and inferior parietal cortex to superior colliculus	Dorsal tegmental decussation to medial longitudinal fasciculus, through ventral funiculus	Cervical spinal cord	Influence muscles of neck, in conjunction with XI accessory (visual orientation)
Corticorubral tract	Precentral gyrus of cerebral cortex, BA 4 and 6	Course with pyramidal tract	Ipsilateral red nucleus in tegmentum of midbrain	Indirect route to spinal cord; give rise to rubrospinal tract
Rubrospinal tract	Red nucleus of midbrain	Decussates at ventral tegmental decussation, descends through lateral tegmentum to lateral funiculus of spinal cord	Terminates at all spinal levels	Indirect route to spinal cord; synapse at all spinal cord levels to facilitate flexor and inhibit extensor neurons (especially distal arms)
Corticoreticular tract	Cerebral cortex; precentral gyrus (BA 4, 6), medial prefrontal cortex, limbic system, including amygdala	Accompany pyramidal tract	Brainstem reticular formation	Mediate reflex systems of micturition, genital function; integrates reflexes into emotional and social behaviors
Pontine reticulospinal tract	Reticular formation of brainstem	Uncrossed pontine (medial) reticulospinal tract; travels with medial longitudinal fasciculus to thoracic level and continues through ventral funiculus	All spinal cord levels	Excitatory for extensor muscles, midline musculature, and proximal extremities; influences posture and locomotion
Medullary (lateral) reticulospinal tract	Reticular formation of brainstem	Primarily uncrossed, through lateral funiculus anterior to rubrospinal tract	All spinal cord levels	Autonomic information to influence respiration, circulation, sweating, shivering, dilation of pupils, sphincter muscles of gastrointestinal tract, cardiovascular function

TABLE 9–2.	*continued*			
Tract	Origination	Pathway	Termination	Function
Lateral vestibulospinal tract	Neurons of vestibular nuclei, medulla	Anterior funiculus of spinal cord	All spinal cord levels	Excitation of muscles of neck, back, arm, and leg; inhibit flexors; affects postural adjustments related to head position and movement
Medial vestibulospinal tract	Neurons of vestibular nuclei, medulla	Anterior funiculus of spinal cord	Combines with medial longitudinal fasciculus and terminates in upper thoracic levels	Excitation and inhibition of neck and back muscles; affects postural adjustments related to head position and movement
Medial longitudinal fasciculus (MLF)	Contains pontine reticulospinal tract, medial vestibulospinal tract, interstitiospinal tract, tectospinal tract	Ascending MLF	Upper cervical levels	Modulates reflex movements of head and neck relative to vision and vestibular stimulation

Source: Based on data of Gilman & Winans (2003).

TABLE 9–3.	Body Region Innervated by Somatic Afferent Cranial and Spinal Nerves			
Spinal or cranial nerve	Body region	Spinal or cranial nerve	Body region
---	---	---	---
V ophthalmic	Upper face, anterior scalp	T10	Umbilical girdle area
V maxillary	Middle face, maxilla, upper dentition	L1	Inguinal area
V mandibular	Lower face, mandible, lower teeth, external ear, and ear canal	L2	Lateral thigh
C2	Occiput	L3	Knee
C3	Neck	L4	Great toe, lateral thigh, medial leg, calf
C4	Neck, upper shoulder	L5	Calf, shin
C5	Upper arm, proximal	S1	Posterior shin, heel
C6	Upper arm, distal	S2	Posterior thigh
C6, C7, C8	Fingers	S3	Medial thigh
T1	Upper thorax; inner lateral arm	S4	Buttocks
T2	Proximal inner arm	S5	Around anus
T4	Nipple area		

Source: Based on data of Noback, Strominger, Demarest, & Ruggiero (2005).

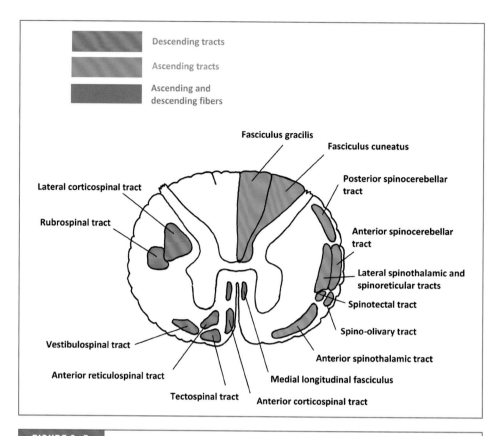

FIGURE 9–5. Major tracts of the spinal cord. This is a composite showing the major pathways of the spinal cord. Note that the dorsal funiculus consists of the fasciculi gracilis and cuneatus. The lateral funiculus includes the posterior and anterior spinocerebellar tracts, the lateral spinothalamic, spinoreticular, spinoolivary and anterior spinothalamic tracts. The ventral funiculus includes the vestibulospinal, anterior reticulospinal, tectospinal and anterior corticospinal tracts. *Source:* After view of Netter (1983).

Ascending Pathways

Ascending pathways are, by their nature, delivering some form of sensory information to higher levels of the CNS. Remember that these pathways get their input from the sensors of the body, such as stretch sensors, pain sensors, and tactile sensors. Your brain is continually creating a "map" of your sensory experience that you call "reality," and here's the input to your reality. Sometimes we refer to "first-order neurons," "second-order neurons," and so on. This refers to the neurons in the chain of communication. First-order neurons are the first neurons in the chain, such as afferent neurons passing information into the spinal cord. The next neuron in this communication chain is the second-order neuron, and so on.

Posterior Funiculus: Fasciculus Gracilis and Fasciculus Cuneatus

Within the posterior funiculus pass the **fasciculus gracilis** and **fasciculus cuneatus**. As shown in Figures 9–5 and 9–6, the fasciculus gracilis conveys information concerning kinesthetic sense (which is the sense of movement) and touch

pressure (touch pressure includes vibration sense, which is pressure that repeats rapidly). The sensation arises from muscle spindles (rate of muscle stretch) and Golgi tendon organs (GTOs; muscle tendon stretch). This sensory information is conveyed within the dorsal root ganglion of the spinal cord by means of unipolar neurons whose axons ascend ipsilaterally through the spinal cord. The fasciculus gracilis mediates information from the lower extremities, while the fasciculus cuneatus serves the cervical regions. The nerve tracts terminate in the medulla oblongata at the nucleus gracilis and nucleus cuneatus. Fibers from these two nuclei decussate and ascend as the medial lemniscus, which terminates in the thalamus. From the thalamus, fibers ascend to the postcentral gyrus of the cerebral cortex, also known as the primary sensory cortex (SI). The relationship between specific parts of the body being stimulated is projected on the cortex in spatiotopic array, so that there is a sensory map developed to represent the body. Damage to these pathways can result in deficits of touch discrimination of the hands and feet, as well as loss of sense of the position of body in space (proprioceptive sense), resulting in a gait impairment.

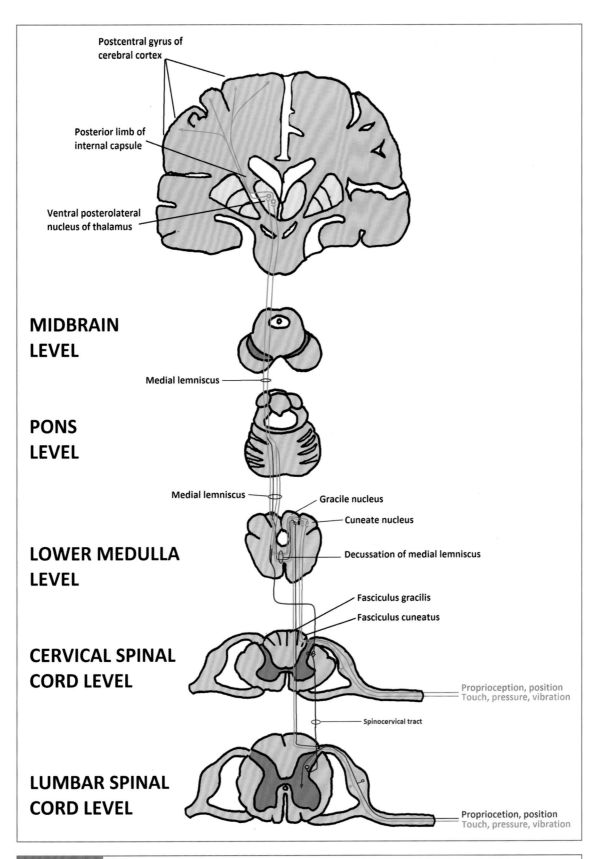

FIGURE 9–6. Ascending pathways for sensation, transiting through the nuclei gracilis and cuneatus. Touch, vibration, pressure, and proprioceptive sensation (combined sensation of muscle spindles and Golgi tendon organs) are mediated by the dorsal column–medial lemniscus pathways terminating in the gracile and cuneate nuclei of the lower medulla.

Anterior Funiculus: Anterior and Lateral Spinothalamic Tracts

The anterior spinothalamic tract is responsible for mediating the sensation of light touch to the thalamus. Axons from the first-order neurons enter the spinal cord and synapse with second-order neurons, whose axons decussate at the level of entry of up to three segments above that point. The axons of the second-order neurons ascend to the level of the pons, enter the medial lemniscus, and finally synapse at the **ventral posterolateral** (VPL) **nucleus** of the thalamus.

Lateral Funiculus

The lateral funiculus contains the lateral spinothalamic tract, the pathway that mediates information about pain and temperature sense from the lower body to the thalamus (Figure 9–7). Dorsal root fibers entering the spinal cord synapse with interneurons, which in turn synapse with third-order neurons that decussate and ascend. The fibers from this pathway terminate in the VPL nucleus and the reticular formation of the brainstem.

Anterior and Posterior Spinocerebellar Tracts

The posterior spinocerebellar tract receives its input from the muscle spindle receptors and GTO of the trunk and lower limb, as shown in Figure 9–8. This information travels ipsilaterally in an uncrossed tract to the level of the cerebellum. Sensory information enters the spinal cord via dorsal root ganglia, with first-order neurons bifurcating to ascend and descend to locations above and below the point of entry. The first-order neurons synapse at the dorsal nucleus of Clarke, with second-order neurons ascending ipsilaterally to the medulla oblongata, entering the inferior cerebellar peduncle, and terminating in the caudal and rostral vermis of the cerebellum. While the information about muscle spindle and GTO activity remains below the level of consciousness, alterations or loss of this sensory information would have a real effect on movement and posture. The anterior spinocerebellar tract carries similar information but ascends as a contralateral pathway to the superior cerebellar peduncle.

In summary,

- The spinal cord is grossly divided into dorsal, lateral, and ventral funiculi made up of white matter, and funiculi are further divided into fasciculi.
- Sensory pathways are in the posterior (dorsal) portion of the spinal cord, and motor pathways tend toward the anterior (ventral) aspect.
- The posterior funiculus contains the fasciculus gracilis and fasciculus cuneatus. The fasciculus gracilis conveys touch pressure and kinesthetic sense arising from muscle spindles and GTOs. The fasciculus gracilis mediates infor-

mation from the lower extremities, while the fasciculus cuneatus serves the cervical regions.
- The fasciculi gracilis and cuneatus nerve tracts terminate in the medulla oblongata at the nucleus gracilis and nucleus cuneatus. Fibers from the nuclei decussate and ascend as the medial lemniscus and terminate in the thalamus before ascending to the primary sensory cortex. Damage to these pathways can result in deficits of touch discrimination of the hands and feet, as well as loss of sense of the position of body in space (proprioceptive sense), resulting in a gait impairment.
- The anterior funiculus includes the anterior and lateral spinothalamic tracts. The anterior spinothalamic tract conveys sensation of light touch to the ventral posterolateral nucleus of the thalamus.
- The lateral funiculus contains the lateral spinothalamic tract that conveys pain and temperature sense from the lower body to the thalamus. The fibers terminate in the ventral posterolateral nucleus of the thalamus and the reticular formation of the brainstem.
- The anterior and posterior spinocerebellar tracts receive their input from muscle spindle and GTO of the trunk and lower limb, conveying information to the cerebellum. The information about muscle spindle and GTO activity remains below the level of consciousness, but alterations or loss of this sensory information has a deleterious effect on movement and posture.

Descending Pathways

Descending pathways provide the means by which we act on the environment. They are the effector pathways that cause muscle function and glandular secretion. Some of these involve voluntary activity, while others serve to moderate or inhibit reflexive activation. We are most interested in those that arise from the cerebral cortex because of their critical importance to speech and language. The major pathways include the pyramidal tracts for voluntary function, as well as several pathways involved in modulation and motor control.

Pyramidal Pathways

The pyramidal pathways are so-named because they arise from pyramid-shaped cells in the cerebral cortex, particularly in the motor cortex. The pyramidal tracts include the corticospinal and corticobulbar tracts. As will be seen, the differentiator between these two pathways is the termination point: spinal cord or brainstem.

Corticospinal Tract

The corticospinal tract arises from the cortex ("cortico") and terminates in the spinal cord ("spinal"). This is a direct pathway to initiation of motor function in areas served

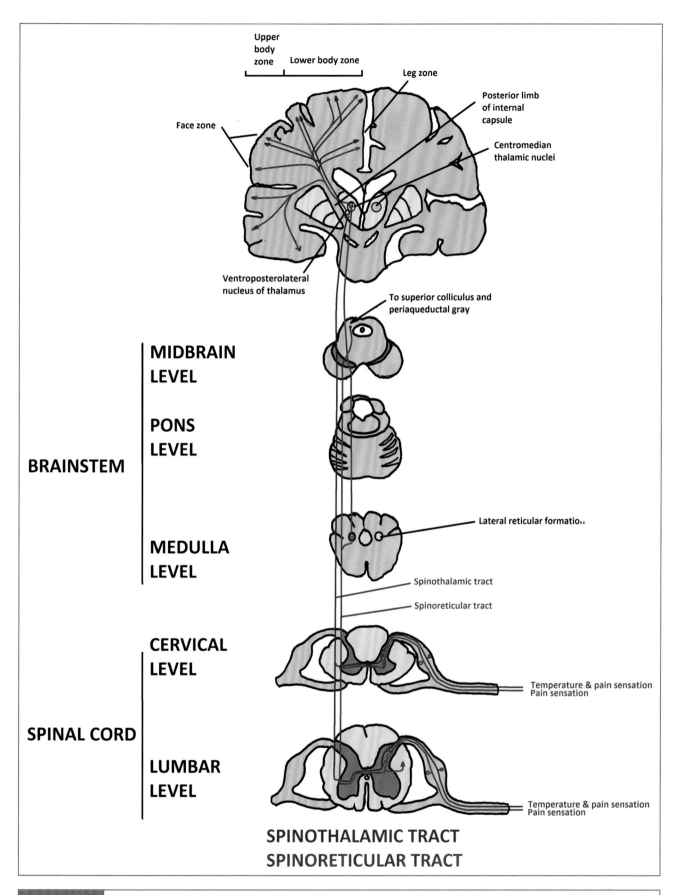

Upper
body
zone
Lower body zone
Leg zone
Face zone
Posterior limb
of internal
capsule
Centromedian
thalamic nuclei
Ventroposterolateral
nucleus of thalamus
To superior colliculus and
periaqueductal gray

**MIDBRAIN
LEVEL**

**PONS
LEVEL**

BRAINSTEM

**MEDULLA
LEVEL**

Lateral reticular formation

Spinothalamic tract

Spinoreticular tract

**CERVICAL
LEVEL**

Temperature & pain sensation
Pain sensation

SPINAL CORD

**LUMBAR
LEVEL**

Temperature & pain sensation
Pain sensation

SPINOTHALAMIC TRACT
SPINORETICULAR TRACT

FIGURE 9–7. Spinothalamic and spinoreticular tracts.

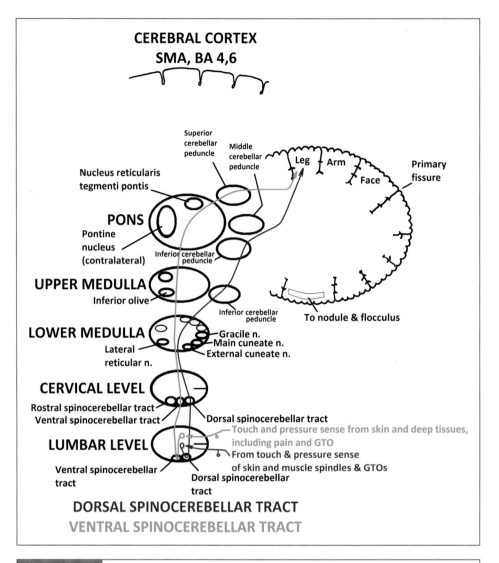

FIGURE 9–8. Dorsal and ventral spinocerebellar pathways.

by the spinal cord, including legs, trunk, and arms (Figure 9–9). The axons of the corticospinal tract are myelinated, greatly enhancing conduction rate of the neural impulse. More than half of the one million fibers of the corticospinal tract arise from the precentral gyrus, while the rest come from the supplementary motor area. The axons of the corticospinal tract descend from the cerebral cortex, condensing as the **corona radiata** (or "radiating crown") and funneling through the internal capsule and crus cerebri at the midbrain level (Figures 9–9 and 9–10). The corticospinal tract descends to the level of the lower medulla, where 75% to 90% of the fibers cross at a region known as the pyramidal decussation, descending as the lateral corticospinal tract. The remaining uncrossed fibers descend as the anterior corticospinal tract.

Spasticity

Spasticity is defined clinically as including increased muscle tone, hyperactive reflexes, and involuntary muscle contraction that creates tightness or stiffness and affects movement (Mayo, DeForest, Castellanos, & Thomas, 2017). When it involves musculature of speech, it is called spastic dysarthria. **Spastic dysarthria** is a frequent result of traumatic brain injury, spinal cord injury, stroke, amyotrophic lateral sclerosis, and multiple sclerosis. In these conditions, the speech-language pathologist will seek to improve intelligibility.

The neuroanatomical basis of spasticity involves bilateral lesions in any course of the pyramidal and extra-

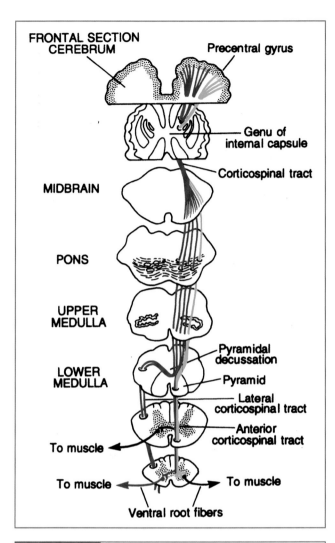

FRONTAL SECTION
CEREBRUM — Precentral gyrus
— Genu of internal capsule
— Corticospinal tract
MIDBRAIN
PONS
UPPER MEDULLA
LOWER MEDULLA — Pyramidal decussation
— Pyramid
— Lateral corticospinal tract
— Anterior corticospinal tract
To muscle
To muscle → ← To muscle
Ventral root fibers

FIGURE 9–9. Corticospinal tract. *Source:* From Seikel/King/Drumright. *Anatomy and Physiology for Speech, Language, and Hearing,* 3E. © 2005 Delmar Learning, a part of Cengage, Inc. Reproduced by permission. http://www.cengage.com/permissions

pyramidal tracts, which are responsible for skilled movements and the regulation of reflexes, posture, and tone. Bilateral lesions create overactivity in the muscles and result in increased muscle tone, spasticity, and slowness of movement.

In addition to speech therapy, oral medications such as baclofen, benzodiazepines, and gabapentin are frequently used for the pharmaceutical management of spasticity. Finally, botulinum toxin injections (Botox®) have been increasingly used to relax the spastic muscles. Since the duration of effectiveness of Botox is about 12 to 16 months, speech therapy done in this window may be most effective.

Axonal fibers descend for the purpose of activating muscle or otherwise communicating with peripheral neurons or tissues. When the fiber reaches its intended level on the spinal cord, it synapses with either a lower motor neuron (LMN) or an interneuron that, in turn, synapses with an LMN. The LMN exits the spinal cord, terminating on muscle at the motor end plate, thus completing the circuit for motor activation. Ultimately, all fibers arising from one cerebral hemisphere terminate on the contralateral side of the spinal cord.

The corticospinal tract is also responsible for inhibition of reflexes, as discussed in Chapter 3. A lesion of the corticospinal tract before the LMN will result in retention of reflexes and spastic conditions for the muscles affected. If the lesion occurs within the LMN, the effect will be a flaccid weakness or paralysis.

Corticobulbar Tract

The corticobulbar tract (Figure 9–11) also arises from the motor strip of the cerebral cortex in the region associated with the face, mouth, and larynx. This tract is extremely important for communication sciences and disorders, as it is the means by which all muscles of the face, mouth, and most of the neck are activated. The corticobulbar tract travels with the corticospinal tract to the level of the brainstem but not beyond. Fibers of the corticobulbar tract terminate in the brainstem to innervate motor cranial nerves. ("Bulb" is an old term for the medulla oblongata but, in this context, refers to the brainstem. You will often hear the term "bulbar" when people refer to the brainstem.) The corticobulbar tract also inhibits and facilitates thalamic transmission of sensory information, so its role extends beyond motor activation.

You will recall the notion of the homunculus, wherein the representation of the parts of the body is arrayed along the precentral and postcentral gyrus as a "map" of activation and sensation (see Figure 4–11). Recalling that map, you may remember that the areas that serve the corticobulbar tract are closely allied with the areas associated with motor speech planning, specifically BA 44, 45 (Broca's area in the dominant hemisphere), and the insular cortex (BA 13, 14). The sensory cortex (postcentral gyrus) also provides fibers for the corticobulbar tract, paralleling the function of the corticospinal tract efferents. The critical difference between the corticospinal and corticobulbar tracts is that the corticobulbar tract terminates in the head and neck region, thereby serving speech and swallowing function.

The course of the corticobulbar tract is very similar to that of the corticospinal tract. The corticobulbar tract descends within the corona radiata, condenses to enter the genu of the internal capsule, and then passes into the brainstem. Unlike the corticospinal tract, corticobulbar tract fibers do not cross at the pyramidal decussation, but rather descend to the level required for innervation of a nucleus, and decussate

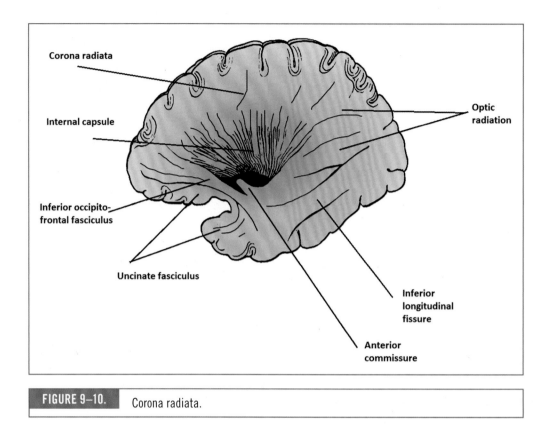

FIGURE 9–10. Corona radiata.

at that level. In this manner, fibers from the left corticobulbar tract descend on the left side of the brainstem to the level of termination, where they cross midline and synapse with the nucleus of a lower motor neuron. Activation of the muscles of mastication arises from an impulse generated at the lower lateral precentral gyrus that descends through axons passing through the internal capsule and the midbrain, decussates at the level of the pons, and synapses with the motor nucleus of the trigeminal nerve. At that point, the lower motor neuron of the V trigeminal nerve is activated, causing the masseter to contract.

So, recognize the parallels and differences between the corticospinal and corticobulbar tracts. Both tracts arise from the precentral (and, to some extent, postcentral) gyrus and supplemental motor area (SMA), both descend through the corona radiata and internal capsule, and both descend through the brainstem. Fibers of the corticobulbar tract decussate at the level of termination, while most of those of the corticospinal tract cross at the pyramidal decussation of the medulla.

In summary,

- Descending pathways are the effector pathways that cause muscle function and glandular secretion.
- The pyramidal pathways arise from pyramidal cells in the motor cortex, and include the corticospinal and corticobulbar tracts.

- The corticospinal tract arises from the cortex and terminates in the spinal cord. It is responsible for activation of motor function in areas served by the spinal cord, including legs, trunk, and arms. The axons of the corticospinal tract descend from the cerebral cortex, condensing as the corona radiata and funneling through the internal capsule and crus cerebri at the midbrain level.
- At the level of the lower medulla, 75% to 90% of the fibers decussate at the pyramidal decussation and descend as the lateral corticospinal tract. The remaining uncrossed fibers descend as the anterior corticospinal tract.
- When the fiber reaches its intended level on the spinal cord, it synapses with either a lower motor neuron (LMN) or an interneuron that synapses with an LMN. The LMN exits the spinal cord and activates muscle. Fibers of the anterior corticospinal tract descend and decussate at the point of termination. The corticospinal tract is also responsible for inhibition of reflexes.
- The corticobulbar tract is the means by which all muscles of the face, mouth, and most of the neck are activated. The corticobulbar tract travels with the corticospinal tract to the level of the brainstem, where fibers terminate in the brainstem to innervate motor cranial nerves. The corticobulbar tract also inhibits and facilitates thalamic transmission of sensory information, so its role extends beyond motor activation.

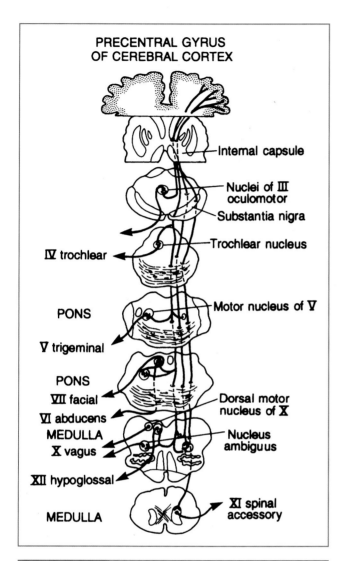

PRECENTRAL GYRUS
OF CEREBRAL CORTEX

—Internal capsule

Nuclei of III
oculomotor

Substantia nigra

—Trochlear nucleus

IV trochlear

PONS

Motor nucleus of V

V trigeminal

PONS
VII facial
VI abducens
MEDULLA
X vagus

Dorsal motor
nucleus of X

Nucleus
ambiguus

XII hypoglossal

XI spinal
accessory

MEDULLA

FIGURE 9–11. Corticobulbar tract serving the brainstem. *Source:* From Seikel/King/Drumright. *Anatomy and Physiology for Speech, Language, and Hearing,* 3E. © 2005 Delmar Learning, a part of Cengage, Inc. Reproduced by permission. http://www.cengage.com/permissions

Other Descending Pathways

There are a number of other pathways whose roles are not direct activation; instead, they provide support or modulation of that activation. These include the tectospinal, rubrospinal, vestibulospinal, and reticulospinal tracts.

Extrapyramidal System

The extrapyramidal system, also known as the indirect pathway, provides several important functions that support the direct, pyramidal pathway. The term "**extrapyramidal**" refers

to the fact that this control pathway lies outside of the pyramidal tract, but its influence is critical to skilled movement. The extrapyramidal system consists of several individual pathways, as discussed below (Figure 9–12). Taken together, the extrapyramidal system controls inhibition of reflexes, maintenance of muscle tone, and control of graded antagonistic contraction in support of fine motor activity. Said another way, failure of the extrapyramidal system can result in dysregulation of muscle tone and reflexes, disinhibition of the basal ganglia control network, and loss of skilled motor function. Tracts within the extrapyramidal system include the tectospinal tract, rubrospinal tract, lateral vestibulospinal tract, and reticulospinal tract.

Tectospinal Tract. The tectospinal tract (not seen in Figure 9–12) arises from the superior colliculus within the brainstem. The superior colliculus is a major reflexive relay for the visual system, providing a mechanism for orientation to a visual stimulus in space (i.e., orienting to movement in the visual field). The fibers of the tectospinal tract course through the tectum of the midbrain and descend to act on the first four or five spinal nerves. These nerves serve the motor function of neck muscles so that the tract can mediate rotation of the head in response to a visual stimulus.

Rubrospinal Tract. The rubrospinal tract ("rubro" refers to red) tract arises from the midbrain red nucleus. These fibers cross in the tegmental decussation of the midbrain to descend with the medial longitudinal fasciculus. The rubrospinal tract is involved in activation of flexor muscles and inhibition of extensors, as well as in maintenance of muscle tone in flexor muscles (Hongo, Jankowska, & Lundberg, 1969). The rubrospinal pathway appears also to be part of a circuit involved in stereotyped, multi-joint movements. Individuals who have suffered stroke that affected the direct pathway (corticospinal tract) may show reduced fine motor movement capability that was replaced by gross, stereotyped multi-joint movement, referred to as flexion synergy or co-activation patterns that are abnormal. An example of this would be shoulder abduction coupled with elbow, wrist, and finger flexion during an attempt to reach for an object. It is hypothesized that loss of the corticospinal control pathway allows the rubrospinal pathway to dominate the movement pattern, reducing skilled movements and replacing them with abnormal synergistic patterns that are more characteristic of the basal ganglia (Cahill-Rowley & Rose, 2014).

Vestibulospinal Tract. As the name suggests, the vestibulospinal tract (not shown in Figure 9–12) arises from the vestibular nuclei of the pons and medulla level. This tract is activated by output from the vestibular mechanism as related to movement and position of the body in space, and is important in mediation of spinal reflexes, as well as in extensor muscle

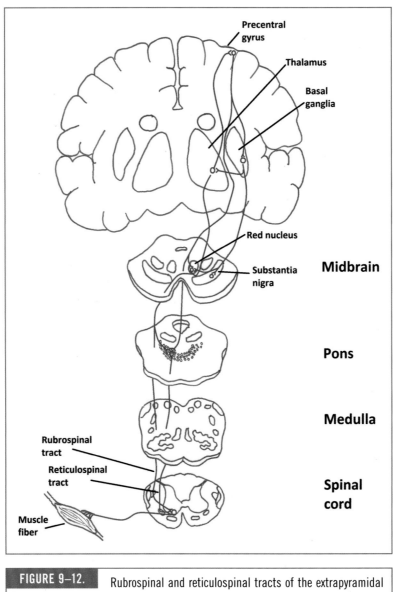

FIGURE 9–12. Rubrospinal and reticulospinal tracts of the extrapyramidal system.

tone. This pathway is part of the extrapyramidal system, and is responsible for maintaining posture and for stabilizing the head. The pathway also projects to the lower body and facilitates contraction of the leg extensors to support the body against gravity.

Pontine and Medullary Reticulospinal Tracts. The pontine reticulospinal tract originates in the medial tegmentum of the pons, while the medullary reticulospinal tract arises at the level of the medulla. The reticulospinal tracts are also part of the extrapyramidal motor control system. Both tracts descend in the spinal cord, with the pontine reticulospinal tract descending near the medial longitudinal fasciculus, and the medullary tract coursing near the lateral funiculus. Both

tracts are responsible for modulation of spinal tract motor activity by inhibiting reflexive responses to facilitate voluntary motor activity.

Corticostriate Pathway

Corticostriate fibers originate in the cerebral cortex and project to the caudate nucleus and putamen in the corpus striatum of the basal ganglia. These fibers are part of a network of modulatory neurons that connect the basal ganglia, prefrontal cortex, and thalamus, and appear to be intimately involved in cognitive and motor functions. Disturbance of these fibers can result in psychiatric and hyperkinetic disorders. These pathways have been implicated in autism, schizophrenia, obsessive-compulsive disorder, Huntington's disease, Parkinson's disease, and others (Cepeda et al., 2003; Shepherd, 2013). The corticostriate tract arises from the orofacial motor cortex, Rolandic operculum, and SMA, and is an important pathway associated with vocal imitation (Belyk, Pfordresher, Liotti, & Brown, 2016).

Corticothalamic Fibers

Corticothalamic fibers originate from layer VI of the cortex (specifically from the visual cortex, somatosensory cortex, and auditory cortex) and project to and from the thalamus via the internal capsule. They provide communication between the cortex and thalamus concerning reciprocal information at the sensory cortices (Briggs & Usrey, 2008).

Corticopontocerebellar Fibers

Corticopontocerebellar fibers originate from the frontal, temporal, and occipital lobes, synapse at the pons, and cross contralaterally to terminate in the cerebellum via the middle cerebellar peduncles. As the name implies, corticopontocerebellar fibers originate in the cerebral cortex, synapse in the pons, and terminate in the cerebellum. These fibers make up a critical component of the feedback loop associated with motor learning and the motor act itself (Brodal, 1978; Schmahmann & Pandya, 1995). The corticopontine fibers arise from the motor cortex, particularly areas 8, 9, 46, and 10 (in rhesus monkeys), and apparently serve what is termed "feed-forward function." We'll discuss feed-forward function in Chapter 11, but the important concept is that feed-forward processes involve previously learned motor actions. We compare our expectations about an action with what really happened, and make corrections when they don't match. This feed-forward control is a cardinal function of the cerebellum. Indeed, individuals with isolated pontine lesions exhibited increased speech, swallowing, and walking difficulties (Kwa, Zaal, Verbeeten, & Stam, 1998).

In summary,

- Corticostriate fibers originate in the cerebral cortex and project to the basal ganglia that appear to be involved in cognitive and motor functions. Disturbance of these fibers can result in psychiatric and hyperkinetic disorders.
- Corticothalamic fibers originate from the sensory layer of the cortex and project to and from the thalamus via the internal capsule. They provide communication between the cortex and thalamus concerning reciprocal information at the sensory cortices.
- Corticopontocerebellar fibers originate in the cerebral cortex, synapse in the pons, and terminate in the cerebellum and are a critical component of the feedback loop associated with motor learning and the motor act itself.

CHAPTER SUMMARY

The spinal cord is suspended by denticulate ligaments that arise from the pia mater and attach the spinal cord to the vertebral column. The conus medullaris is the lower section of the spinal cord, with the final projection called the filum terminale. The filum terminale joins with the dural tube of the spinal cord and becomes the coccygeal ligament, which attaches to the coccyx. There are 31 pairs of spinal nerves related to each vertebra. The spinal cord is shorter than the vertebral column, leaving a space in the lower aspect. Spinal nerves can have both afferent and efferent components. Spinal nerves serve specific body regions, known as dermatomes. The transverse anatomy of the spinal cord includes a central gray area surrounded by white matter. The gray area is made up of neuron cell bodies and the white, myelinated fibers of the neurons. The gray matter is divided into posterior and anterior gray columns. The myelinated fibers make up the tracts of the spinal cord for communication to and from the higher CNS structures. The central canal is continuous with the fourth ventricle of the brain. Dorsal root fibers are sensory in nature, and sensory information from the periphery enters the dorsal root ganglion that lies outside of the spinal cord. The ventral root consists of fibers that are exiting the spinal cord as spinal nerves and that will activate muscle.

Afferent and efferent pathways are responsible for communicating between the periphery and the higher levels of the CNS. Afferent pathways of the spinal cord convey information from peripheral sensors to the CNS, where it can be processed. Efferent pathways convey impulses from the CNS that allow some sort of action by muscles or glands. The pathways of the spinal cord are longitudinal in nature and the spinal cord gets larger as it ascends because more pathways are added. The spinal cord is grossly divided into dorsal, lateral, and ventral funiculi made up of white matter, and funiculi are further divided into fasciculi. Sensory pathways are in the posterior (dorsal) portion of the spinal cord, and motor pathways tend toward the anterior (ventral) aspect. The posterior funiculus contains the fasciculus gracilis and fasciculus cuneatus. The fasciculus gracilis conveys touch pressure and kinesthetic sense arising from muscle spindles and GTOs.

The fasciculus gracilis mediates information from the lower extremities, while the fasciculus cuneatus serves the cervical regions. The fasciculi gracilis and cuneatus nerve tracts terminate in the medulla oblongata at the nucleus gracilis and nucleus cuneatus. Fibers from the nuclei decussate and ascend as the medial lemniscus and terminate in the thalamus before ascending to the primary sensory cortex. Damage to these pathways can result in deficits of touch discrimination of the hands and feet, as well as loss of sense of the position of the body in space (proprioceptive sense), resulting in a gait impairment.

The anterior funiculus includes the anterior and lateral spinothalamic tracts. The anterior spinothalamic tract conveys sensation of light touch to the ventral posterolateral nucleus of the thalamus. The lateral funiculus contains the lateral spinothalamic tract that conveys pain and temperature sense from the lower body to the thalamus. The fibers terminate in the ventral posterolateral nucleus of the thalamus and the reticular formation of the brainstem. The anterior and posterior spinocerebellar tracts receive their input from muscle spindle and GTO of the trunk and lower limb, conveying information to the cerebellum. The information about muscle spindle and GTO activity remains below the level of consciousness, but alterations or loss of this sensory information has a deleterious effect on movement and posture.

Descending pathways are the effector pathways that cause muscle function and glandular secretion. The pyramidal pathways arise from pyramidal cells in the motor cortex and include the corticospinal and corticobulbar tracts. The corticospinal tract arises from the cortex and terminates in the spinal cord. It is responsible for activation of motor function in areas served by the spinal cord, including legs, trunk,

and arms. The axons of the corticospinal tract descend from the cerebral cortex, condensing as the corona radiata and funneling through the internal capsule and crus cerebri at the midbrain level. At the level of the lower medulla, 75% to 90% of the fibers decussate at the pyramidal decussation and descend as the lateral corticospinal tract. The remaining uncrossed fibers descend as the anterior corticospinal tract. When the fiber reaches its intended level on the spinal cord, it synapses with either a lower motor neuron (LMN) or an interneuron that synapses with an LMN. The LMN exits the spinal cord and activates muscle. Fibers of the anterior corticospinal tract descend and decussate at the point of termination. The corticospinal tract is also responsible for inhibition of reflexes. The corticobulbar tract is the means by which all muscles of the face, mouth, and most of the neck are activated. The corticobulbar tract travels with the corticospinal tract to the level of the brainstem where fibers terminate in the brainstem to innervate motor cranial nerves. The corticobulbar tract also inhibits and facilitates thalamic transmission of sensory information, so its role extends beyond motor activation.

CASE STUDY 9–1

Physician's Notes on Initial Physical Examination and History

This is a 68-year-old male who has a history of progressive **spasticity** in all extremities over the last few years (see Table 9–4 for terminology. Note that we are presenting the data of this case in chronological order to show the emerging speech and language signs and symptoms as the condition progresses). The neurologic examination showed increased muscle tone and **hyperreflexia** in all extremities, and the patient walks with a spastic gait. There is no muscle atrophy. The patient presents with **dysarthria**. The **electromyographic (EMG) results** showed normal **right peroneal and tibial motor responses** as well as the right sural sensory response of the calf region. Needle EMG of selected muscles in the right lower limb spanning the **L2–S1 myotomes** showed evidence of moderate chronic denervation in all muscles examined. Selective EMG of the right upper limb muscles showed no significant abnormalities. Spontaneous activity was absent throughout. The clinical impression is of electrophysiological evidence of moderate chronic denervation in the right **L4, L5,** and S1 myotomes, which may indicate **chronic radiculopathies** or a possible slowly evolving motor dysfunction at the corresponding levels. Clinically, he has mostly upper motor neuron dysfunction.

I reviewed this patient who has progressive **spastic paraparesis** with mild cerebellar signs in the lower limbs.

There is also a degree of dysarthria that was noticed by his family. MRI imaging of the brain and cervical spine did not show any structural lesion, but there is some white matter change posteriorly in the cerebrum and therefore it is probably worthwhile checking for long-chain fatty acids. In addition, we are checking for gene abnormalities of **hereditary spastic paraplegia** collection that are currently being done here. So far, we have not been able to document any specific explanation for his spasticity, which is also associated with bilateral optic nerve abnormalities. The MRI is not consistent with **multiple sclerosis (MS)**. Blood tests have shown a **borderline B12 deficiency** for which he is having treatment, and his niece reports some improvement, but not in the underlying signs as such.

One Year, 6 Months Following Intake

The patient with progressive gait disorder the last three years has come for a six-month follow-up. He presents with dysarthria, minimal swallowing difficulties, spastic paraparesis with **hip flexion graded at 4/5**, bilateral **Babinski sign with brisk reflexes**, abnormal joint position sensation in the lower limbs, as well as vibration loss in the left ankle (see Table 9–5 for definitions of muscle testing). In the upper limbs, there was **dysdiadochokinesia** on the left. The patient will probably need to consult our speech therapist in the near future. I was also thinking that the patient had a **lumbar puncture** so far and I asked him to

TABLE 9–4.   **Terminology for Case Study 9–1**

"c" score	Scoring on the *Frenchay Dysarthria Assessment* (FDA). See Table 9–6 for details of the Frenchay scoring.
Acoustic neuroma	Noncancerous tumor that develops on the VIII vestibulocochlear nerve. Pressure from an acoustic neuroma may cause hearing loss, tinnitus in the affected ear, and vestibular dysfunction.
Babinski sign with clonus reflexes	The Babinski reflex is elicited when the sole of the foot is stimulated with a blunt instrument. The response involves an extension of the hallux. The clonus reflex is the result of involuntary rhythmic contraction that activates muscle spindles. The Babinski sign is normal up until approximately 6 months of age, after which it is inhibited by the cerebral cortex. Presence in individuals after 6 months of age is considered abnormal.
Baclofen (active ingredient), Lioresal (generic name)	A muscle relaxant, used to improve spasticity, pain, and stiffness.
bid	Twice a day.
Borderline B12 deficiency	The lack of vitamin B12 may cause numbness, balance problems, anemia, swollen tongue, problems in attention and concentration, weakness and fatigue.
Chronic radiculopathies	Radiculopathy is due to a compressed nerve in the spine causing pain, numbness, or weakness. It is more frequent in the lower back (lumbar radiculopathy) and in the neck (cervical radiculopathy).
Dysarthria	Motor speech disorder involving muscular weakness, dyscoordination, and alteration of muscle tone. It includes slow movement of the muscles used for speech production, including the lips, tongue, vocal folds, and/or muscles of respiration.
Dysdiadochokinesia	Reduced ability to perform rapid, alternating movements (i.e., diadochokinesia).
Electromyographic (EMG) laboratory results	Results of a laboratory technique to record the electrical activity (electric potential) of skeletal muscles.
Evoked potentials	Electrical response from the nervous system after a stimulus is presented.
Hereditary spastic paraplegia	A group of inherited disorders characterized by progressive weakness and spasticity in the legs.
Hip flexion graded at 4/5	See Table 9–5 for details of muscle testing.
Hyperreflexia	Overactive responses of the reflexes.
L2, L4, L5, and S1 myotomes	A myotome is the group of muscles that a spinal nerve innervates. L2 myotome is responsible for hip flexion, L4 myotome is responsible for ankle dorsiflexion, L5 myotome is responsible for great toe extension, and S1 myotome is responsible for ankle plantar-flexion/ankle eversion/hip extension.
Lioresal	See baclofen.
Lumbar puncture	Medical procedure used to collect cerebrospinal fluid (CSF) via a needle that is inserted into the spinal canal. CSF analysis will help in the diagnosis of neurological diseases.
Motor neuron disease	Includes a number of degenerative neurological disorders (amyotrophic lateral sclerosis, hereditary spastic paraplegia, primary lateral sclerosis, progressive bulbar palsy, pseudobulbar palsy, and progressive muscular atrophy).
Multiple sclerosis (MS)	An autoimmune neurodegenerative disease with a range of symptomatology (depending on the area that is damaged in the central nervous system) such as double vision, muscle weakness, and trouble with sensation and/or coordination. It is caused by damage in the myelin sheath of the cells in the brain and spinal cord.

continues

TABLE 9–4.	*continued*
Peroneal and tibial motor responses	Responses of the peroneal and tibial nerves.
Prolonged P100 latencies	Conduction along the optic nerve is measured by the latency of the P100 component of the visual evoked potential (VEP) using electroencephalography.
Small vessel disease (coronary microvascular disease)	A disease in which there is damage in the walls of the small arteries.
Spastic paraparesis	Condition characterized by progressive weakness and spasticity (stiffness) in the legs.
Spasticity	Continuous abnormal contraction in certain muscles that results in stiffness or tightness in movement, speech, and gait.
Tizanidine (active ingredient), Zanaflex (brand name) 2 mg 1/2 tab	Medication used for reducing the symptom of spasticity.

TABLE 9–5.	**Examining Muscle Strength**

When examining a patient, identifying specific areas of muscular weakness helps to localize the site of lesion. Strength testing is completed for each muscle group, making sure that you test one side and then the next for each group, so you can compare strength for the two sides. Here is a muscle strength rating scale.

0/5	No contraction of muscle
1/5	Indication of muscle flicker, but no movement noted
2/5	Movement occurs, but not against gravity when tested in the horizontal plane
3/5	Movement occurs against, but not when there is resistance provided by the the examiner
4/5	Movement occurs against some resistance provided by the examiner
5/5	Normal strength

bring me the MRI scan of the brain. He will continue with vitamin B12 injections, **baclofen 6 daily**, **tizanidine 2 mg 1/2 tab bid** and magnesium for cramps. Review of his MRI of the brain showed evidence of white matter changes involving the frontal and parietal lobes and periventricular areas, which could be related to **small vessel disease**. There is also a focal area of enhancement involving the right acoustic nerve in the intracanalicular part, which could be related to a small **acoustic neuroma**. The **evoked potentials** report showed **prolonged P100 latencies** bilaterally, more so for the right eye. The clinical impression is for bilateral R > L optic pathway dysfunction.

Medical Diagnosis

Motor neuron disease (amyotrophic lateral sclerosis: ALS)

Speech Examination at One Year and Six Months Following Intake

The patient reported slow rate of speech and harsh voice quality one year ago, becoming progressively worse. His speech during dialogue was characterized perceptually by slow rate, harsh voice quality, and imprecise consonants. The *Frenchay Dysarthria Assessment* (FDA) showed moderate difficulty **"c" score** (see Table 9–6 for details of Frenchay scoring):

- Respiration in speech: Patient has to speak quickly because of poor respiratory control with a fading of his voice. Patient requires up to three breaths to complete counting from 1 to 20 (c).
- Palate in speech: Moderate hypernasality with some nasal emission when saying "/may pay/" and "/nay bay/" (c).
- Laryngeal component time: Sustained phonation for /a/ in 7 seconds with phonation interrupted by breaks (c)
- Laryngeal component volume: Changes in volume (vocal intensity) but noticeably uneven progression when the patient counted from 1 to 5 by increasing volume on each number (whisper for number 1, very loud voice for number 5) (c).

TABLE 9–6.	Frenchay Scoring Details

The *Frenchay Dysarthria Assessment* (FDA) utilizes a rating scale for all testing.

a score	Normal for age
b score	Mild abnormality noticeable to skilled observer
c score	Obvious abnormality but the patient can perform task/movements with reasonable approximation
d score	Some production of task but poor in quality, unable to sustain, inaccurate, or extremely labored
e score	Unable to undertake task/movement/sound

- Laryngeal component during speech: Voice production requires effort and attention, deteriorates, and can be unpredictable during monologue. Difficulties with modulation, clarity of phonation, or pitch variation, but patient was able to control these on occasion (c).
- Tongue component (protrusion): Variable ability of the patient to protrude/retract tongue (5 times in 7 seconds) (c). The tongue movement was accompanied by facial grimacing.
- Tongue component (elevation): Patient was able to point the tongue toward the nose and then toward the chin slowly. The tongue moved in both directions, but the movement was incomplete (c).

- Tongue component (lateral): Slow movement of the tongue side to side (5 times) produced in 7 seconds. The tongue moved in both directions, but the movement was labored (c).
- Tongue component alternate: Diadochokinetic rate of the bisyllable /kala/ (10 times) with one sound well articulated but the other poorly presented and the task deteriorated with time. Task took 10 seconds to complete (c).
- Tongue component during speech: Slow alternating movements of the tongue with distorted vowels and several omissions of consonants during dialogue (c).

Speech-Language Diagnosis

Mixed spastic-flaccid dysarthria

Questions Concerning This Case

1. In many progressive neurological diseases, the speech symptomatology starts three to six years after the initial symptomatology, with amyotrophic lateral sclerosis being an exception. What accounts for the lag between medical diagnosis and onset of speech signs and symptoms in these diseases? ALS targets the brainstem early in its course. How does this account for the rapid progression of speech deficits?
2. Limbs of the patient in this case demonstrated spasticity. How are the speech signs of spastic dysarthria associated with the general symptom of spasticity?

Case provided by Dr. Kostas Konstantopoulos, European University Cyprus.

CASE STUDY 9–2

Physician's Notes on Initial Physical Examination and History

This patient was admitted for investigation of a predominantly symmetrical **pyramidal syndrome** with mild cerebellar signs (see Table 9–7 for terminology. Note that we are presenting the data of this case in chronological order to show the emerging speech and language signs and symptoms as the condition progresses.). **Visual evoked responses, brainstem evoked responses**, and upper limb evoked potentials were normal. Lower limb somatosensory responses were unobtainable at both the cortical and the lumbar level. **Electromyography** of selected muscles failed to show any denervation. Previous nerve conduction studies of the same year did not show any evidence of a **peripheral neuropathy**. It appeared therefore that the patient had a pyramidal syndrome of unknown etiology. In view of the cerebellar signs, albeit a bit mild, the differential diagnosis was between **primary lateral sclerosis (PLS)** and **multisystem atrophy**.

Nine Months Following Intake

I reviewed this patient who has **spastic paresis** with a **pseudobulbar affect** and pseudobulbar signs. The working diagnosis was of PLS. He had an additional slight unsteadiness, which may be due to his spasticity. **MRI** of the brain did not show any significant abnormalities. **Bulbar** evaluation has shown that he has **dysphagia** mainly for liquids, but he is able to cope as long as he drinks slowly. Previous

TABLE 9–7.	**Terminology for Case Study 9–2**

"b-c" score	Scoring on the *Frenchay Dysarthria Assessment* (FDA). See Table 9–6 for details on Frenchay scoring.
1 tds to 1½ tds	1 tablet to 1½ tablets 3 times a day.
Amirol	See amitriptyline hydrochloride.
Amitriptyline hydrochloride (active ingredient), Amirol 10 mg (brand name)	Medication used to treat depression. In neurology, it is also sometimes used to reduce saliva production to avoid choking, a sign of dysphagia.
Baclofen (active ingredient), Lioresal (brand name) 10 mg	Medication that works as a muscle relaxer to improve spasticity, pain, and stiffness.
bid	Twice daily.
Brainstem evoked potentials or responses	Electrical potentials of the nervous system recorded following a presentation of a stimulus.
Bulbar	This refers to brainstem, including the medulla, pons, or cerebellum.
Deltoid 4+/5: deltoid muscle rating	See Table 9–5 for details of muscle test scoring.
Denervation	Loss of nerve supply arising from various pathological conditions.
Dysarthria	Motor speech disorder involving muscular weakness, dyscoordination, and alteration of muscle tone. It includes slow movement of the muscles used for speech production, including the lips, tongue, vocal folds, and/or muscles of respiration.
Dysphagia	Difficulty with one of the stages of swallowing.
Electromyography (EMG)	A laboratory technique to record the electrical activity (electric potential) of skeletal muscles.
Evoked potentials	Electrical response arising from the nervous system after a stimulus is presented.
Finger extension and abduction 4+/5	See Table 9–5 for details of muscle testing.
Folic acid	B9 water soluble vitamin.
Frenchay Dysarthria Assessment **(FDA)**	A standardized test to assess nonspeech and speech movements of lips, jaw, tongue, phonation, intelligibility, etc. (see Table 9–6 for details concerning scoring of the FDA).
Gabapentin (active ingredient), Neurontin (brand name) 300 mg	An anti-epileptic medication to treat neuropathic pain and seizures.
Gait	The manner of walking of an individual.
Harshness	Voice that is rough and raspy.
Hip flexion 4/5	See Table 9–5 for details of muscle testing.
Hyperreflexia	Overactive responses of reflexes.
Imprecise consonants	The consonants are slurred and distorted and exhibit inadequate sharpness.
Knee extension 4+/5	See Table 9–5 for details of muscle testing.
Knee flexion 4+/5	See Table 9–5 for details of muscle testing.
Lioresal	See baclofen.
Magnetic resonance imaging (MRI)	A diagnostic technique that uses magnetic fields to show an image of the body's soft tissue and bones.

TABLE 9–7.	*continued*
Monopitch	Voice that lacks normal variation in fundamental frequency.
Multisystem atrophy or multiple system atrophy (MSA)	A neurodegenerative disease involving abnormalities in heart rate, bladder control, etc. (autonomic nervous system), tremor, rigidity, speech difficulties, etc. (central nervous system).
Neurontin	See gabapentin.
Peripheral neuropathy	A disease that is caused by traumatic brain injury, infections, metabolic problems, etc. There is a variability of symptomatology that usually involves weakness, numbness, and pain in the limbs.
Primary lateral sclerosis (PLS)	A neurodegenerative disease that affects voluntary muscle movement. Its symptoms involve stiffness, spasticity, weakness, hoarseness of voice, slow speech rate, and dysphagia.
Pseudobulbar affect	Involuntary crying or uncontrollable laughing caused secondarily by a neurological disorder.
Pyramidal syndrome	A disorder that involves a symptomatology of spasticity, weakness, hyperreflexia, etc. It is caused by a dysfunction in the corticospinal (pyramidal) tract of the spinal cord.
Reduced stress	Loss of stress patterns in speech arising from reduced variability in vocal intensity and fundamental frequency.
Rilutek 50 mg (substance riluzole)	Medication used to protect the nerve cells. It is prescribed in amyotrophic lateral sclerosis.
Rilutek	See riluzole.
Riluzole (active ingredient), Rilutek (brand name) 50 mg	Medication to protect the nerve cells. It is prescribed in amyotrophic lateral sclerosis.
Spastic paresis	Disorder involving symptoms such as progressive weakness, spasticity in the legs, exaggerated reflexes, and hyperreflexia.
Visual evoked response	Electrical response from the nervous system after a visual stimulus is presented.

EMG failed to show any disseminated active **denervation** and therefore he did not fulfill the criteria of motor neuron disease. Nevertheless, he was placed on **Rilutek 50 mg bid** as well as B12 and **folic acid**.

Two and a Half Years Following Intake

I reviewed this 51-year-old patient with what appears to be primary lateral sclerosis. He demonstrated mild pharyngeal dysphagia but nothing significant, in that his weight has gone up by 2 kg. On examination, he showed more spasticity than weakness, and therefore we increased his **baclofen** from **1 tds to 1½ tds**. The rest of the medications remained the same.

Three and a Half Years Following Intake

I reviewed this 52-year-old patient with presumed primary lateral sclerosis. He was complaining that he had harshness in his voice. Dysphonia can occur with motor neuron disease, therefore this was still a possibility. He is also complaining of undue drowsiness during the day, and he is a snorer. We therefore admitted him for a sleep study. His gait remained stable on baclofen 1 tds.

Three Years, 9 Months Following Intake

The patient with PLS came for a follow-up. He stated that he felt weaker and complained of mildly increased salivation. On examination, there was **dysarthria** and harshness of the voice, and the muscle power was as follows: **deltoid 4+/5**, finger extension and abduction 4+/5, hip flexion 4/5, knee flexion 4+/5, **knee extension 4+/5** (see Table 9–5 for definitions of muscle testing). There was **hyperreflexia** throughout. He was continued with the same medication (Rilutek, vitamin E, **gabapentin**, amp vitamin B12, magnesium, and inhalers). He started amitriptyline for hypersalivation. He was referred for physiotherapy in the hospital.

Four Years, 7 Months Following Intake

I saw today this patient with PLS. Over the years, there was a very slow progression and generally he was feeling more weakness in the upper and lower limbs. He was able to eat solids and liquids without difficulties. He had no major complaints of pains, and he is able to live independently. On examination, the spasticity was worse on the right side and generally he was not very weak. I believe that there was no change in his speech, and the palatal movements were not very affected. He was to continue the same medications and he was to be seen again in four months.

Medical Diagnosis

Primary lateral sclerosis

Speech Examination

The *Frenchay Dysarthria Assessment* was administered to the patient (see Table 9–6 for details of Frenchay scoring). The results showed a mild to moderate difficulty, resulting in scores in the **"b-c" range**. The patient complained about slow speech rate, increased effort to speak, fatigue when speaking, and poor control of emotional expression. The most deviant speech characteristics involved imprecise consonants, monopitch, reduced stress, and harshness. More specifically:

- Respiration in speech: When asked to count from 1 to 20 as quickly as possible, the patient exhibited very occasional breaks in fluency due to poor respiratory control. An extra breath was required to complete the task (b).
- Lips seal: Occasional air leakage and breaks in lips seal when the patient was asked to blow air into cheeks and maintain for 15 seconds (b).

- Laryngeal time: Sustained phonation for /a/ with clear voice for 7 seconds (c). Phonation interrupted by intermittent huskiness or breaks in phonation.
- Laryngeal in speech (intonation): Voice during speech was mostly effective—there was occasional inappropriate use of volume and pitch noticeable to the examiner (b).
- Tongue protrusion: Irregular movement accompanied by facial grimace (5 times in 7 seconds) ("c" score).
- Tongue elevation: tongue is gross (d).
- Tongue lateral: Labored or incomplete tongue movement (5 times in 8 seconds) (c").
- Tongue alternate: Diadochokinetic rate of the bisyllable /kala/ (10 times) with observed slight incoordination and slowness of the tongue (7 seconds to complete the task) (b).
- Tongue in speech: Tongue with slow alternating movements that make speech labored. Several omissions of consonants were found, especially the sound /k/ (c).

Speech-Language Diagnosis

Spastic dysarthria

Questions Concerning This Case

1. The physician was ultimately able to diagnose primary lateral sclerosis (PLS). What is the neuropathological basis of primary lateral sclerosis, and did this patient's pattern of degeneration fit the classical presentation of PLS?
2. The patient demonstrated spasticity and some muscular rigidity in limbs. How does this relate to the speech characteristics seen in the FDA?

Case provided by Dr. Kostas Konstantopoulos, European University Cyprus.

CHAPTER 9
STUDY QUESTIONS

1. The notation C1 refers to the _____ _____ nerve.

2. Meningeal linings of the spinal cord are attached to the vertebral column by means of _____ _____.

3. At the lower end of the spinal cord is a cone-shaped projection known as the _____ _____.

4. The projection from the conus medullaris is termed the _____ _____.

5. True or False: There are 31 pairs of spinal nerves.

6. The specific body region served by a spinal nerve is referred to as a _____.

7. Nerves combined for a specific function are called a _____.

8. The gray area of the spinal cord is made up of _____ _____.

9. The _____ _____ is continuous with the fourth ventricle of the brain.

10. A _____ is a band of fibers that make up tracts.

11. Dorsal root fibers of the spinal cord are sensory/motor (circle one).

12. Motor fibers of the spinal cord that activate skeletal muscle exit through the _____ root.

13. True or False: The dorsal root ganglion is a motor ganglion.

14. The spinal cord is suspended by _____ _____ that arise from the pia mater and attach the spinal cord to the vertebral column.

15. Afferent/efferent (circle one) pathways convey information from the cerebrum to the spinal cord.

16. Afferent/efferent (circle one) pathways convey information from the periphery to the brain.

17. Sensory pathways are in the dorsal/ventral (circle one) portion of the spinal cord.

18. The _____ funiculus contains the fasciculus gracilis and fasciculus cuneatus.

19. The fasciculus _____ conveys touch pressure and kinesthetic sense arising from muscle spindles and GTOs of the lower extremities.

20. The fasciculus _____ conveys touch pressure and kinesthetic sense arising from muscle spindles and GTOs of the cervical region.

21. The nuclei for the fasciculi gracilis and cuneatus are found in the medulla/pons/midbrain (circle one).

22. The _____ _____ tract conveys sensation of light touch to the ventral posterolateral nucleus of the thalamus.

23. The _____ _____ tract conveys pain and temperature sense from the lower body to the thalamus.

24. The anterior and posterior _____ tracts receive their input from muscle spindle and GTO of the trunk and lower limb, conveying information to the cerebellum.

25. Descending pathways from the cortex are the effector pathways that cause _____ function.

26. The _____ pathways arise from pyramidal cells in the motor cortex, and include the corticospinal and corticobulbar tracts.

27. The _____ tract arises from the cortex and terminates in the spinal cord. It is responsible for activation of motor function in areas served by the spinal cord, including legs, trunk, and arms.

28. At the level of the lower medulla, 75% to 90% of the fibers of the _____ tract decussate at the pyramidal decussation and descend as the lateral corticospinal tract. The remaining uncrossed fibers descend as the anterior corticospinal tract.

29. The acronym LMN refers to the _____ _____ _____.

30. The _____ tract is the means by which all muscles of the face, mouth, and most of the neck are activated.

31. The _____ system is also known as the indirect pathway.

32. The _____ system controls inhibition of reflexes, maintenance of muscle tone, and control of graded antagonistic contraction in support of fine motor activity.

33. The _____ tract mediates rotation of the head in response to a visual stimulus.

34. The _____ tract arises from the midbrain red nucleus.

35. The _____ tract is involved in activation of flexor muscles and inhibition of extensors, as well as in maintenance of muscle tone in flexor muscles

36. The _____ tract arises from the vestibular nuclei of the pons and medulla level and is important in mediation of spinal reflexes and in extensor muscle tone, as well as maintaining posture and stabilizing the head.

37. The _____ tracts modulate spinal tract motor activity by inhibiting reflexive responses to facilitate voluntary motor activity.

38. _____ fibers originate from the frontal, temporal, and occipital lobes, synapse at the pons, and cross contralaterally to terminate in the cerebellum via the middle cerebellar peduncles.

REFERENCES

Baldi, J. C., Jackson, R. D., Moraille, R., & Mysiw, W. J. (1998). Muscle atrophy is prevented in patients with acute spinal cord injury using functional electrical stimulation. *Spinal Cord, 36*(7), 463–469.

Belyk, M., Pfordresher, P. Q., Liotti, M., & Brown, S. (2016). The neural basis of vocal pitch imitation in humans. *Journal of Cognitive Neuroscience, 28*(4), 621–635.

Briggs, F., & Usrey, W. M. (2008). Emerging views of corticothalamic function. *Current Opinion in Neurobiology, 18*(4), 403–407.

Brodal, P. (1978). The corticopontine projection in the rhesus monkey: Origin and principles of organization. *Brain, 101*(2), 251–283.

Cahill-Rowley, K., & Rose, J. (2014). Etiology of impaired selective motor control: Emerging evidence and its implications for research and treatment in cerebral palsy. *Developmental Medicine & Child Neurology, 56*(6), 522–528.

Carpenter, M.B. (1978). *Core text of neuroanatomy* (2nd ed.). Baltimore, MD: Williams & Wilkins.

Cepeda, C., Hurst, R. S., Calvert, C. R., Hernández-Echeagaray, E., Nguyen, O. K., Jocoy, E., . . . Levine, M. S. (2003). Transient and progressive electrophysiological alterations in the corticostriatal pathway in a mouse model of Huntington's disease. *Journal of Neuroscience, 23*(3), 961–969.

Crewe, N. M., & Krause, J. S. (2009). Spinal cord injury. In M. G. Brodwin, F. A. Tellez, & S. Brodwin (Eds.), *Medical, psychosocial and vocational aspects of disability* (3rd ed., pp. 289–304). Athens, GA: Elliott and Fitzpatrick.

Hongo, T., Jankowska, E., & Lundberg, A. (1969). The rubrospinal tract. II. Facilitation of interneuronal transmission in reflex paths to motoneurones. *Experimental Brain Research, 7*(4), 365–391.

Kwa, V. I., Zaal, L. H., Verbeeten, B., & Stam, J. (1998). Disequilibrium in patients with atherosclerosis: Relevance of pontine ischemic rarefaction. *Neurology, 51*(2), 570–573.

Liu, L. Q., Moody, J., Traynor, M., Dyson, S., & Gall, A. (2014). A systematic review of electrical stimulation for pressure ulcer prevention and treatment in people with spinal cord injuries. *Journal of Spinal Cord Medicine, 37*(6), 703–718.

Mayo, M., DeForest, B. A., Castellanos, M., & Thomas, C. K. (2017). Characterization of involuntary contractions after spinal cord injury reveals associations between physiological and self-reported measures of spasticity. *Frontiers in Integrative Neuroscience, 11*.

Netter, F. H. (1983). *The CIBA collection of medical illustrations. Vol. 1. Nervous system. Part I. Anatomy and physiology*. West Caldwell, NJ: CIBA Pharmaceutical.

Noback, C. R., Strominger, N. L., Demarest, R. J., & Ruggiero, D. A. (Eds.). (2005). *The human nervous system: Structure and function* (No. 744). New York, NY: Springer Science & Business Media.

Proctor, M. R. (2002). Spinal cord injury. *Critical Care Medicine, 30*(11), S489–S499.

Ragnarsson, K. T. (2008). Functional electrical stimulation after spinal cord injury: Current use, therapeutic effects and future directions. *Spinal Cord, 46*(4), 255.

Schmahmann, J. D., & Pandya, D. N. (1995). Prefrontal cortex projections to the basilar pons in rhesus monkey: Implications for the cerebellar contribution to higher function. *Neuroscience Letters, 199*(3), 175–178.

Seikel, J. A., Drumright, D. G., & King, D. W. (2016). *Anatomy and physiology for speech, language and hearing* (5th ed.). Clifton Park, NY: Cengage Learning.

Seikel, J. A., King, D. W., & Drumright, D. G. (2005). *Anatomy and physiology for speech, language and hearing* (3rd ed.). Clifton Park, NY: Thomson Delmar Learning.

Shepherd, G. M. (2013). Corticostriatal connectivity and its role in disease. *Nature Reviews Neuroscience, 14*(4), 278–291.

Stolov, W. C., & Clowers, M. R. (1981). *Handbook of severe disability: A text for rehabilitation counselors, other vocational practitioners, and allied health professionals*. Washington, DC: U.S. Government Printing Office.

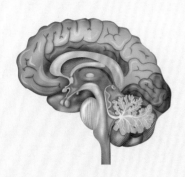

10 CEREBROVASCULAR SUPPLY

INTRODUCTION

The brain is a metabolic giant. While it makes up only 2% of the body's weight, it utilizes 20% of the oxygen of the body! Ischemia (cessation of blood flow) can result in irreversible brain damage within minutes, so a steady supply of blood is essential to the health of the brain. As we will see, the human brain has several redundant features that have the effect of partially protecting the brain from loss of nutrients. It is important for us as speech-language pathologists and audiologists to become well versed in the vasculature of the brain because the damaged brain tissues caused by either ischemia or hemorrhage (ruptured blood vessels) will affect hearing, language, speech, and cognition, causing such disorders as cortical deafness aphasia, apraxia, and dysarthria.

The vascular supply to the brain arises from two major sources: the carotid and vertebrobasilar systems. The dorsal aorta with its ascending and descending branches supplies the head and neck with blood. The branches of the aorta include the left brachiocephalic trunk, the left and right common carotid arteries, and the left and right subclavian arteries. The **common carotid arteries** give rise to the external and internal carotid arteries (Figure 10–1), while the vertebral arteries give rise to the basilar artery, posterior cerebral artery, and cerebellar arteries (Figure 10–2). We'll discuss the cerebrovascular supply based on these two major systems. You may wish to refer to the arterial territories schematically illustrated in Figures 10–2 C–F and Table 10–1 as we discuss them.

CAROTID ARTERY SUPPLY

External Carotid Artery Supply

While our focus will be on the internal carotid artery, the external carotid requires some attention as well. The **external carotid arteries** (see Figure 10–1) deliver blood to the cervical and facial soft tissues, the external ear, the sinonasal cavity of the skull, and the soft tissues of the scalp. The important **middle meningeal branch** (Figure 10–1B) of the external carotid arteries provides blood to the meninges of the brain by way of the **meningeal arteries** in the area superficial to the dura mater.

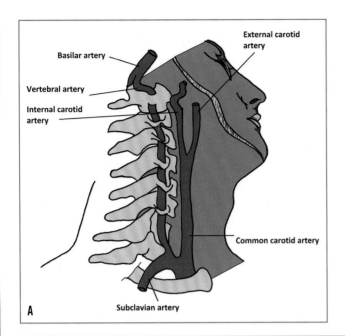

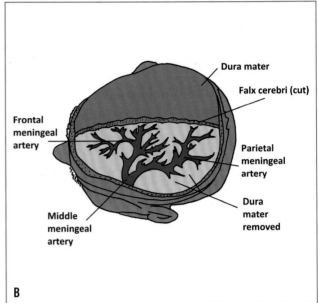

FIGURE 10–1. **A.** Vertebrobasilar sources. The aorta gives rise to the common carotid artery as well as the vertebral artery. The common carotid artery bifurcates into the external and internal carotid supplies. The internal carotid artery enters the brain case, dividing into the middle cerebral and anterior cerebral arteries. The vertebral artery enters the brain case, anastomoses into the basilar artery, and gives rise to the posterior cerebral artery and cerebellar arteries. The internal carotid supply and the vertebrobasilar supply are connected by means of the circle of Willis. **B.** Anterior and middle meningeal arteries.

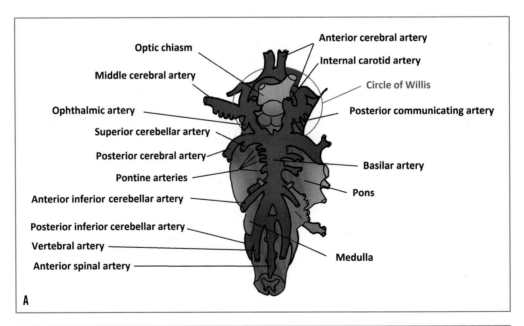

FIGURE 10–2. **A.** Carotid and vertebrobasilar supplies from ventral surface of cerebral cortex.

continues

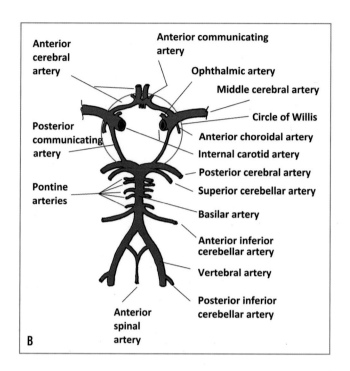

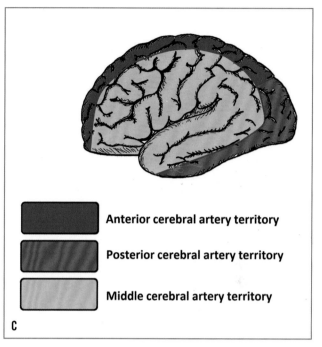

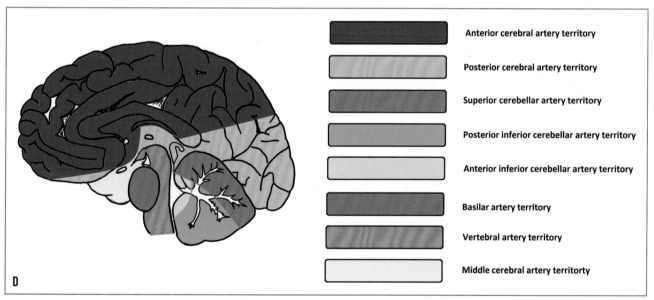

FIGURE 10–2. *continued* **B.** Schematic of vascular supply showing major components. Note that circled area indicates location of circle of Willis. **C.** Arterial coverage of the lateral cerebral cortex. **D.** Medial cerebral cortex. *continues*

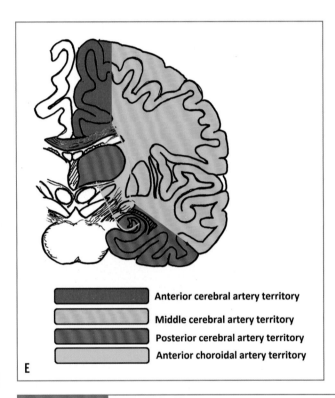

Anterior cerebral artery territory

Middle cerebral artery territory

Posterior cerebral artery territory

Anterior choroidal artery territory

E

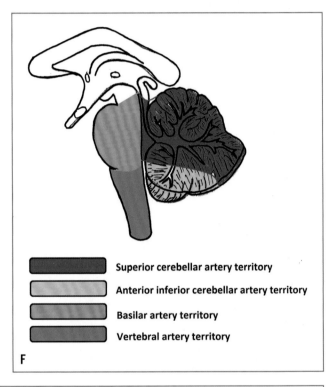

Superior cerebellar artery territory

Anterior inferior cerebellar artery territory

Basilar artery territory

Vertebral artery territory

F

FIGURE 10–2. *continued* **E.** Internal cerebrum (coronal section). **F.** Brainstem and cerebellum.

TABLE 10-1.		Major Arteries of Cerebrovascular System and Areas Supplied		
Internal carotid supply	Major artery	Gives rise to		Serves
	Anterior cerebral artery			Corpus callosum
		Medial orbitofrontal a.		Gyrus rectus, olfactory bulb
		Frontopolar a.		Medial and lateral of anterior superior frontal gyrus
		Callosomarginal a.		Cingulate gyrus and sulcus
		Anterior, posterior and middle internal frontal branch of callosomarginal		Posterior of superior frontal gyrus and medial frontal lobe to precentral gyrus
		Pericallosal a.		Sulcus between corpus callosum and cingulum
		Paracentral a.		Superior precentral and postcentral gyri and paracentral lobule
		Precuneal artery		Anterior precuneus and superior parietal lobe
		Anterior communicating a.		Communication between left and right anterior cerebral arteries
		Recurrent a. of Heubner		Anterior/inferior head of caudate, putamen, anterior limb of internal capsule
		Inferior branches		Optic nerves and chiasm
		Superior branches		Anterior hypothalamus, septum pellucidum, anterior commissure, fornix, anterior/inferior corpus striatum
	Middle cerebral artery			
		Medial lenticulostriate a.		Outer globus pallidus
		Lateral lenticulostriate a.		Putamen, superior internal capsule and adjacent corona radiata, caudate nucleus
		Lateral frontobasal (orbitofrontal) a.		Inferior frontal gyrus
		Lateral frontobasal (orbitofrontal) a.		Lateral orbit and inferior frontal gyri
		Prefrontal a.		Operculum, pars triangularis, inferior frontal gyrus
		Ascending frontal (candelabra) a.		
		Anterior parietal a.		Intraparietal sulcus
		Posterior parietal a.		Posterior parietal lobe

continues

301

TABLE 10–1.   *continued*

Internal carotid supply	Major artery	Gives rise to	Serves
		Precentral (prerolandic) a.	Posterior/middle of inferior frontal gyri, inferior lateral precentral gyrus
		Central (Rolandic) a.	Posterior precentral gyrus and inferior postcentral gyrus
		Temporooccipital	Superior and inferior occipital gyri
		Temporopolar	Temporal pole and anterior temporal lobe
		Anterior temporal	Temporal pole and anterior temporal lobe
		Middle temporal	Superior and middle portions, temporal lobe
		Posterior temporal a.	Posterior temporal lobe, insula
		Anterior choroidal a.	Choroid plexus, optic chiasm, optic tract, internal capsule, lateral geniculate body, globus pallidus, tail of caudate, hippocampus, amygdala, substantia nigra, red nucleus, crus cerebri
Vertebrobasilar supply	Vertebral arteries	Anterior and posterior spinal arteries	Anterior and posterior spinal cord
		Posterior inferior cerebellar a.	Branches into anterior-inferior cerebellar and superior cerebellar branches
Vertebrobasilar supply	Basilar artery		
		Superior cerebellar a.	Upper surface of cerebellum; branches to serve anterior medullary velum, tela chorioidea of third ventricle
		Superior cerebellar a.	Upper surface of cerebellum
		Posterior communicating a.	Connects posterior cerebral and middle cerebral arteries
		Anterior inferior cerebellar a.	Anterior undersurface of cerebellum; gives rise to internal auditory a.
		Internal auditory a. (labyrinthine a.)	Arises from anterior inferior cerebellar artery; serves auditory and vestibular mechanism
		Pontine a.	Pons
		Posterior cerebral a.	Gives rise to thalamoperforating arteries, thalamogeniculate, peduncular perforating, medial posterior choroidial branch, lateral posterior choroidal branch

The Meningeal Artery and Traumatic Brain Injury

The meningeal vessels, located in the sulci of the skull, are susceptible to penetrating traumatic brain injury (TBI). The middle meningeal artery, which covers a large portion of the skull, is frequently affected, with penetrating injury rupturing the artery and causing release of blood into the area above the dura mater (epidural hematoma). Clinically, the development of such a mass creates increased intracranial pressure and a concomitant herniation and swelling of the brain, with symptomatology involving speech, mobility, vision, and consciousness.

Internal Carotid Artery Supply

The internal carotid arteries give rise to the anterior cerebral arteries, posterior communicating arteries, and middle cerebral arteries as well as a number of other smaller branches. For speech-language pathology and audiology, the middle cerebral artery (MCA) is extraordinarily important, as it serves all of the speech, language, and hearing territory of the brain.

(high blood pressure). Further, turbulence at the bifurcation of the common carotid artery increases the likelihood that plaques will become dislodged and become emboli that can lodge elsewhere within the bloodstream. The arterial supply mimics the branching in trees, with larger branches splitting into smaller branches at bifurcations, which then branch again to create even smaller branches. In the vascular supply, arteries give rise to arterioles, which give rise to capillaries, with each successive generation at a branching becoming smaller in diameter. The terminal point of this branching is the union of veins and arteries, with veins showing increasing diameter as the blood makes its way back to the heart for oxygenation. (This is why there are rarely problems with emboli in the venous system, although clots may enter the heart and cause significant problems there.) Thus, any foreign body in the arterial system has a high probability of lodging somewhere downstream of where it is released. The larger a floating clot is, the greater the area it will affect when it does lodge in the bloodstream. Doppler and magnetic arteriography are essential tools for the assessment of blood flow, as they provide a non-invasive and low cost means of determining the presence of plaques and restrictions before they cause ischemic events.

Internal Carotid Artery Branching and Stroke

The internal carotid arteries and the vertebral arteries have tortuous bends and branching, which can lead to problems as we age. One of the most significant problem spots in the cerebrovascular system is at the point of **bifurcation** (dividing) of the common carotid artery into the internal and external carotid arteries. There is a significant narrowing at this branch in the artery, and if an **embolus** (floating blood clot) lodges at this location, it may starve the downstream tissue of oxygen. This is a critical emergency, since irreversible brain damage begins within five minutes of blood stoppage. In this case, blocking the entire internal carotid artery deprives blood to the anterior two-thirds of one entire cerebral hemisphere. An infarct covering this much of the MCA territory can result in profound aphasia if it involves the dominant hemisphere.

This is not the end of the problems with this bifurcation. Atherosclerotic plaques develop as we age as a result of diet, exercise level, and genetics. These plaques plaster themselves to the arterial walls, reducing the flexibility of the wall and thereby promoting hypertension

Arterial Branches from the Carotid Supply

While we tend to focus on the anterior and middle cerebral arteries in our discussion of the carotid supply, it's worth reminding ourselves of other very relevant branches for speech-language pathologists and audiologists. The ophthalmic artery provides oxygenated blood to the eyeball, while the meningeohypophyseal artery supplies the pituitary gland. The inferolateral artery is very important, in that it supplies the III oculomotor, IV trochlear, and VI abducens nerves, and ischemia associated with this blood vessel can result in oculomotor paralysis (Capo, Kupersmith, Berenstein, Choi, & Diamond, 1991). The capsular arteries serve the internal capsule and the basal ganglia. Ischemia affecting the posterior limb of the internal capsule can result in severe paralysis due to the effect on the pyramidal pathway, although recovery can occur (Fries, Danek, Scheidtmann, & Hamburger, 1993), and involvement of the basal ganglia can result in motor control deficit (Boyd, Edwards, Siengsukon, Vidoni, Wessel, & Linsdell, 2009) and cognitive impairment (e.g., Seidel, Gronewold, Wicking, Bellebaum, & Hermann, 2016; Westmacott et al., 2017).

The posterior communicating artery is partially responsible for regulating blood flow and pressure within the cerebrovascular supply. Specifically, this artery connects the internal carotid and vertebrobasilar supplies, so that an occlusion in one supply can be compensated by the other supply. Occlusion of the posterior communicating artery threatens the ability of the circle of Willis to compensate for blood flow fluctuations (Liebeskind, 2003; Schomer et al., 1994). The anterior choroidal artery also serves the internal capsule (posterior limb), thalamus, and optic chiasm, so an infarct involving this artery can result in hemiplegia on the contralateral side of the body.

Anterior Cerebral Artery

As seen in Figure 10–2A, the **anterior cerebral artery (ACA)** comprises a portion of the circle of Willis, coursing through the superior longitudinal fissure along the dorsal surface of the corpus callosum. The **circle of Willis** acts as a vascular backup system. Look at the schematic in Figure 10–2B, and first identify the basilar artery and then the internal carotid arteries so that you have located the two sources of blood for the brain. Now examine the way they are connected. The circle of Willis connects these two vascular supplies, and if the internal carotid artery supply is cut off due to infarct, the vertebrobasilar supply has the potential to supply those areas that are not receiving blood due to the infarct. The circle of Willis includes the anterior cerebral artery and the anterior and posterior communicating arteries. The anterior cerebral artery continues into the superior longitudinal fissure, serving the medial surface of the cerebral cortex, as well as a portion of the dorsal surface of the frontal and parietal lobes (Figures 10–3A, B, and C). The ACA is divided into three major segments. Section A1 includes the portion of the ACA within the circle of Willis and supplies blood to the basal ganglia, while A2 extends distally into the anterior two-thirds of the medial surface of the cerebral hemispheres to the genu of the corpus callosum. Segment A3 extends to the superior surface of the corpus callosum and supplies blood to the medial cerebral cortex.

Ischemia of the Anterior Cerebral Artery

A number of clinical signs arise from an infarction involving the anterior cerebral artery (ACA), depending on the anatomical sites involved, although collateral blood supply often reduces the signs of ACA blockage. The ACA serves the medial surface of the cerebral cortex, which supplies the areas controlling the legs. An infarct involving the ACA

can result in hemiplegia, particularly if the supplementary motor area is involved, as well as cortical sensory loss. With paralysis, a person may also find that inhibited reflexes are released and become active, including grasp and sucking reflexes. If the frontal pole, corpus callosum, and superior frontal gyrus are involved, the patient may have reduced ability to make decisions (hypobulia) or other cognitive involvement (Kang & Kim, 2008). Infarcts of the ACA are related to emotional lability, which is uncontrollable laughing or crying in absence of a relevant stimulus.

Posterior Communicating Artery

The **posterior communicating artery** sends collateral arterioles into the deep tissues of the brain, serving the thalamus, internal capsule, and optic tract. It gives rise to the **anterior choroidal artery**, which supplies the optic tract, posterior internal capsule, cerebral peduncles, medial temporal lobe, thalamus, and a portion of the corpus striatum.

Middle Cerebral Artery

Because of the critical nature of the **middle cerebral artery (MCA)** to speech, language, and hearing, it requires some focused attention. The middle cerebral artery oxygenates the speech and language zones of the brain, including the superolateral temporal as well as the lateral parietal and frontal lobes (see Figures 10–2 C–E and 10–3 A & B).

There are superficial and deep branches of the middle cerebral artery within the cortex. The **orbitofrontal** and **prefrontal superficial cortical branches** oxygenate the frontal lobe laterally and the frontal pole anteriorly. The posterior branches of the MCA (**parietal**, **angular**, **temporal**, and **occipital branches**) oxygenate the lateral surface of the frontal, parietal, occipital, and temporal lobes, including virtually all of the speech and language zones. The insular segment (also known as the Sylvian segment) supplies blood to the insular cortex and gives rise to the opercular segment, which serves the operculum, which is superficial to the insula. The many perforating branches provide blood to the caudate nucleus, the basal ganglia, and the internal capsule.

Infarcts of the Middle Cerebral Artery

Depending on the size of the infarct, lesions in the middle cerebral artery of the dominant hemisphere (typically the left hemisphere) will produce significant effects on motor function. One can expect upper motor hemiparesis on the right side, as well as a nonfluent or fluent aphasia, depending on the site of the lesion.

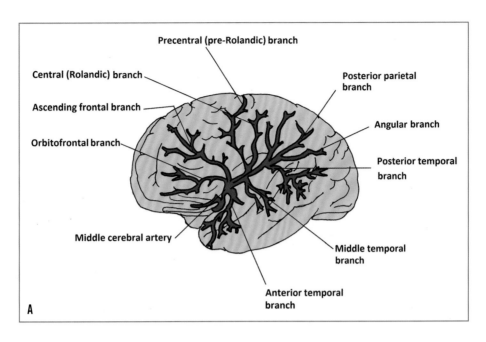

A

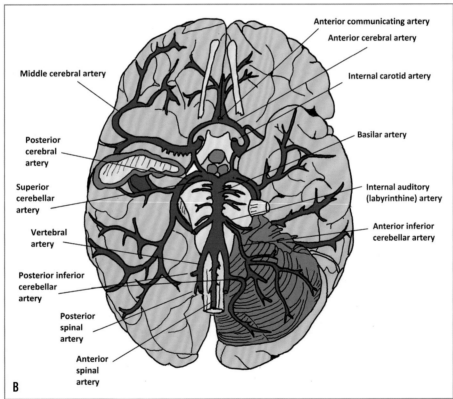

B

FIGURE 10–3. Views of the anterior and middle cerebral arteries. **A.** Lateral view of middle cerebral artery, showing its reach to the frontal, temporal, and parietal lobes. Note the proximity to the language (BA 40, 45, and 22) and cognition (BA 4, 46, and 10) areas. **B.** View of middle cerebral artery territory on inferior surface of the cortex. *continues*

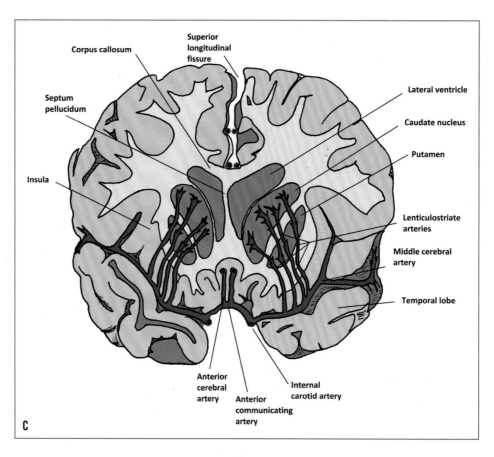

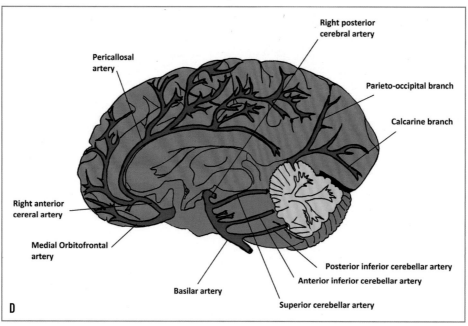

FIGURE 10–3. *continued* **C.** Coronal section showing the middle cerebral artery serving the basal ganglia and thalamus. **D.** Medial view showing anterior cerebral artery.

Lesions in the insular and Sylvian fissure segments of the middle cerebral artery can affect Broca's area, Wernicke's area, and the precentral gyrus, resulting in aphasia, apraxia, and dysarthria. Infarct involving the insula can result in apraxia of speech, as well as loss of thermal sensation (Kodumuri et al., 2016). If the lesion extends to the cortical white matter beneath the insular cortex, one may see sensory disturbances, transcortical motor aphasia, phonatory deficiency, and dysphagia. A lesion in the area of the basal ganglia and internal capsule may create dysfunction in the direct and indirect pathways responsible for the initiation and control of movement, as well as dysfunction of the corticobulbar tract.

In summary, the brain uses a disproportionate volume of blood, and ischemia can result in irreversible brain damage within minutes.

- The vascular supply to the brain arises from two major sources: the carotid and vertebrobasilar systems. The common carotid arteries give rise to the external and internal carotid arteries, and the vertebral arteries give rise to the basilar artery, posterior cerebral artery, and cerebellar arteries.
- The external carotid arteries deliver blood to the cervical and facial soft tissues, the external ear, the sinonasal cavity of the skull, and the soft tissues of the scalp. The middle meningeal branch of the external carotid arteries provides blood to the meninges of the brain by way of the meningeal arteries in the area superficial to the dura mater.
- The internal carotid arteries give rise to the anterior and middle cerebral arteries as well as a number of other smaller branches. The middle cerebral artery is particularly relevant to speech-language pathologists and audiologists because of the territory it serves.
- The anterior cerebral artery courses through the superior longitudinal fissure along the dorsal surface of the corpus callosum. The anterior cerebral artery continues into the superior longitudinal fissure, serving the medial surface of the cerebral cortex, corpus callosum, a portion of the dorsal surface of the frontal and parietal lobes, and basal ganglia.
- The circle of Willis provides vascular redundancy to the blood supply to the brain. The circle of Willis includes the anterior cerebral artery and the anterior and posterior communicating arteries.
- The posterior communicating artery serves the thalamus, internal capsule, and optic tract.
- Superficial branches of the middle cerebral artery serve the superior temporal lobe, as well as the lateral and most of the dorsal surfaces of the frontal and parietal lobes, and the insula and operculum. Perforating branches serve the caudate nucleus, the basal ganglia, and the internal capsule.

VERTEBROBASILAR SYSTEM

Vertebral and Basilar Arteries

The **left and right vertebral arteries**, arising from the anterior vertebral column, join together (anastomose) to form the **basilar artery** at the junction of the pons and medulla in the brainstem (see Figures 10–2B and 10–3B). The vertebral and basilar arteries together deliver blood by means of large and small vessels in the posterior cerebrovascular circulation. Small arteries branch off of the vertebral arteries before the vertebral arteries combine to form the basilar artery. The posterior inferior cerebellar artery serves the base of the posterior cerebellum, while the anterior and posterior spinal arteries serve the spinal cord. The **perforating branches** of the vertebral arteries oxygenate the lower medulla, the upper cervical spinal cord, and the inferior cerebellar peduncles.

The **basilar artery** branches to serve posterior brain structures. The **pontine perforating artery** provides blood to the pons, midbrain, and cerebellar peduncles, while the **anterior inferior cerebellar artery** gives blood to the anterior cerebellar hemisphere, the pons, and the cerebellar peduncles. The anterior inferior cerebellar artery gives rise to the internal auditory artery (also known as the labyrinthine artery), which serves the auditory and vestibular mechanisms. The **superior cerebellar arteries** oxygenate the superior and lateral aspects of the cerebellar hemispheres, the superior cerebellar peduncle, and the superior cerebellar vermis.

Posterior Cerebral Artery

The basilar artery gives rise to the left and right **posterior cerebral arteries** (see Figures 10–2A & B and 10–3B). As with the other arteries, the posterior cerebral arteries branch to form a number of smaller arteries that serve the cerebral cortex. The anterior temporal branch oxygenates the inferior surface of the temporal lobe, specifically the anterior fusiform gyrus and the uncus, while the posterior temporal artery oxygenates the posterior fusiform gyrus and the inferior temporal gyrus. The parietal branch serves the medial surface of the parietal lobe, including the cuneus and precuneus. The medial occipital branch serves the occipital lobe. The splenial branch serves the splenium of the corpus callosum, while the posterior medial choroidal branch oxygenates the choroidal plexus of the lateral and third ventricles, the thalamus and hypothalamus, and the posterior internal capsule and midbrain.

VENOUS DRAINAGE OF THE CEREBROVASCULAR SUPPLY

A number of veins drain the cerebrum, cerebellum, and brainstem, subsequently emptying into the dural venous sinuses. Figure 10–4 shows the superficial venous system of the brain.

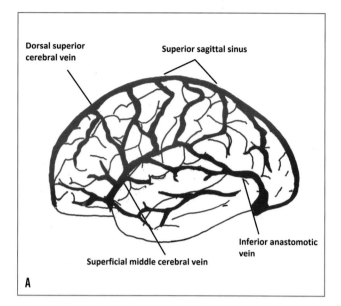

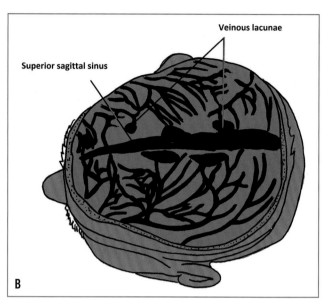

FIGURE 10–4. Venous drainage of the cerebral cortex. **A.** Lateral cortex, showing major veins and superior sagittal sinus drainage. **B.** Superior view, showing superior sagittal sinus and lacunar drains.

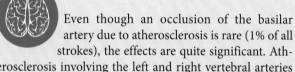

Ischemia of the Vertebrobasilar System

Even though an occlusion of the basilar artery due to atherosclerosis is rare (1% of all strokes), the effects are quite significant. Atherosclerosis involving the left and right vertebral arteries affects all downstream structures served by the basilar, cerebellar, and posterior cerebral arteries. Signs of vertebral artery infarct can include reduced consciousness due to involvement of the reticular formation of the brainstem, dysarthria, dysphagia, and horizontal gaze paresis. Dysarthria and dysphagia may also be initial signs of transient ischemic attacks or minor strokes, even though the most common initial signs are vertigo and headaches (Mattle et al., 2011). Dysarthria and dysphagia are caused by lesions in the corticobulbar tracts, cerebellum, and caudal cranial nerve nuclei (Mattle et al., 2011).

Large pontine strokes will result in either hemiplegia or quadriplegia. An embolus involving the basilar artery will affect the blood flow through the superior cerebellar artery, affecting function of the midbrain and thalamus. The result can be decreased consciousness and **tetraparesis** (paralysis affecting all four limbs). **Locked-in syndrome** is associated with basilar artery infarct. In this syndrome, a person is fully conscious but unable to accomplish any voluntary motor act except for vertical eye movement (Smith & Delargy, 2005).

Strokes involving the posterior cerebral artery can have broad-ranging effects (e.g., Cereda, & Carrera, 2012).

Infarcts that affect the thalamoperforating branch may produce **hypersomnolence** (a sleep disorder involving excessive sleepiness during the day), cognitive deficits, and vertical oculomotor paresis. Infarction in the thalamogeniculate branch produces severe contralateral diminished sensation (**hypesthesia**) and ataxia. A unilateral infarct in the posterior cerebral artery affecting the occipital lobe will produce contralateral **hemianopsia** (visual field cut). If it affects the dominant occipital lobe plus the splenium of the corpus callosum, it will produce difficulty reading (alexia) without difficulty writing (agraphia). A bilateral lesion in the posterior cerebral artery may produce cortical blindness with normal ophthalmological clinical findings (Benson, Marsden, & Meadows, 1974; Brandt, Steinke, Thie, Pessin, & Caplan, 2000; Szabo, Förster, Jäger, Kern, Griebe, Hennerici, & Gass, 2009).

Infarct in the border zone between the posterior cerebral artery and the middle cerebral artery will produce different stroke syndromes. A bilateral lesion of the fusiform gyrus will result in inability to recognize familiar faces (**prosopagnosia**). A unilateral lesion in the left temporal-parietal region will produce fluent speech with impaired comprehension but preserved repetition, a syndrome that is called transcortical sensory aphasia.

Chronic hypertension will often affect the median and paramedian pontine perforating arteries, resulting in lacunar infarcts. **Lacunar** means "little lakes," and lacunar infarcts are so-called because they leave "lakes" of necrotic or dead tissue in the deep tissues of the brain. Lacunar strokes are particularly problematic because they arise from hypertension and deep arteriole hemorrhage but don't typically result in acute emergencies. Lacunar strokes are often referred to as "silent strokes" for this reason, but the long-term effects can be quite significant. Lacunar infarcts often affect the basal ganglia and related structures and can be the cause of vascular dementia (Fisher, 1982).

The superior sagittal sinus receives blood from the veins from varying sources. The cortical surface is drained from the **superficial** cerebral veins, and the meninges are drained from the **meningeal** veins, ultimately draining into the venous sinuses. Blood from deep tissue of the brain, including subcortical structures, is received by the basal veins of Rosenthal and the internal cerebral veins. These veins anastomose to become the great vein of Galen, ultimately draining into the superior sagittal sinus. The superior sagittal sinus is the product of the union of the dura mater and the skull, with the sinus being immediately superior to the falx cerebri. In the posterior aspect at the tentorium cerebelli, the superior sagittal sinus joins the straight sinus, and subsequently the transverse sinuses. The blood passes consecutively through the sigmoid and cavernous sinus, where it ultimately drains into the jugular veins.

In summary, the left and right vertebral arteries arise from the anterior vertebral column and join to form the basilar artery.

- The posterior inferior cerebellar artery serves the base of the posterior cerebellum, while the anterior and posterior spinal arteries serve the spinal cord. The perforating branches of the vertebral arteries oxygenate the lower medulla, the upper cervical spinal cord, and the inferior cerebellar peduncles.
- The basilar artery serves the pons, midbrain, and cerebellar peduncles, and the anterior inferior cerebellar artery serves the anterior cerebellar hemisphere and the cerebellar peduncles. The superior cerebellar arteries oxygenate the superior and lateral aspects of the cerebellar hemispheres, the superior cerebellar peduncle, and the superior cerebellar vermis.
- The posterior cerebral artery indirectly serves the inferior temporal lobe, including the fusiform gyrus and the uncus, the inferior temporal gyrus, medial surface of the parietal lobe, and the occipital lobe. Branches also serve the splenium of the corpus callosum, the choroidal plexus of the lateral and third ventricles, the thalamus/hypothalamus, and the posterior internal capsule and midbrain.
- The cortical surface is drained by the superficial cerebral veins, and the meninges are drained by the meningeal veins. Blood from deep tissue of the brain is received by the basal veins of Rosenthal and by the internal cerebral veins. These veins anastomose and ultimately drain into the superior sagittal sinus. The superior sagittal sinus drains into other sinuses, finally issuing blood into the jugular vein.

CHAPTER SUMMARY

The brain uses a disproportionate volume of blood, and ischemia can result in irreversible brain damage within minutes. The vascular supply to the brain arises from the carotid and vertebrobasilar systems. The common carotid arteries give rise to the external and internal carotid arteries, and the vertebral arteries give rise to the basilar artery, posterior cerebral artery, and cerebellar arteries. The external carotid arteries deliver blood to the cervical and facial soft tissues, the external ear, the sinonasal cavity of the skull, and the soft tissues of the scalp. The middle meningeal branch of the external carotid arteries provides blood to the meninges of the brain by way of the meningeal arteries in the area superficial to the dura mater. The internal carotid arteries give rise to the anterior and middle cerebral arteries as well as a number of other smaller branches. The middle cerebral artery is particularly relevant to speech-language pathologists and audiologists because of the territory it serves. The anterior cerebral artery courses through the superior longitudinal fissure along the dorsal surface of the corpus callosum. The anterior cerebral artery continues into the superior longitudinal fissure, serving the medial surface of the cerebral cortex, corpus callosum, a portion of the dorsal surface of the frontal and parietal lobes, and basal ganglia. The circle of Willis provides vascular redundancy to the blood supply to the brain. The circle of Willis includes the anterior cerebral artery and the anterior and posterior communicating arteries. The posterior communicating artery serves the thalamus, internal capsule, and optic tract. Superficial branches of the middle cerebral artery serve the superior temporal lobe, as well as the lateral and most of the dorsal surfaces of the frontal and parietal lobes, and the insula and operculum. Perforating branches serve the caudate nucleus, the basal ganglia, and the internal capsule.

The left and right vertebral arteries arise from the anterior vertebral column and join to form the basilar artery. The posterior inferior cerebellar artery serves the base of the posterior cerebellum, while the anterior and posterior spinal arteries serve the spinal cord. The perforating branches of the vertebral arteries oxygenate the lower medulla, the upper cervical spinal cord, and the inferior cerebellar peduncles. The basilar artery serves the pons, midbrain, and cerebellar peduncles, and the anterior inferior cerebellar artery serves the anterior cerebellar hemisphere and the cerebellar peduncles. The superior cerebellar arteries oxygenate the superior and lateral aspects of the cerebellar hemispheres, the superior cerebellar peduncle, and the superior cerebellar vermis. The posterior cerebral artery indirectly serves the inferior temporal lobe, including the fusiform gyrus and the uncus, the inferior temporal gyrus, medial surface of the parietal lobe, and the occipital lobe. Branches also serve the splenium of the corpus callosum, the choroidal plexus of the lateral and third ventricles, the thalamus/hypothalamus, and the poste-rior internal capsule and midbrain. The cortical surface is drained by the superficial cerebral veins, and the meninges are drained by the meningeal veins. Blood from deep tissue of the brain is received by the basal veins of Rosenthal and by the internal cerebral veins. These veins anastomose and ultimately drain into the superior sagittal sinus. The superior sagittal sinus drains into other sinuses, finally issuing blood into the jugular vein.

CASE STUDY 10–1

Physician's Notes on Initial Physical Examination and History

Today I first saw this 64-year-old right-handed male patient with gait difficulties and unsteadiness that had begun seven years ago. His condition was of slow progression, and over the last five years he has had only minor speech changes. He has no complaints of dysphagia or pain (see Table 10–2 for terminology. Note that we are presenting the data of this case in chronological order to show the emerging speech and language signs and symptoms as the condition progresses). He did not complain of symptoms in the upper limbs. Past medical history included a diagnosis for **diabetes mellitus** two years ago, and he is currently controlling his blood sugar with **Glucophage** 500 mg **prn**. There was no family history of neurological disease. On examination he was walking with a wide-based gait and bilateral lower limb **spasticity** (see Table 10–3 for definitions of muscle testing). He could neither walk in a straight line nor walk on his toes and heels. The **Romberg** was negative. Ocular movements were full but had rather **slow saccades**. There was no **nystagmus** and diplopia. The pupils were equal in reacting to light. Mild dysarthria was noted of rather spastic origin. The rest of the cranial nerves were normal. In the upper and lower limbs there was no wasting and the **muscle tone** was increased especially in the lower limbs. The **reflexes** were brisk diffusely bilaterally with **upgoing plantars**. The **heel-to-knee** examination in the lower limbs could not be evaluated due to the increased spasticity. In the upper limbs he had no **dysmetria** and no **dysdiadochokinesia**. I referred him for hematological and biochemical examinations, and scheduled a follow-up when the results are in hand.

Three Years, 2 Months Following Intake

This 67-year-old right-handed patient has been followed in our clinic for 3 years now. The patient reported that he developed gait difficulties 10 years previously. His condition has slowly progressed, and over the past 5 years he has developed speech changes. He had no complaints of **dysphagia**, **diplopia**, or pains. He never had difficulties using his hands. The patient has been fully tested with EMG and nerve conduction studies, and these were not suggestive for **peripheral neuropathy**. The **BAEP** was normal. The upper and lower limb somatosensory **evoked potentials** were suggestive of dysfunction of the somatosensory pathways from the upper and lower limbs. Vitamin E and vitamin B12 were within the normal limits. The clinical picture of the patient with progressive spinocerebellar condition was suggestive of a **spinocerebellar syndrome**. He has no family history of cerebellar problems. The genetic investigation at the beginning of treatment was at the **alsin (ALS2) gene** in order to rule out this condition due to the major symptom of slow progressive spasticity. The genetic investigation was negative. The patient is under genetic investigation to rule out the known spinocerebellar ataxia (SCA) loci but also the **spastic paraplegias** loci. He began treatment for spasticity with **tetrabenazine** and baclofen, but he could not tolerate high doses because it caused muscular weakness. He was currently on treatment with tetrabenazine but also **coenzyme Q10** and vitamin E.

Five Years, 1 Month Following Intake

The patient was seen for follow-up for spastic **tetraparesis** and **dysarthria**. The patient reported that there was deterioration in his spasticity even though he exercises regularly and follows a physiotherapy schedule. He is on treatment with **baclofen** 10 mg **x2**, **tizanidine** 4 mg **1-1/2-1/2**. He also takes vitamin E and coenzyme Q10. On examination, there was spastic gait and the patient was able to walk with the help of a stick. There was increased tone in the lower limbs with mild proximal weakness bilaterally. He recently had blood analysis, full blood count, and **biochemistry**, which were satisfactory with mild elevation of the glucose. The dosage of baclofen was increased to 10 mg x3 and he continued his current treatment and physiotherapy. He was scheduled for a re-examination in four months.

| TABLE 10–2. | Terminology for Case Study 10–1 |

"b-c" score	Scoring on the *Frenchay Dysarthria Assessment* (FDA). See Table 10–4 for information concerning Frenchay scoring.
1-1/2-1/2	Medical shorthand for 1 tablet in the morning, half tablet in midday, and half tablet in the evening.
Alsin (ALS2) gene	Alsin is a protein signaled by the ALS2 gene for production. Alsin is abundant in motor neurons.
Baclofen (active ingredient), Lioresal (brand name)	Medication that works as a muscle relaxer to improve spasticity, pain, and stiffness.
Biochemical examination (biochemistry)	Methods used to analyze substances of organisms and their chemical reactions.
BAEP (brainstem auditory evoked potentials)	These are electrical potentials that are recorded as a response of the nervous system following a presentation of an auditory stimulus (a sound).
Co-enzyme Q10	Coenzyme is an antioxidant used to protect cells from free radicals by facilitating specific proteins (enzymes) to speed up the rate of chemical reactions in the body.
DAB	Classification system for dysarthria, referring to the pioneering work of Darley, Aronson, and Brown at Mayo Clinic. For further information, see Darley, Aronson, & Brown (1969).
Diabetes mellitus	An autoimmune disease in which the pancreas does not produce the hormone insulin and so there are high blood sugar levels in the body.
Diplopia (double vision)	A single object seen as two images.
Dysarthria	Motor speech disorder involving muscular weakness, dyscoordination, and alteration of muscle tone. It includes slow movement of the muscles used for speech production, including the lips, tongue, vocal folds, and/or muscles of respiration.
Dysdiadochokinesia	Reduced ability to perform rapid, alternating movements.
Dysmetria	Incoordination of movement or inability to judge distance. The result is that the hand, arm, or leg undershoots or overshoots an intended position. It is considered to be the result of ataxia and is caused by impairment in the cerebellum.
Dysphagia	Difficulty with one or more stages of swallowing.
EMG (electromyography)	A laboratory technique to record electrical activity (electric potential) of skeletal muscles.
Evoked potentials	Electrical response from the nervous system after a stimulus is presented.
Excess and equal stress	A perceptual feature in the DAB classification in which there is excessive stress on unstressed syllables, arising from lack of variation in vocal intensity or fundamental frequency.
Frenchay Dysarthria Assessment (FDA)	A standardized test to assess nonspeech and speech movements of lips, jaw, tongue, phonation, intelligibility, etc. (see Table 10–4 for details concerning scoring of the FDA).
Glucophage	See metformin.
Glucose (sugar)	Energy source for muscles and neurons arising from food intake (fruit, cereals, etc.).
Heel-to-knee examination	A neurological test that is used to examine coordination (after ipsilateral cerebellar lesion) by having the patient be in the supine position and place his/her right heel on his/her left shin. The patient is then instructed to slide the heel down the shin on the top of the foot as quickly as possible.
Imprecise consonants	Consonants are slurred and distorted and have inadequate sharpness.

continues

TABLE 10–2.   *continued*

Lioresal	See baclofen.
Metformin (active ingredient), Glucophage (brand name) 500 mg	Medication used to treat type 2 diabetes and control blood sugar levels.
Monoloudness	Phonation that lacks normal variations of intensity.
Monopitch	Phonation that lacks normal variation in frequency.
Muscle tone	The continuous state of tension in muscle fibers. In relaxation, the tension is low, while in stretching the tension is high.
Nystagmus	Involuntary saccadic movement of the eye.
Peripheral neuropathy	Disease caused by traumatic brain injury, infections, metabolic problems, etc. Symptomatology is variable but usually involves weakness, numbness, and pain in the limbs.
Plantar response or reflex	The plantar reflex in infants is stimulated by rubbing a blunt object on the sole of the foot with moderate force. Normal plantar reflexive response includes extension (dorsiflexion) of the big toe and abduction or fanning of the other toes. This reflex is inhibited by cortical control around 6 months of age and is seen in only pathological conditions in adults.
prn	As needed.
Reflexes	Involuntary automatic movements in response to a stimulus (not involving a conscious effort).
Romberg (negative)	Test used to assess balance. In this test, the patient stands with feet together, eyes open and hands by the sides and then closes the eyes while the examiner observes him/her. Negative in this case means "normal."
Slow saccades	The eye movements exhibit abnormally slow speed.
Spastic dysarthria	Motor speech disorder produced by bilateral damage to the direct and indirect pathways of the central nervous system. The patient complains of slow speech rate, increased effort to speak and fatigue while speaking. See Duffy (2013) for the speech characteristics of spastic dysarthria.
Spastic paraplegias	A group of inherited neurological disorders characterized by stiffness in the legs and gait abnormalities.
Spasticity	Continuous abnormal contraction in certain muscles that results in stiffness or tightness in movement, speech, and gait.
Spinocerebellar syndrome	A progressive, genetic degenerative neurological disease with many different types and genes involved. Its symptomatology involves incoordination in the movement of the limbs (feet and hands) as well as speech and eye movements. The main neuroanatomical site that is affected is the cerebellum (atrophy).
Tetrabenazine (active ingredient), Xenazine (brand name)	Medication used to alleviate and decrease the uncontrollable movements in the body (chorea) caused by Huntington's disease. It decreases the levels of dopamine, serotonin, and norepinephrine.
Tetraparesis	Paralysis or weakness of all four limbs.
Tizanidine (active ingredient), Zanaflex (brand name) 2 mg 1/2 tab	Medication used for daily use to reduce the signs and symptoms of spasticity.
Upgoing plantars	See plantar. The normal response is downward movement of the hallux.
x2	Two times.

TABLE 10–3.	Examining Muscle Strength

When examining a patient, identifying specific areas of muscular weakness helps to localize the site of lesion. Strength testing is completed for each muscle group, making sure that you test one side and then the next for each group, so you can compare strength for the two sides. Here is a muscle strength rating scale.

0/5	No contraction of muscle
1/5	Indication of muscle flicker, but no movement noted
2/5	Movement occurs, but not against gravity when tested in the horizontal plane
3/5	Movement occurs against, but not when there is resistance provided by the the examiner
4/5	Movement occurs against some resistance provided by the examiner
5/5	Normal strength

Medical Diagnosis

Progressive spinocerebellar degeneration of unknown etiology

Speech Examination at Five Years, Five Months Post Intake

The **Frenchay Dysarthria Assessment** was administered to the patient (see Table 10–4 for details of Frenchay scoring). The results showed a moderate difficulty with **"b-c" score**. The **DAB** classification shows most deviant speech characteristics for **spastic dysarthia**, including **imprecise consonants**, **monopitch**, **monoloudness**, and slow rate (Darley, Aronson, & Brown, 1969; Duffy, 2013). The most deviant speech characteristic for ataxic dysarthria is **excess and equal stress** and prolonged phonemes. More specifically:

- Reflexes cough: Patient had occasional difficulty with choking, or food sometimes going down the wrong way (b).
- Reflexes swallow: Patient observed drinking ½ cup of water and eating a cookie and it was slow during eating/drinking with pauses while drinking (b).
- Respiration in speech: When asked to count from 1 to 20 as quickly as possible, the patient had to speak quickly because of poor respiratory control and it took him 3 breaths to complete the task (c).
- Lips seal: Occasional air leakage and breaks in lips seal when the patient was asked to blow air into cheeks and maintain for 15 seconds (b).

TABLE 10–4.	Frenchay Scoring Details

The *Frenchay Dysarthria Assessment* (FDA) utilizes a rating scale for all testing.

a score	Normal for age
b score	Mild abnormality noticeable to skilled observer
c score	Obvious abnormality but the patient can perform task/movements with reasonable approximation
d score	Some production of task but poor in quality, unable to sustain, inaccurate, or extremely labored
e score	Unable to undertake task/movement/sound

- Lips alternate: Labored movement when the patient was asked to repeat "oo ee" 10 times. One movement was within normal limits, while other movements were severely distorted (c).
- Laryngeal time: Sustained phonation for /a/ with clear voice only for 10 seconds (b).
- Laryngeal pitch: Minor difficulty with pitch breaks when the patient was asked to sing a scale (b).
- Laryngeal volume: Changes in volume when the patient counted from 1 to 5 showed noticeably uneven progression (c).
- Laryngeal in speech (intonation): Voice during speech was mostly effective—there was occasional inappropriate use of volume and pitch noticeable to the examiner (b).
- Tongue protrusion: Irregular movement accompanied by facial grimace (5 times in 7 seconds) (c).
- Tongue elevation: Labored gross movement of the tongue (d).
- Tongue lateral: Slow labored or incomplete tongue movement (5 times in 8 seconds) (c).
- Tongue alternate: Diadochokinetic rate of the word /kala/ (10 times), with one sound well articulated and the other poorly presented (10 seconds to complete the task) (c).
- Tongue in speech: Grossly distorted movement and severe changes in tongue function. Vowels distorted and consonants frequently omitted (d).

Speech-Language Diagnosis

Mixed spastic/ataxic dysarthria

Questions Concerning This Case

1. This patient presented with progressive discoordination and spasticity, secondary to likely spinocerebellar pathway degeneration. Knowing what you do about swallowing function, how would dysphagia arise from these symptoms? That is, how would discoordination and spasticity increase his risk for aspiration?

Case provided by Dr. Kostas Konstantopoulos, European University Cyprus.

1. Please identify arteries and landmarks indicated on the figure.

   a. _____ _____ artery

   b. _____ _____ artery

   c. _____ artery

   d. _____ _____ artery

   e. _____ _____ _____
      (landmark)

   f. _____ _____ artery

   g. _____ _____ artery

   h. _____ _____ artery

   i. _____ _____ artery

   j. _____ artery

   k. _____ _____ _____ artery

   l. _____ artery

   m. _____ _____ _____ artery

   n. _____ _____ artery

   o. _____ arteries

   p. _____ _____ artery

2. The artery that supplies the middle cerebral artery is the _____ _____ _____.

3. The artery that supplies the anterior cerebral artery is the _____ _____ _____.

4. The artery that supplies the posterior cerebral artery is the _____ _____.

5. The _____ carotid arteries deliver blood to the cervical and facial soft tissues, the external ear, the sinonasal cavity of the skull, and the soft tissues of the scalp.

6. The _____ _____ branch of the external carotid arteries provides blood to the meninges of the brain by way of the meningeal arteries in the area superficial to the dura mater.

7. The _____ _____ arteries give rise to the anterior cerebral arteries, posterior communicating arteries, and middle cerebral arteries.

8. The _____ cerebral artery serves the areas of the brain associated with speech, language, and hearing.

9. The _____ of _____ is a redundant circuit of vascular supply that connects anterior, middle, and posterior cerebral arteries.

10. The _____ cerebral artery courses through the superior longitudinal fissure along the dorsal surface of the corpus callosum.

11. The _____ cerebral artery serves the medial surface of the cerebral cortex.

12. The _____ communicating artery sends collateral arterioles into the deep tissues of the brain, serving the thalamus, internal capsule, and optic tract.

13. The _____ communicating artery gives rise to the anterior choroidal artery, which supplies the optic tract, posterior internal capsule, cerebral peduncles, medial temporal lobe, thalamus, and a portion of the corpus striatum.

14. The _____ cerebral artery oxygenates the speech and language zones of the brain, including the superolateral temporal as well as the lateral parietal and frontal lobes.

15. Please identify arteries indicated in this figure.

a. _____ _____ artery

b. _____ _____ artery

c. _____ _____ artery

d. _____ artery

e. _____ _____ _____ artery

f. _____ _____ artery

g. _____ _____ artery

h. _____ _____ artery

i. _____ _____ artery

j. _____ _____ artery

k. _____ artery

l. _____ _____ artery

m. _____ _____ _____ artery

16. The vascular supply to the brain arises from two major sources: the _____ and _____ systems.

17. The _____ carotid arteries give rise to the external and internal carotid arteries.

18. The _____ arteries give rise to the basilar artery, posterior cerebral artery, and cerebellar arteries.

19. The _____ _____ arteries give rise to the anterior and middle cerebral arteries as well as a number of other smaller branches.

20. The _____ cerebral artery continues into the superior longitudinal fissure, serving the medial surface of the cerebral cortex, corpus callosum, a portion of the dorsal surface of the frontal and parietal lobes, and basal ganglia.

21. The _____ communicating artery serves the thalamus, internal capsule, and optic tract.

22. Superficial branches of the _____ cerebral artery serve the superior temporal lobe, as well as the lateral and most of the dorsal surfaces of the frontal and parietal lobes, and the insula and operculum.

23. Perforating branches of the _____ cerebral artery serve the caudate nucleus, the basal ganglia, and the internal capsule.

24. The left and right vertebral arteries join together to form the _____ artery at the junction of the pons and medulla in the brainstem.

25. The _____ _____ cerebellar artery serves the base of the posterior cerebellum.

26. The perforating branches of the _____ arteries oxygenate the lower medulla, the upper cervical spinal cord, and the inferior cerebellar peduncles.

27. The _____ artery branches to serve posterior brain structures.

28. The _____ _____ cerebellar artery gives blood to the anterior cerebellar hemisphere, the pons, and the cerebellar peduncles.

29. The _____ cerebellar arteries oxygenate the superior and lateral aspects of the cerebellar hemispheres, the superior cerebellar peduncle, and the superior cerebellar vermis.

30. The _____ cerebral arteries oxygenate the inferior surface of the temporal lobe, including the anterior fusiform gyrus and the uncus.

31. The _____ cerebral artery serves the occipital lobe, as well as the splenium of the corpus callosum.

REFERENCES

Benson, D. F., Marsden, C. D., & Meadows, J. C. (1974). The amnesic syndrome of posterior cerebral artery occlusion. *Acta Neurologica Scandinavica, 50*(2), 133–145.

Boyd, L. A., Edwards, J. D., Siengsukon, C. S., Vidoni, E. D., Wessel, B. D., & Linsdell, M. A. (2009). Motor sequence chunking is impaired by basal ganglia stroke. *Neurobiology of Learning and Memory, 92*(1), 35–44.

Brandt, T., Steinke, W., Thie, A., Pessin, M. S., & Caplan, L. R. (2000). Posterior cerebral artery territory infarcts: Clinical features, infarct topography, causes and outcome. *Cerebrovascular Diseases, 10*(3), 170–182.

Capo, H., Kupersmith, M. J., Berenstein, A., Choi, I. S., & Diamond, G. A. (1991). The clinical importance of the inferolateral trunk of the internal carotid artery. *Neurosurgery, 28*(5), 733–738.

Cereda, C., & Carrera, E. (2012). Posterior cerebral artery territory infarctions. *Frontiers of Neurology and Neuroscience, 30*, 128–231.

Darley, F. L., Aronson, A. E., & Brown, J. R. (1969). Clusters of deviant speech dimensions in the dysarthrias. *Journal of Speech and Hearing Research, 12*(3), 462–496.

Duffy, J. R. (2013). *Motor speech disorders-E-book: Substrates, differential diagnosis, and management*. Elsevier Health Sciences.

Fisher, C. M. (1982). Lacunar strokes and infarcts: A review. *Neurology, 32*(8), 871–876.

Fries, W., Danek, A., Scheidtmann, K., & Hamburger, C. (1993). Motor recovery following capsular stroke: Role of descending pathways from multiple motor areas. *Brain, 116*(2), 369–382.

Kang, S. Y., & Kim, J. S. (2008). Anterior cerebral artery infarction. Stroke mechanism and clinical-imaging study in 100 patients. *Neurology, 70*(24), 2386–2393.

Kodumuri, N., Sebastian, R., Davis, C., Posner, J., Kim, E. H., Tippett, D. C., . . . Hillis, A. E. (2016). The association of insular stroke with lesion volume. *Neuroimage: Clinical, 11*, 41–45.

Liebeskind, D. S. (2003). Collateral circulation. *Stroke, 34*(9), 2279–2284.

Mattle, H. P., Arnold, M., Lindsberg, P. J., Schonewille, W. J., & Schroth, G. (2011). Basilar artery occlusion. *Lancet Neurology, 10*, 1002–1014.

Schomer, D. F., Marks, M. P., Steinberg, G. K., Johnstone, I. M., Boothroyd, D. B., Ross, M. R., . . . Enzmann, D. R. (1994). The anatomy of the posterior communicating artery as a risk factor for ischemic cerebral infarction. *New England Journal of Medicine, 330*(22), 1565–1570.

Seidel, U. K., Gronewold, J., Wicking, M., Bellebaum, C., & Hermann, D. M. (2016). Vascular risk factors and diseases modulate deficits of reward-based reversal learning in acute basal ganglia stroke. *PloS One, 11*(5), e0155267.

Seikel, J. A., Drumright, D. G., & King, D. W. (2016). *Anatomy & physiology for speech, language and hearing* 5th ed. Clifton Park, NY: Cengage Learning.

Smith, E., & Delargy, M. (2005). Locked-in syndrome. *British Medical Journal, 330*(7488), 406–409.

Szabo, K., Förster, A., Jäger, T., Kern, R., Griebe, M., Hennerici, M. G., & Gass, A. (2009). Hippocampal lesion patterns in acute posterior cerebral artery stroke. *Stroke, 40*(6), 2042–2045.

Westmacott, R., McDonald, K. P., deVeber, G., MacGregor, D., Moharir, M., Dlamini, N., . . . Williams, T. S. (2017). Neurocognitive outcomes in children with unilateral basal ganglia arterial ischemic stroke and secondary hemidystonia. *Child Neuropsychology*, 1–15.

11 NEURAL CONTROL OF SPEECH AND SWALLOWING

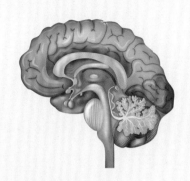

Learning Outcomes for Chapter 11

• Discuss the differences and interconnection between central pattern generators and reflexes.

• Discuss the difference between feedback and feed-forward processes and their role in learning and execution of the speech act.

• Discuss the differences among motor theories, psycholinguistic theories, and the hierarchical state feedback control models of speech production.

• Discuss the anatomical substrate of motor speech control.

• Discuss the neurophysiological underpinnings of each stage of swallowing, including the swallowing patterns apparent in early development.

• Discuss the role of afferent input to the swallowing process, including sensory stimulation concerning the quality of the bolus as well as stimulation involved in triggering various reflexes.

INTRODUCTION

Motor control of speech and other actions share common elements, but speech adds some significant complexity to the motor act. We've discussed reflexes at length, so you should be familiar with the notion of a motor response arising from a simple environmental stimulus, such as tapping on the patellar tendon to get a knee-jerk. In the section that follows on swallowing function, we'll introduce the notion of **central pattern generators** (CPGs) that take groups of reflexes and bring them together in a coordinated, highly orchestrated, complex action sequence. Reflexes and CPGs are execution-stage constructs: they are involved in the activation of muscles in either simple or complex fashion. Voluntary movement takes these concepts to an entirely new level, and voluntary movement for speech is even more complex. Let's examine what we think are essential components of motor control.

NEURAL CONTROL OF SPEECH

You know that motor control requires the "motor" part, which is contracting muscle, but this can be accomplished through a simple reflex circuit. A more complex motor act, such as reaching for a glass on a table top, requires that you see where the glass is (**visual input**); know where your body, arm, and hand are in space; know the state of your joints and muscles at the moment (**proprioceptive input**); and have a plan to activate muscles to achieve your goal. All of this sensory information needs to be integrated with the motor plan before execution, and indeed, it must be updated once the action is initiated in order to account for variables that arise in the course of reaching for the glass (such as your dog bumping you or the wind picking up). Integration of the sensory information with the plan makes this a skilled motor activity. Those of you pursuing speech-language pathology will work with people who have problems with this **sensorimotor integration**, resulting in significant speech production problems.

Feedback and Correction

Two essential elements of skilled motor control are feedback and correction. In his landmark text *Cybernetics*, Norbert Wiener set out the mechanisms of feedback and control that govern physical systems (Wiener, 1948), and this model has served as the basis for discussion of motor control ever since. In living organisms,

- Discuss the oral, pharyngeal, and respiratory reflexes, including the physical triggers and responses involved in these reflexes.

- Discuss mediation of gustation in the processes of mastica-

tion and deglutition, including the pathways involved in the sense of taste, olfaction, and chemesthesia.

- Discuss the role of mechano-receptors, proprioceptors, and

thermal receptors in the acts of mastication and deglutition.

- Discuss the specific neural components of the CPG for swallowing.

feedback for motor function takes the form of information from multiple sensors. When we reach for an object, muscles are contracted and information about the position of joints, tension of the muscle, and rate of contraction is conveyed rapidly and continuously to the cerebellum for integration with other sensory information (such as vestibular input) and the motor plan. The cerebellum compares the planned motor act with the ongoing reality and makes rapid, ongoing changes to the plan to correct for errors in the process. Thus, our nervous system continuously compares the state of its sensors with motor plans and corrects the plan to meet the reality of the action itself.

If you can remember the last time your tongue was deadened for dental work, you will recognize the results of faulty feedback. When the dentist injects anesthetic into the trigeminal nerve, sensory information about position of the tongue in space, tongue muscle tension, and rate of movement are muted. When you attempt to speak, your speech is slurred, and when you attempt to chew, there's an unfortunately high probability that your tongue and teeth will have a bad interaction. Note that the dentist didn't paralyze the muscle, but rather the injection eliminated important information about what your body was doing so that the motor plan could not be corrected based on that information.

There are two important forms of feedback and correction: closed-loop and open-loop systems. In a **closed-loop system**, there is a set reference or target, and the correction comes from comparing accuracy in hitting the target with the standard. This is the feedback and correction system just described. One of the limitations of a closed-loop system is that it takes a great deal of time to integrate sensory information with the motor act. Closed-loop systems do not work for rapid movements because the movements are faster than the integration and correction process of the nervous system. **Open-loop systems** do not operate on sensory feedback and correction and are termed feed-forward processes. Open-loop control does not use feedback for correction, but is used to accomplish tasks rapidly. Correction of errors in open-loop systems cannot depend on a sensory feedback mechanism because the motor act is complete before sensory stimuli can be analyzed and compared with a model.

These two mechanisms work together in the motor act. When we are learning a new task, we must use closed-loop feedback and correction to gain the skill required. Once we know the limits of the system that will accomplish the task, we can shift to an open-loop system. Motor learning requires slow movement, but skilled execution can occur at a much faster pace. These feed-forward processes combine the current state of the system with a motor program that already accounts for your knowledge of how the action was accomplished in the past. Since the action is based upon prediction of how it will turn out, if you perceive that the action did not meet your expectation, you'll very likely slow down and try again!

The act of speaking adds another significant level of complexity to the process. We must first have an idea or concept that we wish to convey, and that concept must be encoded into language by our linguistic system. The lateral frontal lobe of the dominant hemisphere is deeply involved in this process. Grammatical encoding occurs largely within Broca's area, while phonetic encoding occurs within the left insular cortex and left supramarginal gyrus. Riecker and associates (2005) have shown there are two distinct loops involved in the motor act for speech. A "preparative" loop includes the left dorsolateral prefrontal cortex, anterior insular cortex, supplementary motor area, and the superior cerebellum. The "executive" loop is made up of the motor cortex, thalamus, putamen and caudate, and the inferior cerebellum. It should be noted that these would be considered open-loop components for speech, since the elements under study were well known to the participants.

In summary, motor control of speech adds complexity to the motor act.

- Central pattern generators (CPGs) take groups of reflexes and bring them together into a complex action sequence.
- The motor act requires visual input, proprioceptive input, and a motor plan. This sensory information is integrated with the motor plan before execution.
- In a closed-loop feedback system, there is a set reference or target, and correction comes from comparing accuracy in hitting the target with a standard.
- Open-loop systems do not operate on direct sensory feedback and correction and are termed feed-forward processes. Speaking requires an idea or concept we wish to

convey that must be encoded into language. Grammatical encoding occurs largely within Broca's area, and phonetic encoding occurs within the left insular cortex and left supramarginal gyrus.

- There are two distinct loops involved in the motor act for speech. A "preparative" loop includes the left dorsolateral prefrontal cortex, anterior insular cortex, supplementary motor area, and the superior cerebellum. The "executive" loop is made up of the motor cortex, thalamus, putamen and caudate, and the inferior cerebellum.

MODELS OF SPEECH PRODUCTION

Historically, two major models have been proposed to explain the production of speech. The **psycholinguistic view** sees speech as, quite literally, the oral manifestation of language. The **motor view** relates to how the manifestation occurs.

Hickok (2012) proposed a model that integrated these two approaches called the **Hierarchical State Feedback Control model**. This model recognizes the hierarchical nature of speech production and acknowledges the importance of the linguistic input (Figure 11–1). In this model, the initial stimulus for speech is a concept or idea that triggers a verbal manifestation (known as the **lemma**). Recognize that the word at this stage has no production nature (i.e., does not have phonological form), but rather is conceptual, and this stage directly parallels the psycholinguistic model. The word that was generated in response to the idea is projected to the highest cortical processing areas, including Broca's area (BA 44) and the juncture of the parietal and temporal lobes, the **temporoparietal juncture** (TPJ). This Broca's–TPJ loop projects to centers that govern the motor plan, including the somatosensory (BA 1, 2, 3), motor strip (BA 4, 6), and cerebellum. Thus, phonological representation occurs at both higher levels (Broca's–TPJ loop) and lower levels (motor strip, somatosensory integration, and cerebellum) simultaneously.

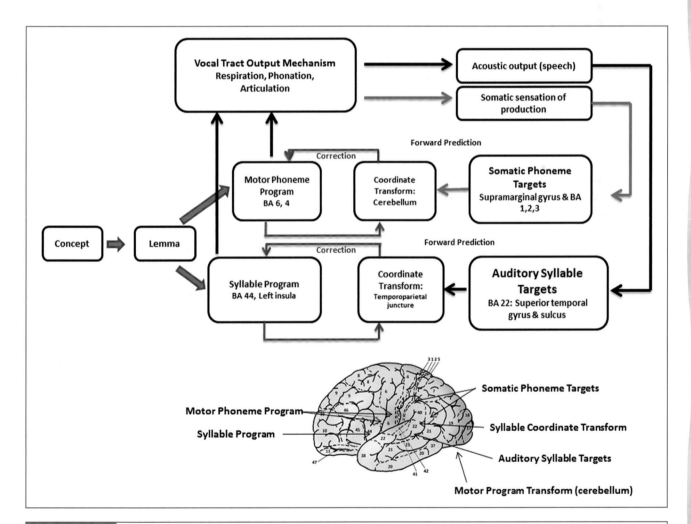

FIGURE 11–1. Hickok's hierarchical state feedback control model. *Source:* Modified from Hickok, G. (2012). Computational neuroanatomy of speech production. *Nature Reviews Neuroscience, 13*(2), 135–145.

If you examine Figure 11–1, you'll see that the Broca's–TPJ circuit produces a prediction of the outcome that is checked by the auditory system (superior temporal gyrus and superior temporal sulcus). If the target is met auditorily, the output of those centers is not used as feedback, but if an acoustic error is sensed, a correction is fed back to the TPJ and Broca's motor plan region. In the same way, programs for phonemes arising from the premotor region (BA 6) are sent to the cerebellum, and a prediction of resulting sensory states of articulators is created. The supramarginal gyrus (superior BA 6) and primary sensory cortex (BA 1) receive the sensory output resulting from articulation, and a mismatch between prediction and production will result in feedback to the cerebellum and premotor region.

This model builds on the **Directions into Velocities of Articulation** (DIVA) model of speech production that has arisen from the work of Guenther and others (Guenther, Hampson, & Johnson, 1998; Callan, Kent, Guenther, & Vorperian, 2000). The DIVA model utilizes sensory inputs as checks for the accuracy of the executed speech (feed-forward), as well as sensory feedback to support the learning process in speech production. The model clearly differentiates learning from learned execution of a motor act (Guenther, Ghosh, & Tourville, 2006; Guenther & Vladusich, 2012), specifying that the learning stage requires much slower and more deliberate production based on the laborious integration of ongoing sensory states. If you ever tried to play the piano, you may remember how slowly you had to play when first learning the scales, but how you could play much more quickly once you had mastered them. Even then, when you made a mistake and hit the wrong key, you experienced a mismatch between expectation and reality that caused you to stop and try again. Feed-forward does not integrate immediate sensory information into the motor act, but rather uses the sensory information to validate accuracy of production in a learned skill. Feedback, on the other hand, is an essential component of motor learning, a process that is inherently slow because of the slow nature of real-time sensory feedback.

In the DIVA model, the auditory model for the desired phoneme is generated and conveyed to the auditory cortex and somatosensory cortex so that the word that is produced can be validated against the target. When an error is detected, it will result in a correction in the following articulatory trial.

In all cases, it is clear that the process of learning an articulatory act is markedly different from the execution of an act that has been previously learned. The feedback mechanisms for learning use the same elements that control the feed-forward system, but the result is markedly different.

In summary, two major models have been proposed to explain the production of speech.

- In the psycholinguistic view, speech is the oral manifestation of language. The motor view relates to how the manifestation occurs.

- The Hierarchical State Feedback Control model views speech production in a hierarchical fashion that acknowledges the linguistic input. The initial stimulus for speech is a concept or idea that triggers a verbal manifestation (lemma).
- The word is directed to the Broca's–temporoparietal juncture loop that projects to lower centers that govern the motor plan, including the somatosensory area, motor strip, and cerebellum. Phonological representation occurs at both higher levels and lower levels simultaneously.
- The Broca's–TPJ circuit produces a prediction of the outcome that is checked by the auditory system, and if an acoustic error is sensed, a correction is fed back to the TPJ and Broca's motor plan region.
- The DIVA model of speech production utilizes sensory inputs as checks for the accuracy of the executed speech (feed-forward), as well as sensory feedback to support the learning process in speech production. In the DIVA model, the auditory model for the desired phoneme is generated and conveyed to the auditory cortex and somatosensory cortex so that the word that is produced can be validated against the target.

NEURAL CONTROL OF MASTICATION AND DEGLUTITION

As you now know, motor control for speech is not only complex but capitalizes on both voluntary and involuntary motor patterns. We exercise voluntary control in development of the plan for articulation and its execution, but the actual implementation of the plan involves a feed-forward process that capitalizes on existing reflexes and stereotyped motor function. Swallowing follows a similar pattern, with components that can be governed by voluntary action but which don't require a great deal of active conscious thought.

The process of preparing food for swallowing is termed **mastication**, while the term for swallowing the **bolus** (or "ball") of food is termed **deglutition**. The nervous system components involved in mastication and deglutition span all of the motor functions for speech, including the articulatory, phonatory, and respiratory systems. The processes of mastication and deglutition integrate the motor function of the velum, tongue, pharyngeal musculature, larynx, face, and respiration. First, let's define the movements associated with swallowing, and then we can elaborate on the motor control elements.

Development of Swallowing Function

As you may be aware, swallowing function begins *in utero*. By 15 weeks of gestational age, the fetus can be seen through ultrasound to exhibit **non-nutritive sucking behavior**. Reflexes present at birth, such as rooting, sucking, and orienting, allow the infant to get nutrition. The rooting reflex is stimulated by light tactile contact on the cheek, which causes the infant to turn toward the stimulus (orient) and the mouth to open. The sucking reflex is elicited by tactile contact with the lips, producing a piston-like protrusion and retraction movement of the tongue. The early movement pattern is termed "suckling" and involves simple protrusion and retraction, while the more mature pattern entails a stronger labial seal coupled with raising and lowering of the tongue as it retracts. Rooting and sucking involve muscles of the face (particularly the lips) as well as the muscles of the tongue and mandible. These reflexive movements will ultimately be replaced by voluntary movements that will, nonetheless, utilize the gross reflexive patterns seen in these early stages. When the bolus is swallowed, the infant suspends respiration (referred to as the apneic period) to allow passage of the bolus through the pharynx into the esophagus.

Adult mastication and deglutition patterns begin to emerge around 6 months of age. As the infant dentition erupts and solid food is introduced, use of teeth to grind and chew the bolus will develop. This mature pattern of mastication is supported by contraction of the muscles of mastication (masseter, temporalis, pterygoids), and the mature retropulsive movement of the tongue replaces the tongue protrusion that was used to express milk from the breast or bottle.

In summary, reflexes present at birth such as rooting, sucking, and orienting allow the infant to get nutrition.

- The rooting reflex causes the infant to turn toward the stimulus and the mouth to open. The sucking reflex results in a piston-like protrusion and retraction movement of the tongue.
- Adult mastication and deglutition patterns emerge around 6 months of age. As dentition erupts and solid food is introduced, teeth start to grind and chew the bolus, and this requires use of the muscles of mastication.

Disorders of the Oral Stage

The oral stage of swallowing involves the processes of bolus preparation (oral preparation) and movement of the bolus to the pharyngeal cavity (oral transit). Mastication of a bolus requires an individual to move the bolus to the molars using the tongue, which is a relatively complex process. In order to do this, a person needs to move the tongue tip laterally and deliver the bolus by twisting the tongue and scraping the bolus off, onto the molars. To perform this task, a person has to have very refined bilateral and differential control of the intrinsic muscles of the tongue. Twisting the tongue while elevating it requires a great deal of coordination because the intrinsic and extrinsic

muscles of the two sides of the tongue have to be differentially activated to perform this task. Once the bolus is on the molars, the masseter, temporalis, and internal and external pterygoids have to contract in alternating fashion to grind the bolus (shift the mandible side-for-side as well as front-back, to get rotation).

Deficits of this stage arise from loss of motor control, as well as muscle weakness. Low strength can cause difficulties in elevating the tongue and make the process of moving the bolus difficult. Strength is also an issue with the muscles of mastication, as chewing requires a great deal of effort. Both of these stages can be affected by neuromuscular conditions that cause muscular weakness. Degenerative diseases such as amyotrophic lateral sclerosis and later stages of Parkinson's disease cause progressive muscle weakness, making chewing and swallowing not only difficult but dangerous. Impaired muscle function in the oral cavity can lead to spillage and pocketing of food in the buccal cavity and premature spillage into the pharyngeal cavity. Weak muscles can also cause slow transit of the bolus to the pharynx, which can disrupt coordination of the pharyngeal swallow.

Reduced sensation is not uncommon in neurological conditions, particularly those related to cerebrovascular accident. If sensation is reduced, the oral feedback provided by pressure sensors in the mouth will not provide the sensory information necessary for monitoring the lingual pressure against the roof of the mouth, which can result in poor oral transit of the bolus. Reduced sensation can also lead to appetite loss, as olfactory and gustatory senses provide motivation for food intake. People with Alzheimer's disease show a progressive loss of appetite due to reduced taste and olfactory sensor function, and caretakers may increase the sweetness of the food to improve palatability, since sweet sensation is retained longer in the degenerative process.

ADULT PATTERNS OF MASTICATION AND DEGLUTITION

In the adult there are three identifiable stages involved in mastication and deglutition: oral, pharyngeal, and esophageal.

Oral Stage

The oral stage is further broken into the oral preparation and oral transit stages. In the **oral preparation stage**, the bolus is prepared for swallowing, a process that involves receipt of the bolus of food or liquid by the tongue and movements that prepare the bolus for swallowing. If the bolus is solid food, it will be moved to the molars by the tongue for crushing and mixed with saliva on the tongue for bolus preparation before swallowing. During this process you will utilize taste sensors (see Chapter 3) to identify the food being masticated, a process that (hopefully) increases the pleasure of the process and supports the desire to increase the intake of food. When we sense that the bolus is ready to be swallowed, the tongue pushes against the roof of the mouth and squeezes the bolus toward the pharynx, defining the oral transit stage.

Salivation is accomplished through three glands: the sublingual, submandibular, and parotid glands. The **sublingual** and **submandibular glands** are innervated by the VII facial nerve, while the **parotid gland** is innervated by the IX glossopharyngeal nerve.

In the oral stage of swallowing, the VII facial nerve innervates the facial muscles and anterior digastricus, while the muscles of mastication and the posteriordigastricus are innervated by the V trigeminal nerve, which also mediates oral sensation. The XI accessory nerve innervates the sternocleidomastoid for head rotation, while the IX glossopharyngeal, X vagus, and XI accessory nerves innervate the velum. Lingual muscles are innervated by the XII hypoglossal nerve. (See Table 11).

Pharyngeal Stage

The pharyngeal stage is initiated when the tongue and/or bolus contact the posterior region of the mouth (Table 11–2). The stimulus site for triggering the pharyngeal stage appears to be pressure on mechanoreceptors of the anterior fauces, the posterior tongue, velum, or even posterior pharyngeal wall (Ertekin, Kiylioglu, Tarlaci, Truman, Secil, & Aydogdu, 2011;

Lang, 2009; Martin-Harris, Brodsky, Michel, Lee, & Walters, 2007; Mendell & Logemann, 2007; Stephen, Taves, Smith, & Martin, 2005). Pressure sensors in one or more of these sites provide the input to the motor program that will simultaneously protect the airway and propel the bolus through the upper esophageal sphincter (UES). The pharyngeal stage is entirely reflexive in nature (although we can reproduce all of the actions of the pharyngeal stage voluntarily, as in therapy techniques such as the effortful swallow). Each component of the pharyngeal stage is governed by individual reflexes that are organized by assemblies of neurons termed **central pattern generators** (CPGs). The CPG is responsible for organizing the sequence and timing of the reflexive responses in order to accomplish a complex (yet involuntary) motor function. Once initiated, a CPG will produce a motor sequence from start to finish, triggering the motor pattern of numerous reflexes sequentially and with precise timing.

Disorders of the Pharyngeal Stage of Swallowing

The pharyngeal stage of swallowing is highly orchestrated for good reason. At least 27 muscles governed by 5 cranial nerves must fire in an organized effort to move the bolus to the awaiting esophagus. A misfire of any of these muscles can cause a dysfunction of timing, loss of control, or reduced force generation, all of which can disrupt the swallowing process and place the individual at risk. Here are a few examples of problems that can occur as a result of neurological insult.

TABLE 11–1.	Cranial Nerves Involved in the Oral Stage of Swallowing	
Nerve	Function	Muscle
V trigeminal	Elevates mandible	Masseter, temporalis muscles, internal pterygoid muscle
	Elevates hyoid and floor of mouth	Mylohyoid muscle
XII hypoglossal	Elevates tongue tip	Superior longitudinal muscle
	Cups and grooves tongue	Verticalis muscle, genioglossus muscle
	Elevates and retracts posterior tongue	Styloglossus muscle
IX glossopharyngeal X vagus XI accessory	Elevates posterior tongue	Palatoglossus muscle

Source: Based on data of Seikel, Drumright, & King (2016).

TABLE 11–2.	Cranial Nerves Involved in the Pharyngeal Stage of Swallowing	
Nerve	**Function**	**Muscle**
V trigeminal	Elevates hyoid and tongue	Mylohyoid
XII glossopharyngeal	Elevates hyoid and larynx, depresses mandible	Geniohyoid
V trigeminal VII facial	Digastricus anterior and posterior	Elevates hyoid, elevates larynx
XII hypoglossal	Genioglossus	Retracts tongue
XII hypoglossal	Styloglossus	Elevates posterior tongue
XII hypoglossal	Palatoglossus	Narrows fauces, elevates posterior tongue
XII hypoglossal	Stylohyoid	Elevates hyoid and larynx
XII hypoglossal	Hyoglossus	Elevates hyoid
XII hypoglossal	Thyrohyoid	Elevates hyoid
XII hypoglossal	Superior longitudinal	Depresses tongue
XII hypoglossal	Inferior longitudinal	Depresses tongue
XII hypoglossal	Transversus	Narrows tongue
XII hypoglossal	Verticalis	Flattens tongue
X, XI	Levator veli palatini	Elevates soft palate
V trigeminal	Tensor veli palatini	Dilates auditory tube
X vagus XI accessory	Musculus uvulae	Shortens velum
X vagus XI accessory	Palatopharyngeus	Constricts oropharynx to channel bolus
XI accessory	Salpingopharyngeus	Elevates pharynx
XI accessory	Stylopharyngeus	Elevates larynx
X vagus XI accessory	Cricopharyngeus	Relaxes esophageal sphincter
X vagus XI accessory	Superior pharyngeal constrictor	Narrows pharynx
X vagus XI accessory	Middle pharyngeal constrictor	Narrows pharynx
X vagus XI accessory	Inferior pharyngeal constrictor	Narrows pharynx
X vagus	Lateral cricoarytenoid	Adducts vocal folds
X vagus	Transverse arytenoids	Adducts vocal folds
X vagus	Oblique arytenoids	Adducts vocal folds
X vagus	Aryepiglotticus	Retracts epiglottis and constricts aditus
X vagus	Thyroepiglotticus	Dilates airway

Source: Based on data of Seikel, Drumright, & King (2016).

Cerebrovascular accident is a frequent cause of oro-pharyngeal dysphagia. One significant contributor to dysphagia is loss of sensation. While we often think of stroke as resulting in muscular weakness, loss of sensation mediated by the V trigeminal can result in delayed or absent triggering of the pharyngeal swallow. Because the swallow response includes elevation of the larynx, deflection of the epiglottis, and adduction of the true and false vocal folds to protect the airway, food and liquid may enter the laryngeal aditus (penetration) or make it past the vocal folds (aspiration), leading potentially to aspiration pneumonia. If you had an accidental penetration or aspiration, you would likely cough in response, eliminating the unwanted and dangerous material from the airway. A person with low or absent sensation might not feel the food in the airway and not cough in response (silent aspiration). We are well armed with protective devices to keep this from happening, but sensation is at the forefront of all of them because reflexive responses (e.g., coughing) are triggered by sensations.

Cerebrovascular accident and neuromuscular conditions can easily cause muscle weakness as well. The X vagus and XI accessory work together in many swallowing functions. Deficits affecting these two nerves can result in weak velar function and poor or absent velopharyngeal seal. Without this seal, adequate swallowing pressure can't be generated to move the bolus into the esophagus, resulting in slowed pharyngeal transit. Because the swallow is so precisely timed, the bolus might not reach the esophagus before the cricopharyngeus closes, leaving food residue in the pyriform sinuses. This food, if not swallowed, can be aspirated at a later time, for instance when a person is supine. Likewise, lesions affecting the function of these two nerves can cause reduced laryngeal elevation. When the larynx elevates, it stimulates the X vagus superior or recurrent laryngeal nerve to inhibit the tonic contraction of the cricopharyngeus muscle, thereby opening up the UES (Uludag, Aygun, & Isgor, 2016). This sphincter separates the pharyngeal from esophageal cavities and when it opens, the bolus can pass through it after moving through the pharynx. Again, failure to open the sphincter can allow residue to pool in the pyriform sinuses. Further, elevation of the larynx helps invert the epiglottis to cover the airway. Without the inversion of the epiglottis, the airway is open to penetration and aspiration. The vagus is the nerve responsible for adduction of the vocal folds, and a lesion that affects this nerve places the individual at significant risk for aspiration because adduction of the vocal folds is the primary defense against aspiration.

This is truly a case of "the list goes on and on," because a functioning nervous system is a prerequisite for a safe swallow. Anything that intrudes on the function of the cranial nerves or the central pattern generator that orchestrates their sequential activities places an individual at risk for aspiration and serious illness.

The pharyngeal stage accomplishes three important functions: laryngeal elevation, pressure generation, and airway protection. **Laryngeal elevation** is accomplished through movement of the hyoid and larynx by means of the suprahyoid and lingual musculature, and involves the V trigeminal (mylohyoid, digastricus), VII facial (digastricus, stylohyoid), XII hypoglossal (geniohyoid, styloglossus, hyoglossus, thyrohyoid), and the combination of the IX glossopharyngeal, X vagus, and XI accessory nerves (palatoglossus). Similarly, **airway protection** depends on the elevation of the larynx, but also involves laryngeal adduction through the recurrent laryngeal nerve of the vagus (lateral cricoarytenoid, oblique and transverse arytenoids, aryepiglotticus, and thyroepiglotticus muscles). In addition to laryngeal elevation, **pressure generation** requires velar elevation and tongue retraction, which involve the X vagus and XI accessory (levator veli palatini and musculus uvulae), V trigeminal (tensor veli palatini), and X vagus recurrent and superior laryngeal nerves (inhibition of cricopharyngeus).

The cricopharyngeus is innervated by the pharyngeal plexus. The primary innervation is by means of the recurrent and superior laryngeal nerves of the X vagus, as well as the pharyngoesophageal nerve, the cervical sympathetic system, and the glossopharyngeal nerve (Lang & Shaker, 1997; Uludag, Aygun, & Isgor, 2016).

Relaxation of the Upper Esophageal Sphincter

The muscular component of the UES is the cricopharyngeus muscle, which is part of the inferior pharyngeal constrictor.

An important part of the pharyngeal stage is opening of the passageway to the esophagus. The muscular component of the **upper esophageal sphincter** is the cricopharyngeus muscle, which is part of the inferior pharyngeal constrictor. The cricopharyngeus stays in tonic contraction except when required to relax during the swallow (Lang & Shaker, 1997). The UES relaxes upon elevation of the larynx, allowing the bolus to pass unimpeded into the esophagus. Relaxation of the cricopharyngeus is accomplished through inhibition, mediated variously by the X vagus, superior laryngeal nerve, or recurrent laryngeal nerve (Uludag et al., 2016).

Esophageal Stage

The esophageal stage is outside of voluntary control, consisting of the period during which the swallowed bolus passes through the esophagus to the stomach. This stage is governed by peristaltic action: rings of smooth muscle contract in sequence to propel the bolus. The esophagus is innervated by the X vagus and the sympathetic trunk of the cervical and thoracic region (Goyal, Padmanabhan, & Sang, 2001).

In summary, in the adult there are three identifiable stages involved in mastication and deglutition: oral (oral preparation and oral transit), pharyngeal, and esophageal.

- In the oral preparation stage, the bolus is prepared for swallowing. This involves movements such as chewing and crushing. Movement of the bolus is accomplished during the oral transit stage.
- The sublingual and submandibular glands are innervated by the VII facial nerve, while the parotid gland is innervated by the IX glossopharyngeal nerve.
- Cranial nerves used in the oral stage include VII facial nerve, V trigeminal nerve, IX glossopharyngeal, X vagus, and XI accessory nerves and XII hypoglossal nerve.
- The pharyngeal stage is initiated when the tongue and/or bolus contact the posterior region of the mouth. Pressure sensors at the trigger site provide input to the motor program that will simultaneously protect the airway and propel the bolus through the upper esophageal sphincter.
- The pharyngeal stage is entirely reflexive in nature and each component of the pharyngeal stage is governed by individual reflexes that are organized by assemblies of neurons termed central pattern generators (CPGs).
- Once initiated, a CPG will produce a motor sequence from start to finish, triggering the motor pattern of numerous reflexes sequentially and with precise timing.
- The pharyngeal stage accomplishes laryngeal elevation, pressure generation, and airway protection. Laryngeal elevation requires the V trigeminal, VII facial, XII hypoglossal and IX glossopharyngeal, X vagus, and XI accessory nerves.
- Airway protection depends on the X vagus recurrent laryngeal nerve, X vagus pharyngeal nerve, XI accessory, V trigeminal, and X vagus superior laryngeal nerves.
- The upper esophageal sphincter is inhibited by the X vagus, superior laryngeal nerve. The esophageal stage is outside of voluntary control. The esophagus is innervated by the X vagus and the sympathetic trunk of the cervical and thoracic region.

REFLEXES AND THEIR INTEGRATION INTO CENTRAL PATTERN GENERATORS

As mentioned previously, the basic elements of mastication and deglutition are reflex circuits. These circuits can operate as both primary stimulus-response mechanisms, or serve as components of centrally governed programs, known as cen-tral pattern generator circuits (Ertekin & Aydogdu, 2003). Following are critical reflexes that serve the mastication and deglutition processes.

Oral Stage Reflexes

Orienting, Rooting, and Sucking

When the cheek of an infant is lightly stroked, the infant will turn toward the stimulus in what is termed the **orienting reflex**. When the lips are touched or stroked, the infant will begin **sucking** in response. Cheek or lip contact stimulates the V trigeminal nerve via light pressure sensors in the skin, with subsequent mediation by a brainstem region between the trigeminal motor nucleus and facial nucleus of the brainstem, a region responsible for rhythmic movements of the mandible and lips (Barlow & Estep, 2006; Chandler & Tal, 1986; Miller, 2002). The orienting component presumably involves the XI accessory nerve.

Chewing Reflex

The **chewing reflex** is stimulated by deep pressure to the roof of the mouth and results in rhythmic contraction of the muscles of mastication. Pressure sensation is conveyed by the V trigeminal nerve to the **chewing CPG** of the brainstem, located between the V trigeminal motor nucleus and the VII facial nucleus within the pons. Information is also conveyed to the nucleus pontis caudalis of the reticular formation, which is also involved in tongue movements during chewing (Baehr & Frotscher, 2012; Lund & Kolta, 2006).

Pharyngeal Stage Reflexes

Palatal Reflex and Gag Reflex

The **palatal reflex** (also known as the uvular reflex) and **gag reflex** are mediated through similar circuitry. The palatal reflex occurs via the IX glossopharyngeal nerve as a result of tactile contact with the uvula. The gag reflex is also elicited by tactile contact, typically with the posterior pharyngeal wall or fauces, but also with the posterior tongue in some individuals. Tactile sensation (or taste, mediated by the IX glossopharyngeal nerve) is conveyed to the nucleus solitarius and solitary fasciculus by means of the inferior and superior ganglia of the IX glossopharyngeal nerve. Interconnection with the X vagus ensures that the abdominal, velar, and pharyngeal muscles are involved in the process .

Vomit Reflex

The **vomiting reflexes** share many of the same components of the palatal and gag reflexes. Vomiting arises from a number of stimuli and requires a dense set of muscular actions.

Stimuli can include olfactory (I olfactory), taste (typically IX glossopharyngeal), vestibular disturbance (VIII vestibulocochlear), and gastrointestinal distress (X vagus). It can also be internally generated by disturbing thoughts or visual or auditory stimuli. The **vomiting and retching center** is located in the reticular formation at the level of the medulla oblongata. The response itself involves near-simultaneous adduction of the vocal folds, depression of the epiglottis, elevation of the larynx, relaxation of the upper and lower esophageal sphincters, elevation of the velum, and protrusion of the tongue (Miller, 2002).

Cough Reflex

Stimulation of the upper airway by a foreign object is a typical stimulus for the **cough reflex**, although irritation of the airway through disease conditions certainly occurs. The general visceral afferent component of the X vagus nerve conveys information concerning stimulation to the nucleus solitarius at the level of the medulla oblongata of the brainstem. Interconnection with the expiratory center within the reticular formation of the medulla activates abdominal musculature, while the motor nucleus of the X vagus (nucleus ambiguus) facilitates adduction of the vocal folds.

Reflexes of Respiration and Apnea

Respiration control consists of a complex of reflexive responses. The amount of oxygen, carbon dioxide, and acidity in the blood is sensed within the carotid sinus, resulting in decreases or increases of respiratory rate. The nucleus solitarius, activated by the IX glossopharyngeal nerve, signals the **brainstem respiratory center** to increase the rate of respiration. The rhythms of **inspiration and expiration** are controlled through separate centers within the medulla oblongata, with the inspiratory center activating the muscles of inspiration, and the expiratory center being responsible for the muscles of expiration. When the nasopharynx is mechanically stimulated, a sniff reflex is triggered, while forced expiration can be triggered by mechanical stimulation of the pharyngeal wall.

The **apneic reflex** is elicited by stimulation of the oral, pharyngeal, or laryngeal spaces (Thach, 2001) and results in adduction of the vocal folds, elevation of the larynx, and inversion of the epiglottis (Miller, 2002). This reflex is clearly protective (Thach, 2001), although simply terminating respiration without laryngeal protection will not prevent aspiration.

In summary, the basic elements of mastication and deglutition are reflex circuits.

- The orienting, rooting, and sucking reflexes are stimulated by light contact with the cheek and lips, mediated by the V trigeminal. Orienting is accomplished through the XI accessory nerve.
- During the chewing reflex, pressure sensation is conveyed by the V trigeminal nerve to the chewing CPG of the brainstem, then to the nucleus pontis caudalis of the reticular formation for rhythmic tongue movements.
- The palatal reflex and gag reflex are mediated through the IX glossopharyngeal nerve, conveyed to the nucleus solitarius and solitary fasciculus by means of the inferior and superior ganglia of the IX glossopharyngeal nerve.
- The vomiting reflex arises from a number of stimuli mediated by the I olfactory, IX glossopharyngeal, VIII vestibulocochlear, or X vagus. The vomiting and retching center is located in the reticular formation at the level of the medulla oblongata.
- The X vagus nerve conveys information concerning stimulation for the cough reflex to the nucleus solitarius. Interconnection in the reticular formation activates abdominal musculature and the motor nucleus of the X vagus adducts the vocal folds.
- Carbon dioxide and acidity in the blood is sensed within the carotid sinus, which triggers a response at the nucleus solitarius to increase the rate of respiration. Rhythms of respiration are controlled through separate inspiratory and expiratory centers within the medulla oblongata.
- The apneic reflex results in adduction of the vocal folds, elevation of the larynx, and inversion of the epiglottis.

SENSATION IN MASTICATION AND DEGLUTITION

As can be seen from the discussion of reflexes above, sensation related to mastication and deglutition is critical for stimulation of the processes involved. While each reflex has its stimulus, you should be aware that many of the same stimuli trigger a cascade of responses through the CPG circuits (Broussard & Altschuler, 2000; Ertekin & Aydogdu, 2003; Jean, 2001). Thus, sensory mechanisms, cranial nerve nuclei, and the CPG work together to accomplish the swallow. A failure of any of these elements will result in dysphagia, a deficit of swallowing.

Sensation

Sensors in mastication and deglutition include gustation (taste), olfaction, thermal, tactile, and pressure sensors (Kandel, Schwartz, Jessell, Siegelbaum, & Hudspeth, 2013; Møller, 2003).

Gustation

Gustation, or the sense of taste, is mediated by two separate systems in the oral cavity, and two more for the pharyngeal and laryngeal spaces. Taste sensors are **chemoreceptors** that respond to specific molecular complexes within a sampled food (Buck, 2000). Food molecules are broken down by saliva, and the molecular product binds with the taste receptor (typically in the oral cavity) to activate specific taste responses within the nervous system. Taste sensors are found within the epithelia of the mouth and the papillae of the tongue. The sampled molecules are isolated by taste pores in the sensor, held in place by small hair-like fibers termed microvilli. The variety of taste sensations arise from stimulation of combinations of five basic taste sensors (sweet, sour, salty, bitter, and umami).

Taste sense from the anterior two-thirds of the tongue and palate is mediated by the VII facial nerve, while the posterior one-third of the tongue is served by the IX glossopharyngeal nerve (Geran & Travers, 2011; Ninomaya, Imoto, & Sugimura, 1999). Note that the anterior salivary glands are innervated by the VII facial, while the posterior gland is innervated by the IX glossopharyngeal as well. The X vagus mediates the sense of taste for the epiglottis and esophagus, as well as within the trachea. (While it may seem odd to have taste receptors in the airway, it could well serve to signal the presence of a foreign body by means other than tactile stimulation.) **Chemesthetic sense** (such as the sensation arising from capsaicin or quinine) is mediated by the V trigeminal nerve (Cometto-Muñiz, Cain, & Abraham, 2004; Green, 2011, 2012; Krival & Bates 2012). Sensation mediated by the VII facial nerve passes to the solitary tract nucleus of the medulla within the gustatory center in the brainstem. The sensation mediated by the IX glossopharyngeal nerve also terminates on the solitary tract nucleus. Taste sense of the X vagus nerve is conveyed via the nodose ganglion, but also terminates on the solitary tract nucleus. This information is conveyed from that nucleus to the ventral posterior medial nucleus of the thalamus, and ultimately terminates in the insular cortex.

If you examine Figure 11–2, you will see the circuit for these taste sensations, including chemesthetic sense, which is mediated by the V trigeminal nerve (Sørensen, Møller, Flint, Martens, & Raben, 2003). Chemesthetic sense is perceived

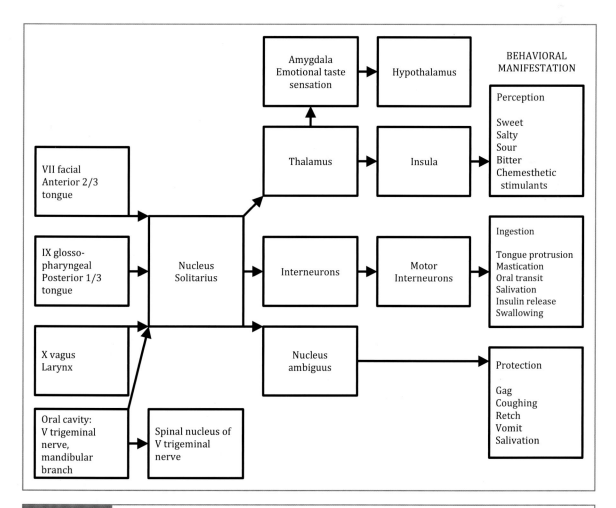

FIGURE 11–2. Neural pathways of taste. Note that chemesthetic sense is mediated by the V trigeminal nerve, terminating in both the spinal nucleus of trigeminal nerve and nucleus solitarius. *Source:* Based on data of Rudenga, Green, Nachtigal, and Small (2010); Seikel, Drumright, and King (2016); Whitehead and Frank (1983).

through the tactile system, with afferents going to both the spinal nucleus of the trigeminal and the solitary tract nucleus (Cowart, 1998; Dessirier, Simons, Carstens, O'Mahony, & Carstens, 2000). The chemesthetic sense ultimately activates the insular cortex (Rudenga et al., 2010; Whitehead & Frank, 1983). Taste and smell are integrated at the insula (Møller, 2003). Output from the insula projects to both the motor regions of the brainstem and the limbic system.

Olfaction

Olfaction, which refers to the sense of smell, is mediated by the I olfactory nerve. This nerve is phylogenetically quite old and does not pass through the brainstem. Olfactory sensors are embedded in the epithelia of the nasal cavity and sense the presence of molecules. The information concerning olfactory stimulation is transmitted to the olfactory bulb within the braincase. The olfactory tract conveys the information to the amygdala, anterior olfactory nucleus, pyriform cortex, hippocampus, and entorhinal cortex. Ultimately, the information arrives at the orbital region of the frontal lobe. The amygdala information is conveyed to the hypothalamus, while the information from the entorhinal cortex is transmitted to the hippocampus.

Tactile, Proprioceptive, and Thermal Sensation

Mechanoreceptors convey sensation concerning bolus movement in the oral and pharyngeal cavities. **Meissner's corpuscles** within the epithelia of the tongue sense movement of the bolus, while Merkel disk receptors sense pressure. **Pacinian corpuscles** sense deep pressure that changes over time, while **Ruffini endings** sense tissue stretch. These sensations are transmitted via the V trigeminal nerve to the trigeminal semilunar ganglion and then to the principal sensory nucleus of the trigeminal nerve. This nucleus also processes pain and thermal sense, which is also mediated by the trigeminal nerve. Joint and muscle sense of the oral, lingual, and pharyngeal structures are also mediated by the trigeminal nerve, with information terminating in the mesencephalic nucleus of the trigeminal.

Complex Motor Responses

The complex processes associated with mastication and deglutition are governed by the highly orchestrated interaction of lower-level reflexes. This is accomplished by means of central pattern generators (CPGs). The **CPG for swallowing** involves two separate networks that provide both excitatory and inhibitory influences on the brainstem nervous system. The **dorsal swallowing group** (DSG) is found in the medulla oblongata near the solitary tract nucleus, while the **ventral swallowing group** (VSG) is near the nucleus ambiguus. The V trigeminal, maxillary branch, IX glossopharyngeal nerve,

and X vagus all provide input arising from the tongue dorsum, epiglottis, faucial pillars, and posterior pharyngeal wall to the VSG. Input from the DSG to the hypoglossal nucleus results in rhythmic tongue movements, such as those involved in bolus preparation (Cunningham & Sawchenko, 2000). The respiratory CPGs reside in the posterior brainstem reticular formation, interacting with the phrenic nerve (diaphragm contraction), X vagus recurrent laryngeal nerve (vocal fold abduction), and intercostal nerves for inspiration. There are separate inspiratory and expiratory networks (Janczewski & Feldman, 2006).

In summary, sensory mechanisms, cranial nerve nuclei, and the CPG work together to accomplish swallowing, and failure of any of these elements will result in dysphagia.

- Gustation is mediated by four separate systems. Chemoreceptors respond to a variety of taste sensations mediated by the five basic taste sensors: sweet, sour, salty, bitter, and umami.
- Taste sense from the anterior two-thirds of the tongue and palate is mediated by the VII facial nerve, while the posterior one-third of the tongue is served by the IX glossopharyngeal nerve. Anterior salivary glands are innervated by the VII facial, and the posterior gland is innervated by the IX glossopharyngeal.
- The X vagus mediates the sense of taste for the epiglottis and esophagus, as well as within the trachea.
- Chemesthetic sense is mediated by the V trigeminal nerve. Chemesthetic sense is perceived through the tactile system, with afferents going to both the spinal nucleus of trigeminal and the solitary tract nucleus and ultimately activates the insular cortex. Taste and smell are integrated at the insula, and output from the insula projects to both the motor regions of the brainstem and the limbic system.
- Olfaction is mediated by the I olfactory nerve. Olfactory information is transmitted to the olfactory bulb and tract, which conveys information to the amygdala, anterior olfactory nucleus, pyriform cortex, hippocampus, and entorhinal cortex, and ultimately to the orbital region of the frontal lobe.
- Mechanoreceptors convey sensation concerning bolus movement in the oral and pharyngeal cavities. Meissner's corpuscles sense movement, and Merkel disk receptors sense pressure. Pacinian corpuscles sense deep pressure, and Ruffini endings sense tissue stretch. These sensations are transmitted via the V trigeminal nerve to the trigeminal semilunar ganglion and then to the principal sensory nucleus of the trigeminal nerve.
- The central pattern generator for swallowing involves two separate networks that provide both excitatory and inhibitory influences on the brainstem nervous system. The dorsal swallowing group (DSG) is found in the medulla oblongata near the solitary tract nucleus, while the ventral swallowing group (VSG) is near the nucleus ambiguus.

- The VSG receives input from V trigeminal, IX glossopharyngeal, and X vagus. The DSG output results in rhythmic tongue movements, such as those involved in bolus preparation. Respiratory CPGs reside in the posterior brainstem reticular formation, interacting with the phrenic nerve, X vagus recurrent laryngeal nerve, and intercostal nerves for inspiration. There are separate inspiratory and expiratory networks.

CHAPTER SUMMARY

Central pattern generators (CPGs) take groups of reflexes and bring them together into a complex action sequence. The motor act requires visual input, proprioceptive input, and a motor plan, and this sensory information is integrated with the motor plan before execution. In a closed-loop feedback system, there is a set reference or target and correction comes from comparing accuracy in hitting the target with some standard. Open-loop systems do not operate on sensory feedback and correction and are termed feed-forward processes. Speaking requires an idea or concept that we wish to convey that must be encoded into language. Grammatical encoding occurs largely within Broca's area, and phonetic encoding occurs within the left insular cortex and left supramarginal gyrus. There are two distinct loops involved in the motor act for speech. A "preparative" loop includes the left dorsolateral prefrontal cortex, anterior insular cortex, supplementary motor area, and the superior cerebellum. The "executive" loop includes the motor cortex, thalamus, putamen and caudate, and the inferior cerebellum.

Two major models have been proposed to explain the production of speech. In the psycholinguistic view, speech is the oral manifestation of language; the motor view relates to how the manifestation occurs. The Hierarchical State Feedback Control is a blended model that views speech production in a hierarchical fashion that acknowledges the linguistic input. The initial stimulus for speech is a concept or idea that triggers a verbal manifestation (lemma). The word is directed to the Broca's–temporoparietal juncture (TPJ) loop that projects to lower centers that govern the motor plan, including the somatosensory area, motor strip, and cerebellum. Phonological representation occurs at both higher levels and lower levels simultaneously. The Broca's–TPJ circuit produces a prediction of the outcome that is checked by the auditory system, and if an acoustic error is sensed, a correction is fed back to the TPJ and Broca's motor plan region. The DIVA model of speech production utilizes sensory inputs as checks for the accuracy of the executed speech (feed-forward), as well as sensory feedback to support the learning process in speech production. In the DIVA model, the auditory model for the desired phoneme is generated and conveyed to the auditory cortex and somatosensory cortex so that the word that is produced can be validated against the target.

Reflexes present at birth such as rooting, sucking, and orienting allow the infant to get nutrition. The rooting reflex causes the infant to turn toward the stimulus and the mouth to open. The sucking reflex results in a piston-like protrusion and retraction movement of the tongue. Adult mastication and deglutition patterns emerge around 6 months of age. As dentition erupts and solid food is introduced, teeth start to grind and chew the bolus, and this requires use of the muscles of mastication.

In the adult there are three identifiable stages involved in mastication and deglutition: oral (oral preparation and oral transit), pharyngeal, and esophageal. In the oral preparation stage, the bolus is prepared for swallowing. This involves movements such as chewing and crushing. Movement of the bolus is accomplished during the oral transit stage. The sublingual and submandibular glands are innervated by the VII facial nerve, while the parotid gland is innervated by the IX glossopharyngeal nerve. Cranial nerves used in the oral stage include VII facial nerve, V trigeminal nerve, IX glossopharyngeal, X vagus, and XI accessory nerves and XII hypoglossal nerve. The pharyngeal stage is initiated when the tongue and/or bolus contact the posterior region of the mouth. Pressure sensors at the trigger site provide input to the motor program that will simultaneously protect the airway and propel the bolus through the upper esophageal sphincter. The pharyngeal stage is entirely reflexive in nature and each component of the pharyngeal stage is governed by individual reflexes that are organized by assemblies of neurons termed central pattern generators (CPGs). Once initiated, a CPG will produce a motor sequence from start to finish, triggering the motor pattern of numerous reflexes sequentially and with precise timing. The pharyngeal stage accomplishes laryngeal elevation, pressure generation, and airway protection. Laryngeal elevation requires the V trigeminal, VII facial, XII hypoglossal and IX glossopharyngeal, X vagus, and XI accessory nerves. Airway protection depends on the X vagus recurrent laryngeal nerve, X vagus pharyngeal nerve, XI accessory, V trigeminal, and X vagus superior laryngeal nerves. The upper esophageal sphincter is inhibited by the X vagus, superior laryngeal nerve. The esophageal stage is outside of voluntary control. The esophagus is innervated by the X vagus and the sympathetic trunk of the cervical and thoracic region.

The basic elements of mastication and deglutition are reflex circuits. The orienting, rooting, and sucking reflexes are stimulated by light contact with the cheek and lips, mediated by the V trigeminal. Orienting is accomplished through the XI accessory nerve. During the chewing reflex, pressure sensation is conveyed by the V trigeminal nerve to the chewing CPG of the brainstem, then to the nucleus pontis caudalis of the reticular formation for rhythmic tongue movements. The palatal reflex and gag reflex are mediated through the IX glossopharyngeal nerve, conveyed to the nucleus solitarius and solitary fasciculus by means of the inferior and superior ganglia of the IX glossopharyngeal nerve. The vomiting reflex arises from a number of stimuli mediated by the I olfactory, IX glossopharyngeal, VIII vestibulocochlear, or X vagus. The vomiting and retching center is located in the reticular formation at the level of the medulla oblongata. The X vagus nerve conveys information concerning stimulation for the cough reflex to the nucleus solitarius. Interconnection in the reticular formation activates abdominal musculature, and the motor nucleus of the X vagus adducts the vocal folds. Carbon dioxide and acidity in the blood is sensed within the carotid sinus, which triggers a response at the nucleus solitarius to increase the rate of respiration. Rhythms of respiration are controlled through separate inspiratory and expiratory centers within the medulla oblongata. The apneic reflex results in adduction of the vocal folds, elevation of the larynx, and inversion of the epiglottis.

Sensory mechanisms, cranial nerve nuclei, and the CPG work together to accomplish swallowing, and failure of any of these elements will result in dysphagia. Gustation is mediated by four separate systems. Chemoreceptors respond to a variety of taste sensations mediated by the five basic taste sensors: sweet, sour, salty, bitter, and umami. Taste sense from the anterior two-thirds of the tongue and palate is mediated by the VII facial nerve, while the posterior one-third of the tongue is served by the IX glossopharyngeal nerve. Anterior salivary glands are innervated by the VII facial and the posterior gland is innervated by the IX glossopharyngeal. The X vagus mediates the sense of taste for the epiglottis and esophagus, as well as within the trachea. Chemesthetic sense is mediated by the V trigeminal nerve. Chemesthetic sense is perceived through the tactile system, with afferents going to both the spinal nucleus of the trigeminal and the solitary tract nucleus and ultimately activates the insular cortex. Taste and smell are integrated at the insula, and output from the insula projects to both the motor regions of the brainstem and the limbic system. Olfaction is mediated by the I olfactory nerve. Olfactory information is transmitted to the olfactory bulb and tract, which conveys information to the amygdala, anterior olfactory nucleus, pyriform cortex, hippocampus, and entorhinal cortex, and ultimately to the orbital region of the frontal lobe. Mechanoreceptors convey sensation concerning bolus movement in the oral and pharyngeal cavities. Meissner's corpuscles sense movement, and Merkel disk receptors sense pressure. Pacinian corpuscles sense deep pressure and Ruffini endings sense tissue stretch. These sensations are transmitted via the V trigeminal nerve to the trigeminal semilunar ganglion and then to the principal sensory nucleus of the trigeminal nerve. The central pattern generator for swallowing involves two separate networks that provide both excitatory and inhibitory influences on the brainstem nervous system. The dorsal swallowing group (DSG) is found in the medulla oblongata near the solitary tract nucleus, while the ventral swallowing group (VSG) is near the nucleus ambiguus. The VSG receives input from V trigeminal, IX glossopharyngeal, and X vagus. The DSG output results in rhythmic tongue movements, such as those involved in bolus preparation. Respiratory CPGs reside in the posterior brainstem reticular formation, interacting with the phrenic nerve, X vagus recurrent laryngeal nerve, and intercostal nerves for inspiration. There are separate inspiratory and expiratory networks.

CASE STUDY 11–1

Physician's Notes on Initial Physical Examination and History

I reviewed this patient demonstrating reduction in cognitive capacity following multiple cerebrovascular accidents (CVAs, or strokes) with subsequent seizures. (See Table 11–3 for terminology. Note that we are presenting the data of this case in chronological order to show the emerging speech and language signs and symptoms as the condition progresses.) Since his last stroke in August of this year, he has become more cognitively impaired. He is apathetic, restless at times, and disoriented. He has sleep apnea, but he does not cooperate with treatment for the apnea. He has not had further seizures. He is currently on **Exelon** 3 mg **bid**, **Trileptal** 600 mg bid, **Plavix** 75 mg once daily for his neurological conditions, and I added 0.5 mg of **Risperdal** at 6 p.m. so he would be more cooperative in the evening, which might also help with acceptance of the ventilator. The electrophysiological report revealed an abnormal EEG with findings of moderate diffuse background slowing and organization, and an absence of epileptiform activity. The MRI findings showed extensive focal and diffuse signal alteration of the periventricular white matter and centrum semiovale bilaterally on **T2W and FLAIR** images, consistent with a **small vessel disease**.

Seven Years Following Intake

Type II diabetes mellitus and **vascular dementia** were diagnosed in this patient seven years ago. Now, he has been injected with **Mixtard** 30 units a.m. along with 12 units at supper time. His laboratory findings show fasting **hypoglycemia**. He doesn't have his sugars checked in the afternoon. I have reduced the dose of Mixtard to 26 units in the morning and 6 units in the evening. His wife will inform me about his blood sugar profile next week.

TABLE 11–3.   **Terminology for Case Study 11–1**

Aspiration	Pathological admission of food or liquid into the airway below the level of the vocal folds.
bid	Twice daily.
Blood pressure (BP)	The systolic blood pressure is the pressure that the heart pumps blood, while the diastolic blood pressure is the pressure that the heart relaxes and refills with blood. Normal blood pressure is lower than 120 (systolic) over 80 (diastolic) millimeters of mercury (mmHg).
Clopidogrel (active ingredient), Plavix (brand name) 75 mg	Used to prevent blood clots after a heart attack or stroke.
Diabetes mellitus	A disease in which the pancreas does not produce the hormone insulin, resulting in high blood sugar levels in the body.
EEG (electroencephalogram)	Neurophysiological test that shows electrical activity in the brain.
Exelon	See rivastigmine.
Human insulin (active ingredient), Mixtard (brand name)	An injected medication that includes the hormone insulin. It is used in patients diagnosed with diabetes mellitus.
Hypoglycemia	A condition in which the blood sugar is below the normal levels.
In situ	Located in the normal or initial position; literally "in place".
Isosorbide mononitrate (active ingredient), Monoket (brand name)	Drug used to dilate the blood vessels and thus reduce blood pressure.
i.v. antibiotics	Intravenous (into the veins) antibiotics.
Lactulose (active ingredient), Duphalac (brand name) 20 mL	Used to treat constipation.
Mixtard	See human insulin.
Multi-infarct dementia (vascular dementia)	One type of vascular dementia arising from many small strokes in the brain. The early symptoms of multi-infarct dementia may involve difficulty with everyday tasks, naming problems, disorientation, and loss of interest in hobbies.
Nocte	Every night.
Oxcarbazepine (active ingredient), Trileptal (brand name) 600 mg	An anti-epileptic drug.
Penetration	This is the passage of food or liquid into the larynx but not through the vocal folds.
Phenytoin (active ingredient), Dilantin (brand name) 100 mg	Used to control epilepsy (anti-epileptic drug) and seizures.
Plavix	See clopidogrel.
Risperdal	See risperidone.
Risperidone (active ingredient), Risperdal (brand name)	An antipsychotic medication used mainly to treat schizophrenia and bipolar disorders.
Rivastigmine (active ingredient), Exelon (brand name) 3 mg	A medication used to improve memory, awareness, and ability for daily functions.
Small vessel disease (coronary microvascular disease)	A disease in which there is damage in the walls of the small arteries in the heart.

continues

TABLE 11–3.	*continued*
T2-weighted (T2W) and fluid-attenuated inversion recovery (FLAIR) images	A technique of analysis in MRI.
Tachycardia	A type of arrhythmia in which the heart works faster than normal not only during exercise but also at rest.
Trileptal	See oxcarbazepine.
Type II diabetes mellitus	A second type of diabetes mellitus in which the body does not use the effects of insulin or does not produce enough insulin.
Vascular dementia	See multi-infarct dementia.
Videofluoroscopy (VFSS)	X-ray technique that is used to assess swallowing function by visualizing the stages of swallowing function.

Eight Years, 10 Months Following Intake

The patient now lives at a nursing home. He recently had a probable pneumonia for which he received intravenous antibiotics and even more recently urinary tract infection, again treated with **i.v. antibiotics**. He is very difficult to assess, as he does not cooperate. However, his saturation is good at 95% and he has no **tachycardia**. I have given him a referral for a chest x-ray, which they will try to do at the local hospital in the next few days. The patient has a gastrostomy **in situ** and is receiving nutrition by this means. Clinically, he is totally anarthric and dependent, and I am not sure that he recognizes his wife. **BP: 95/60.** He is to continue with the rest of his medications, which include isosorbide mononitrate, **phenytoin** 100 mg daily, Plavix 75 mg daily, and **lactulose** 20 mL **nocte**.

Medical Diagnosis

Multi-infarct dementia and **diabetes mellitus**

Speech Examination and VFSS Study

The patient was not cooperative and was able to follow only simple commands. A **VFSS** study showed the following results.

Procedure

The patient was assessed in a sitting position, viewed in lateral and in an antero-posterior plane. Oral, pharyngeal, and esophageal phases of swallow were examined. Given orally were 3 cc, 5 cc, thin, and thickened liquid consistencies via a spoon and small syringe, as well as ½ spoon pureed consistency mixed with barium suspension. Larger volumes via a cup were not attempted so as not to place patient in danger of **aspiration**.

Oral Phase

Oral management was moderately impaired with reduced bolus control, difficulty with bolus formation and transfer for liquid and pureed consistencies. Reduced lingual coordination resulted in premature spillage into the hypopharynx to the level of the valleculae. During the swallow, tongue base posterior motion and retraction toward the pharyngeal wall was significantly reduced, which resulted in moderate residue coating on the tongue base and bolus stasis in the oral cavity which eventually cleared with multiple swallows.

Pharyngeal Phase

The pharyngeal phase was moderately impaired, characterized by significant difficulty in triggering the pharyngeal swallow. Tracheal aspiration of thin liquid and trace **penetration** of thick liquid in the laryngeal vestibule were noted due to the delay in the initiation of the swallow response (6–10 seconds variable), which resulted in material spilling into the pharynx at the level of the valleculae prior to swallow initiation. Mild residue was noted after the swallow in the valleculae and on the posterior pharyngeal wall due to reduced hyolaryngeal elevation and poor pharyngeal contraction.

Esophageal Phase

Bolus clearance from proximal and distal esophagus to the stomach through the gastroesophageal juncture was successful and timely. No structural or functional esophageal abnormalities were noted.

Speech-Language Diagnosis

Moderate oral and pharyngeal dysphagia characterized by significant difficulty in triggering the pharyngeal swallow, difficulty in formation, control and transfer of bolus posteriorly in the oral cavity, aspiration of thin liquids without spontaneous cough production to clear aspirate, and laryngeal penetration with thick liquid. This patient is at high risk of chronic micro aspiration of liquids. He can still manage blended foods orally relatively safely.

Questions Concerning This Case

1. What is the neuropathological basis of multi-infarct dementia? From the information, can you determine if these are lacunar or ischemic strokes? Consider the typical site of lesion of lacunar strokes and the presence of dementia in this patient as you make your decisions.
2. One of the most consistent risk factors for dysphagia is dysarthria (Duffy, 2013). Why is this the case (i.e., how are the systems affected by dysarthria and the functions associated with swallowing related)?

Case provided by Dr. Kostas Konstantopoulos, European University Cyprus.

CASE STUDY 11–2

Physician's Notes on Initial Physical Examination and History

This was a 64-year-old male who probably had a genetic midline cerebellar ataxia syndrome (see Table 11–4 for terminology. Note that we are

presenting the data of this case in chronological order to show the emerging speech and language signs and symptoms as the condition progresses). The patient was also seen two years prior for an MRI-confirmed acute stroke in the right parietal lobe. MRI did not show any evidence of a source of emboli, as neither did the carotid duplex, as

TABLE 11–4.	Terminology for Case Study 11–2
"c" or "d" scores	Scoring on the *Frenchay Dysarthria Assessment* (FDA). See Table 11–5 for details of Frenchay scoring.
1 tds to 1½ tds	1 tablet to 1½ tablets 3 times a day
Acute ischemic infarct	An occlusion of a cerebral artery, either thrombotic (blood clot in a blood vessel) or embolic (piece of material inside a blood vessel), which results in reduction or loss of blood circulation in the brain.
Ataxic dysarthria (cerebellar dysarthria)	A motor speech disorder characterized by abnormalities in all subsystems for speech (respiration, phonation, resonation, articulation, and prosody), but it is more prominent in articulation and prosody. In this disorder the movement for speech is slow and inaccurate due to the incoordination caused by cerebellar damage.
Ataxic gait	This gait is described as abnormally unsteady, staggering, and uncoordinated.
bid	Twice daily.
Carbidopa-levodopa (active ingredient, Sinemet (brand name)	Drug that is used for the conversion of the neurotransmitter dopamine and helps in the alleviation of symptomatology in Parkinson's disease.
Carotid duplex	An ultrasound procedure that tests the movement of blood cells through the carotid arteries.
Enzyme Q10 (Coenzyme Q10)	Produces energy for cell growth and helps in the mitochondria . It works as an antioxidant to protect cells from enemies such as the free radicals.
Sinemet	See carbidopa-levodopa

confirmed by the cardiologist. More specifically, the MRI findings showed multiple areas of **acute ischemic infarct** on the right cerebral hemisphere without signs of underlying hemorrhage. No stenosis was seen in the right internal carotid artery. The possibility of multiple embolic infarcts of cardiac origin should be considered according to the radiologist. In the last month, the patient exhibited some difficulties putting on his clothes, including the trousers and shirt, due to the right parietal defect. On examination, the patient had a mild to moderate truncal ataxia but no sensory inattention or loss of joint position sense. I scheduled a follow-up with him in 4 months. The patient was referred for physiotherapy to improve his gait function.

One Year, 8 Months Following Intake

I reviewed this patient. The patient was seen nearly two years ago at about the age of 60 when he had mild cerebellar ataxia in the midline that has progressed in the last six years to the degree that he is now using a Zimmer frame to walk without falling. Interestingly, the patient reported that his mother had a similar condition, which she developed at the age of 40, and she has been clinically normal up to now. DNA testing has failed to show any of the known causes of ataxia, but my clinical impression is that there was clearly an autosomal dominant heredity in this man. On today's examination, he presented mild cerebellar dysarthria and bilateral dysdiadochokinesia, but he was reasonably good with finger-to-nose coordination. The patient presented an **ataxic gait** even while using a Zimmer frame and maintained reflexes. There was no nystagmus or atrophy in the hands. He is on co-enzyme **Q10** 100 mg **bid** and vitamin E once daily, and I recommended continuation of the treatment.

Two Years, 1 Month Following Intake

I reviewed this 67-year-old patient who appeared to have an autosomal dominant form of cerebellar syndrome in that his mother was similarly affected in terms of speech and mobility. The patient exhibited cerebellar speech manifestations and has extrapyramidal signs and possibly pyramidal signs with a superimposed right parietal stroke. When we last saw him in March, we decided to increase his **Sinemet** from **1 tds to 1½ tds**, but saw no significant improvement. He currently exhibits difficulties swallowing tablets and therefore we decided to gradually terminate Sinemet altogether. He was unable to walk and was wheelchair bound. On examination, there was cerebellar speech, a mask-like face, impaired up gaze, slow saccades but fall-down gaze. In the arms, there was extrapyramidal rigidity but no cogwheel or any tremor. There were no significant cerebellar signs.

Medical Diagnosis

Unknown medical diagnosis

Speech Examination

The *Frenchay Dysarthria Assessment* was administered to the patient (see Table 11–5 for details of Frenchay scoring). The results showed a moderate difficulty, with scores in the **"c-d"** range. The DAB classification shows a cluster of abnormal speech characteristics for articulatory inaccuracy and more specifically imprecise consonants, irregular articulatory breakdowns, distorted vowels, and slow rate (Darley, Aronson, & Brown, 1969). More specifically:

- Reflexes cough: Patient has occasional difficulty with choking, or food sometimes showing signs of penetration and aspiration (b).
- Reflexes swallow: Patient observed drinking 1/2 cup of water and eating a cookie; slowness during eating/drinking with pauses while drinking (b).
- Respiration in speech: When asked to count from 1 to 20 as quickly as possible, the patient exhibited shallow breath, managing only a few words. There was also poor coordination and marked variability, and the patient required six breaths to complete the task (d).
- Lips seal: Occasional air leakage and breaks in lips seal when the patient was asked to blow air into cheeks and maintain for 15 seconds (b).
- Lips alternate: Labored movement when the patient was asked to repeat "oo ee" 10 times. One movement was within normal limits, while other movements were severely distorted (c).
- Laryngeal time: Sustained phonation for /a/ with clear voice only for 4 seconds (e).
- Laryngeal pitch: Minor difficulty with pitch breaks when the patient was asked to sing a scale (b).

TABLE 11–5.	Frenchay Scoring Details

The *Frenchay Dysarthria Assessment* (FDA) utilizes a rating scale for all testing.

a score	Normal for age
b score	Mild abnormality noticeable to skilled observer
c score	Obvious abnormality but the patient can perform task/movements with reasonable approximation
d score	Some production of task but poor in quality, unable to sustain, inaccurate, or extremely labored
e score	Unable to undertake task/movement/sound

- Laryngeal volume: Changes in volume when the patient counts from 1 to 5 showed noticeably uneven progression (c).
- Laryngeal in speech (intonation): Voice during speech was mostly effective—there may be occasional inappropriate use of volume and pitch noticeable to the examiner (b).
- Tongue protrusion: Irregular movement accompanied by facial grimace (5 times in 7 seconds) (c).
- Tongue elevation: Labored gross movement of the tongue ("d" score).
- Tongue lateral: Labored or incomplete tongue movement (5 times in 8 seconds) (c).
- Tongue alternate: Diadochokinetic rate of the word /kala/ (10 times) with tongue changes in position and misidentification by the examiner of the phoneme attempted (11 seconds to complete the task) (d).
- Tongue in speech: Grossly distorted movement and severe changes in tongue potential. Vowels distorted and consonants frequently omitted (d).

Speech-Language Diagnosis

Mixed type **ataxic-hypokinetic dysarthria**

Questions Concerning This Case

1. The physician was unable to provide a diagnosis, and yet the speech-language pathologist could provide a diagnosis of mixed ataxic-hypokinetic dysarthria. How could the SLP provide a diagnosis without a medical diagnosis?
2. The physician noted that there was a hypokinetic component, which is typically associated with Parkinson's disease. In this case, however, Sinemet did not help the condition. Sinemet provides a precursor for dopamine, which replaces the neurotransmitter lost due to damage to the substantia nigra and is used by the basal ganglia for motor control. Is there another way to have signs of Parkinson's disease without damage to the substantia nigra?

Case provided by Dr. Kostas Konstantopoulos, European University Cyprus.

CASE STUDY 11–3

Physician's Notes on Initial Physical Examination and History

This is a 66-year-old female who presented with a history of long-standing **blepharospasm** as well as **dysphagia** and **ptosis**, which is probably secondary at least partially due to botulinum toxin (**Botox**) injections (see Table 11–6 for terminology. Note that we are presenting the data of this case in chronological order to show the emerging speech and language signs and symptoms as the condition progresses). The question was raised in the past whether the patient presented with **ocular pharyngeal muscular dystrophy**. A left biceps muscle biopsy did not show any **vascular myopathy** suggestive of such a diagnosis, and there was no evidence of **mitochondrial dysfunction**. On examination, the patient did not exhibit significant weakness. She stated that she has frequent excessive saliva, for which **Amirol 10 mg nocte** was started. An MRI scan previously this year showed moderate dilatation of the frontal horns of the lateral ventricles in relation to the peripheral sulci; however, the possibility of early normal pressure **hydrocephalus** was excluded. The dilatation at this point was controlled by medication given by the neurosurgeon (Lyrica and Noritren) and the patient showed some improvement. In addition, there were found some spotty hyperintensities involving the subcorti-

cal areas, and they are probably due to small vessel disease. **Blood pressure** was 145/80 at the time of assessment. The next appointment was scheduled for six months later.

Six Months Following Intake

The patient had complaints of increased frequency to empty her urinary bladder. She also has diabetes and was not controlling her blood sugar effectively. The eyelid blinking was better and no blepharospasm was found on examination. The patient had Botox injections last Monday. Her swallowing ability also remained unchanged. She also exhibited mild unsteadiness while walking and hypomimia. She was scheduled for re-examination in six months.

Medical Diagnosis

Blepharospasm

Speech Examination: One Year Following Intake

Her speech during dialogue was found to be normal. The *Frenchay Dysarthria Assessment* (FDA) showed mild difficulty, with scores in the "b" range for most of the tongue movements produced (see Table 11–5 for details of Frenchay scoring):

TABLE 11–6.	**Terminology for Case Study 11–3**
Amitriptyline (active ingredient), Amirol/Elavil (brand name)	Drug used to treat major depression, anxiety disorder, bipolar disorder, etc. One of its side effects is dry mouth. For this reason, it is used by neurologists to control excessive saliva in patients with different neurological diseases
Blepharospasm	Uncontrollable contraction of eye muscles.
Blood pressure (BP)	The systolic blood pressure is the pressure that the heart pumps blood, while the diastolic blood pressure is the pressure that the heart relaxes and refills with blood. Normal blood pressure is lower than 120 (systolic) over 80 (diastolic) millimeters of mercury (mmHg).
Botox (botulinum toxin, BTX) injection	Botulinum toxin a neurotoxic protein that does not allow the release of the neurotransmitter acetylcholine. There are 8 types of botulinum toxin. Types A and B have a medical use to produce flaccidity in various spasms and hyperkinesias that exist in different neurological diseases.
Dysphagia	Disorder in one of the stages of swallowing.
Hydrocephalus	Excessive cerebrospinal fluid within ventricles of the brain.
Mitochondrial dysfunction	Dysfunction of mitochondria, the organelles involved in energy production in the cell.
MRI (magnetic resonance imaging)	Imaging technique that uses changes in molecular activity when tissue is exposed to electromagnetic energy. A diagnostic technique that uses magnetic fields to show an image of the body's soft tissue and bones.
Nocte	Every night
Ocular pharyngeal muscular dystrophy (OPMD)	Genetic disorder involving myopathy (muscle disease) in the eyelids and throat, resulting in eyelid drooping and difficulty in swallowing.
Ptosis	Drooping of upper eyelid.
Vascular myopathy	Muscular weakness due to vascular etiology.
Videofluoroscopic study of swallowing (VFSS)	Test used for the assessment of swallowing dysfunction through x-ray.

- Laryngeal component time: Sustained phonation for /a/ in 10 seconds (b).
- Tongue component (protrusion): Slow protrusion/retraction of the tongue (5 times in 5 seconds) (c).
- Tongue component (elevation): Patient was able to move her tongue toward the nose and then toward the chin slowly (7 seconds) (b).
- Tongue component (lateral): Slow movement of the tongue side to side (5 times) produced in 5 seconds (c).
- Tongue component alternate: Diadochokinetic rate of the bisyllable /kala/ (10 times) with slight incoordination and slowness. Task took 6 seconds to complete (b).

A videofluoroscopy study of swallowing (**VFSS**) was administered after referral of the neurologist and after patient's complaints of persisting swallowing difficulties, particularly with solids. Her perception is that solids "get stuck" in the upper throat.

Procedure

The patient was assessed in a standing position, viewed in lateral and anterior-posterior planes. Oral, pharyngeal, and esophageal stages of swallowing were examined. Thin liquid, pureed and solid consistencies mixed with barium suspension were given to the patient by spoon, via a cup and bite boluses.

Oral Phase

Lingual propulsion and pumping were mildly impaired and minimal residue and tongue coating with material was noted after each trial.

Pharyngeal Phase

Pharyngeal transit was mildly impaired with slower hyolaryngeal elevation and reduced tongue retraction to the posterior pharyngeal wall. This resulted in mild residue in the valleculae but not in the pyriform sinuses for liquids and pureed consistencies. Oral transit time for liquids and initiation of the swallow response were mildly delayed (1 second), which resulted in spilling of liquid prior to the initiation of swallow at the level of pyriform sinuses when given in sequential sips via a cup. No aspiration or vestibular penetration of any liquid or solid consistencies was observed.

Esophageal Phase

Esophageal emptying was normal.

Speech-Language Diagnosis

Mild oral and pharyngeal dysphagia characterized by somewhat ineffective mastication, and slower hyolaryngeal elevation resulting in mild valleculae and pharyngeal residue. Recommendations for soft diet, finely chopped and moist with thin liquids to be given by a cup in small sips. The patient needs to alternate liquids and solids, chew well, avoid hard foods, and practice dry swallows in between bites.

Questions Concerning This Case

1. The patient presented with some muscular weakness but also signs of hyperkinesia (extraneous movements), as manifested in blepharospasm. The patient had undergone Botox injections to ameliorate the blepharospasm. What is the mechanism of botulinum toxin injections (Botox) with relation to muscular weakness, and could that have caused the swallowing difficulty?
2. Hypomimia is mask-like facies or facial presentation. This is typically seen in Parkinson's disease or conditions with muscular rigidity. In your opinion, could this have been caused by the Botox injections?
3. The patient had multiple comorbidities, and the SLP ultimately diagnosed oropharyngeal dysphagia. Could this be the result of Botox, or could it be an additional comorbidity of unknown etiology?

Case provided by Dr. Kostas Konstantopoulos, European University Cyprus.

CASE STUDY 11–4

Physician's Notes on Initial Physical Examination and History

This 58-year-old woman visited the neurosurgery outpatient department, complaining about gait disturbances, tremor of upper extremities, and abnormal speech. Neurological evaluation revealed **ataxic gait**, **positive Romberg sign**, **dysmetria**, tremor, and incoordination, primarily in the left arm (see Table 11–7 for terminology related to this case. Note that we are presenting the data of this case in chronological order to show the emerging speech and language signs and symptoms as the condition progresses). Additionally several speech difficulties were noted, including nasal voice and poor phonation, and slow and slurred speech with decreased prosody. The patient's voice was trailing off to whispering while speaking without remarkable hoarseness initially. None of the lower cranial nerves showed deficit during neurological assessment. Notwithstanding, there was a great difficulty in expressing consonants, including /t,d,l,r,n/. The patient had difficulty using the hard palate to articulate individual words. An **MRI-MRA-MRV** scan of the brain was performed, revealing a very large meningioma located on the left cerebellopontine angle (Figure 11–3). Associated disorders included **ataxic dysarthria**, cranial nerves X and XII involvement, apraxic agraphia without ideomotor apraxia (distorted and imprecise letter formation; retained ability to spell aloud). Location of the lesion was the left cerebellopontine angle, compressing the left cerebellar hemisphere and lateral brainstem.

Medical Diagnosis

Cerebellopontine angle tumor (meningioma)

Treatment

The patient underwent microsurgical resection of the lesion. Histopathology confirmed the diagnosis of meningioma. Retrosigmoid approach was chosen for this case. Patient did very well with gradual improvement of ataxic gait, dysarthria, tremor, vocal and speech disturbances in approximately six months time.

Speech-Language Implications

Cerebellopontine angle tumor compresses one hemisphere of the cerebellum, as well as the pons (and often medulla) of the brainstem. Depending upon the size of the tumor, cranial nerves VIII vestibulocochlear, V trigeminal, and

TABLE 11–7. **Terminology for Case Study 11–4**

Ataxic dysarthria (cerebellar dysarthria)	A motor speech disorder that is characterized by abnormalities in all subsystems for speech (respiration, phonation, resonation, articulation, and prosody), but it is more prominent in articulation and prosody. In this disorder the movement for speech is slow and inaccurate due to the incoordination that is caused by cerebellar damage.
Ataxic gait	Gait described as abnormal, unsteady, staggering, and uncoordinated.
Cerebellopontine angle tumor	The most common tumor of the posterior cranial fossa; tumor involving the region of the juncture of the cerebellum and pons, often also including the internal auditory meatus.
Dysmetria	Incoordination of movement or inability to judge distance. The result is that the hand, arm, or leg undershoots or overshoots an intended position. It is considered to be the result of ataxia and is caused by impairment in the cerebellum.
MRI (magnetic resonance imaging)	Imaging technique that uses changes in molecular activity when tissue is exposed to electromagnetic energy.
MRA (magnetic resonance imaging–angiography)	MRI to visualize cardiac issues.
MRV (magnetic resonance imaging–vascular)	MRI for vascular system.
Positive Romberg sign	The Romberg test asks a patient to stand upright and close his/her eyes. Loss of balance with eyes closed is a positive sign.
Retrosigmoid approach	Surgical approach to the cerebellopontine angle by means of entry at the foramen magnum.

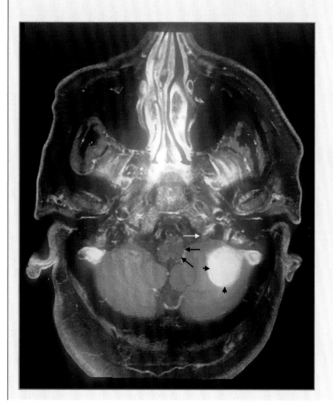

FIGURE 11–3. Contrast-enhanced T1-weighted MR. Axial view of the brain shows left cerebellar hemisphere meningioma (*black arrowheads*), compression of lateral brainstem (*black arrows*), and superior margin of hypoglossal canal (*white arrow*). *Source:* Figure courtesy of Dr. Kyriakos Paraskeva, MD, Resident of Neurosurgery, Nicosia General Hospital, Cyprus.

VII facial nerves will be affected, but compression can involve other cranial nerves as well. The present tumor extended to involve the X vagus and XII hypoglossal nerves in the medulla region. The physician's notation of slowed and slurred speech with hypernasality makes a case for involvement of the XI accessory as well. The X vagus component was manifest in dysphonia. All of the phonemes listed (except the /r/) by the physician imply poor superior lingual force for the purpose of articulation of tongue with hard palate. While not mentioned, it is possible that there would be oral and pharyngeal phase dysphagia arising from the weakened lingual musculature and phonatory involvement. Poor laryngeal elevation and laryngeal adduction would likely ensue, placing the patient at risk for aspiration. The site of lesion would clearly explain the ataxic gait and discoordination of speech.

Questions Concerning This Case

1. Cerebellopontine angle tumors often involve the VIII vestibulocochlear nerve. What would you expect to find if this nerve were involved?
2. Unilateral involvement of the XII hypoglossal nerve should cause unilateral tongue paralysis. What would you expect to happen upon protrusion of the tongue?

From the case book of Dr. Kyriakos Paraskeva, MD, Resident of Neurosurgery, Nicosia General Hospital, Cyprus.

CHAPTER 11
STUDY QUESTIONS

1. _____ _____ generators take groups of reflexes and bring them together into a complex action sequence.

2. _____ information is integrated with the motor plan before execution.

3. In a closed-loop feedback system, there is a set reference or target and correction comes from comparing accuracy in hitting the target with a _____.

4. _____ _____ systems do not operate on sensory feedback and correction and are termed feed-forward processes.

5. _____ language encoding occurs largely within Broca's area and phonetic encoding occurs within the left insular cortex and left supramarginal gyrus.

6. A _____ loop in motor planning includes the left dorsolateral prefrontal cortex, anterior insular cortex, supplementary motor area, and the superior cerebellum.

7. The _____ loop for motor action is made up of the motor cortex, thalamus, putamen and caudate, and the inferior cerebellum.

8. The _____ model of speech production views speech as the oral manifestation of language.

9. The _____ _____ _____ Control model views speech production in a hierarchical fashion that acknowledges the linguistic input.

10. The initial stimulus for speech is a _____ that triggers a verbal manifestation.

11. The _____ _____ loop projects to lower centers that govern the motor plan, including the somatosensory area, motor strip, and cerebellum.

12. The _____ model of speech production utilizes sensory inputs as checks for the accuracy of the executed speech (feed-forward), as well as sensory feedback to support the learning process in speech production.

13. In the DIVA model, the _____ model for the desired phoneme is generated and conveyed to the auditory cortex and somatosensory cortex so that the word that is produced can be validated against the target.

14. A newborn can't voluntarily control motor function, so _____ that are present at birth such as rooting, sucking, and orienting allow the infant to get nutrition.

15. The _____ reflex causes the infant to turn toward the stimulus and the mouth to open.

16. The _____ reflex results in a piston-like protrusion and retraction movement of the tongue.

17. Adult mastication and deglutition patterns emerge around _____ months of age.

18. In the adult there are three identifiable stages involved in mastication and deglutition: _____, _____, and _____.

19. The _____ _____ stage involves movements that prepare the bolus for swallowing, including chewing and crushing.

20. The sublingual and submandibular glands are innervated by the _____ _____ nerve.

21. The parotid gland is innervated by the _____ _____ nerve.

22. Pressure sensors at the trigger site of the _____ stage provide input to the motor program that will simultaneously protect the airway and propel the bolus through the upper esophageal sphincter.

23. The _____ stage is entirely reflexive in nature and is designed to protect the airway and propel the bolus to the esophagus.

24. Each component of the pharyngeal stage is governed by individual reflexes that are organized by assemblies of neurons termed _____ _____ generators.

25. The upper esophageal sphincter is inhibited by the _____ _____, _____ _____ nerve.

26. The sensory component of the orienting, rooting, and sucking reflexes are mediated by the _____ _____ nerve.

27. During the chewing reflex, pressure sensation is conveyed by the _____ _____ nerve to the chewing CPG of the brainstem, then to the nucleus pontis caudalis of the reticular formation for rhythmic tongue movements.

28. The palatal reflex and gag reflex are mediated through the _____ _____ nerve, conveyed to the nucleus solitarius and solitary fasciculus.

29. The vomiting and retching center is located in the reticular formation at the level of the _____ _____ in the brainstem.

30. Rhythms of respiration are controlled through separate inspiratory and expiratory centers within the _____ _____.

31. The _____ reflex results in adduction of the vocal folds, elevation of the larynx, and inversion of the epiglottis.

32. Taste sense from the anterior two-thirds of the tongue and palate is mediated by the _____ _____ nerve.

33. Taste function for the posterior one-third of the tongue is served by the _____ _____ nerve.

34. Anterior salivary glands are innervated by the _____ _____ nerve.

35. Posterior salivary glands are innervated by the _____ _____ nerve.

36. The _____ _____ mediates the sense of taste for the epiglottis and esophagus, as well as within the trachea.

37. _____ sense is perceived through the tactile system, with afferents going to both the spinal nucleus of the trigeminal and the solitary tract nucleus, and ultimately activates the insular cortex.

38. Olfaction is mediated by the _____ _____ nerve.

39. _____ corpuscles sense movement of the bolus.

40. _____ disk receptors sense pressure of the bolus in the mouth.

41. Pressure and movement sensations are transmitted via the _____ _____ nerve to the trigeminal semilunar ganglion and then to the principal sensory nucleus of the trigeminal nerve.

42. The _____ swallowing group receives input from V trigeminal, IX glossopharyngeal, and the X vagus.

43. The _____ swallowing group output results in rhythmic tongue movements, such as those involved in bolus preparation.

REFERENCES

Baehr, M., & Frotscher, M. (2012). *Topical diagnosis in neurology.* New York, NY: Thieme.

Barlow, S. M., & Estep, M. (2006). Central pattern generation and the motor infrastructure for suck, respiration, and speech. *Journal of Communication Disorders, 39*(5), 366–380.

Broussard, D. L., & Altschuler, S. M. (2000). Brainstem viscerotopic organization of afferents and efferents involved in the control of swallowing. *American Journal of Medicine, 108*(4A), 79S–86S.

Buck, L. B. (2000). Smell and taste: The chemical senses. In E. R. Kandel, J. H. Schwartz, & T. M. Jessell (Eds.), *Principles of neural science* (4th ed.). New York, NY: McGraw-Hill.

Callan, D. E., Kent, R. D., Guenther, F. H., & Vorperian, H. K. (2000). An auditory-feedback-based neural network model of speech production that is robust to developmental changes in the size and shape of the articulatory system. *Journal of Speech, Language, and Hearing Research, 43*(3), 721–736.

Carpenter, M. B. (1991). *Core text of neuroanatomy* (4th ed.). Baltimore, MD: Williams & Wilkins.

Chandler, S. H., & Tal, M. (1986). The effects of brain stem transections on the neuronal networks responsible for rhythmical jaw muscle activity in the guinea pig. *Journal of Neuroscience, 6*(6), 1831–1842.

Cometto-Muñiz, J. E., Cain, W. S., & Abraham, M. H. (2004). Chemosensory additivity in trigeminal chemoreception as reflected by detection of mixtures. *Experimental Brain Research, 158*, 196–206.

Cowart, B. J. (1998). The addition of CO2 to traditional taste solutions alters taste quality. *Chemical Senses, 23*(4), 397–402.

Cunningham, E. T., & Sawchenko, P. E. (2000). Dorsal medullary pathways subserving oromotor reflexes in the rat: Implications for the central neural control of swallowing. *Journal of Comparative Neurology, 417*(4), 448–466.

Darley, F. L., Aronson, A. E., & Brown, J. R. (1969). Clusters of deviant speech dimensions in the dysarthrias. *Journal of Speech and Hearing Research, 12*(3), 462–496.

Dessirier, J. M., Simons, C. T., Carstens, M. I., O'Mahony, M., & Carstens, E. (2000). Psychophysical and neurobiological evidence that the oral sensation elicited by carbonated water is of chemogenic origin. *Chemical Senses, 25*(3), 277–284.

Duffy, J. R. (2013). *Motor speech disorders-e-book: Substrates, differential diagnosis, and management.* St. Louis, MO: Elsevier.

Ertekin, C., & Aydogdu, I (2003). Nerophysiology of swallowing. *Clinical Neurophysiology, 114*, 2226–2244.

Ertekin, C., Kiylioglu, N., Tarlaci, S., Truman, A. B., Secil, Y., & Aydogdu, I. (2011). Voluntary and reflex influences on the initiation of swallowing reflex in man. *Dysphagia, 16*, 40–47.

Geran, L. C., & Travers, S. P. (2011). Glossopharyngeal nerve transection impairs unconditioned avoidance of diverse bitter stimuli in rats. *Behavioral Neuroscience, 125*(4), 519.

Goyal, R. K., Padmanabhan, R., & Sang, Q. (2001). Neural circuits in swallowing and abdominal vagal afferent-mediated lower esophageal sphincter relaxation. *The American Journal of Medicine, 111*(8A), 1–11.

Green, B. G. (2011). Chemesthesis and the chemical senses as components of a "chemosensor complex." *Chemical Senses, 37*, 201–206.

Guenther, F. H., Ghosh, S. S., & Tourville, J. A. (2006). Neural modeling and imaging of the cortical interactions underlying syllable production. *Brain and Language, 96*(3), 280–301.

Guenther, F. H., Hampson, M., & Johnson, D. (1998). A theoretical investigation of reference frames for the planning of speech movements. *Psychological review, 105*(4), 611.

Guenther, F. H., & Vladusich, T. (2012). A neural theory of speech acquisition and production. *Journal of Neurolinguistics, 25*(5), 408–422.

Hickok, G. (2012). Computational neuroanatomy of speech production. *Nature Reviews Neuroscience, 13*(2), 135–145.

Janczewski, W. A., & Feldman, J. L. (2006). Distinct rhythm generators for inspiration and expiration in the juvenile rat. *Journal of Physiology, 570*(2), 407–420.

Jean, A. (2001). Brain stem control of swallowing: Neuronal network and cellular mechanisms. *Physiological Reviews, 81*(2), 929–969.

Kandel, E. R., Schwartz, J. H., Jessell, T. M., Siegelbaum, S. A., & Hudspeth, A. J. (2013). *Principles of neural science* (5th ed.). New York, NY: McGraw-Hill.

Krival, K., & Bates C. (2012). Effects of club soda and ginger brew on linguapalatal pressures in healthy swallowing. *Dysphagia, 27*(2), 228–239.

Lang, I. M. (2009). Brain stem control of the phases of swallowing. *Dysphagia, 24*, 333–348.

Lang, I. M., & Shaker, R. (1997). Anatomy and physiology of the upper esophageal sphincter. *American Journal of Medicine, 103*(5A), 50s–55s.

Lund, J. P., & Kolta, A. (2006). Generation of the central masticatory pattern and its modification by sensory feedback. *Dysphagia, 21*, 167–174.

Martin-Harris, B., Brodsky, M. B., Michel, Y., Lee, F. S., & Walters, B. (2007). Delayed initiation of the pharyngeal swallow: Normal variability in adult swallows. *Journal of Speech, Language, and Hearing Research, 50*(3), 585–594.

Mendell, D. A., & Logemann, J. A. (2007). Temporal sequence of swallow events during the oropharyngeal swallow. *Journal of Speech, Language, and Hearing Research, 50*(5), 1256–1271.

Miller, A. (2002). Oral and pharyngeal reflexes in the mammalian nervous system: Their diverse range in complexity and the pivotal role of the tongue. *Critical Reviews in Oral Biology and Medicine, 13*, 409–425.

Møller, A. R. (2003). *Sensory systems: Anatomy and physiology.* New York, NY: Academic Press.

Ninomaya, Y., Imoto, T., & Sugimura, T. (1999). Sweet taste responses of mouse chorda tympani neurons: Existence of Gurmarin-sensitive and insensitive receptor components. *Journal of Neurophysiology, 81*(6), 3087–3091.

Riecker, A., Mathiak, K., Wildgruber, D., Erb, M., Hertrich, I., Grodd, W., & Ackermann, H. (2005). fMRI reveals two distinct cerebral networks subserving speech motor control. *Neurology, 64*(4), 700–706.

Rudenga, K., Green, B., Nachtigal, D., & Small, D. M. (2010). Evidence for an integrated oral sensory module in the human anterior ventral insula. *Chemical Senses, 35*(8), 693–703.

Seikel, J. A., Drumright, D. G., & King, D. W. (2016). *Anatomy & physiology for speech, language and hearing* (5th ed.). Clifton Park, NY: Cengage Learning.

Sørensen, L. B., Møller, P., Flint, A., Martens, M., & Raben, A. (2003). Effect of sensory perception of foods on appetite and food intake: A review of studies on humans. *International Journal of Obesity, 27*(10), 1152–1166.

Stephen, J. R., Taves, D. H., Smith, R. C., & Martin, R. E. (2005). Bolus location at the initiation of the pharyngeal stage of swallowing in healthy older adults. *Dysphagia, 20*(4), 266–272.

Thach, B. T. (2001). Maturation and transformation of reflexes that protect the laryngeal airway from liquid aspiration from fetal to adult life. *American Journal of Medicine, 111*(8), 69–77.

Uludag, M., Aygun, N., & Isgor, A. (2016). Motor function of the recurrent laryngeal nerve: sometimes motor fibers are also located in the posterior branch. *Surgery, 160*(1), 153–160.

Whitehead, M. C., & Frank, M. E. (1983). Anatomy of the gustatory system in the hamster: Central projections of the chorda tympani and the lingual nerve. *Journal of Comparative Neurology, 220*(4), 378–395.

Wiener, N. (1948). *Cybernetics*. Paris, France: Hermann.

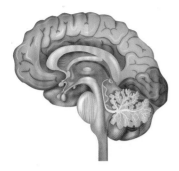

APPENDIX: ANSWERS TO STUDY QUESTIONS

CHAPTER 1

1. neurons
2. dendrite
3. axon
4. soma
5. neurotransmitter
6. organ
7. ganglia
8. nuclei
9. central nervous
10. peripheral nervous
11. cerebral cortex
12. efferent
13. afferent
14. reflexes
15. agonists
16. antagonists
17. superficial
18. deep
19. somatic
20. kinesthetic
21. special
22. anatomy
23. physiology
24. peripheral
25. autonomic
26. sympathetic
27. parasympathetic
28. embryonic
29. fetal
30. telencephalon; diencephalon
31. metencephalon (hindbrain); myelencephalon
32. diencephalon
33. neural crest
34. skeletal
35. sagittal
36. coronal or frontal
37. transverse
38. anterior; posterior
39. superior
40. inferior
41. superficial
42. pronation
43. same
44. decussation
45. aphasia
46. apraxia of speech

CHAPTER 2

1. enzymes
2. mitochondria
3. dendrites
4. axons
5. axon hillock

6. myelin

7. nodes of Ranvier

8. saltatory

9. end *bouton* or end "button"

10. neurotransmitter

11. unipolar

12. bipolar

13. multipoloar

14. Golgi type I

15. Golgi type II

16. microglia

17. microglia

18. astrocytes

19. astrocytes

20. astrocytes

21. astrocytes

22. astrocytes

23. astrocytes

24. oligodendrocytes

25. Schwann cells

26. saltatory conduction

27. radial glia

28. satellite cells

29. ependymal cells

30. synapse

31. a. dendrite

   b. soma

   c. axon hillock

   d. node of Ranvier

   e. axon

   f. myelin sheath

   g. telodendria

   h. end *boutons*

32. a. presynaptic axon

   b. synaptic vesicle

   c. mitochondria

   d. synaptic cleft (synapse)

   e. neurotransmitter substance

   f. postsynaptic ion channels

33. synapse

34. end bouton

35. synaptic

36. synaptic vesicles

37. False (Remember, it is the ions that move into and out of the postsynaptic neuron. The neurotransmitter is just the key to the lock.)

38. excitatory postsynaptic potential (EPSP)

39. action

40. action

41. voltage

42. resting

43. ion channel

44. absolute refractory

45. excitatory

46. inhibitory

47. summation

48. temporal

49. spatial

50. neurotransmitters

51. glutamate or aspartate

52. gamma-aminobutyric acid (GABA) or glycine

53. glutamate

54. GABA

55. acetylcholine (ACH)

56. dopamine (DA)

CHAPTER 3

1. Muscle

2. intrafusal

3. Golgi tendon organs

4. nuclear bag

5. nuclear chain

6. extrafusal

7. Golgi tendon

8. a. afferent fiber

   b. alpha motor neuron

   c. gamma motor neuron

   d. Golgi tendon organ

   e. nuclear bag fiber

   f. muscle spindle

   g. extrafusal muscle fiber

   h. efferent fiber

9. Dermatome

10. plexus

11. Retinal

12. pigment

13. True

14. True

15. passive

16. Extrafusal

17. gamma

18. Golgi tendon organ

19. transduction

20. Somatosensors

21. exteroceptors

22. Interoceptors

23. False (They are responsible for mediating external forces, so they'd be considered exteroceptors.)

24. Mechanoreceptor

25. Thermoreceptors

26. chemoreceptors

27. Meissner's corpuscles

28. Merkel disk receptors

29. Pacinian corpuscles

30. Ruffini endings

31. nociceptor

32. proprioception

33. dermatone

34. first cervical

35. Olfactory

36. Gustation

37. papillae

38. Inner

39. Outer

40. 3,500

41. 12,000

42. Cilia

43. tip links

44. outer hair cells

45. vestibular system

46. semicircular canals

47. acceleration

CHAPTER 4

1. cortex

2. gyri

3. sulci

4. a. central sulcus

   b. postcentral gyrus

   c. postcentral sulcus

   d. superior parietal lobule

   e. intraparietal sulcus

   f. inferior parietal lobule

   g. supramarginal gyrus

   h. parieto-occipital notch

   i. angular gyrus

   j. Wernicke's area

   k. preoccipital notch

   l. inferior temporal gyrus

   m. middle temporal sulcus

   n. middle temporal gyrus

   o. superior temporal sulcus

   p. superior temporal gyrus

   q. Sylvian (or lateral) fissure

   r. operculum

s. Broca's area

t. middle frontal gyrus

u. superior frontal sulcus

v. superior frontal gyrus

w. precentral sulcus

x. precentral gyrus

y. calcarine sulcus

z. frontal lobe

aa. occipital pole

5. precentral

6. postcentral

7. superior longitudinal

8. Sylvian (or lateral) fissure

9. dura mater

10. pia mater

11. arachnoid

12. falx cerebri

13. falx cerebelli

14. tentorium cerebelli

15. diaphragma sella

16. cerebrospinal fluid

17. choroid

18. anterior

19. posterior (or occipital)

20. third

21. interventricular foramen of Monro

22. interthalamic adhesion

23. fourth

24. cerebral aqueduct

25. a. lateral ventricle

b. third ventricle

c. anterior horn

d. interventricular foramen of Monro

e. inferior horn

f. fourth ventricle

g. cerebral aqueduct

h. posterior horn

26. C
A
B
F
E
D

27. central

28. A
C
D
B
B
B
B
C
D
A
A
D
A
B
A
D
D
C
D

29. 4
44, 45
22
39
40
46, 9
6
6
11
1, 2, 3
41
34
17
13, 14

30. operculum

31. dorsolateral prefrontal cortex

32. precentral

33. True

34. True

35. True

36. Broca's

37. Wernicke's

38. orbitofrontal

39. True

40. False (This is the seat of receptive visual language, reading.)

41. True

42. Heschl's

43. calcarine

44. insular

45. insular cortex

46. corpus callosum

47. cingulate

48. fusiform

49. parahippocampal

50. projection

51. corona radiata

52. posterior

53. genu

54. precentral

55. medulla

56. short

57. long

58. commissural

59. cingulate

CHAPTER 5

1. caudate nucleus, globus pallidus, putamen

2. a. interthalamic adhesion

   b. thalamus

   c. head

   d. anterior

   e. corticobulbar

   f. globus pallidus

   g. corticospinal

   h. putamen

   i. lateral

   j. pulvinar

   k. medial

   l. third

3. head

4. claustrum

5. hyperkinesia

6. GABA

7. striate body

8. indirect

9. hippocampus

10. thalamus; epithalamus; hypothalamus; subthalamus

11. thalamus

12. olfaction

13. pulvinar

14. lateral geniculate

15. medial geniculate

16. intralaminar nuclei

17. subthalamic

18. hypothalamus

CHAPTER 6

1. midbrain

2. medulla oblongata

3. a. midbrain

   b. pons

   c. medulla oblongata

   d. anterior median fissure

   e. pyramidal decussation

4. fourth

5. pontocerebellar

6. basal

7. middle

8. inferior

9. cerebellopontine

10. cerebral

11. reticular

12. decussation; pyramids

13. medulla

14. VIII vestibulocochlear

15. spiral

16. cochlear

17. anteroventral cochlear nucleus

18. anteroventral cochlear nucleus

19. dorsal cochlear nucleus; posteroventral cochlear nucleus

20. lateral superior olive

21. medial superior olive

22. olivocochlear

23. medial geniculate

24. True

25. True

26. efferent

CHAPTER 7

1. mixed nerves

2. somatic

3. general

4. E
   B
   D
   F
   A
   G

5. True

6. False (A lesion to the optic chiasm would produce this deficit.)

7. Ptosis

8. a. V trigeminal; maxillary branch

   b. I olfactory

   c. I olfactory

   d. I olfactory

   e. II optic

   f. I olfactory

   g. II optic

   h. III oculomotor

   i. IV trochlear

   j. VI abducens

   k. V trigeminal, ophthalmic branch

   l. II optic

   m. V trigeminal, mandibular branch

   n. V trigeminal; mandibular branch

   o. VII facial

   p. VII facial

   q. VIII vestibulocochlear, auditory branch

   r. VIII vestibulocochlear, vestibular branch

   s. IX glossopharyngeal

   t. IX glossopharyngeal

   u. VII facial

   v. X vagus, recurrent laryngeal nerve

   w. X vagus, superior laryngeal nerve

   x. VII facial

   y. X vagus, pharyngeal branch

   z. XI accessory

   aa. XII hypoglossal

9. outer

10. inner

11. outer

CHAPTER 8

1. inferior

2. middle

3. flocculonodular

4. posterior

5. fourth

6. True

7. True

8. molecular

9. Purkinje

10. False (Purkinje cells inhibit the nuclei when the Purkinje is activated.)

11. vestibular

12. pontine

13. True

14. dentate

15. fastigial

16. emboliform; globose

17. emboliform; globose

18. dentate

19. fastigial

20. True

21. True

22. ventral spinocerebellar

23. rostral spinocerebellar

24. pontocerebellar

25. olivocerebellar

26. olivocerebellar

27. spinocerebellar

28. True

29. False (The cerebellum is the means by which we achieve fine motor control.)

CHAPTER 9

1. first cervical

2. denticulate ligaments

3. conus medullaris

4. filum terminale

5. True

6. dermatome

7. plexus

8. cell bodies

9. central canal

10. funiculus or fasciculus

11. sensory

12. ventral

13. False (It is sensory.)

14. denticulate ligaments

15. efferent

16. afferent

17. dorsal

18. posterior

19. gracilis

20. cuneatus

21. medulla

22. anterior spinothalamic

23. lateral spinothalamic

24. spinocerebellar

25. muscle

26. pyramidal

27. corticospinal

28. corticospinal

29. lower motor neuron

30. corticobulbar

31. extrapyramidal

32. extrapyramidal

33. tectospinal

34. rubrospinal

35. rubrospinal

36. vestibulospinal

37. reticulospinal

38. corticopontocerebellar

CHAPTER 10

1. a. anterior cerebral artery

   b. anterior communicating artery

c. ophthalmic artery

d. middle cerebral artery

e. circle of Willis

f. anterior choroidal artery

g. internal carotid artery

h. posterior cerebral artery

i. superior cerebellar artery

j. basilar artery

k. anterior inferior cerebellar artery

l. vertebral artery

m. posterior inferior cerebellar artery

n. anterior spinal artery

o. pontine arteries

p. posterior communicating artery

2. internal carotid artery

3. internal carotid artery

4. basilar artery

5. external

6. middle meningeal

7. internal carotid

8. middle

9. circle; Willis

10. anterior

11. anterior

12. posterior

13. posterior

14. middle

15. a. middle cerebral artery

b. posterior cerebral artery

c. superior cerebellar artery

d. vertebral artery

e. posterior inferior cerebellar artery

f. posterior spinal artery

g. anterior spinal artery

h. anterior communicating artery

i. anterior cerebral artery

j. internal carotid artery

k. basilar artery

l. internal auditory artery

m. anterior inferior cerebellar artery

16. carotid; vertebrobasilar

17. common

18. vertebral

19. internal carotid

20. anterior

21. posterior

22. middle

23. middle

24. basilar

25. posterior inferior

26. vertebral

27. basilar

28. anterior inferior

29. superior

30. posterior

31. posterior

CHAPTER 11

1. central pattern

2. sensory

3. standard

4. open-loop

5. grammatical

6. preparative

7. executive

8. psycholinguistic

9. Hierarchical State Feedback

10. concept or idea

11. Broca's–temporoparietal juncture

12. DIVA

13. auditory

14. reflexes

15. rooting

16. sucking

17. six

18. oral (oral preparation and oral transit); pharyngeal; esophageal

19. oral preparation

20. VII facial

21. IX glossopharyngeal

22. pharyngeal

23. pharyngeal

24. central pattern

25. X vagus; superior laryngeal

26. V trigeminal

27. V trigeminal

28. IX glossopharyngeal

29. medulla oblongata

30. medulla oblongata

31. apneic

32. VII facial

33. IX glossopharyngeal

34. VII facial

35. IX glossopharyngeal

36. X vagus

37. chemesthetic

38. I olfactory

39. Meissner's

40. Merkel

41. V trigeminal

42. ventral

43. dorsal

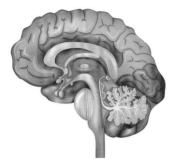

GLOSSARY

Abduction: The process of moving a structure away from midline.

Absolute refractory period: The time during which no application of a stimulus will cause discharge of a neuron.

Acetylcholine (ACH): Excitatory cholinergic neurotransmitter, utilized extensively in the CNS for memory, cognition, and motor control functions. In the PNS acetylcholine is an excitatory neurotransmitter of the neuromuscular junction.

Acoustic reflex: Middle ear reflex triggered by high intensity sounds and mediated by brainstem nuclei, resulting in contraction of the stapedius and tensor tympani muscles.

Action potential: Change in electrical potential of a cell membrane resulting in conduction of neural impulse along the membrane or in contraction of muscle.

Adduction: The process of bringing a structure toward midline.

Adendritic: Neuron without dendrites.

Adenosine triphosphate (ATP): Complex organic molecule involved in energy generation at the cellular level. As a neurotransmitter, ATP is released when tissue is traumatized and is involved in transmitting the sense of pain from that trauma.

Adequate stimulus: Property of a sensor that determines threshold of response for the sensor.

Afferent: Also known as sensory neurons or neurons that convey information toward the central nervous system.

Agnosia: Inability to identify a sensory stimulus.

Agonist: Also known as prime mover; the predominant muscle performing an action.

Agraphia: An acquired neurological disorder that results in inability to write or spell.

Airway protection: In swallowing function, the processes of adduction of vocal folds, elevation and forward movement of the larynx, and depression of the epiglottis during the pharyngeal stage.

Alerting attention: The subtype of attention associated with physiological arousal to the presence of a stimulus.

Alexia: Acquired neurological disorder that results in inability to read.

Alpha motor neurons: Large neurons of the PNS that innervate skeletal muscle, with conduction velocities up to 120 meters/second.

Ampulla: Flask-like structure. In the vestibular system, the enlargement that houses the crista ampularis.

Amygdala (amygdaloid body): Structure of the limbic system involved in emotion response, particularly related to fear.

Anatomy: Study of the structure of the organism.

Aneurysm: Enlargement of blood vessel due to weakening of the arterial wall.

Angular gyrus: Gyrus of the posterior parietal lobe associated with reading, as well as with tactile gnosis and mathematical calculation.

Anomia: Word-finding difficulty, a primary feature of all forms of aphasia.

Anomic aphasia: Acquired language disorder in which the dominant feature is word-finding difficulty.

Antagonists: In movement, muscles that oppose the action of the prime mover.

Anterior: Referring to the front surface of a body.

Anterior cerebral artery: Artery arising from the internal carotid supply of the brain, serving medial surface of the cerebrum and superior corpus callosum.

Anterior choroidal artery: Artery arising from the internal carotid artery that serves the basal ganglia, hippocampus, internal capsule, and other subcortical structures.

Anterior cingulate cortex: Long association fibers associated with limbic control of impulse control and decision processes.

Anterior commissure: Commissural fibers connecting left and right temporal lobes of the brain.

Anterior funiculus: Bundle of fibers in anterior spinal cord.

Anterior horn: Of spinal cord, the ventral gray matter component that is composed of motor neuron cell bodies.

Anterior median fissure: Anterior-most groove of the spinal cord or medulla oblongata.

Aphasia: Acquired deficit of language expression and/or comprehension.

Apneic reflex: Involuntary cessation of respiration, typically seen during pharyngeal stage of swallowing.

Appendage: Arm or leg.

Apraxia: Deficit in planning and programming for execution of a motor act in the absence of paralysis or paresis.

Apraxia of speech (AOS): Also known as verbal apraxia; deficit in the planning and programming of the articulators of speech.

Arachnoid mater: Middle meningeal lining, deep to the dura mater and superficial to the pia mater.

Arcuate fasciculus: Portion of superior longitudinal fasciculus that connects temporal and inferior parietal lobes.

Aspartate: Amino acid; is excitatory amino acid neurotransmitter, stimulating NMDA receptors.

Astrocytes: Glial cell in CNS with broad range of functions, including structural support, regulation of ions and neurotransmitters, and long-term memory.

Ataxic dysarthria: Motor speech disorder resulting in loss of coordination of articulators, often with low muscle tone.

Autonomic nervous system (ANS): Portion of central nervous system responsible for involuntary functions of the body, including contraction of smooth muscle, glandular secretion, and digestive and cardiac function.

Axon: The cellular process from which neural impulses pass and that synapses with downstream neurons.

Axon hillock: Specific site of axon that is the site of generation of the action potential.

Ballism: Hyperkinetic motor disorder involving large, flailing movements of arms or legs.

Basal ganglia: Group of nuclei within the subcortex involved in motor initiation and control.

Basal sulcus: Sulcus of medulla oblongata in which basilar artery rests.

Basilar artery: Artery forming from anastomosis of left and right vertebral arteries.

Bell's palsy: Facial paralysis caused by inflammation or damage to the facial nerve resulting in weakness or paralysis on one side of the face.

Bipolar neurons: Neurons with two processes extending from the body.

Blood-brain barrier: Functional separation of cerebrovascular supply from somatic vascular supply, mediated by astrocytes.

Bolus formation: In swallowing, the ball of food or liquid that is to be swallowed.

Broca's area: Area on the inferior frontal lobule, located in the third frontal convolution above the Sylvian fissure, and involved in linguistic expression; BA 44,45.

Brodmann brain map: Cytoarchitectural map of the cortex, with areas delineated numerically and known as Brodmann areas.

Calcarine sulcus: On the occipital lobe, the primary visual reception area.

Caudate nucleus: Nucleus of the basal ganglia, consisting of head, body, and tail; involved in motor initiation and termination, procedural learning, reward, associative learning, and inhibition of action.

Cell processes: Prominences arising from a cell; in neurons, the axon and dendrite.

Central canal: In the spinal cord, the inferior extension of the ventricular system through which cerebrospinal fluid passes.

Central gray matter: Also known as periaqueductal gray; cell bodies surrounding the cerebral aqueduct of the brainstem, within the tegmentum.

Central nervous system (CNS): Structures of the nervous system including cerebral cortex, brainstem, basal ganglia, cerebellum, spinal cord, thalamus and subthalamus, nuclei, and tracts within these structures.

Central pattern generators (CPGs): Neuronal circuits made up of simple reflexes, combined to create a complex motor pattern sequence.

Central sulcus of the insular cortex: The sulcus of the insula separating the short and long gyri of insula.

Central sulcus of the cerebral cortex: Also known as the Rolandic fissure; the major sulcus separating parietal and frontal lobes of the brain.

Cerebellopontine angle: Point of union of the cerebellum and pons.

Cerebellum: Anatomical structure responsible for regulation of posture, balance, and coordination.

Cerebral aqueduct: Passageway through which cerebrospinal fluid passes from third ventricle to the fourth ventricle.

Cerebral cortex: Outer layer of the cerebrum.

Cerebral longitudinal fissure: Fissure separating left and right cerebral hemispheres.

Cerebral peduncles: Stalk-like group of projection pathways connecting cerebral cortex with brainstem and spinal cord.

Cerebrospinal fluid: Watery fluid produced by the choroid plexuses of the ventricles of the brain.

Cerebrum: Superior portion of the brain, consisting of two cerebral hemispheres.

Cervical flexure: Embryologic flexure between structures that will be the medulla oblongata and spinal cord.

Chemical gradient: At cellular level, condition in which there is a concentration difference across a cell membrane; the chemical gradient is established when there are more of one molecule type outside of the cell than inside or vice versa.

Chemoreceptors: Sensory receptors that are sensitive to molecular structure of a substance; examples are olfactory and gustatory sensors.

Chewing CPG: Central pattern generator coordinating the complex process of mastication.

Chewing reflex: Reflexive response to stimulation of hard palate that results in initiation of mastication.

Choroid plexuses: Groups of cells within cerebral ventricles that produce cerebrospinal fluid.

Cilia (singular, cilium): Fine protuberances from a cell body.

Cingulate gyrus: On medial surface of cerebrum, set of long association fibers, consisting of BA 23, 24, 26, 29, 30, 31, 32, and 33.

Circle of Willis: The specific loop of interconnecting arteries including the anterior cerebral, posterior cerebral, anterior communicating, and posterior communicating arteries, hypothesized to provide redundant vascular supply to the brain to protect against micropressure variation or ischemic event.

Circular sulcus: Sulcus of insular cortex separating the insula from adjacent cortical tissue.

Claustrum: Nucleus located deep to insular cortex and between external and extreme capsules that is thought to be the mechanism by which the disparate areas of the cortex are synchronized for the unitary perception of consciousness.

Clinical anatomy: Study of the pathological entity that often includes discussion of altered or pathological physiology.

Closed-loop system: Feedback loop typically involved in motor learning, in which there is a set reference or target; correction comes from comparing accuracy in hitting the target with the standard.

Cochlear nucleus: First nucleus of the auditory brainstem pathway.

Co-contraction: Contraction of both agonist and antagonist muscles simultaneously.

Cognition: The means of acquiring knowledge and understanding through thought, perception, and experience; it includes processes such as short-term memory and long-term memory, linguistic processes, perception, visuospatial processes, and attention.

Conduction aphasia: Acquired language deficit considered to arise from lesion to the arcuate fasciculus and the left parietal region; its characteristics involve fluent speech with relatively intact comprehension, but deficit in repetitions.

Conduction velocity: Rate at which information is conducted by neurons, and specifically by the axons of neurons.

Confabulation: Condition in which the individual fabricates information such as recalled memories of events without the intention to deceive.

Conjugate eye movement: Movement of eyes in coordinated effort to maintain focus and fixation.

Connotative meaning: Associative meanings.

Contra: Opposite.

Contralateral: Opposite side.

Convergence: In vision, simultaneous inward movement of both eyes in order to maintain fixation on an object.

Corneal blink reflex: Involuntary blinking of eyelid in response to stimulation of the cornea of the eye.

Corona radiata: Structure of the brain consisting of ascending and descending white matter projection fibers.

Coronal section: Also known as a frontal section; a section that is more or less in parallel to the coronal suture of the head, dividing the body into front and back portions.

Corpora quadrigemina: Structures of the superficial tectal midbrain region consisting of 4 nuclei (paired superior colliculi and inferior colliculi).

Corpus callosum: Commissural fibers connecting left and right cerebral hemispheres.

Corticobulbar tract: Motor pathway arising primarily from the precentral gyrus and premotor regions, but also from the somatosensory cortex, parietal lobe, and cingulate gyrus and terminating in the brainstem, and serving cranial nerves.

Corticopontine fibers: Projection fibers arising in the cerebral cortex from frontal, parietal, temporal, or occipital lobes and terminating in the pontine nuclei.

Corticospinal tract: Motor pathway arising primarily from the precentral gyrus and premotor regions, but also from the somatosensory cortex, parietal lobe, and cingulate gyrus and terminating in the spinal cord.

Corticostriate pathway: Projection fibers arising from cerebral cortex and terminating in caudate nucleus, ventral striatum, and putamen of basal ganglia.

Corticothalamic fibers: Any fibers originating in the cerebral cortex that terminate at the thalamus.

Cough reflex: Reflexive expulsive respiratory response to noxious stimulation of the larynx, pharynx, or other area of the airway.

CPG for swallowing: Also known as Central Pattern Generator; coordinating structure for organization of swallowing function, consisting of dorsal swallowing group of interneurons in the nucleus solitarius and ventral swallowing group in the medulla.

Cranial: Toward the skull.

Crus cerebri: Anterior portion of cerebral peduncle, containing motor fibers.

Cuneus: Wedge-shaped portion of occipital lobe associated with visual reception; BA 17.

Cytoplasm: Material within living cell, excluding the nucleus.

Decussation: Crossing.

Decussation of the pyramids: The point in the medulla oblongata where the corticospinal tract divides to become the anterior corticospinal tract and the decussated lateral corticospinal tract.

Deep: Away from the surface or closer to the middle of the body.

Deglutition: The act of swallowing.

Dementia: Condition arising from brain disease and resulting in cognitive decline secondary to neural degeneration.

Dementia of Alzheimer's Disease (DAT): Neurological condition resulting in progressive cognitive decline, including deficits in memory, behavior, language, and thought processes.

Dendrite: The receptive component of a neuron.

Denotative meaning: Literal or "dictionary" meaning of a word.

Dermatome: Region of the skin innervated by a single spinal nerve.

Diaphragma sella: Dura mater component surrounding the hypophysis.

Diencephalon: Posterior component of the forebrain, including the epithalamus, hypothalamus, thalamus, and third ventricle.

Distal: Away from the root.

Dominant hemisphere: With reference to the cerebral hemispheres, the hemisphere involved in fine motor activity, language, and cognitive analysis.

Dorsal: Posterior surface of the body or superior surface of the head, oral structures, and cerebrum.

Dorsal cochlear nucleus: Component of cochlear nucleus where first level of signal analysis occurs.

Dorsal spinocerebellar tract: Afferent pathway conveying information from skeletal muscle proprioceptors to the cerebellum.

Dorsal swallowing group (DSG): Group of interneurons in the solitary tract nucleus responsible for generating patterns for swallowing.

Dura mater: The outer meningeal lining of the brain and spinal cord.

Dysarthria: Difficulty speaking arising from loss of muscle strength, alteration in muscle tone, or reduced coordination.

Efferent: movement away from the CNS; synonymous with motor.

Embryonic: In neural development, weeks 1 through 8 following fertilization of the egg.

End bouton (end button): Distal-most portion of axon containing synaptic vesicles.

Entorhinal cortex: Region of brain in medial temporal lobe involved in memory, olfaction, and navigation through space.

Ependymal cells (ependymocytes): Secreting glial cells found in the ventricles of the brain

Epithalamus: Part of dorsal forebrain, including the pineal gland and roof of the third ventricle.

Excitatory neurotransmitters: Chemical within neuron that causes an excitatory response in the postsynaptic neuron.

Excitatory postsynaptic potential (EPSP): Postsynaptic potential that makes the postsynaptic neuron more likely to depolarize.

Executive function: Cognitive processes involved in controlling behavior; generally considered to be metacognitive actions that involve manipulation of cognitive functions for the purpose of orienting attention, planning, organization, management of time, etc.

Expiration: In respiration, exhalation.

Extension: Process of increasing the angle between two structures.

Exteroceptors: Class of sensory receptors designed to sense environmental stimuli, such as thermal or tactile stimulation.

Extrafusal fibers: Skeletal muscle fibers innervated by alpha motor neurons.

Extrapyramidal system: Also known as the indirect system; neural pathways involved in background movements and maintenance of muscle tone.

Falx cerebelli: Dura mater component that separates the left and right cerebellar hemispheres.

Falx cerebri: Dura mater component that separates the left and right cerebral hemispheres.

Fasciculus: Bundle of axons.

Feature detector: Neurons or networks of neurons that detect and extract features within a specific modality.

Fetal period: In prenatal development, weeks 9 through 37 of gestation.

Final common pathway: Also known as lower motor neurons; in the brainstem and the spinal cord, the spinal and cranial nerves involved in direct activation of muscle.

Flaccid dysarthria: Dysarthria involving muscular weakness and low muscle tone of the affected articulators or speech system.

Flaccidity: Muscular weakness involving low muscle tone.

Flexion: Moving structures so that the angle between them is decreased.

Fluent aphasia: Acquired language disturbance resulting in deficit of language comprehension but relatively fluid speech output that is dominated by jargon.

Fourth ventricle: Diamond-shaped cerebral ventricle located between the pons and the upper part of the medulla and the cerebellum.

Frontal operculum: Region of the frontal lobe overlying the insular cortex.

Funiculi: Bundle of axons.

Fusiform gyrus: Gyrus associated with face recognition.

Gag reflex: Reflexive response stimulated by tactile contact with the posterior pharyngeal wall, tonsils, or back of the tongue, resulting in contraction of the pharyngeal wall, protrusion of the tongue, laryngeal elevation, and vocal fold adduction.

Gamma-amino butyric acid (GABA): Primary inhibitory neurotransmitter of the CNS.

Gamma motor neurons: Lower motor neuron involved in muscle contraction.

Glial cells: Non-neuronal cells of the nervous system that are involved in numerous functions, including nutrient delivery, the blood-brain barrier, and the glymphatic system.

Global aphasia: Acquired language deficit arising from widespread damage to the cerebral cortex, and resulting in significant expressive and receptive deficits.

Globose nuclei: Deep cerebellar nucleus associated with the spinocerebellum, receiving input from the spinocerebellar tracts and projecting to the ventrolateral thalamic nucleus.

Globular cells: Cells found in cerebellum and cochlear nucleus; in the cochlear nucleus globular cells sharpen high-frequency auditory information.

Globus pallidus: Also known as the dorsal pallidum; medial-most component of basal ganglia, working with subthalamic nucleus to serve as the output structure of the basal ganglia in extrapyramidal function.

Glutamate: Amino acid; most common excitatory neurotransmitter of nervous system.

Glycine: Amino acid; Inhibitory neurotransmitter in cerebrum, brainstem, and spinal cord, and is responsible for inhibitory postsynaptic potential (IPSP).

Gnosis: Knowing.

Golgi apparatus: Within cellular cytoplasm, facilitates secretion of proteins synthesized in endoplasmic reticulum.

Golgi tendon organ (GTO): Proprioceptor that senses change in muscle tension.

Golgi type I neuron: Neuron within gray matter of central nervous system having long axonal processes.

Golgi type II neurons: Neurons of the CNS having short axons.

Gracilis tubercle: Within the medulla oblongata, terminal point of fasciculus gracilis, mediating sense of fine touch and proprioception from the legs and trunk.

Graded potential: Cell membrane potentials that are graduated along a continuum of intensity, as opposed to being all-or-none.

Gustation: Sense of taste.

Gyrus rectus: Also known as straight gyrus; on the inferior frontal lobe of the cerebral cortex and continuous with the superior frontal gyrus, with connections to the medial orbitofrontal cortex.

Gyrus: Ridge on the cerebral or cerebellar cortex.

Habenula perforata: Within the medial osseous cochlear wall, perforation through which dendrites of VIII vestibulocochlear nerve pass as they enter the modiolus.

Hemianopsia (hemianopia): Loss or diminished vision in one-half of the visual field.

Hemispatial neglect: Condition caused by damage to the non-dominant hemisphere, resulting in loss of awareness and attention to the left visual and spatial fields.

Heschl's gyrus: Receptive region of the cerebral cortex for audition (BA 41).

Heteronymous hemianopsia: Visual field cut in different fields of the two eyes.

Homonymous hemianopsia: Loss or diminished vision in the same half of the visual field in both eyes.

Homunculus: Literally, "little man" in Latin; representation of the sensory or motor innervation along the precentral or post-central gyri of the cortex.

Hyperactive reflexes: Overactive reflexes.

Hyperextension: Extension beyond the normal limits.

Hyperkinesias: Group of disorders characterized by excessive, uncontrollable movements.

Hyperkinetic dysarthria: Motor speech disorder resulting in excessive, uncontrollable movement of speech structures.

Hypoactive reflexes: Reflexes that are low in intensity or difficult to stimulate.

Hypoglossal nucleus: Motor cranial nerve nucleus of the XII hypoglossal nerve within medulla oblongata, with visible prominence in posterior brainstem as the hypoglossal trigone.

Hypokinetic dysarthria: Motor speech disorder characterized by paucity of movement in the context of high muscle tone.

Hypothalamus: Region of the diencephalon responsible for coordination of the autonomic system.

I olfactory nerve: Afferent cranial nerve responsible for the sense of smell.

II optic nerve: Afferent cranial nerve responsible for visual sense.

III oculomotor: Motor cranial nerve responsible for most movement of the eyeball as well as pupillary contraction via the Edinger-Westphal nucleus.

Indirect pathway: Also known as the extrapyramidal system; neural pathways involved in control of background movements and muscle tone.

Indusium griseum: Thin layer of gray matter continuous with dentate gyrus of the hippocampus.

Inferior: Lower surface or region of a structure.

Inferior cerebellar peduncle: Within posterior medulla oblongata, connects the spinal cord with the cerebellum via the dorsal spinocerebellar tract, fibers from the inferior olivary nucleus, and other pathways.

Inferior colliculus: Within the midbrain, midbrain nucleus of the auditory pathway associated with localization of sound in space, specifically working in conjunction with superior colliculus as visual relay; mediates rotation of head toward auditory and visual stimulus by means of XI accessory nerve connection.

Inferior frontal gyrus: Within the frontal lobe of the cerebral cortex, the lateral-inferior region encompassing the frontal operculum, Broca's area, and inferior aspects of the precentral gyrus; BA 44, 45, 47.

Inferior longitudinal fasciculus: Long association fibers connecting temporal and occipital lobes.

Inferior medullary velum: Also known as the posterior medullary velum; layer of white matter forming the inferior aspect of the 4th ventricle.

Inferior olivary nucleus: Within the medulla oblongata, coordinating communication between spinal cord and cerebellum.

Inferior parietal lobule: Within the parietal lobe of cerebral cortex, region inferior to intraparietal sulcus and including the supramarginal gyrus and angular gyrus.

Inferior pontine sulcus: Sulcus on inferior superficial pons.

Inferior salivatory nuclei: Within the tegmentum of the pons, nuclei of IX glossopharyngeal nerve providing general visceral efferent innervation to the parotid gland.

Inferior temporal gyrus: Gyrus of the temporal lobe of the cerebrum, inferior to medial temporal gyrus, serving as the temporal lobe component of the ventral "what" visual stream, and a location of audio-visual interaction with afferents from the auditory belt region.

Inferior vestibular nucleus: Nucleus of the medulla oblongata serving as the termination of the lateral vestibulospinal tract and the vestibular branch of the VIII vestibulocochlear nerve.

Inferior vestibular nucleus: Nucleus of the vestibular nuclei lying near 4th ventricle within both pons and medulla oblongata.

Inhibitory interneuron: Interneuron that inhibits the postsynaptic neuron.

Inhibitory postsynaptic potentials (IPSP): Synaptic potential that makes a postsynaptic neuron less likely to discharge.

Initial segment: Of the axon hillock, the first segment of the myelinated axon.

Inner hair cells: Hair cells of cochlea responsible for mediation of frequency information.

Inspiration: In respiration, inhalation.

Insular cortex: Deep to the frontal lobe, underlying the frontal, parietal and temporal operculum; lobe of brain involved in articulatory programming within the dominant insular cortex, and with development of interpersonal elements such as empathy, compassion, and insight in the non-dominant insular cortex.

Intermediate layer: Also known as the Purkinje layer; of the cerebellar cortex, the layer containing Purkinje cells.

Internal acoustic meatus (IAM): The passageway for the VIII vestibulocochlear nerve as it enters the cranial vault on its way to the brainstem.

Internal capsule: White matter structure at the base of the corona radiata separating the caudate nucleus and thalamus from the putamen and globus pallidus, and containing motor and sensory fibers projected from and to the cerebral cortex.

Internal carotid artery supply: One of two major vascular supplies to the cerebrovascular system.

Internal granular: Layer IV of the cerebral cortex.

Internal pyramidal: Layer V of the cerebral cortex.

Interneurons: Neurons that convey impulses between neurons.

Interoceptors: Sensory organ that mediates sensation from within the body, particularly from the visceral organs.

Interthalamic adhesion: Also known as the massa intermedia: the band of tissue spanning the 3rd ventricle and connecting the right and left thalami.

Interventricular foramen of Monro: The cerebrospinal fluid channel connecting the lateral and third ventricles.

Intracellular potential: Electrical potential within a cell.

Intraparietal sulcus: Sulcus on superior-lateral surface of parietal lobe, related to the dorsal visual stream and manual apprehension of a target.

Ion channels: Membrane proteins that allow gated movement of ions across a membrane.

Ipsi: Combining form meaning same.

Ipsilateral: Same side as a referent.

Isometrically: Contraction in which joint angle and muscle length do not change due to fixation or co-contraction.

IV trochlear nerve: Cranial nerve of brainstem involved in activation of the superior oblique muscle of the eye.

IX glossopharyngeal nerve: Mixed cranial nerve of the brainstem involved in sensation of taste, activation of the parotid gland, afferent visceral information from the carotid sinus, and general somatic information from the tympanic membrane, pharynx, and posterior tongue.

Jaw jerk reflex: Reflexive mandibular elevation triggered by activation of muscle spindles in muscles of mastication.

Kinesthetic sense: Sense of movement, mediated by integrated sensation from the proprioceptors of the body.

Lacrimal glands: Glands of the eye region that secrete tears.

Laminar radiation: Dendritic formation in which dendrites radiate away from the soma, but in a single plane.

Lateral: Situated away from midline.

Lateral and anterior corticospinal tracts: Primary motor innervation pathways for skeletal muscle, forming after the pyramidal decussation of the corticospinal tract.

Lateral apertures: Also known as the foramina of Luschka; the paired lateral openings from the 4th ventricle that allow circulation of cerebrospinal fluid from the cerebral ventricular system to the spinal cord and extracortical space.

Lateral geniculate body: Visual relay of the thalamus.

Lateral lemniscus: Brainstem pathway rostral to the superior olivary complex carrying auditory information to the inferior colliculus.

Lateral olivocochlear bundle: Component of the auditory efferent system arising from the region of the lateral superior olive, with fibers coursing ipsilaterally to terminate in the cochlear nucleus and hair cells.

Lateral spinothalamic tracts: Afferent pathways bringing pain, touch, and temperature information from the spine to thalamus.

Lateral sulcus: Also known as the Sylvian fissure; the fissure separating the temporal lobe from the parietal and frontal lobes. In swallowing, the buccal cavity.

Lateral superior olive (LSO): The nucleus of the superior olivary complex of the brainstem involved in localization of sound by means of identifying interaural intensity differences.

Lateral ventricles: Largest ventricles of the cerebrum, occupying regions of the temporal, occipital, frontal, and parietal lobes, and containing cerebrospinal fluid.

Lateral vestibular nucleus: Nucleus of the vestibular nuclei within the pons, and with output to the medial longitudinal fasciculus.

Left visual neglect: The component of hemispatial neglect that involves lack of awareness of the left visual field, arising from damage to the temporoparietal juncture and dorsolateral prefrontal cortex of the right cerebral hemisphere.

Lemniscal pathway: Dorsal spinal cord pathway conveying sense of fine touch, vibration, tactile discrimination, and proprioception from skin and joints to posteroventral nucleus of thalamus and ultimately to the postcentral gyrus of the cerebral cortex.

Lentiform nucleus: Also known as the lenticular nucleus; literally "lens-shaped;" consisting of the putamen and globus pallidus of the basal ganglia.

Limbic association area: Cortical association area that includes the orbitofrontal cortex (BA 11, 10) and the structures of the limbic system.

Lingual: Referring to the tongue.

Lingual gyrus: Gyrus visible on the medial and inferior cerebral cortex involved in visual processing, particularly letter recognition; BA 19.

Lower motor neurons (LMN): Neurons arising from motor cranial nerve nuclei of the brainstem or anterior nerve roots in the spinal cord and that send their axons to skeletal muscles.

Low-threshold free receptors: Free non-encapsulated receptors of the epithelium that respond to mechanical forces of light touch.

Lysosomes: Intracellular enzymes involve in degradation of molecules.

Macroglia: Glial cells including astrocytes and oligodendrocytes that are involved in neuron support, nutrient supply, and myelin generation.

Macula: Of the eye, pigmented area surrounding the fovea of the retina.

Mandibular nerve: Mixed cranial nerve of the V trigeminal nerve, involved in activation of muscles of mastication, tensor tympani, anterior digastricus, buccinators, and tensor veli palatini, as well as somatic sensory perception of the area of the mandible, posterior 2/3 of tongue (not taste), inferior dentition, inferior lip, and lateral scalp region.

Mastication: The process of chewing.

Maxillary nerve: Branch of the V trigeminal cranial nerve that mediates somatic sense from the maxillary nasal cavities, sinuses, palate, mid-face, and upper dentition.

Mechanoreceptors: Sensory receptors that mediate physical force, such as pressure on the skin or stretching of the muscle spindle.

Medial: Also known as mesial; being situated toward the middle or near the median plane.

Medial geniculate body: Auditory nucleus of the thalamus, being the terminal point for auditory information before being relayed to the auditory cortex.

Medial lemniscus: Afferent fibers that decussate in the brainstem before terminating on the nucleus gracilis and cuneatus, and which convey sense of vibration, touch, and pressure from upper and lower body regions.

Medial longitudinal fasciculus: Crossed pathway of the brainstem, connecting the III oculomotor nerve, IV trochlear nerve, VI abducens nerve with the tectospinal and vestibulospinal tracts, for the purpose of mediating the optokinetic reflexes of the eye that dictate eye movement.

Medial nucleus of the trapezoid body (MNTB): Set of brainstem nuclei within the pons receiving input from the cochlear nucleus, continuing as the lateral lemniscus of the auditory pathway.

Medial superior olive: Nucleus of the superior olivary complex involved in localization of sound by comparing interaural temporal (frequency) information.

Medial vestibular nucleus: Nucleus of the medulla oblongata serving as the termination of the lateral vestibulospinal tract and the vestibular branch of the VIII vestibulocochlear nerve.

Medial vestibular nucleus: Nucleus of the vestibular nuclei within the pons.

Median aperture: Also known as the foramen of Magendie; the midline opening from the 4th ventricle that allows circulation of cerebrospinal fluid from the cerebral ventricular system to the spinal cord and extracortical space.

Median raphe: Medial nuclei of the reticular formation of the brainstem.

Medulla oblongata: Lower part of the brainstem that is continuous with the spinal cord, and which contains nuclei of the IX glossopharyngeal, X vagus, XI accessory, and XII hypoglossal nerves.

Medullary reticulospinal tract: Extrapyramidal pathways descending from the reticular formation to the trunk and extremities for the purpose of locomotion and posture control.

Meissner's corpuscles: Mechanoreceptors of the superficial epidermis that are sensitive to stretch and light touch.

Membrane potential: Also known as resting potential; the potential within a membrane prior to depolarization.

Meningeal arteries: Branches of the maxillary artery arising from the external carotid artery, and serving the meningeal linings of the brain.

Meningeal linings: Membranes that overlay the cerebral cortex, consisting of the dura mater, arachnoid mater, and pia mater.

Merkel disk receptors: Mechanoreceptors of the epidermis that sense deep static pressure.

Metencephalon: Also known as the hindbrain; portion of embryonic brain that will differentiate into the pons and cerebellum, and give rise to the 4th ventricle, V trigeminal nerve, VI abducens nerve, VII facial nerve, and VIII vestibulocochlear nerve.

Microglia: Glial cells serving as macrophages, being responsible for removing waste products, the immune defense through release of cytokines in inflammatory conditions such as infections, tumors, and trauma.

Microvilli: Hair-like fibers within the taste pore that hold molecules for sampling by the gustatory sensors.

Midbrain: Superior-most portion of the brainstem, known as the embryonic mesencephalon, and includes the cerebral peduncles, corpora quadrigemina, the cerebral aqueduct, a portion of the reticular activating system, as well as cranial nerve nuclei for the III oculomotor and IV trochlear nerves.

Middle cerebellar peduncle: Also known as the brachia pontis; connecting the cerebellum to the pons and consisting entirely of sensory fibers to the cerebellum; fibers of the peduncle arise from the pontine nuclei and convey information from the cerebral cortex.

Middle cerebral artery: Artery of cerebrovascular system arising from the internal carotid artery and supplying the lateral surface of the brain, including the inferior and lateral frontal lobe, the lateral parietal lobes, and superior temporal lobe, including all of the speech, language, and hearing zones of the cerebrum.

Middle frontal gyrus: Region of the anterior frontal lobe consisting of more than one gyrus, bounded by the precentral sulcus, inferior frontal sulcus, and superior frontal sulcus.

Middle meningeal artery: Branch of the external carotid artery supplying the dura mater of the brain.

Middle temporal gyrus: Gyrus the temporal lobe (BA 21) between inferior and superior temporal gyri, and involved in language comprehension.

Miniature excitatory postsynaptic potentials (mEPSP): Excitatory potential generated at local region of the postsynaptic membrane as a result of release of neurotransmitter from presynaptic axon.

Miniature postsynaptic potential (MPSP): Potential generated at local region of the postsynaptic membrane as a result of release of neurotransmitter from presynaptic axon.

Mitochondria: Organelle of the nucleus responsible for energy production in the cell.

Mixed laterality: In the context of hemispheric specialization, the condition in which dominant functions normally attributed to one or the other hemisphere (e.g., language, calculation) are distributed between the two hemispheres.

Mixed nerve: With reference to cranial nerves, a nerve that has both motor and sensory components.

Modiolus: Central bony axis of the cochlea containing the spiral ganglion.

Monoamines: Amino acid neurotransmitters, including dopamine, norepinephrine and noradrenaline, epinephrine, and serotonin.

Monocular blindness: Loss of vision in one eye.

Motor activity: Contraction of muscle or gland by means of neural action.

Motor nerves: Neurons within the cerebral cortex, brainstem, or spinal cord responsible for direct activation of muscle or glands.

Motor nucleus of the facial nerve: Also known as the facial motor nucleus; located within pontine tegmentum, with axons of the VII facial nerve coursing around the abducens nucleus and exiting the brainstem in the ventral pons.

Motor speech system: System of cortical, subcortical, and brainstem structures involved in the complex planning and execution of the speech act.

Motor strip: Also known as the precentral gyrus; of the frontal lobe of the cerebral cortex, the point of primary activation of the motor act; BA 4.

Motor trigeminal nucleus: Within the pons, the motor nucleus for the V trigeminal nerve arising from the first branchial arch, supplying innervation for muscles of mastication, tensor tympani, tensor veli palatini, mylohyoid, and anterior digastricus.

Multiform: The deepest layer of the cerebral cortex, containing predominantly pyramidal cells that project to the thalamus.

Multipolar neuron: Neuron with single axon and multiple dendrites.

Muscle spindle: Stretch receptors within intrafusal muscle.

Muscle tone: Continuous and partial contraction of muscle, providing resistance to passive stretch when at rest.

Myelencephalon: Also known as the afterbrain; most posterior region of the embryonic hindbrain from which medulla oblongata arises.

Myelin: Fatty substance of nervous system serving as insulating layer on axons.

Myelinated fibers: Axons with myelin.

Nasal portions of the visual field: The mesial portion of the left and right visual fields.

Negative afterimages: Also known as afterimage; in visual processes, perception of an image that is retained after the image terminates, arising from stimulation of visual feature detectors within the retina or cerebral cortex.

Neocerebellum: Also known as the cerebrocerebellum; portion of cerebellum receiving input from the cerebral cortex via the pontine nuclei, and whose output is directed to the thalamus and subsequently the premotor and motor cortex for the purpose of modifying the motor plan.

Neural crest cells: In embryonic development, cells arising from the border of the neural plate and non-neural ectoderm that migrate to differentiate into a set of branchial arches, ultimately giving rise to the sensory neurons, glia of the dorsal root ganglia, ganglia of the VII facial, V trigeminal, IX glossopharyngeal, and X vagus cranial nerves, dental primordia, ossicles, hyoid, and other structures.

Neurofibrils: Threadlike structures located in the cytoplasm.

Neurology: The study of the diseases of the nervous system.

Neurons: Also known as nerve cells; cells within the nervous system that are specialized for communication.

Neuropeptides: Proteins acting as neurotransmitters and that include hormones and neurotransmitters, including opioids, oxytocin, and insulin; involved in sensory perception, emotion, pain, and stress responses.

Neurotransmitter: Chemical messenger substances that permit the chemical synapse between two neurons.

Nociceptors: Pain receptors; receptor at termination of axon that responds to damage.

Node of Ranvier: On a myelinated axon, an area devoid of myelin but typically having ion channels that facilitate saltatory conduction.

Nodes: Area of localized swelling.

Nodule: Also known as nodulus; within the cerebellum, the medial component of the flocculonodular lobe.

Non-dominant hemisphere: Within the cerebral cortex, the cerebral hemisphere not responsible for language and calculation, typically the right hemisphere.

Non-fluent aphasia: Also known as Broca's aphasia or expressive aphasia; acquired language disorder resulting in short utterances, limited vocabulary, and/or production of few words.

Non-pyramidal cells: Within the fourth internal granular layer of the cerebral cortex, cells receiving primarily sensory information from the thalamus.

Norepinephrine (NE): Also known as noradrenaline; as neurotransmitter within the CNS, serves to arouse the cerebral cortex, and known as the "stress hormone."

Nuclear bag fibers: Intrafusal muscle fiber within the muscle spindle, relating information about passive movement of muscle by means of Group Ia nerve fibers.

Nuclear chain fibers: Intrafusal fibers responsible for detecting passive movement of muscle.

Nucleolus: Location within the cell nucleus in which there is synthesis of ribosomal and ribonucleic acid (RNA).

Nucleus: In cellular structure, the large, spherical structure found at the center of a soma containing genetic deoxyribonucleic acid (DNA), which controls the synthesis of the proteins and enzymes in a cell.

Nucleus ambiguus: Group of motor neurons associated with the X vagus and IX glossopharyngeal nerve within the medulla oblongata sending efferents to the velum, pharynx, and larynx.

Nucleus gracilis: Also known as the gracile nucleus; within the medulla oblongata, terminal point for the fasciculus gracilis conveying proprioceptive and kinesthetic information from the lower body.

Nucleus solitarius: Also known as solitary tract nucleus; within the medulla oblongata, mediating sensation of taste, somatic sensation, chemoreception from the vascular supply, lungs, gastrointestinal system, and VII facial, IX glossopharyngeal and X vagus nerves, and projecting to the reticular formation, hypothalamus, and thalamus; mediates activation of the gag reflex, carotid sinus reflex, cough reflex, and respiratory reflexes.

Nucleus: Within the CNS, a group of cell bodies with functional unity.

Nystagmus: Involuntary oscillatory ocular movements.

Obex: Inferior-most point within the 4th ventricle on dorsal brainstem surface that marks narrowing of the ventricle.

Occipital horn: Also known as posterior horn; of lateral ventricles, the aspect found within the occipital lobe region.

Occipitofrontal fasciculus: Association fibers of the medial corona radiata passing from the frontal lobe to the occipital and temporal lobes.

Octopus cells: Within the posteroventral cochlear nucleus, cells involved in processing of neural timing.

Olfaction: Sense of smell.

Olfactory bulb: Sensory element of the olfactory nerve, sending olfactory nerve axons through the perforated plate of the ethmoid bone into the nasal cavity mucosal lining.

Olfactory epithelium: Specialized epithelial tissue within the nasal cavity involved in sense of smell.

Olfactory sulcus: On the inferior surface of the cerebral cortex, the midline sulcus on which the olfactory tract resides.

Oligodendrocytes: Glial cells of the CNS responsible for generation of myelin.

Olivary nuclei: Within the medulla oblongata lateral to the pyramidal decussation, part of the olivocerebellar system, including the inferior and superior olivary nuclei.

Olivocerebellar tract: Fibers originating at the olivary nucleus and passing through the inferior cerebellar peduncle of the opposite side and terminating on the Purkinje cells.

Olivocochlear bundle: Fibers originating within the periolivary nuclei of the superior olivary complex involved in attenuation of cochlear output.

Ontogeny: Development of the organism.

Operculum: Cortical region overlying the insular cortex.

Ophthalmic nerve: Of the V trigeminal, the nerve mediating somatic sense from the region above the level of the eyes and including the forehead.

Optic radiation: Also known as the geniculocalcarine tract or pathway; pathway made up of axons from the lateral geniculate body projecting to the calcarine sulcus of the occipital lobe (BA 17).

Oral apraxia: Deficit in planning and programming of the articulators for non-speech activities.

Oral preparation stage: First of the stages of swallowing in which the food is masticated into a cohesive bolus through chewing, mixing with saliva, and positioning on the tongue.

Orbital gyri: On the inferior (orbital) surface of the frontal lobe, involved in processing of emotion; BA 10.

Orbitofrontal branch: Of the anterior cerebral artery, providing supply to the inferior cerebral hemisphere in the area around the gyrus rectus.

Organ: Group of cells with functional unity.

Orienting attention: Attention that results in physical or perceptual orientation to a novel stimulus.

Orienting reflex: Reflexive orientation to a novel stimulus, typically by an infant in response to stimulation of cheek or lips.

Otoliths: Also known as statoconia, otoconia, or statolith; calcium structure of the saccule and utricle involved in stimulating the vestibular mechanism during movement.

Outer hair cells: Of the cochlea, hair cells involved in mediating the intensity of an auditory signal.

Outermost molecular layer: Outermost layer of the cerebral cortex, consisting primarily of glial cells and axons from other layers.

Pacinian corpuscles: Also known as lamellar corpuscles; subcutaneous sensors within glabrous skin responsible for sensation of vibration and deep pressure.

Pain sense: Nociception, mediated by traumatized nerve endings.

Palatal reflex: Also known as uvular reflex; elevation of the velum in response to tactile stimulation of the uvula, posterior pharyngeal wall, or faucial pillars.

Paleocerebellum: Also known as the spinocerebellum; medial region of the anterior and posterior lobes of the cerebellum, responsible for coordination of limb and body movements, receiving afferents from the spinal cord via the spinocerebellar tract, as well as V trigeminal and VIII vestibulocochlear nerves.

Palmar grasp reflex: Grasp reflex of the hand in which there is flexion of the fingers in a grasping manner; seen in infants prior to 6 months of age.

Palmar surface: Of the hand, the ventral surface.

Papillae: Prominences of the tongue surface, with taste buds being in the filiform papillae.

Paracentral lobule: Inflected continuation of the precentral and postcentral gyri on the medial cerebral cortex.

Parahippocampal gyrus: Of the inferior cerebral cortex, the gyrus surrounding the hippocampus.

Paralysis: Loss of the ability to move a muscle.

Parasympathetic nervous system: The component of the autonomic nervous system that counteracts sympathetic nervous system responses such as stress responses.

Paresis: Muscular weakness.

Parieto-occipital suture: On the inferior-lateral cerebral surface, the boundary of the parietal and occipital lobes.

Parkinson's disease: Progressive neurological disease involving degeneration of the substantial nigra, resulting in signs such as rest tremor, rigidity, bradykinesia, difficulty with walking, and hypokinetic dysarthria.

Parotid gland: Major salivary gland located around the mandibular ramus, secreting serous saliva.

Pars opercularis: On the frontal lobe, the region of the inferior frontal gyrus overlying the insular cortex; BA 44.

Pars orbitale: Orbital part of the inferior frontal gyrus; BA 47.

Pars triangularis: Of the frontal lobe, the region of the inferior frontal gyrus making up part of Broca's area; BA 45.

Perforating arteries: Branches of the middle cerebral artery providing vascular supply to the basal ganglia and internal capsule.

Periolivary region: Region surrounding the major nuclei of the superior olivary complex, giving rise to the olivocochlear bundle of the auditory system.

Peripheral nervous system (PNS): Portion of nervous system consisting of the 31 spinal nerves and the 12 cranial nerves.

Perpendicular fasciculus: Association fibers connecting the fusiform gyrus (BA 37) with the superior parietal lobule (BA 5 and 7).

Pes hippocampus: Lower, enlarged end of the hippocampus.

Pharyngeal branch: Of the X vagus nerve, providing motor innervation of the pharynx.

Photoreceptors: Specialized retinal receptors that are sensitive to light.

Phylogeny: Evolution of a species.

Physiology: Study of the function of an organ.

Pia mater: Deepest of the meningeal linings, surrounding the cerebrum, brainstem, and spinal cord.

Plantar: Sole of the foot.

Plantar grasp: Reflex characterized by flexion of the toes when the dorsum of the foot is stimulated, typically by deep, moving pressure; reflex is present in first 6 months of life.

Plexus: Branching network of nerves.

Pons: Middle component of brainstem, containing cranial nerve nuclei for the V trigeminal sensory and motor components, the nucleus abducens for the VI abducens nerve, the facial nerve nucleus for the VII facial nerve, and the vestibular and cochlear nuclei for the VIII vestibulocochlear nerve.

Pontine nuclei: Nuclei of pons that receive information from the premotor and motor cortex and convey that information via the middle cerebellar peduncle to the cerebellum.

Pontine perforating artery: Collateral arteries arising from the basilar artery that serve the pons deep tissue.

Pontine reticulospinal tract: Extrapyramidal pathways descending from the reticular formation to the trunk and extremities for the purpose of locomotion and posture control.

Pontocerebellar tract: Fibers from the pontine nuclei receiving cortical efferent and conveying motor planning information to the cerebellum.

Pontocerebellum: Portion of cerebellum served by pontine fibers.

Postcentral gyrus: Gyrus of parietal lobe immediately posterior to central sulcus, being the primary somatosensory reception area, SI; BA 1, 2, 3, 5.

Postcentral sulcus: Sulcus of parietal lobe immediately posterior to the postcentral gyrus.

Posterior: The back of an organ.

Posterior branches of the middle cerebral artery: The parietal, angular, temporal, and occipital branches of the middle cerebral artery.

Posterior cerebral artery: Artery arising from the vertebrobasilar supply and serving the occipital lobe.

Posterior cingulate cortex: Caudal portion of cingulate gyrus, involved in spatial and autobiographical memory, learning, and emotional valence.

Posterior communicating artery: Artery of the circle of Willis that provides communication between middle cerebral artery and vertebrobasilar system.

Posterior horn: Also known as occipital horn; of lateral ventricles, the aspect found within the occipital lobe region.

Posterior lobe: Of the cerebellum, part of the spinocerebellum (paleocerebellum) responsible for coordination of limb movements.

Posterior tegmentum: In the pons, the upper extension of the reticular formation.

Posteroventral cochlear nucleus (PVCN): The component of the cochlear nucleus performing analysis of the auditory input and conveying it to the intermediate stria.

Postsynaptic neuron: Neuron that receives communication signal from another upstream neuron.

Precentral gyrus: Also known as the motor strip; in the frontal lobe, the gyrus immediately anterior to the central sulcus, responsible for direct activation of skeletal muscle; BA 4.

Precuneus: In the superior parietal lobe, immediately anterior to the cuneus of the occipital lobe, and involved in episodic and visual memory, visuospatial attention, and conscious information processing; considered integral to the default mode network.

Prefrontal superficial branch: Of the middle cerebral artery, serving the frontal lobe and frontal pole.

Premotor region: Of the frontal lobe, the region immediately anterior to the precentral gyrus, involved in motor planning and complex motor execution, BA 6; may be extended to include the supplementary motor area (SMA, BA6).

Preoccipital notch: Inferior landmark indicating boundary between occipital and parietal lobes.

Prepyriform cortex: Portion of rhinencephalon considered the primary olfactory cortex.

Pressure generation: In swallowing function, generation of positive air pressure within the pharynx through the combination of anterior lingual-oral seal and retropulsion and elevation of the velum; essential for bolus transport through the upper esophageal sphincter.

Presynaptic neuron: The neuron conveying information to a following neuron in a chain.

Primary fissure: In the cerebellum, the fissure separating anterior and posterior lobes.

Primary olfactory cortex: Portion of cortex made up of the uncus and lateral stria.

Prime mover: Also known as agonist; the predominant muscle performing an action.

Principal inferior olivary nucleus: Within the medulla oblongata, nucleus involved in motor function.

Pronation: Of the foot, rotation of the foot so that it turns out; of the hand, rotation of the hand so that the palm of the hand is turned upward.

Prone: Position of lying on the belly.

Proprioception: Sensory perception related to the musculoskeletal system, including sensory information concerning joints, muscles, muscle spindle afferents, and Golgi tendon afferents.

Prosencephalon: Also known as forebrain; in embryology, the portion of the embryonic brain that will differentiate into the diencephalon (including thalamus, hypothalamus, and subthalamus) and the telencephalon (cerebrum).

Proximal: Toward the root of a free extremity.

Pseudo-unipolar neurons: Neurons in PNS whose axon divides into two branches, with one directed to the spinal cord and one directed to the periphery.

Psycholinguistic view of speech production: View that speech is the oral manifestation of language.

Pulvinar: Nucleus of the thalamus associated with language function.

Purkinje cells: Cells of the cerebellum and cerebrum characterized by stereotypical radiation arborizations, which, in the cerebellum, are responsible for taking inputs from parallel fibers in the cerebellum and translating that input into inhibitory output responses for fine motor control.

Putamen: Nucleus of the basal ganglia involved with motor planning, execution, and motor sequences; together with the caudate nucleus forms the striatum.

Pyramidal cells: Multipolar neurons found in cerebral cortex involved in motor activation.

Pyramidal tract: Tract arising from the precentral and premotor gyrus of the cerebral cortex, responsible for motor activation.

Pyriform lobe: Component of rhinencephalon within cerebrum, consisting of the amygdala, uncus, and parahippocampal gyrus.

Radial glial cells: Bipolar-shaped glial cells serving as scaffolds for neuron migration during development, as well as progenitor cells for generation of neurons, astrocytes, and oligodendrocytes.

Receptor: Protein responsive to a neurotransmitter.

Reciprocal inhibition: Process by which muscles on one side of a joint are inhibited from contracting when the muscle on the other side is contracting.

Recurrent laryngeal nerve: Branch of X vagus cranial nerve responsible for activation of all of the intrinsic muscles of the larynx except the cricothyroid muscle.

Red nucleus: Nucleus of the rostral midbrain involved in motor activation and control by means of the rubrospinal tract.

Reflexes: An involuntary movement in response to a stimulus, mediated by reflex arcs or stimulus-response pathways.

Relative refractory period: Period during which a neuron can be stimulated, but requires greater intensity of stimulation for to discharge that at resting membrane potential.

Resting state of a neuron: Also known as resting membrane potential; one in which the electrical potential within the cell is between −50 and −70 mV (millivolts) relative to the outside of the cell.

Retching center: Within the dorsal medulla oblongata in the reticular formation and the area postrema of the inferior 4th ventricle; the area responsible for sensation of toxic or noxious stimuli and conveying efferent information to the solitary tract nucleus for the purpose of initiating the central pattern generator sequence for retching.

Reticular activating system (RAS): Also known as extrathalamic control modulatory system; set of nuclei responsible for regulating wakefulness and sleep-state transitions.

Reticular formation: A group of nuclei located in the brainstem, playing a major role in consciousness and cortical wakefulness.

Reticulospinal tract: Extrapyramidal tract arising in the reticular formation of the brainstem and terminating in the spinal cord, serving to regulate muscle tone and contraction of limb flexors and extensors.

Retinal cells: Also known as retinal ganglion cells; cells located within the retina of the eye and sensitive to light stimulation.

Rhombencephalon: Embryonic neural component from which the medulla, pons and cerebellum will differentiate.

Ribosomes: Organelles within the cellular protoplasm responsible for production of proteins.

Right hemisphere damage: Lesions to the right hemisphere resulting in a constellation of problems, including personality changes, loss of sense of humor, loss of affect, and loss of social skills.

Rolandic fissure: Also known as Rolandic sulcus or central sulcus; sulcus dividing parietal and frontal lobes of the cerebral cortex.

Rostral: Toward the oral or nasal regions.

Rostral spinocerebellar tract: Pathway transmitting information from Golgi tendon organs of the upper trunk region to the cerebellum.

Rostral system: Of the olivocochlear pathway, the portion of the efferent auditory system directed by cerebral cortex efferents to the superior olivary complex, inferior colliculus, and medial geniculate body, implying some degree of cognitive control over signal identification and separation performed by the olivocochlear bundle.

Rostrum: Beak or structure resembling a beak.

Rubrospinal tract: Tract arising from the red nucleus of the midbrain forming part of the extrapyramidal tract, serving to maintain background movement in support of pyramidal excitation.

Ruffini endings: Also known as Ruffini's corpuscles; exteroceptors within cutaneous layer responsible for sensing deep stretch.

Saccule: Of the vestibular system, the bed of sensory cells within the vestibular mechanism that senses acceleration.

Sagittal: Section or view that divides a structure into left and right components.

Saltatory conduction: Neural propagation in which impulses jump from node to node in the myelin.

Satellite cells: In the CNS, glial cells responsible for regulation of ions and re-uptake of neurotransmitter substance.

Schwann: Glial cells of the PNS responsible for myelin generation on axons.

Semantic processing deficits: Difficulties understanding word meaning.

Semicircular canals: In the vestibular system, any of the three canals responsible for mediating sense of position in space.

Sensors: Structure responsible for sensing change.

Sensory alpha fibers: Sensory neural fibers differentiated by sense being mediated, including pain, touch, pressure, thermal sense.

Sensory nerves: Nerves mediating sensation to the central nervous system.

Sensory nucleus: Nucleus from which sensory dendrite arises.

Septum pellucidum: Thin membranous structure separating the anterior horns of the left and right lateral ventricles.

Serotonin: Monamine neurotransmitter important for regulation of mood and depression and involved in regulation of appetite, memory, sleep, and learning.

Shearing action: In the cochlea, the action produced by movement of the basilar membrane relative to the pendulous tectorial membrane, causing deflection of the cilia of the outer hair cell.

Solitary tract nucleus: Also known as nucleus solitarius; A set of sensory nuclei within the medulla oblongata, with inputs arising from the VII facial, IX glossopharyngeal, and X vagus nerves and projecting to the reticular formation, preganglionic neurons, hypothalamus, and thalamus.

Soma: Also known as body; cell body.

Somatic nerves: Nerves that serve skeletal muscle.

Somatic sense: Also known as body sense or somesthetic sense; sensations including those associated with deep and light pressure, thermal stimulation, joint position sense, muscle tension, and tendon tension.

Somatosensory receptors: Cells mediating somatic sensation, including mechanoreceptors, chemoreceptors, and nociceptors found in skin, epithelial tissue, muscles, bones, joints, and internal organs.

Spastic dysarthria: Motor speech disorder arising from upper motor neuron lesion and resulting in high muscle tone, muscular weakness, and loss of fine motor control.

Spasticity: Increased resistance to movement due to high muscle tone

Spatiotopic representation: In the somatosensory system, representation at the cortical level in a spatial array representing the physical region from which the sensation arose.

Special sense: Senses of special receptors, including the sense of hearing, vision, smell, and taste.

Special visceral afferent: Afferent fibers carrying special senses of smell and taste.

Spherical radiation: Dendritic formation of stellate cells, in which dendrites radiate from all areas of the soma.

Spinal component of the XI accessory nerve: Portion of XI accessory nerve serving the sternocleidomastoid and trapezius muscles.

Spinal meningeal linings: Meningeal linings of the spinal cord.

Spinal nucleus of the V trigeminal: In the medulla oblongata, the nucleus of the trigeminal nerve mediating the sense of touch, pain, and thermal sense from the ipsilateral face.

Spinal reflex arc: Reflexive circuit at level of spinal segment that controls a reflex; typically consisting of a sensor, afferent pathway, interneuron, effector, and muscle.

Spindle radiation: Neural dendritic configuration in which dendrites emerge from opposite poles of the soma, as in bipolar neurons of the cerebral cortex.

Spinocerebellum: Also known as the paleocerebellum; the medial region of the anterior and posterior lobes of the cerebellum, responsible for coordination of limb and body movements, receiving afferents from the spinal cord via the spinocerebellar tract, as well as V trigeminal and VIII vestibulocochlear nerves.

Spiral ganglion: In the cochlea, the aggregate of cell bodies making up the nucleus of the cochlear component of the VIII vestibulocochlear nerve.

Splenium of the corpus callosum: Posterior aspect of the corpus callosum.

Stapedial reflex: Reflexive contraction of the stapes in response to sounds of high intensity.

Stellate cells: Neurons with a star-like, spherical dendritic shape, responsible for integrating input from many different sources.

Stereocilia: In the auditory system, prominence from surface of hair cells of the vestibular mechanism, closely related to cilia.

Striate body: Also known as the corpus striatum, neostriatum, striate nucleus; nucleus of the basal ganglia involved in motor function and reward systems.

Subdural hematoma: Accumulation of blood collecting between the dura mater and arachnoid mater, often arising from traumatic brain injury.

Subliminal: Below the threshold of detection.

Sublingual glands: Salivary glands beneath the tongue that release mucoid saliva.

Submandibular glands: Also known as submaxillary glands; salivary glands beneath the tongue that release a combination of serous and mucoid saliva.

Submaxillary salivary glands: Also known as submandibular glands; salivary glands beneath the tongue that release a combination of serous and mucoid saliva.

Substantia nigra: Nucleus of dopamine-secreting cells located in the midbrain within the cerebral peduncle, often considered a part of the basal ganglia.

Subthalamic nucleus: Nucleus of the subthalamus that functions with the globus pallidus as output system of basal ganglia.

Subthalamus: Structure of the diencephalon often considered part of the basal ganglia, responsible for modulation of motor function.

Sucking reflex: In infants, the reflexive protrusion and retraction of lips and tongue in response to stimulation of the lips through light stroking movement.

Sulcus: Groove.

Superficial: Toward the surface.

Superficial cerebral veins: Veins of the cranium, including superior cerebral veins, superficial middle cerebral vein, inferior cerebral vein, inferior anastomotic vein, and superior anastomotic vein.

Superficial sensations: Sensations from the periphery of the body.

Superior cerebellar artery: Artery arising from the basilar artery serving the superior surface of the cerebellum.

Superior: Upper surface of a structure.

Superior cerebellar peduncles: Also known as the brachia conjunctiva; pathway connecting the cerebellum to the midbrain, consisting of efferent fibers of the cerebellothalamic tract and cerebellorubral tract, as well as the afferent ventral spinocerebellar tract and others.

Superior colliculus: Nucleus of midbrain involved in visual processing and visual orientation.

Superior frontal gyrus: Region of the frontal lobe bounded by the superior frontal sulcus laterally, and implicated in self-awareness.

Superior laryngeal nerve: Branch of X vagus nerve involved in contraction of the cricothyroid muscle for vocal fundamental frequency control as well as inhibition of the cricopharyngeus for relaxation of the upper esophageal sphincter during swallowing.

Superior longitudinal fasciculus: Association fiber tract of the cerebrum consisting of three components, SLF I, SLF II and SLF III; responsible for connecting frontal, occipital, parietal, and temporal lobes.

Superior longitudinal fissure: Also known as cerebral longitudinal fissure and longitudinal fissure; fissure separating the two cerebral hemispheres.

Superior medullary velum: Also known as anterior medullary velum; white matter between superior cerebellar peduncles, forming the roof of the 4th ventricle.

Superior olivary complex (SOC): Also known as the superior olive; within the pons, nuclei including the lateral superior olive, medial superior olive, and periolivary nuclei, involved in localization of sound in space as well as cochlear output attenuation through the olivocochlear bundle.

Superior parietal lobule: Lobe of parietal lobe bounded inferiorly by the intraparietal sulcus, and being part of the dorsal visual stream.

Superior salivatory nucleus: Also known as nucleus salivatorius superior; nucleus of the VII facial nerve within the pontine tegmentum, responsible for innervation of submandibular and sublingual salivary glands.

Superior temporal gyrus: Of the temporal lobe of the cerebral cortex, the gyrus containing a portion of Heschl's gyrus (primary auditory reception) and Wernicke's area; BA 22.

Superior vestibular nucleus: Dorsolateral portion of vestibular nucleus of pons, receiving input from the vestibular nerve.

Supination: Of the foot, involving rotation of the foot medially; of the hand, turning the palm superiorly.

Supine: Lying on the back.

Supplementary motor area (SMA): Region of the superior frontal gyrus and premotor region involved in motor preparation and rehearsal; BA 6.

Supramarginal gyrus: Within the inferior parietal lobule, involved in phonetic processing and language perception; BA 40

Sympathetic system: Also known as the thoracolumbar system; component of the autonomic system responding to stimulation by expenditure of energy.

Synapses: The physical connections between neurons, and point at which stimulation of postsynaptic neuron occurs.

Synaptic cleft: The gap between a pre- and postsynaptic neuron into which neurotransmitter is released.

Synergists: Muscles that support movement of the prime mover or agonist.

Tactile agnosia: Loss of the ability to know the nature of an object through the sense of touch.

Target muscle length: In muscle spindle function, the criterion established through contraction of intrafusal muscle.

Taste receptors: Also known as taste buds and taste cells; chemoreceptors involved in sensing molecules of food.

Tectospinal tract: Also known as colliculospinal tract; tract of the extrapyramidal system arising from the midbrain tectum and terminating in the cervical spinal cord regions, and responsible for postural adjustments of the head, particularly in response to auditory and/or visual stimulation.

Tectum: Also known as quadrigeminal plate; dorsal component of midbrain, and including superior and inferior colliculi.

Tegmentum: In the brainstem, the region anterior to the 4th ventricle, mediating numerous reflexes, inhibiting many motor responses, controlling eye movement, and maintaining cortical wakefulness. Contains the red nucleus and substantia nigra.

Tela choroidea: Region of the pia mater of the meningeal linings that gives rise to the choroid plexus of each ventricle.

Telencephalon: In fetal development, the telencephalon develops from the prosencephalon or forebrain, and develops into the cerebral cortex.

Telondendria: Of the axon, the terminal process to which the end bouton is attached.

Temporal operculum: Portion of the temporal lobe overlying the insular cortex.

Temporal pole: The anterior-most region of the temporal lobe; BA 38.

Temporal portion of the visual field: The lateral portion of the left and right visual fields.

Tentorium cerebelli: Also known as cerebellar tentorium; dura mater shelf separating the cerebrum from the cerebellum.

Thalamus: Diencephalon structure located superiorly to the midbrain in the forebrain, receiving most afferent input from the body and projecting to the cerebral cortex.

Thermoreceptors: Non-specific sensors for temperature sensation.

Third ventricle: Of the cerebral hemisphere, the ventricular space between the paired thalami.

Threshold: In sensation, the weakest sensation that can cause a physiological response.

Tip links: On cochlear hair cells, links between the cilia of the hair cell, ensuring that the cilia move as a unit.

Transcortical motor aphasia: Acquired language disorder arising from damage to the anterior superior frontal lobe of the dominant hemisphere, characterized by non-fluent aphasia with good comprehension.

Transcortical sensory aphasia: Acquired language disorder characterized by fluent speech, intact repetition and poor auditory comprehension.

Transduce: To convert energy from one form to another.

Transverse section: Section dividing the structure into upper and lower portions.

Trapezoid body: Ventral acoustic stria of the auditory pathway, between the cochlear nucleus and superior olivary complex.

Traveling wave: Of the cochlea, the action of the basilar membrane in response to auditory stimulation that is wavelike, with maximum perturbation of the wave arising at a location on the basilar membrane corresponding to the frequency of excitation.

Trigeminal ganglion: Also known as Gasserian ganglion and semilunar ganglion; sensory ganglion of the V trigeminal nerve.

Trigeminal neuralgia: Severe pain arising from trigeminal nerve damage.

Tuber cinereum: Part of the hypothalamus, between the optic chiasm and the mammillary body.

Type Ia sensory fibers: Afferent fibers of the muscle spindle.

Type Ib sensory fibers: Afferent sensory fibers for Golgi tendon organs.

Type II afferent fibers: Afferent sensory fibers conveying touch and pressure information.

Type II, III, and IV sensory fibers: Fibers conveying information about somatic sense.

Type III afferent fibers: Fibers conveying pain, pressure, touch, and cool thermal sense.

Type IV afferent fibers: Fibers conveying pain and warm thermal sense.

Types Ia and Ib sensory alpha fibers: Fibers conveying kinesthetic sense.

Umami: Taste sense categorized as savory, or with the quality of meat.

Uncinate fasciculus: Association fiber tract connecting hippocampus and amygdala with orbitofrontal gyrus of the frontal lobe.

Uncus: On the inferior cerebral cortex, the structure overlying the amygdaloid body.

Unipolar neurons: Neurons with one process extending from the body.

Upper esophageal sphincter (UES): The sphincter made up of the cricopharyngeus muscle and the upper esophagus.

Upper motor neurons: Neurons arising from the cortex, generally from the precentral and premotor regions.

Utricle: Of the vestibular system, organ sensing acceleration.

V trigeminal nerve: Cranial nerve arising from pons, consisting of two afferent branches (ophthalmic and maxillary) and one mixed afferent-efferent nerve (mandibular), and being responsible for mediation of somatic sense for face and oral cavity, as well as activation of the muscles of mastication and other muscles.

Venous drainage of the cerebrovascular supply: Drainage of the vascular supply of the brain into the dural venous sinuses and the inferior sagittal and straight sinuses.

Ventral nucleus of lateral lemniscus: Nucleus of the lateral lemniscus of the auditory pathway receiving input from the contralateral anteroventral and posteroventral cochlear nuclei and ipsilateral medial nucleus of trapezoid body, and projecting to the inferior colliculus.

Ventral posterolateral (VPL) nucleus of the thalamus: Nucleus of thalamus receiving input concerning touch and pressure sense, and whose output projects to the somatosensory cortex (BA 1, 2, 3).

Ventral spinocerebellar tract: Tract from spinal cord conveying proprioceptive information from the lumbar and sacral levels to the cerebellum by means of the superior cerebellar peduncle.

Ventral surfaces: Surface of the body in humans that includes the anterior abdomen, anterior thorax, etc. The ventral surface of the cerebrum is the inferior surface.

Ventral swallowing group (VSG): Located in the ventral medulla oblongata near the nucleus ambiguus and receiving input from the V trigeminal, maxillary branch, IX glossopharyngeal nerve, and the X vagus; the central pattern generating unit that serves as a switching mechanism, ordering the activation of pools of neurons within the swallowing central pattern generator.

Ventrolateral sulcus: Midline sulcus on spinal cord and medulla oblongata.

Verbal agnosia: Loss of ability to identify verbal stimulation.

Vermis: Structure in medial superior surface of the cerebellum, and is involved in coordination of body posture and locomotion.

Vertebral arteries: Major arteries of the neck, coursing through the transverse foramena of the cervical vertebrae, and anastomosing to form the basilar artery.

Vertebrobasilar system: Cerebrovascular supply arising from the anastomosing of the vertebral arteries into the single basilar artery, which serves the brainstem, cerebellum, and occipital lobes of the brain.

Vertigo: Perception of movement of self or external objects in absence of physical movement, often with a sense of spinning, and often accompanied by nausea.

Vestibular ganglion: Ganglion containing the cell bodies of the vestibular branch of the VIII vestibulocochlear nerve, housed in the internal auditory meatus.

Vestibular nuclei: Nuclei of the vestibular nerve of the VIII vestibulocochlear nerve and consisting of the medial vestibular nucleus (medulla), lateral vestibular nucleus (medulla), inferior vestibular nucleus (medulla), and superior vestibular nucleus (pons).

Vestibular pathway: Sensory pathway providing sensation concerning the sense of balance, as well as position and movement in space.

Vestibular system: Sensory system associated with maintenance of the sense of balance and position in space, including the labyrinth of the inner ear, vestibular branch of the VIII vestibulocochlear nerve, vestibular nuclei, and vestibulocerebellar tract.

Vestibulocerebellum: Also known as the archicerebellum; portion of cerebellum consisting of the flocculonodular lobe and adjacent vermis, being responsible for ocular movement relative to head orientation as well as control of gait.

Vestibulocochlear nerve: The combined auditory and vestibular branches of the VIII vestibulocochlear nerve, responsible for mediation of the sense of auditory and vestibular sense.

Vestibulospinal tract: Tract of the extrapyramidal system involved in maintaining neck and limb muscle tone and head position relative to position and movement of the body in space.

VI abducens nerve: Cranial nerve within the pons that controls abduction of the eyeball through activation of the lateral rectus muscle.

VII facial nerve: The cranial nerve arising from the junction of the pons and medulla that controls the muscles of the face as well as conveys the sense of taste from the anterior 2/3 of the tongue.

VIII vestibulocochlear nerve: The combined auditory and vestibular branches of the VIII vestibulocochlear nerve, responsible for mediation of the sense of auditory and vestibular sense.

Visceral nerves: Nerves of the autonomic nervous system.

Visual agnosia: Inability to identify a visual stimulus.

Visual field: Perceived field of visual reception.

Visual neglect: Visual component of hemispatial neglect, in which the left visual field is not attended to by the individual; typically arising from right hemisphere damage to right dorsolateral prefrontal cortex and temporoparietal juncture.

Voltage sensitive ion channels: Proteins that respond to voltage change in the environment by allowing ions to pass.

Vomiting center: Within the dorsal medulla oblongata in the reticular formation and the area postrema of the inferior 4th ventricle; the area responsible for sensation of toxic or noxious stimuli and conveying efferent information to the solitary tract nucleus for the purpose of initiating the central pattern generator sequence for vomiting.

Vomiting reflexes: Complex expulsive response, mediated by central pattern generator, of the gastrointestinal system in which abdominal muscles contract, the larynx elevates and vocal folds adduct, the velum elevates, and the tongue protrudes.

Wernicke's aphasia: Acquired language disorder resulting in language comprehension deficit and fluent speech output with significant jargon.

Wernicke's area: The region of the posterior superior temporal gyrus (BA 22) in the dominant cerebral hemisphere that is involved in receptive language and language comprehension.

X vagus: Cranial nerve involved in multiple functions, notably including vocal fold action of adduction, abduction, tension and relaxation (recurrent laryngeal nerve), cricothyroid contraction for changing the fundamental frequency, relaxation of the cricopharyngeus muscle to open the upper esophageal sphincter (superior laryngeal nerve), and innervation of the muscles of the pharynx (pharyngeal nerve).

XI accessory nerve: Nerve of the medulla oblongata and upper spinal cord responsible for innervation of the sternocleidomastoid and trapezius muscles, but also working in conjunction with the IX glossopharyngeal and X vagus on other innervations.

XII hypoglossal nerve: Motor cranial nerve of the medulla oblongata responsible for innervation of all tongue muscles except the palatoglossus.

Zonal microcomplexes (MZMC): Zones of sensation within the cerebellum, which monitor different sensory/motor subunits for errors.

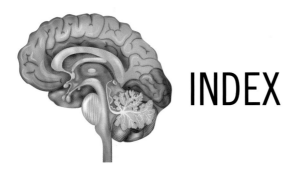

INDEX

Note: Page numbers in **bold** reference non-text material.